DR. SUSAN LOVE'S BREAST BOOK

FOURTH EDITION
FULLY REVISED

DR. SUSAN LOVE'S BREAST BOOK

FOURTH EDITION
FULLY REVISED

Susan M. Love, M.D.

with Karen Lindsey

Illustrations by Marcia Williams

A MERLOYD LAWRENCE BOOK
DA CAPO LIFELONG

Set in 10 point Palatino

Cataloging-in-Publication Data for this book is available from the Library of Congress.

ISBN 0-7382-0973-2
ISBN-13 978-0-7382-0973-9

First Da Capo Press edition 2005

Published by Da Capo Press
A Member of the Perseus Books Group
www.dacapopress.com

20 19 18 17 16 15 14 13 12 11 10

To Katie, Kim and Nina,
and all the girls in the next generation,
with the hope that for them breast cancer will be history.

Contents

PART EIGHT: WHAT IS COMING

APPENDICES

Acknowledgments

This book, which started out more than fifteen years ago, has become a joint effort of many people working hard to make it accurate and up-to-date. We began in Boston, and Karen Lindsey and I met once a week to move it along. We now work digitally, with her as often as not in the Netherlands while I am at my computer in Los Angeles. Connie Long, my assistant, works tirelessly at the formatting and coordinating. She is truly the guardian angel of this book.

As in the past, I have many friends and associates who read through the drafts to make sure I have not missed something. This edition they did it with a tight deadline and with particular grace. I especially need to thank Sanford Barsky MD, Larry Bassett MD, Leslie Bernstein PhD, William Dooley MD, Irene Gage MD, Hester Hill Schnipper LICSW, Judi Hirschfield-Bartek RN, Ellen Mahoney MD, Musa Mayer, Hyman Muss MD, Olufunmilayo Olapade MD, Joyce O'Shaughnessy MD, Lori Pierce MD, Julia Rowland PhD, Sumner Slavin MD, and Susan Troyan MD. Any errors that may have snuck in are despite their hard work.

As always it is important to me to mention the people who work with me and without me as I spend the year it takes to get a new edition done. The Dr. Susan Love Research Foundation could not run without the hard work of Kate McLean, Alice Gillaroo, Helene Brown,

Chris Hershey, Nina Merrill, and our new "goddess," Meghan Brennan RN. The board of directors, including Kay Coleman, Anne Levin, Elizabeth Browning, Brock Vinton, and Don Franchesini, has given its support through thick and thin. As we move forward with the intraductal research, I need to mention that team as well: Dave Licata, Julian Nikolchev, Howard Palefsky, and David Wilson. Our goal is to have that project done for the next edition.

This book would not exist without the work of my agent, Jill Kneerim, and my patient editor, Merloyd Lawrence. Karen Lindsey, cowriter, puts up with my crazy schedule and always finds a way to get things done. Marcia Williams is wonderful with the art often on a moment's notice, and Christine Marra did an amazing job with the cliffhanging moments of final production.

And then there is my family. My life partner, Helen Cooksey, has put up with every edition of this book and still supports me in all things! Katie, our seventeen-year-old, is fast becoming a better writer than I. This year, as I was working on this edition, our old cocker spaniel Brownie died. He had been at my feet for several editions helping me through the night. Charlie, our new cocker spaniel, has been much less helpful. He is much more interested in having his toy thrown for him than the intricacies of breast cancer. Still he has become part of the team.

This book in the end belongs to the women with breast cancer and their families, who crave the information and understanding necessary to get through one of the toughest times in their lives. I continue to work toward the day when it will no longer be necessary.

Introduction to the Fourth Edition

As I was working on this fourth edition of the *Breast Book*, I had to upgrade my Mac computer to the new operating system. Suddenly I realized that this book is also an upgrade to a new operating system. While it remains a guide for the newly diagnosed, it is also an upgrade of the previous editions for all the survivors out there who had an older version on the shelf. So much has changed over the years! Often when I am doing a speaking engagement, women bring their tattered and torn first or second edition to be signed. "This is what got me through my experience with breast cancer," they say. I am moved and glad to sign the book—but I always advise them to regard these earlier editions as mementos of their journey with breast cancer, not current tools. For that, they need the most up-to-date version as well. I say this not to keep my royalty fees coming in but because for survivors, new questions will always arise as new information comes in. Further, each of these women has become an expert, to whom many women new to the experience will turn for advice. This book, along with their firsthand accounts, provides the most current information.

For a long time I felt discouraged at our lack of progress in treating breast cancer. But in writing this edition, I've been blown away with how far we've come.

Screening with imaging—whether digital mammography, MRI, or

ultrasound—has improved, while prevention using hormone interventions has become an established part of working with high-risk women. Most exciting to me is the hint that local intraductal therapy will indeed be able to prevent breast cancer someday. This has been my dream for decades, and as I describe in Chapter 13, it is close to becoming a reality. Some day in the not too distant future, a doctor will squeeze a drop of fluid from a woman's breast and dip a stick into it. If it turns blue, the doctor will send her to another doctor who will go duct to duct and figure out which one is abnormal and then squirt the treatment down the duct and it will be taken care of.

Today not only are carriers of the mutations in the BRCA 1 and 2 genes easier to detect on a blood test, but there are options for intervention, ranging from surveillance with MRI, mammography, and ultrasound to prophylactic mastectomy and/or oophorectomy. These women could be the biggest beneficiaries of a chemical version of mastectomy that will be done down the ducts, leaving the breast intact. They will lead the way in the search for prevention.

And meanwhile we can incorporate lifestyle changes to reduce our chances of getting breast cancer in the first place.

While we are feverishly working on that reality, there are already many improvements in the standard approaches to treatment.

To begin with, we have the first of what should be many tests to help determine which women will benefit from which therapies. Although we have used hormone receptor tests for a while to tell us who can benefit from hormones, we now can take that to a new level. The Oncotype Dx test will tell hormone-positive women whether they are in the subgroup for whom tamoxifen has little benefit and chemotherapy works very well, or in the larger group for whom chemotherapy has little benefit and tamoxifen does well. A different type of test being developed in Europe based on patterns of mutations (MammaPrint) shows promise in better determining prognosis and therefore need for therapy. The move towards individualized therapy is well under way.

Although we are still treating breast cancer with surgery, radiation therapy, and drugs, we have had major advances in each one of those areas.

In surgery we are doing almost all biopsies in a minimally invasive fashion with core biopsies, and often we can remove the tumor the same way. Cryoablation is being used for benign tumors and it won't be long before we are ablating cancers as well with either cryosurgery, microwave, laser, or radiofrequency. Wide excisions are being done with oncoplastic surgery, which merges oncology and plastic surgery to get the best cosmetic results. And sentinel node biopsies, which had just been introduced when the third edition was written, have become the standard of care.

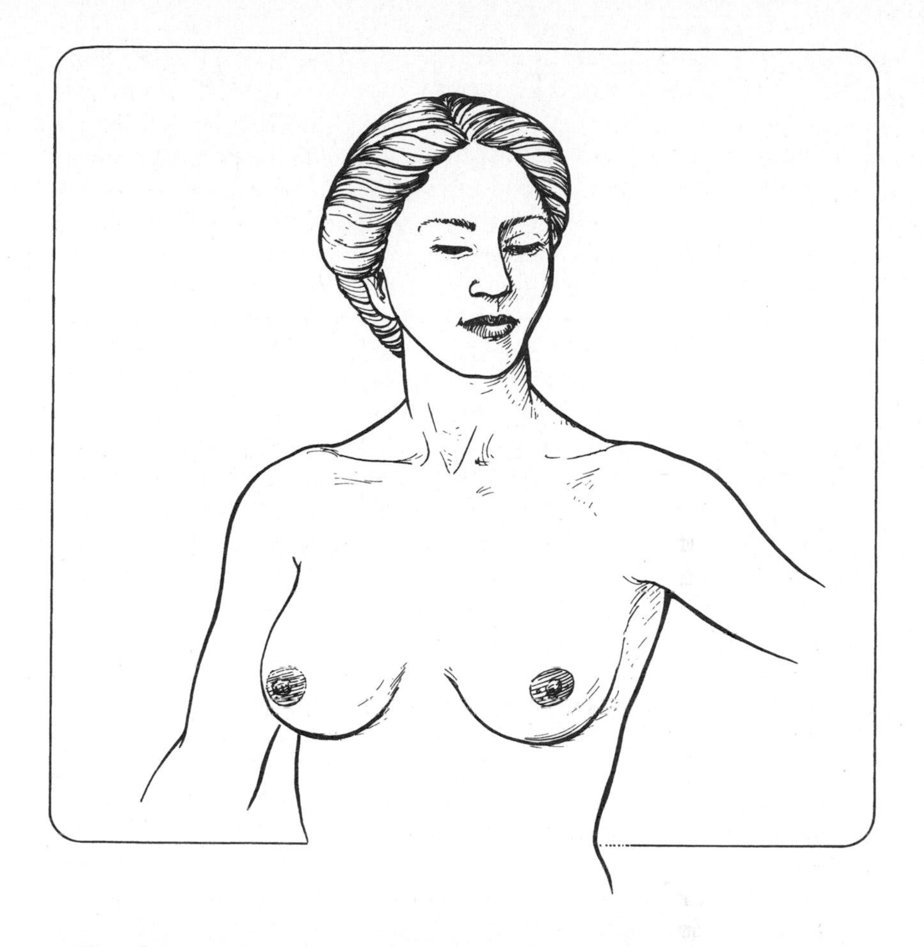

Big changes in radiation therapy will markedly improve women's quality of life. What used to take six weeks with daily visits to the hospital is being replaced by partial breast radiation therapy given either in the operating room or through tubes or "balloons" for at most a few days. This will make radiation therapy much more available to women who do not live near a metropolitan area.

And the drugs are getting better. First we have had an enormous advance in the area of hormone therapy. Once restricted to tamoxifen, it now includes the new aromatase inhibitors that reduce recurrences with different side effects. These drugs have now been shown to work not only in treating metastatic disease but also as adjuvant therapy for original cancer. They are now being tested as prevention.

On the nonhormone side, the targeted therapies alluded to in the previous edition are becoming clinically established. Trastuzumab, or Herceptin, works in women with metatstatic disease and Her-2/neu overexpressing tumors: the news came in as the book was near completion that it also works in women with newly diagnosed node positive Her-2/neu overexpressing tumors in conjunction with chemotherapy. Bevacizumab (Avastin), the first antiangiogenesis factor treatment, has been shown to benefit women with metastatic disease when given with chemotherapy. It will undoubtedly be tested in the adjuvant setting as well. These two drugs are the results of over ten years of laboratory work, and it is wonderful to see them emerge in the clinic.

To me, the biggest change of all is the growing attention to what is being called "survivorship." The norm has been to simply study the treatments and then tell women they're lucky to survive and shouldn't complain about such side effects as premature menopause, lymphedema, or "chemo brain." Now large research projects have given us lots of information regarding the experiences of therapy and its aftermath. Research on nonhormone drugs for hot flashes has exploded.

One of the biggest findings, in my mind, is the evidence that weight is a major factor in recurrence. Women who are overweight (often a side effect of therapy) have a higher rate of recurrence. Physical activity, along with sensible eating, is looking more important than any specific diet in improving survival. This fits with the idea that gene environment has a large effect on breast cancer survival, as discussed in the last chapter. It is not only carcinogens causing mutations that do us in, but the environment that either blunts or accelerates their effects.

In the world of software all upgrades are new and revolutionary. In breast cancer research, we aren't quite there yet. But this fourth edition of the *Breast Book,* fifteen years after the first, documents the progress we have made and the hope for the future. The Dr. Susan Love Research Foundation has as its goal the eradication of breast cancer in ten years. This is an audacious goal, but one that is doable. And if we don't set this as the ultimate goal—not only cure or containment but eradication—we will never reach it. It has happened before with polio and to a certain degree with cervical cancer in the Western world. I think by getting to the root of breast cancer deep in the milk ducts, we indeed have a chance to accomplish this. And I will not rest until it happens. I guess you'd better buy this upgrade: it may one day be a collector's item that reflects the history of a defunct disease.

PART ONE

THE HEALTHY BREAST

1

The Breast and Its Development

What do "normal" breasts look like? It's hard to say: the actual range of size and shape of breasts is so wide. Most of us haven't seen many other women's breasts, and we've all grown up with the "ideal" image of breasts that permeates our society. But few of us fit that image, and there's no reason we should. The wide range in size and shape of breasts makes it hard to say what's "normal." Not only are there very large and very small breasts, but in most women one breast is slightly larger than the other. Breast size is genetically determined and depends chiefly on the percentage of fat to other tissue in the breasts. Usually about a third of the breast is composed of fat tissue; the rest is milk ducts and supportive fibrous tissue. The amount of fat varies as you gain or lose weight; the amount of breast tissue remains constant. A "flat-chested" woman's breasts will grow as she gains weight, just as her stomach and thighs do; if she loses the weight, she'll also lose her larger breasts.

Breasts of every size can make milk, and breast size has nothing to do with vulnerability to cancer or other breast disease. Very large breasts, however, can be physically uncomfortable, and, like very small or very uneven breasts, they can be emotionally uncomfortable as well. We'll discuss this at length in Chapter 3.

The breast itself is usually tear-shaped (Fig. 1-1). There's breast tissue

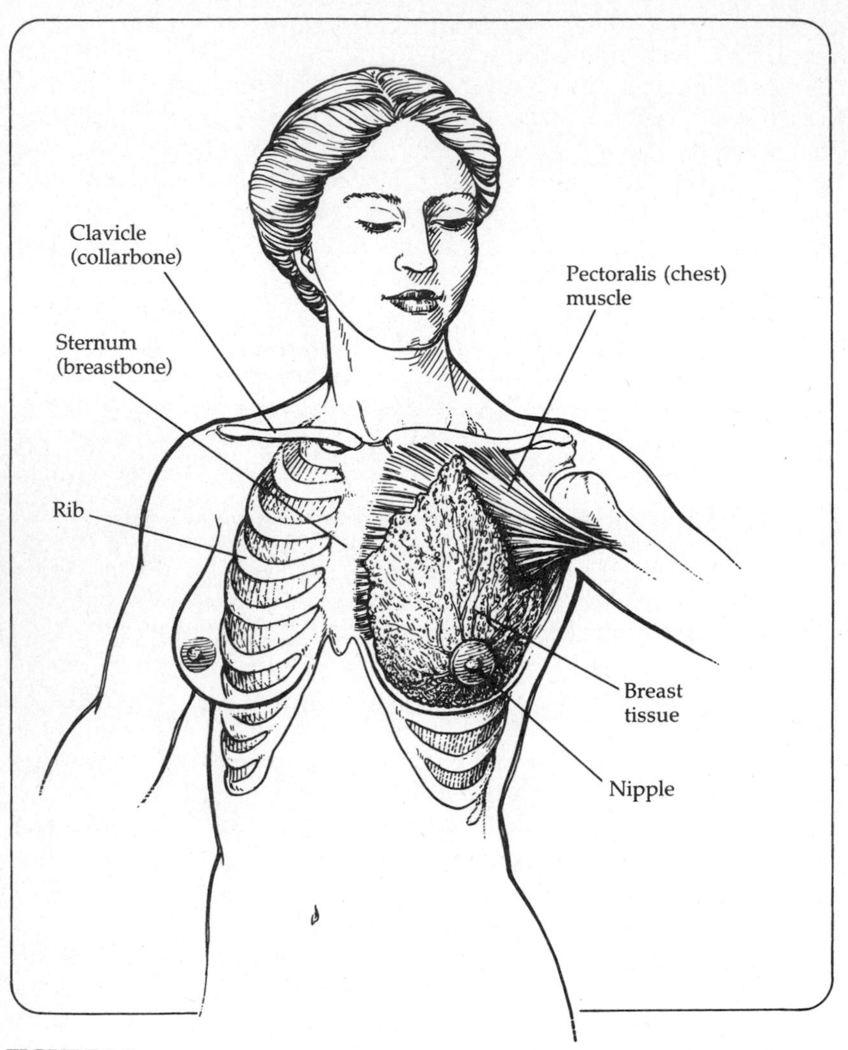

FIGURE 1-1

from the collarbone all the way down to the last few ribs, and from the breastbone in the middle of the chest to the back of the armpit. Your ribs lie behind the breast, and sometimes they may feel hard and lumpy. When I was in medical school I embarrassed myself horribly when I found a "lump" in my breast, and frantically ran to one of the older doctors to find out if I had cancer. I found out I had a rib.

Often there's a ridge of fat at the bottom of the breast—the inframammary ridge. This ridge is perfectly normal. Because we walk upright, our breasts fold over themselves, creating the ridge of fat.

The areola is the darker area of the breast surrounding the nipple (Fig. 1-2). Its size and shape vary from woman to woman, and its color varies according to complexion. In blondes it tends to be pink, in brunettes it's browner, and in dark-skinned people it's brown to black. In most women it gets darker after the first pregnancy. Its color also changes during the various stages of sexual arousal and orgasm.

Many women find their nipples don't face front; they stick out slightly toward the armpits. There's a reason for this. Picture yourself holding a baby you're about to nurse. The baby's head is held in the crook of your arm—a nipple pointing to the side is comfortably close to the baby's mouth (Fig. 1-3).

There are hair follicles around the nipple, so most women have at least some nipple hair. It's perfectly natural, but if you don't like it, don't worry. You can shave it off, pluck it out, use electrolysis, or get rid of it any sensible way you want—it's just like leg or armpit hair. And, as with leg or armpit hair, if it doesn't bother you, you can just ignore it. You may also notice little bumps around the areola that look like goose pimples. These are the little glands known as Montgomery's glands. The nipple also has sebaceous glands, which I talk about later on in this chapter.

Sometimes nipples are "shy": when they're stimulated they retreat into themselves and become temporarily inverted. This is nothing to worry about; it has no effect on milk supply, breast-feeding, sexual pleasure, or anything else. (Permanently inverted nipples are discussed in Chapter 3.)

Inside, as already noted, the breast is made up primarily of fat and breast tissue (Fig. 1-4). The breast tissue is sandwiched between layers

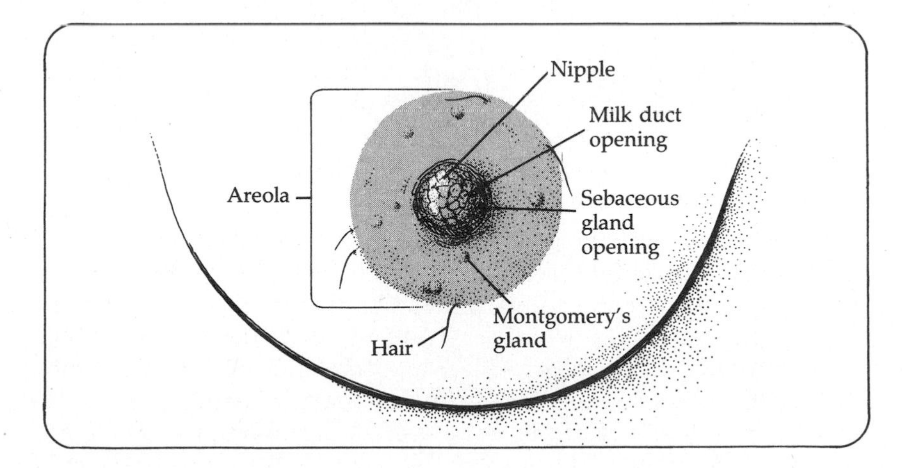

FIGURE 1-2

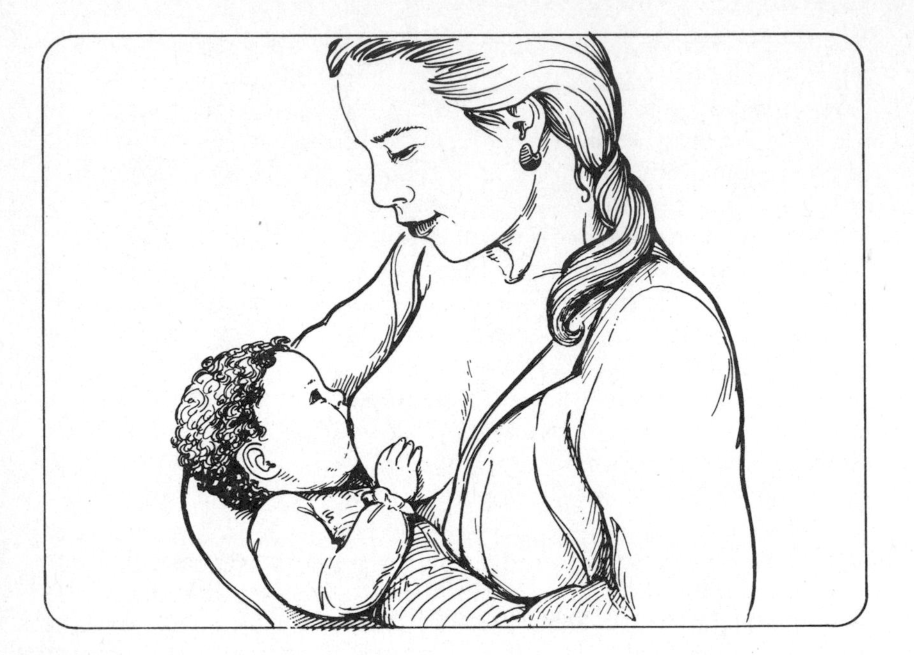

FIGURE 1-3

of fat, behind which is the chest muscle. The fat has some give to it, which is why we bounce. The breast tissue is firm and rubbery. One of my patients told me while I was operating on her that she thought the breast was constructed like a woman—soft and pliant on the outside, and tough underneath. The breast also has its share of the connective tissue that holds the entire body together. This material creates a solid structure—like gelatin—in which the other kinds of tissues are loosely set.

Like the rest of the body the breast has arteries, veins, and nerves. As you probably know, the arteries carry blood rich with oxygen and fuel to the cells, while the veins carry the depleted blood full of carbon dioxide back to the lungs. Another, almost parallel, network of vessels called the lymphatic system (or *lymphatics*) works like recyclers. The job of these vessels is to collect the garbage from the cells and strain it through the lymph nodes found scattered in nests throughout the body; they then send the filtered fluid back into the bloodstream to be reused (Fig. 1-5). They do more than just recycle, however. In the process of filtering the discarded fluid, they register what is in it. If there is anything threatening—a bacterial cell, a piece of suture material, or a virus—they hold on to it and use it to develop an immune response. They send cells to the site to identify the invader and make antibodies to combat it. The lymph nodes are important when we talk about

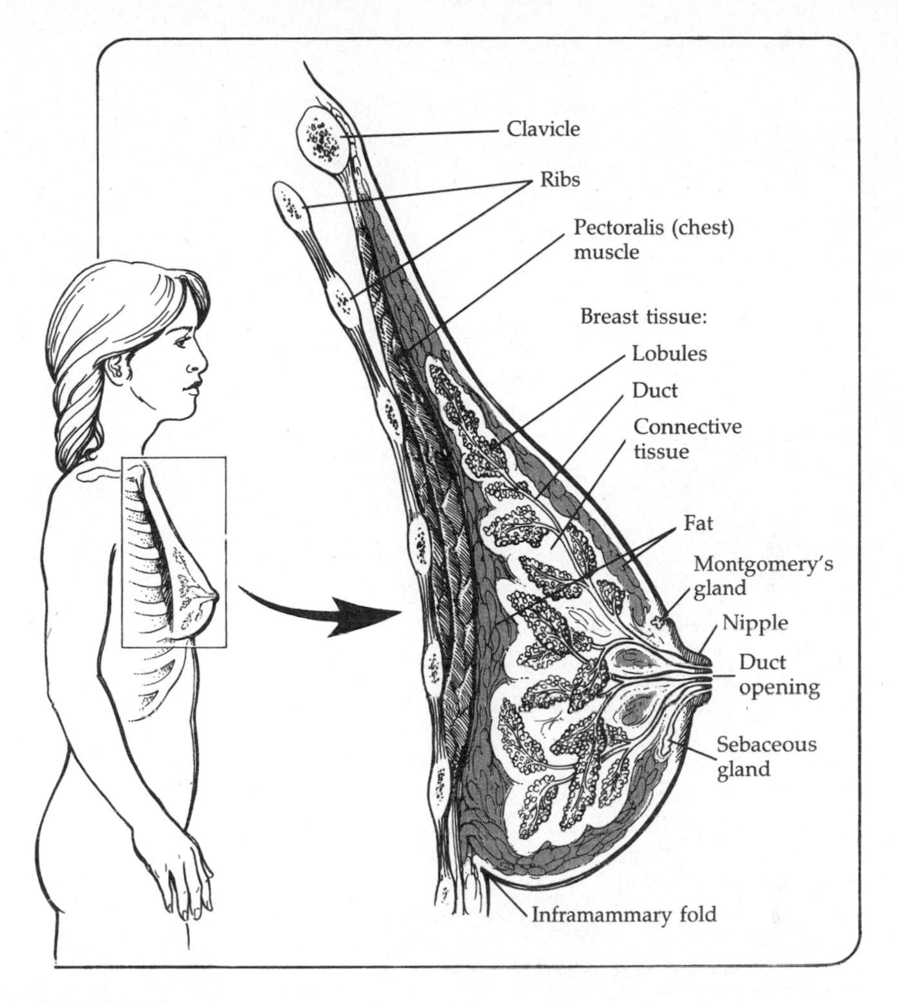

FIGURE 1-4

breast cancer later in the book. It is crucial to identify which lymphatic and which lymph node drain a particular area of the breast so that the correct lymph nodes can be removed and examined for signs of cancer.

There's very little muscle in the breast. There's a bit of muscle in the areola, which is why it contracts and stands out with cold, sexual stimulation, and, of course, breast-feeding. This too makes sense: if the nipple stands out, it's easier for the baby's mouth to get a good grip on it. There are also tiny muscles around the lobules that help deliver milk, as we will discuss later in this chapter. But the major muscles in the area are behind the breasts—the pectorals. Because there is so little

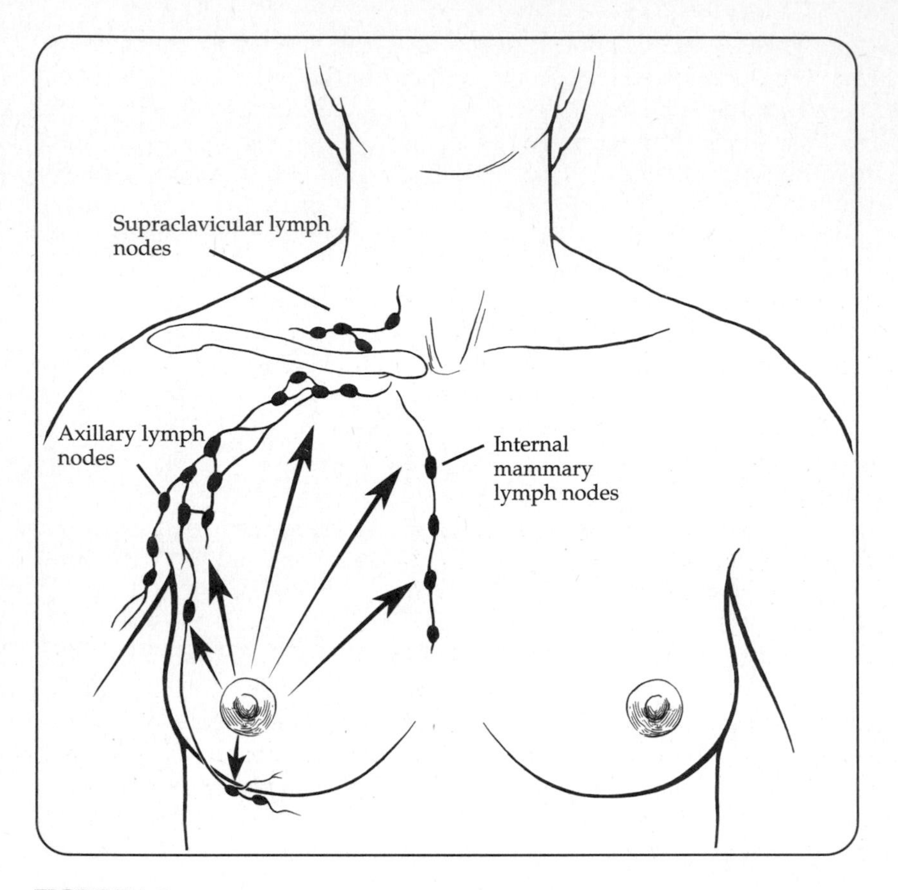

FIGURE 1-5

muscle inside the breasts, the idea that you can grow larger breasts through exercise is false. You can grow stronger pectorals—as bodybuilders do—but all that means is that your breasts will rest on an expanded chest.

THE DUCTAL ANATOMY

All of this structure surrounds and supports the critical ductal system. Curiously, although the ducts and lobules are the main "business" part of the breast, their anatomy has largely been ignored.

Years ago, when I began my own research, I was amazed to find how little basic information was available on the milk ducts—such as how many there were, where they were, which little holes in the nipple were ducts and which weren't. The only study I could find had been done by Sir Astley Cooper in 1839.[1] Experimenting on cadavers, he injected soft wax into the ducts through the nipple and made casts when the wax hardened. He discovered that the ducts did not connect to one another; there were separate ductal systems. Though he mentioned that the nipple contained between 15 and 20 holes, he found that he could only get wax into between five and eight milk duct openings.

From then on all the textbooks dutifully reported the existence of 15 to 20 ductal systems. No one followed up on Dr. Cooper's research, and no one thought to investigate the issue further.

So when I began to explore the possibility of an intraductal approach to the detection of precancerous cells (see Chapter 13), I had to start at the beginning. My team and I tried to figure out an easy way to determine how many holes there were in the nipple. One of my research assistants, Jean Chou, came up with a wonderful idea: we could undoubtedly see the ductal openings best when women were breast-feeding, so why not go to meetings of La Leche League? This organization promotes breast-feeding, and with its help Jean was able to examine the women who were breast-feeding and map the holes in the nipple that were squirting milk.

She examined the breasts of 219 amiable women who had agreed to have their breasts catalogued by a stranger. Examining both breasts, she mapped out the openings. She found that there were about six to eight per breast, arranged in a fairly consistent pattern. It's possible that she missed a few. If you've ever breast-fed, you know that once the milk starts coming out, it's like a watering can—and of course it immediately becomes one big blob of milk on your nipple. Still, if she was undercounting, it was probably by two or three, not by 10 or more.

Usually, we learned, there are two or three milk duct orifices in the center of the nipples, with others scattered around them (Fig. 1-6). The middle ones were consistent in all the women we examined. The number and placement of the openings around the periphery tended to be more variable: one woman might have three on the outside, and another, five. However, they never varied in an individual woman: if she had three in her left breast, she had three in her right breast.

What, then, were those other holes Dr. Cooper found back in 1839—the ones that everybody's been calling "ducts" ever since? We think they're little glands that make a sebaceous material—a white, oily substance. These sebaceous glands are found all over the body. We don't know what they're for, or why there are so many around the nipple. My own theory is that the body produces them to provide a coating that protects the skin—sort of your own little skin-care system. The nipple, designed to be sucked on, is especially vulnerable to getting chapped and sore, so having a lot of these glands makes sense.

We then studied the anatomy beyond the nipple, using cadavers

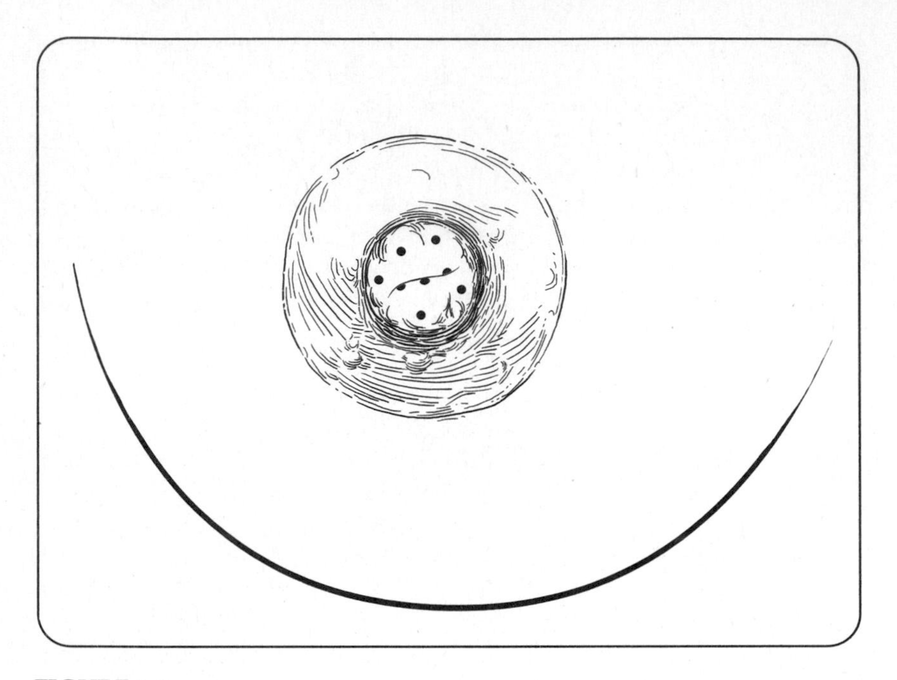

FIGURE 1-6

and breasts that had been removed by mastectomy. We learned that the duct opening in the nipple leads into the breast in a straight line for a very short distance—only about a centimeter. It has a small amount of keratin—dead skin—that forms a kind of plug. There's a little sphincter muscle here that prevents milk from squirting out when a breast-feeding woman is not feeding her baby. Behind that is a little antechamber called the *lactiferous sinus.* From there, the ductal system, like a tree, breaks up into little branches that go to the back of the breast. These branches are the ducts. Leafing out at the end of each branch are the lobules, which make the breast milk and then send it through the ducts to the nipple. Each ductal system is independent of all the others; each creates milk separately. They coexist, but they don't connect with one another.

We explored the pattern of the ducts themselves. In the 1970s and 1980s Dr. Otto Sartorius, a breast surgeon in Santa Barbara, did many ductograms—a procedure in which he put a tiny catheter into a woman's nipple, ran dye through it, then took X rays. He did about 2,000 of these procedures. When he died in 1994, I inherited the X rays and continued his work. My research team and I analyzed the X rays, which gave us a good idea of where ducts tended to be within the breast. We discovered a few surprises. Until now, we'd visualized the

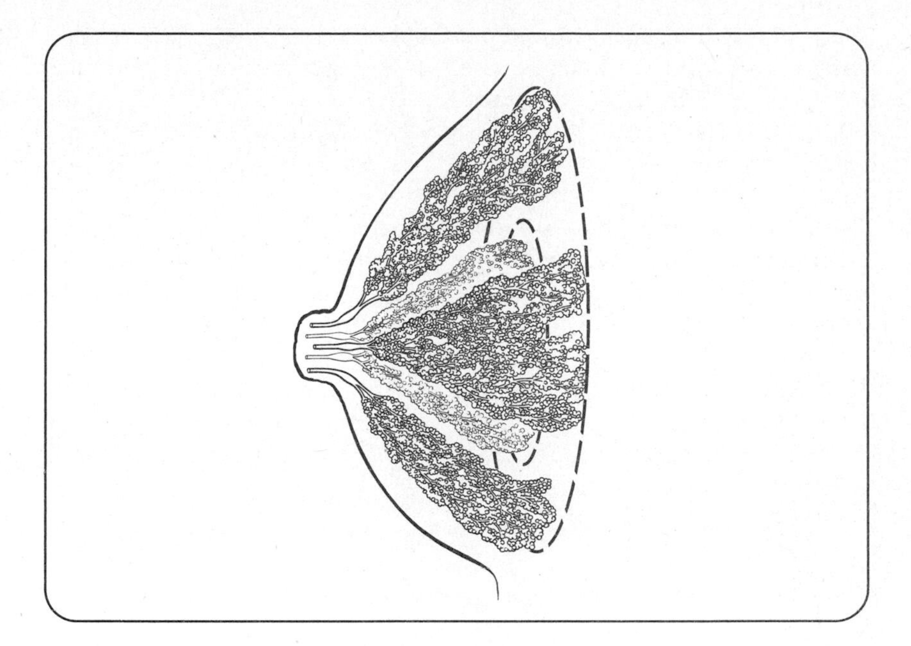

FIGURE 1-7

breast as though it were a pie, with each ductal system radiating from the center like equal slices. Finally the obvious occurred to us—the breast isn't two-dimensional! Anatomy exists in three dimensions, though it appears two-dimensional in photographs and x-ray images. The breast is in reality shaped like a giant gumdrop. What this means is that the ductal systems go from the nipple toward the chest wall (Fig. 1-7). And the ductal systems are not all the same size. One system might cover the whole upper part of the breast, or perhaps there are two or three. In addition, the ductal systems run throughout the breast, often as far up as the collarbone or as far down as the lower ribs. Our x-ray studies of the ducts matched the findings from La Leche League, even though they involved different patients. Medically, then, perhaps we should be thinking not of a breast but of six to nine ductal systems.[2]

HOW THE BREAST DEVELOPS

To understand how the breast typically develops, we need to know what it's for. The breast is an integral part of a woman's reproductive system. It actually defines our biological class: mammals derive their name from the fact that they have mammary glands and feed their young at their breasts. Different mammals have different numbers and sizes of breasts, but human females are the only ones to develop full breasts long before they are needed to feed their young. We are also the only animals who are actively sexual when we're not fertile. This suggests that our breasts have an important secondary function as contributors to our sensual pleasure.

Although women have traditionally been thought of as "other" (to use Simone de Beauvoir's word) in our male-dominated culture, biologically we're the norm. The genitalia of all embryos are female. When the hormone testosterone is produced at the direction of the Y chromosome, the fetus starts to develop male genitalia. If the testes are destroyed early in fetal development, the male fetus will develop breasts and retain female genitalia. It makes sense to suggest that the basis of "mankind" is, in fact, woman. To me that is confirmed by the fact that men have rudimentary nipples.

Early Development

Human breast tissue begins to develop remarkably early—in the sixth week of fetal life. It develops across a line known as the milk ridge, which runs from the armpit down to the groin (Fig. 1-8). In most cases the milk ridge soon regresses, and by the ninth week it's just in the chest area. (Other mammals retain the milk ridge, which is why they have multiple nipples.) So you already have breast tissue at birth, and it's sensitive to hormones even then (your mother's sex hormones have been circulating through the placenta). Infants may even have nipple discharge. This "witch's milk," as it's called, goes away in a couple of weeks, since the infant is no longer getting the mother's hormones. Between 80 and 90 percent of all infants of both genders have this discharge on the second or third day after birth.

Puberty

After early infancy, not much happens to the breast until puberty (Fig. 1-9). Then the ductal tissue begins to grow and create the beginnings of ducts. Though they aren't yet capable of making milk, the general outline of the ductal system is there. The cells that make this happen are called stem cells—cells capable of turning into other cells. They're sort of great-grandmother progenitor cells that can become a lot of things. The stem cells can become duct cells or lobular cells growing along a complex branching system. Some stem cells remain to replenish in-

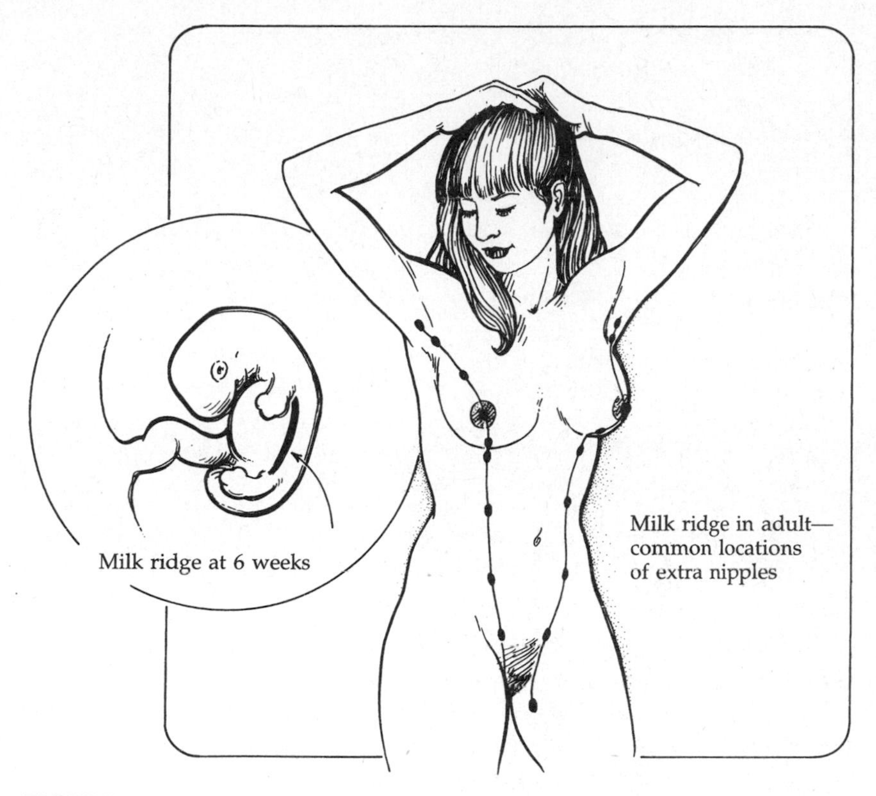

FIGURE 1-8

jured ductal or lobular cells. A new hypothesis is focusing on these cells as the eventual origin of cancer.[3]

Soon after the pubic hair begins to grow, the breasts start responding to the hormonal changes in the girl's body. (Typically her periods start a year or two after her breasts begin growing.) They begin with a little bud of breast tissue under the nipple—it can be itchy and sometimes a bit painful. The rudimentary ducts begin to grow, and the breasts expand until they've reached their full growth—usually by the time menstruation begins. One little girl quoted in *Breasts,* a book of photos and text about women's relationship to their breasts, described it beautifully: "At first they were flat, then all of a sudden the nipples came out like mosquito bites. And three or four days ago I noticed that my breasts were coming out from the sides. When I first started they were just little lumps by the nipple."[4]

The first tiny breasts can be confusing to children and to their parents as well. One of my patients was an 11-year-old girl whose mother

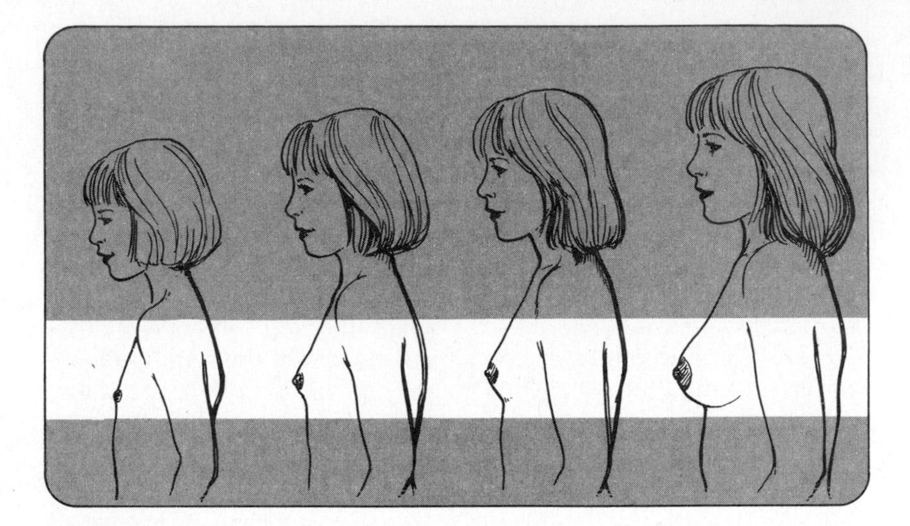

FIGURE 1-9

had breast cancer, and they found what they were sure was a lump under the girl's nipple. I was certain it was just the beginning of her breast development and was able to reassure them. It's never advisable to remove newly forming breast tissue, since it won't grow back and the child will never have that breast.

The rate at which breasts grow varies greatly from girl to girl; some start off very "flat-chested" and end up with large breasts; others have large breasts at an early age. Often one breast grows more quickly than the other. (We'll discuss this and other variations in breast development in Chapter 3.)

The emotional confusion around all of puberty can be intensified for the girl growing up in a society that both mystifies and obsesses about breasts. For the adolescent girl, the growth of her breasts can be a source of extreme pleasure or extreme dismay—and often both at once. In a 1980 British survey researchers learned that 56 percent of the women they questioned had been pleased with their breast development, while 33 percent were shy and 24 percent, embarrassed. Ten percent had been "worried" or "unhappy."[5] In 1986, I did an informal survey among my own patients, with similar results. Of 165 patients who filled out a questionnaire in my office, 70 recalled having been happy or proud of their budding breasts; 61 had been embarrassed and angry; 20, confused; and 9, ambivalent. One had been "amazed." Not surprisingly, only four were "indifferent."

I also talked with a number of my patients about their memories of how they felt when their breasts began to develop. Again, I found a range of feelings. Two of my youngest patients had opposite reactions to their breast growth. One, 13, said that when her breasts began to grow, "I felt older and I felt mature, that I was becoming a woman." She was proud of her new breasts: "I think that for my age, my boobs are just right," she said. But a 16-year-old patient told me she was embarrassed when her breasts began to grow because she "always felt as if people were staring at me and talking about me." She didn't like her breasts, which she saw as "too hard and lumpy, and triangular, not round."

Similar differences of attitude appeared in the recollections of my older patients. One 48-year-old recalled the first day she wore her bra to school: "I was so proud—I was the second girl in the sixth grade to have one. All the other girls gathered around me and I showed them my bra." Others were less delighted. A 39-year-old remembered thinking, "Oh, shit, now I'm supposed to be a girl!" To her, developing breasts represented confusion and "the world getting much worse." A 65-year-old patient said that she hadn't been "ready for this sign of growing up. It was like going down a roller coaster and not being able to stop it." A middle-aged mother recalled that for many years she wore overlarge sweaters to hide the breasts that embarrassed her. "My teenage daughter does the same thing now," she said, "and it makes me a bit sad to remember that stage of my life." For many women, breasts represented enforced femininity: they could no longer play ball with the boys and felt they had lost forever a kind of freedom boys still had.

On the other hand, a delay in the appearance of breasts can be equally upsetting. One of my friends, whose breasts didn't begin developing until her midteens, recalled her feelings of inadequacy. "I was so upset," she said. "My grandmother had told me that I'd get breasts if I rubbed cocoa butter on my chest. So for months, every night, before I went to sleep, I rubbed cocoa butter on my flat little chest, hoping I'd wake up with breasts."

Sometimes, because of their hormonal development, adolescent boys develop a condition called *gynecomastia*—which translates to "breasts like a woman." This can be in one breast or both. For obvious reasons, the boys' reactions don't parallel the ambivalence of the developing girls—for them, breast development is uniformly embarrassing. I remember my seventh-grade boyfriend was so humiliated by it that he paid another boy to push him into the swimming pool so he wouldn't have to take off his shirt to swim or explain to the other kids why he was swimming with his shirt on. I occasionally had patients suffering from gynecomastia. Their mental anguish, as well as their acute embarrassment at having to show me their chests, was really painful to see. Fortunately the condition usually regresses on its own in about 18 months; if it doesn't, it can easily be helped through surgery.

The Menstruating Years

A girl's initial breast development is soon followed by the establishment of the menstrual cycle as her body begins to prepare for reproduction. Hormones play a crucial part in this development, as they do in all aspects of reproductive growth. On the ovary are follicles with eggs encased in their developmental sacs (Fig. 1-10). These, stimulated by FSH (follicle stimulating hormone) in the pituitary gland, produce estrogen. The resulting high levels of estrogen in the blood tell the pituitary to turn off the FSH and start secreting LH (luteinizing hormone). When the estrogen and LH are both at their peak, you ovulate—the follicle bursts and releases its egg into the fallopian tube.

The follicle is now an empty sac, but it still has a job to do: it becomes the *corpus luteum* and starts producing progesterone, which prepares the lining of the uterus for pregnancy ("progesterone" means "pro-pregnancy"). Usually the egg doesn't get fertilized. Then the progesterone level falls off, the lining of the uterus is shed, and you start all over again. If the egg is fertilized, the corpus luteum starts to produce HCG (human choriogonadotropin), which maintains the progesterone level until the placenta takes over producing it, and you're well on your way to a baby.

In addition to maintaining fertility, these cyclical hormones are preparing the breast for a potential pregnancy each month. In a very general sense, estrogen causes the ductal tissue in the breast to grow, and progesterone the lobular tissue. This obviously has something to do with the cyclical changes women's breasts go through—swelling, pain, tenderness—but exactly what is still unclear.

Breast-Feeding

The purpose of the breast is to make milk, and so a woman's breast doesn't reach its full potential until she's been through a nine-month pregnancy. This stage of the breast's development becomes evident soon after conception. Even before she misses her period, a woman may notice that her breasts are unusually tender or her nipples are unusually sore. I've had a few patients coming to me complaining of strange breast pain that turns out to be an early sign of pregnancy.

Breasts enlarge rapidly and become very firm during pregnancy. The Montgomery's glands—those little glands around the areola—become darker and more prominent, and the areola darkens. The nipples become larger and more erect, preparing themselves for future milk production (Fig. 1-11).

The development of the breast into a milk-producing machine is

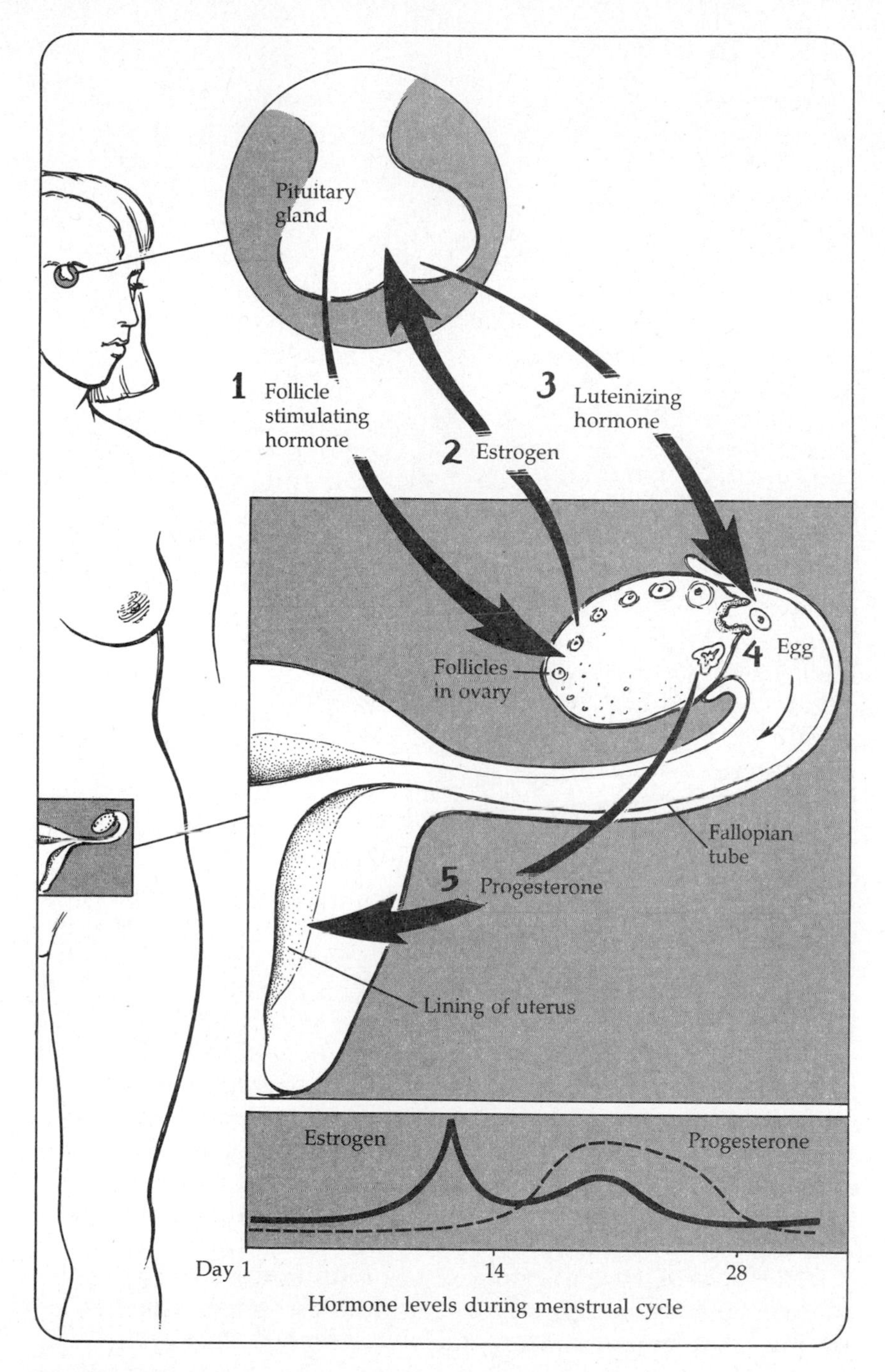
Pituitary gland
1 Follicle stimulating hormone
2 Estrogen
3 Luteinizing hormone
Follicles in ovary
4 Egg
Fallopian tube
5 Progesterone
Lining of uterus
Estrogen
Progesterone
Day 1
14
28
Hormone levels during menstrual cycle

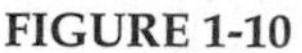
FIGURE 1-10

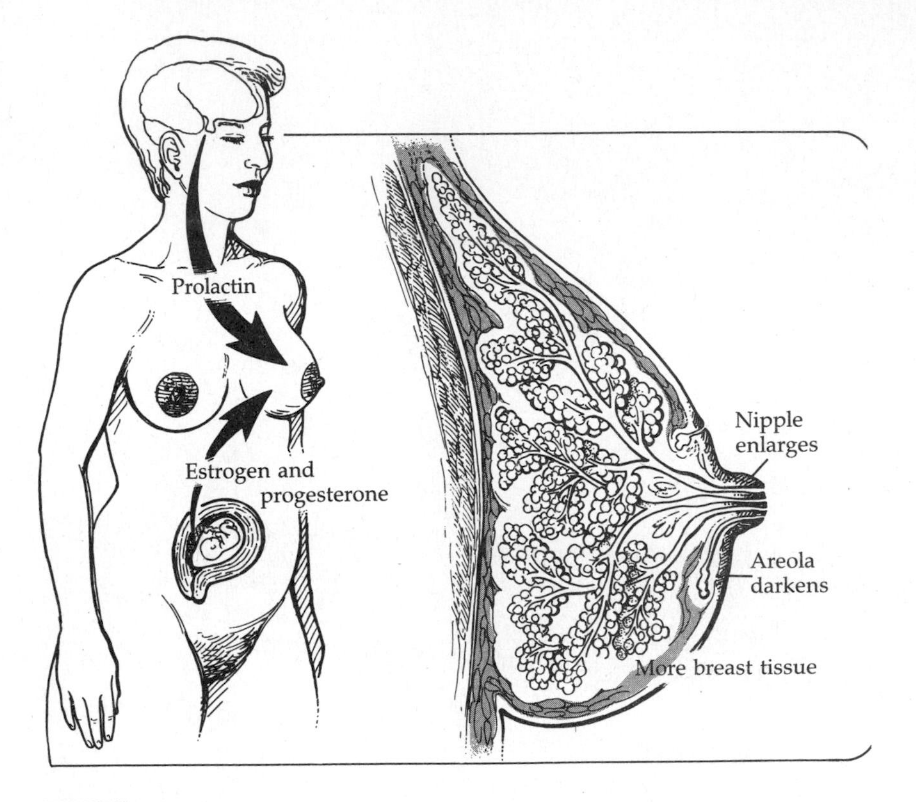

FIGURE 1-11

orchestrated by several hormones, including estrogen and progesterone as well as prolactin and oxytocin. Meanwhile, other hormones are at work—insulin, thyroid, and cortisol, as well as background nutritional hormones. These take part of the food the pregnant woman eats and remanufacture it so that it can become part of the baby's milk.

Once the baby is born and the placenta has been delivered, the woman's estrogen and progesterone levels plummet, while prolactin levels begin a much slower decline. This is the sign for the breasts to begin producing milk. The milk, however, doesn't come right away, and for three and five days the breasts make another liquid, a sort of premilk called *colostrum,* which the baby can drink while waiting for the milk to come in. Colostrum is filled with antibodies that help the infant fight off infection.

While some milk is sucked out by the baby, some simply gushes into the baby's mouth, squeezed out by the tiny muscles lining the lobules. The mother experiences this as "letdown": her milk is literally being let down inside her breasts. The other surprise to most new parents is that the milk comes out of many holes in the nipple—like a watering can.

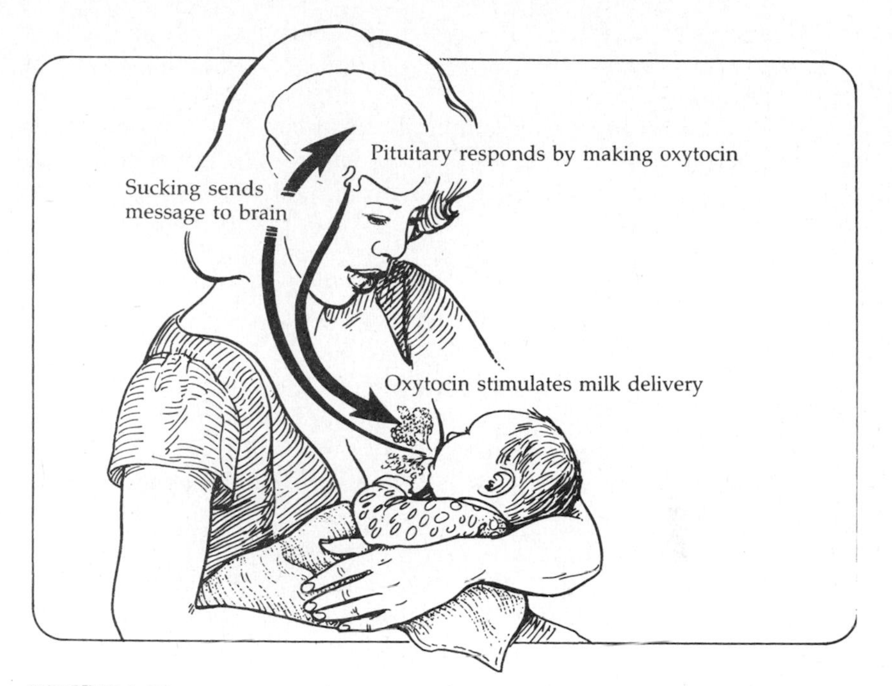

FIGURE 1-12

As noted earlier, these holes are the openings of the six to nine milk ducts.

If a new mother is not producing milk within a week of the baby's birth, something is wrong and a clinician should be consulted. Aside from deliberate attempts to inhibit milk, several things can prevent breasts from producing milk. The woman may have a problem in her pituitary gland—she may have hemorrhaged into it, or it may be otherwise damaged, and she won't be able to produce the necessary prolactin and oxytocin (see Fig. 1-12). Sometimes the milk comes into the breast but can't get out. This is caused by damage to the duct system, usually by surgery around the nipple or perhaps by breast reduction surgery (see Chapter 3). Sometimes the ducts can be unblocked but often they can't, and in that case the baby will have to be bottle-fed instead of breast-fed. (The milk is reabsorbed into the mother's body.) Sometimes the baby has a problem coordinating tongue motions, or the shape of a woman's nipples makes it hard for the baby to latch on. Insufficient milk needs to be evaluated by a clinician expert in breastfeeding: a pediatrician, family doctor, or lactation consultant.

After the mother stops breast-feeding she'll continue to have some secretions for two or three months, and sometimes as long as a year or two.

Breast-feeding has some contraceptive effect, but only in the first three or four months—and even then, it's important to realize that it isn't 100 percent effective.

Some women have too little milk. In most cases this can be alleviated by feeding more often—a feeding every two hours generally helps. If such a rigorous schedule proves impossible for you, it may be time to stop breast-feeding and turn to formula—or at least combine breast- and bottle-feeding. Sometimes even frequent feeding doesn't help: for some reason, the woman's body simply doesn't make enough milk, no matter what she does. Many women feel an irrational guilt when this happens, as though they've failed in their "motherly duties." They haven't—it's a biological idiosyncrasy, not a cosmic flaw.

What are the advantages of breast-feeding? Probably the most important is the nutritional composition of breast milk. It's tailor-made for the human baby's needs—it has the perfect combination of water, protein, carbohydrates (mainly lactose), immunoglobin (which helps create immunity against disease), lots of cholesterol (which, though unhealthy for adults, is great for babies), and vitamins and minerals. Cow's milk, on the other hand, is tailor-made for the needs of baby cows, which are obviously somewhat different from those of the human baby.

Formula is our attempt to modify cow's milk to make it as close as possible to human milk. We've done a pretty impressive job, but it's not perfect. For one thing, cow's milk isn't as digestible as human milk. It takes a baby four hours to digest formula, and only two to digest human milk. No formula has been able to duplicate the immunity-providing properties of colostrum.

Breast-feeding also creates a unique bonding between mother and infant, which some psychologists feel is essential to the child's later well-being. While there are plenty of emotionally healthy people who were bottle-fed and many neurotics who were breast-fed, the particular bonding created by breast-feeding can't be wholly duplicated in bottle-feeding. On the other hand, breast-feeding can create difficulties for the mother that may outweigh the advantages to the child—difficulties that proselytizers for breast-feeding sometimes underrate. Breast-feeding every two or three hours may be very difficult for a woman who has a job outside her home, and it's not always that easy for the woman at home who has primary responsibility for raising other children and/or doing housework. Sometimes a combination of breast-feeding and bottle-feeding (using either formula or breast milk expressed by the mother at an earlier time) can be a useful compromise. (See Fig. 1-13.)

Lactation can cause problems, even for the mother combining breast and bottle feeding. Oxytocin can be produced by emotional as well as

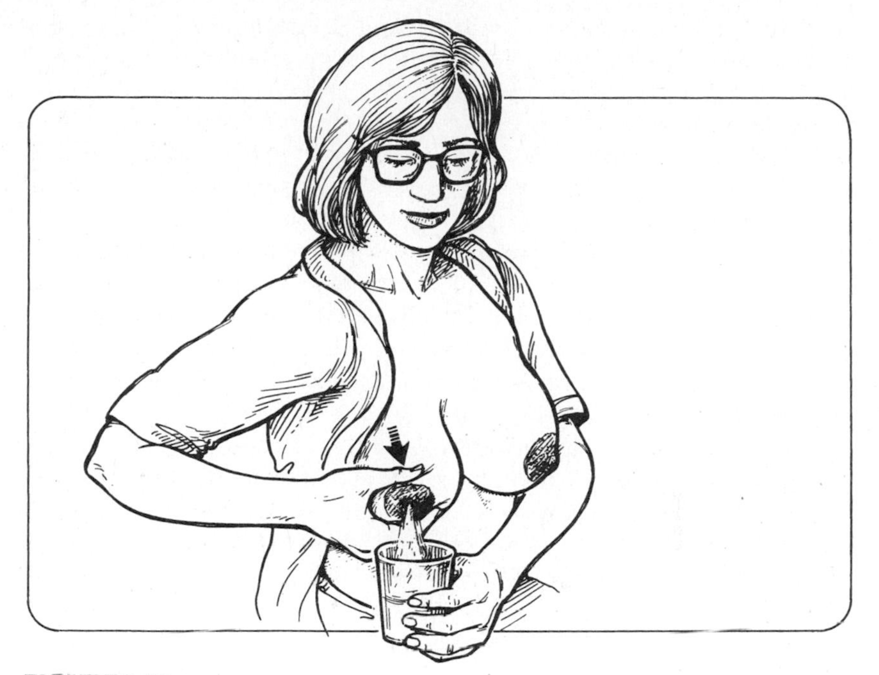

FIGURE 1-13

direct physical responses to the baby, and many mothers will find to their embarrassment that milk will suddenly begin to flow when they think about the baby. A surgeon colleague of mine decided to stop breast-feeding when the thought of her baby came to her during an operation and milk started dripping onto her patient.

There are also women whose own eating habits or medications can make breast-feeding a problem. It's true that the baby will consume, through your milk, everything you consume, and many women really cherish their cups of coffee or their evening martinis. It's probably safest to remain drug- and alcohol-free while breast-feeding. For some women this is easy; for others, it's not. Some mothers are on medication for chronic health problems, and some (though certainly not all) medication will harm a breast-feeding baby. Sacrificing your own health or comfort may not be the best thing for either you or your child.

Menopause

We've got the menstruating years figured out, but our understanding of the process is a little fuzzier when we come to the end of the fertile years. The standard line in the textbooks is that when you run out of eggs and you're no longer ovulating, your body stops making estrogen. This causes your FSH to go up as your pituitary tries to kick-start the ovary into producing more eggs. When that doesn't work, everything just shuts down.

Yet often the symptoms of perimenopause (right before menopause)—breast tenderness, headaches, increased vaginal lubrication—are symptoms of high, not low, estrogen. Sometimes your estrogen levels are high and your progesterone is low, and you might get symptoms of PMS (premenstrual syndrome), while other times your estrogen levels shift and you get hot flashes. Then for several months you're back to normal. So the common explanation is wrong: your symptoms aren't due to low estrogen. They're caused by fluctuations of high and low estrogen.

Sometimes doctors test FSH levels in the blood to decide whether you are in menopause. The problem is that just as estrogen and progesterone fluctuate widely, so does FSH. It could be high at one time and low a month later. If you've stopped menstruating for several months, the FSH tests might be a little more useful for determining if you've really gone into menopause. But even then, it's not 100 percent accurate. One study found that 20 percent of women who had no period for three months started having their cycles again.[6] Breast cancer patients who were thrown into menopause by their chemotherapy treatments missed three or four months of periods, showed high FSH levels—and then got their periods back. There's no foolproof test to determine menopause. The only way we can really do that is the good old-fashioned way. If you haven't menstruated for a year, you're considered menopausal. However, don't assume you're totally out of the woods even then. Some women will get another period after the magic year has passed.

The Role of the Ovary

Throughout most of medical history we have not really understood the ovary. And because we haven't grasped the full complexity of this intricate organ, doctors have assumed that after menopause, when it is no longer capable of making eggs, the ovary shrivels up, dries out, and becomes completely useless.

But egg making isn't the ovary's whole function anymore than reproduction is a woman's whole function. The ovary is more than just an egg sack. It's an endocrine organ—one that produces hormones. And it produces them before, during, and after menopause. With menopause, the ovary goes through a shift. It changes from a follicle-rich producer of estrogen and progesterone into a stromal-rich producer of estrogen and androgen (a male hormone). Stroma is the glue

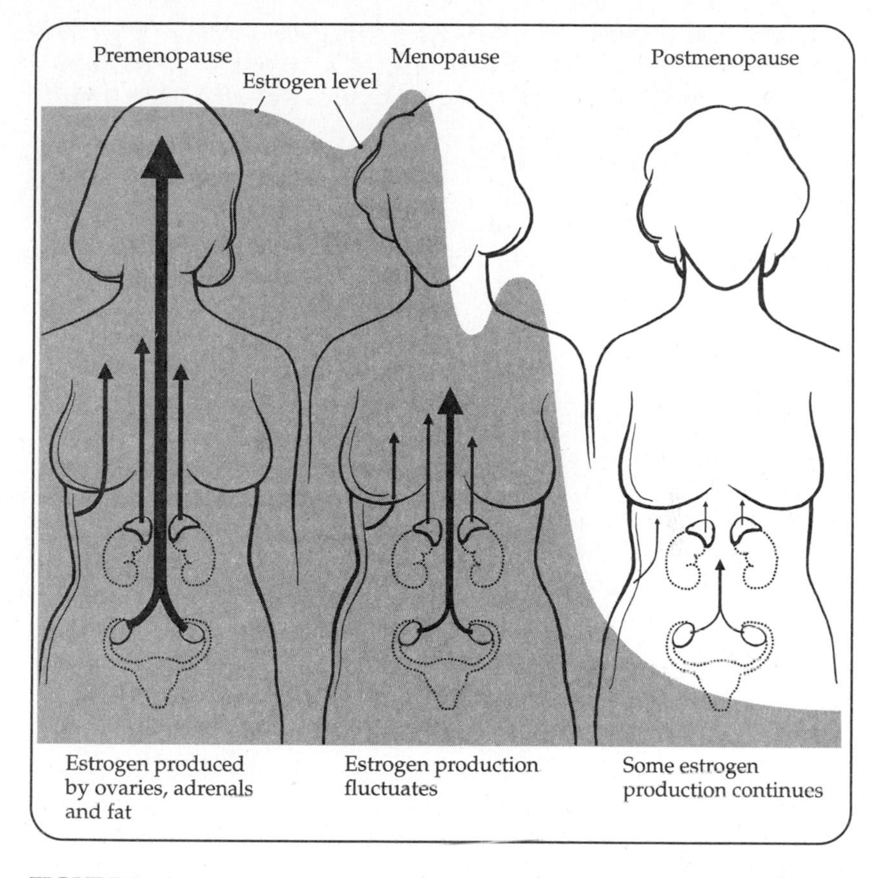

FIGURE 1-14

or background tissue in which eggs are embedded. In youth, you have more eggs and less stroma. As time goes on, you have fewer and fewer eggs and more and more stroma. In its hormonal dance with the hypothalamus and pituitary, the postmenopausal ovary continues to respond to the call of the pituitary. It responds to the high levels of FSH and LH with increased production of testosterone as well as lower levels of estrone and estradiol (two forms of estrogen) and androstenedione (a male hormone).[7,8] The hormonal dance doesn't end; the band just strikes up a different tune. (See Fig. 1-14.)

Testosterone, of course, is a male hormone. But don't panic: you're not going to grow a beard. Every human being produces both male and female hormones; the proportion differs according to gender. Much of the testosterone and androstenedione is converted to estrone by fat and muscle. This continued production of hormones varies somewhat from one woman to the next and may well explain some of the individual differences in symptoms after menopause. It also explains why women who have both ovaries removed surgically, losing all of these hormones, have worse symptoms of menopause and increased vulnerability to cardiovascular disease and osteoporosis.[9]

What all this means is that the ovaries have more than one function. Reproduction is their most dramatic function, but it isn't the only one. These organs have as much to do with the maintenance of the woman's own life as they do with her role in bringing other lives into the world. The menopausal ovary is neither failing nor useless. It's simply beginning to shift from its reproductive to its maintenance function. It's doing in midlife exactly what many people do—changing careers.

As we learn more about hormone levels in women after menopause, we begin to understand their effects on the breast. We have observed, for example, that women with osteoporosis have 60 percent less breast cancer than women with normal bone density have. This is probably due to natural estrogen levels. If you have relatively high levels of estrogen in your body postmenopausally you will have good bones and bad breasts; on the other hand, if your estrogen levels are lower you will have good breasts and bad bones.

The postmenopausal breast is even more complex. Giving women hormones postmenopausally increases estrogen (and usually progestins), resulting in hormone-sensitive tumors (see Chapter 16). Yet not every woman who takes postmenopausal hormones gets breast cancer. Also, women on postmenopausal hormones often, but not always, experience an increase in breast density, known to be a risk factor for breast cancer (see Chapter 9). It is likely that some women are more sensitive to postmenopausal hormones than others. Which ones and why is a subject of much research. In addition, recent studies have shown that breast tissue itself has the enzyme aromatase, which can convert testosterone and androstenedione into estrogen. This means that estrogen levels in the breast may indeed be higher than those in the rest of the body after menopause and may explain the estrogen-sensitive cancers that occur at this age. Our increasing understanding of the postmenopausal breast's response to hormones will give us insight into the cause of breast cancer after menopause.

Bras

In our society breasts and their coverings have become almost a fetish. The bra, a relatively recent invention, became popular in the 1920s as a replacement for the uncomfortable and often mutilating corsets of the nineteenth century. While wearing a bra is never physically harmful, it has no medical necessity whatsoever. Many of my large-breasted patients feel more comfortable wearing a bra, especially if they run or engage in other athletic activities. As one patient said, "These babies need all the support they can get!"

Many women, however, find bras uncomfortable. Interestingly, I had one patient who got a rash underneath her breasts when she didn't wear a bra and her breasts sagged, and another who had very sensitive skin and got a rash when she did wear a bra, because of the elastic, the stitching, and the metal hooks (she switched to camisoles). Except for the women who find bras especially comfortable or uncomfortable, the decision to wear or not wear one is purely aesthetic—or emotional.

For some women, bras are a necessity created by society. One of my patients told me she enjoyed going without a bra, but, she said, "Men made nasty and degrading comments as I walked down the street." Another patient, a high school teacher, felt obligated to wear a bra, although she described it as "a ritual object, like a dog collar. . . . I take it off immediately after work."

But other women like the uplift and the different contours a bra provides. A woman quoted in *Breasts* said she was "crazy about bras—I think of them as jewelry."[10] She and others find them sexy and enjoy incorporating them into their lovemaking rituals.

A mistaken popular belief maintains that wearing a bra strengthens your breasts and prevents sagging. But you sag because of the proportion of fat and tissue in your breasts, and no bra changes that. Furthermore, breast-feeding and lactation increase the size of the breast, and when the tissue returns to its normal size the skin is stretched out and saggy. As I noted earlier, except for the small muscles of the areola and lobules, the muscles are behind your breast—and are unaffected by whether or not you wear a bra. If you've been wearing a bra regularly and decide to give it up, you may find that your breasts hurt for a while. Don't be alarmed. The connective tissue in which the ducts and lobules are suspended is suddenly being strained. It's the same tissue that hurts when you jog or run. Once your body adjusts to not wearing a bra, the pain will go away.

No type of bra is better or worse for you in terms of health. Some of my patients who wear underwire bras have been told they can get cancer from them. This is total nonsense. It makes no difference medically whether your bra opens in the front or back, is padded or not padded, is made of nylon, cotton, or anything else, or gives much support or little support. The only time I recommend a bra for medical reasons is after breast surgery. Then the pull from a hanging breast can cause more pain, slow the healing of the wound, and create larger scars. For this purpose, I recommend a firmer rather than a lighter bra during the immediate postoperative period.

Otherwise, if you enjoy a bra for esthetic, sexual, or comfort reasons, by all means wear one. If you don't enjoy it, and job or social pressures don't force you into it, don't bother. Medically, it's all the same.

Breast Sensitivity

Breasts are usually very sensitive—as you'll notice if you get hit in the breasts. It's very painful, but if you've been told being injured in the breast leads to cancer, ignore it. All a bruised breast causes is temporary pain. Similarly, scar tissue that results from an injury to the breast won't cause cancer. Breast sensitivity changes during the menstrual cycle. During the first two weeks of the cycle the breasts are less sensitive; they are very sensitive around ovulation and after, and less sensitive again during menstruation. There are also changes during the larger development process. There's little sensitivity before puberty, much sensitivity after puberty, and extreme sensitivity during pregnancy and perimenopause. After menopause, the sensitivity diminishes but never fully vanishes. As in most aspects of the normal breast, sensitivity varies greatly among women. There's no "right" or "healthy" degree of responsiveness.

Breasts also vary greatly in their sensitivity to sexual stimuli. Physiologic changes in the breasts are an integral part of female sexual response. In the excitement phase the nipples harden and become more erect, the breasts plump up, and the areola swells. In the plateau just before orgasm breasts, nipples, and areola get larger still, peaking with the orgasm and then gradually subsiding. For most women, breast stimulation contributes to sexual pleasure. Many who enjoy having their breasts stroked or sucked by their lovers have been told that this can lead to cancer. It can't. Breasts, after all, are made to be suckled, and your body won't punish you because it's a lover rather than a baby doing it. Some women's breasts are so erogenous that breast stimulation alone can bring them to orgasm; others find breast stimulation uninteresting or even unpleasant. Neither extreme is more "normal." Different people have different sexual needs and respond to different sexual stimuli. Patients ask me whether a lack of sexual responsiveness around their breasts means something is wrong with them. It doesn't. There is an unfortunate tradition in our culture to label as "frigid" women whose sexual needs don't correspond to those of their (usually) male partners. Ironically, the converse of this persists in our supposedly liberated era: a woman who is easily sexually stimulated is seen as a "slut." All such stereotypes are unfortunate and destructive. If your breasts contribute to your sexual pleasure, enjoy it. If not, focus on what you do like and don't worry.

2

Getting Acquainted with Your Breasts

Babies, as yet unconditioned by social inhibitions, are wiser than their elders. Watch a baby gleefully playing with its toes. We smile at this but often stop smiling when the baby's joyful self-discovery focuses on the genitals. Then children learn that body parts associated with sexuality are taboo. We need to reverse this process, to teach little children to respect and cherish their bodies. And as adults, we need to reclaim that lesson for ourselves.

This is as true for breasts as for any other part of the body. Little girls should be encouraged to know their breasts, so that when the changes of puberty come about, they can experience their growing breasts with comfort and pride, and continue to do so for the rest of their lives. Most of us have not been raised that way, however, and it's often hard for an adult woman to begin feeling comfortable with her breasts. Yet it's important to become acquainted with your breasts—to know what they feel like and what to expect from them. No part of your body should be foreign to you.

This chapter helps you get acquainted with your breasts and teaches you how to explore them. It isn't as easy as it might seem because of all the taboos about "erogenous zones." Our culture both overemphasizes and negates sexual arousal, and that makes it difficult to allow yourself to touch your breasts unself-consciously.

There are two things to remember as you read this chapter. One is that breasts are a body part, just as elbows and ribs are, and there's nothing shameful about exploring them. The other is that for many women they are centers of erotic feeling, and in the process of exploring them you might experience some sexual arousal. So what? That's a perfectly reasonable response. We've finally come to realize that it's a bad idea to teach kids to be ashamed of their sexual feelings; rather, we need to help them understand and cherish them. Similarly, we need to give ourselves permission to feel the entire range of reactions—sexual and nonsexual—to our own bodies.

To begin getting acquainted with your breasts, look at them. Stand in front of a mirror and look at yourself. See how your breasts hang and get a sense of how they project. If you're young they'll tend to stick out; if you're older they'll tend to be more droopy. In Chapter 1, I mentioned the inframammary ridge, where the breast folds over itself, and the underlying muscles, the pectorals. Look at your nipple—what color is it? Does it have hairs or little bumps on it? If so, that's perfectly normal. You might want to swing your arms around and watch how your breasts move, or don't move, with the motion. Put your hands on your hips; flex your muscles; stretch your arms up. How do your breasts look with each change of position?

It's important to do this nonjudgmentally. You're not trying out for a *Playboy* centerfold; you're learning about your body. Forget everything you've learned about what breasts are supposed to look like. These are your breasts, and they look fine.

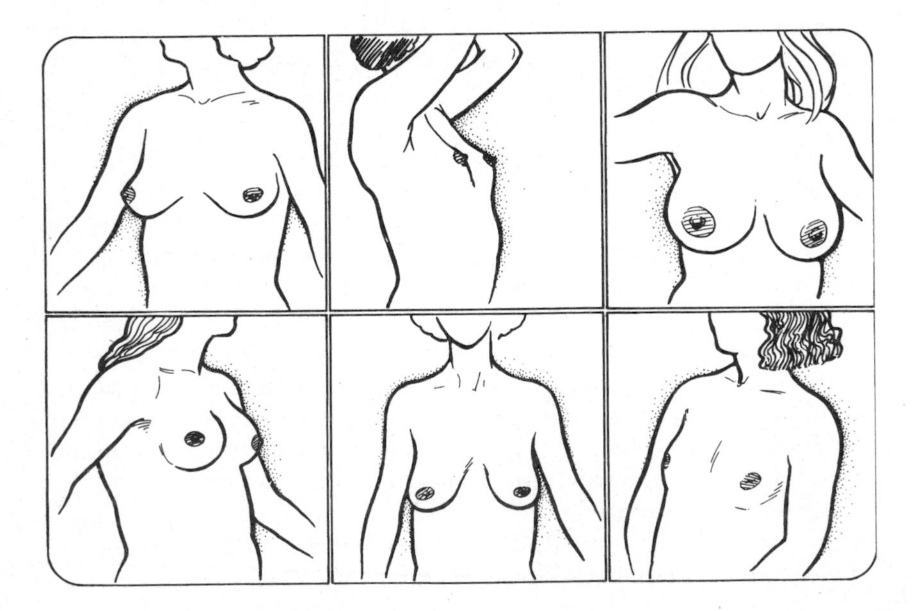

The next step is to feel your breasts. It's best to do this soaped up in the shower or bath. Your hands slip very easily over your skin. Put the hand of the side you want to explore behind your head. This shifts the breast tissue that's beneath your armpit to over your chest wall. Since the tissue is sandwiched between your skin and your chest bones you have good access to it. If you're very large-breasted you may want to do it lying down, in the bathtub or even in bed. You can then roll on one side and then the other to shift the breast closer to your chest wall so you can get a better feel for it.

Breast tissue generally has a texture that is finely nodular or granular, like large seeds. A lot of this more or less bumpy feeling is the normal fat that intermingles with the breast tissue. Lumpy breasts have inspired some of the most unfortunate misconceptions about our bodies. Often this lumpiness gets confused with actual breast lumps, as discussed in Chapter 6. But lumpiness itself often gets bad press. Women have been told their lumpy breasts are symptoms of "fibrocystic disease" (see Chapter 4) and have suffered from needless anxiety, fear, and even disfiguring surgery.

Lumpy breasts are caused by the way the breast tissue forms itself. In some women the breast tissue is fairly fine and thus not perceived as "lumpy." Others clearly have lumpy breasts, which can feel somewhat like cobblestone paving. Still others are somewhere between the extremes—just a bit nodular. There's nothing unusual about this—breasts vary as much as any other part of the body. Some women are tall and some short; some are fair-skinned and some dark; some have lumpier breasts and some have smoother breasts. There can even be differences within the same woman's breasts. Your breasts might be a little more nodular near your armpit or at the top, for example, and the pattern may be the same in both breasts or may occur only in one. You'll find, if you explore your breasts, that there's a general, fairly consistent pattern. It's important to become acquainted with your breasts and get a sense of what your pattern is.

In the middle part of your chest you can feel your ribs. They jut out from your breastbone. If your ribs are very prominent or if you are thin or small-breasted, you may feel them under the breast tissue. Many women have congenital deformities in their ribs, which affect the flatness of the rib cage. This can show in different ways. When the ribs arch outward, a so-called chicken-breasted condition is produced. Then there's a sunken chest, in which the breastbone is depressed. Women can have either of these conditions and not realize it because their breasts camouflage their chest structure.

Another common variation in the rib cage occurs with scoliosis. Many women have minor scoliosis and never realize it. As you feel your breast tissue you may notice that your ribs are more prominent on one

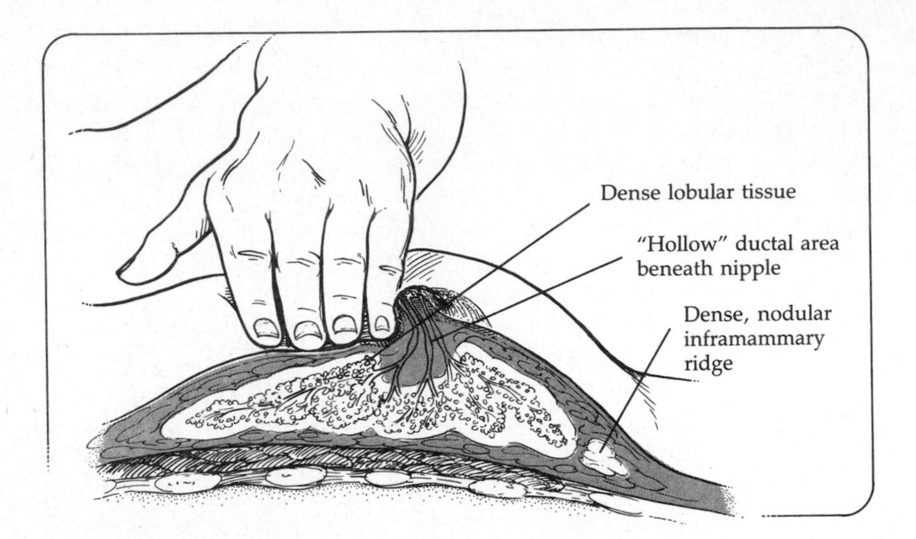

FIGURE 2-1

side or the other. This occurs because your back is not entirely straight. It has no real significance except that it can cause your ribs to be asymmetrical. Like the breasts, the rib cage is a little different in everyone, and it affects the feel of the breast area differently in different women.

Usually you'll feel more tissue up toward your armpit than in the middle of the breast. As I said in Chapter 1, the breast is really tear-shaped. The tissue toward the armpit is often the part that tends to get lumpier premenstrually and less lumpy after your period. There are lymph nodes in the armpits, as there are in many other parts of the body, and if you've had any sort of infection you might feel these nodes. The inframammary ridge, described in Chapter 1, is an area of thickening, and the older you get, the thicker that area gets. It usually has some fat globules that are larger than in other areas. There's a hollow spot under the nipple, where the ducts join together to exit the nipple. Around this area is a ridge of tissue—shaped rather like the crater edge of a volcano.

All of this you can easily get to know with the pads of your fingers just by running your hand over your breast area, getting a sense of how it feels (Fig. 2-1). There's no point in grabbing at the breast. You won't get a good idea of its texture because you're pulling it forward into a big wad.

You can squeeze your nipple if you're curious about how that feels. Don't be surprised if there's some discharge—squeezing the nipple can produce discharge in many women. (If you're concerned about it, see Chapter 5.)

To become thoroughly acquainted with your breasts, explore them at different times of the month. Hormones affect your breasts and they'll feel different at different points in your menstrual cycle. It's interesting to be aware of these changes. Are they lumpier or more tender before your period? If you've had a hysterectomy but still have your ovaries, the hormone patterns continue: monitoring your breasts may help you know where you would have been in your menstrual cycle. If you're postmenopausal or if you've had your ovaries out and aren't taking hormones, the changes no longer occur. Your breast tissue in general will be less sore, less full, less lumpy. If you take hormones—conjugated estrogen (Premarin), or conjugated estrogen and medroxyprogesterone acetate (Provera)—postmenopausally, that too will affect your breasts. They often become enlarged and sore, although not necessarily firmer. Similarly, if you're on birth control pills, your breasts may respond to those hormonal changes by becoming more sore or less lumpy.

There's a good practical as well as psychological reason for knowing your breasts. Such knowledge can help prevent needless biopsies. In our mobile era, you rarely have the same doctor all your life. If you've got a lump from, say, silicone injections or scar tissue from a previous operation, and you go to a new doctor who doesn't know your medical history, the doctor may well feel a biopsy is necessary. If you can say with conviction, "Yes, I know about that lump: it formed right after my operation ten years ago, and it's been there ever since," the doctor will know the lump is okay. I've often been through this with patients. If a doctor thinks a lump is okay, but the patient doesn't know whether or not it's been there a long while, the doctor has to assume it might be dangerous and will want to operate. If you know it's an old lump, your doctor won't have to worry.

If the doctor argues with you, argue back. Remember that you are a perfectly valid observer of your own body. You don't need to be a medical expert to know that you've had the same lump in the same place and it hasn't grown at all in 10 years. I had one 80-year-old patient who came to me after her doctors insisted that she'd been wrong about a lump in her breast that looked troublesome on her mammogram. Sexism and ageism can unite into a potent force, and obviously the doctors had decided that the "little old lady" didn't know what she was talking about when she told them her breast had been that way since her last child was born, 50 years earlier. They intimidated her, and she decided they must be right and had me do a biopsy. What I found was a congenital condition, perfectly harmless, that she'd probably had all her life and noticed after breast-feeding. She knew her body in a way that her doctors couldn't.

Women with disabilities may have a more difficult time getting to know their bodies. Often they have less mobility and thus don't reach all areas of their bodies when they bathe. Some women use adaptive equipment to help them bathe—which is wonderful for its purpose but can't feel lumps, the way one's hand does. (For those who wish to do breast self-exam, this is also a problem.) In such cases, more frequent physician examination is a good idea.

Is This Breast Self-Examination?

This may all sound a bit like breast self-examination, but there's a crucial difference. In breast self-examination (BSE) you're hunting for something. What I'm talking about is different—knowing your body, apart from anything ominous that may or may not occur there. For example, advocates of BSE tell you to examine your breasts once a month at the same time each month to see if there's a lump. What I'm suggesting, however, is that you check out your breasts at different times of the month to know how they feel at all times. Once you do know, you don't have to keep checking on a rigid schedule every month, unless that pleases you. (Do keep in mind that breasts, like the rest of your body, change over time, so that it's worth exploring your breasts regularly, every couple of months, even after you feel fully acquainted with them. But again, this isn't on any particular timetable.)

As you can see, I am consciously not presenting the idea of getting to know your breasts in terms of breast self-examination. The idea is to become familiar with your breasts as one significant part of your body, and to experience all their variations. Breast self-exam, on the other hand, has been set up as a way to monitor your breasts for cancer. Why am I making such a big point of this? I have very strong feelings about the concept of breast self-exam and its overuse. I think it alienates women from their breasts instead of making them more comfortable with them. It puts you in a position of examining yourself once a month to see if your breast has betrayed you. It pits you against your breast: can you find the tiniest lump that may be cancer?

Admittedly, breast cancer is scary, and it has become almost an epidemic. At the same time, the majority of women will never get breast cancer. To set up this alienation is a mistake. I get particularly alarmed when I hear people talk about teaching breast self-exam in the high schools. This takes young girls just developing breasts and, instead of teaching them to revel in their changing bodies, teaches them to see the breast as an enemy, something alien that has the ability to hurt them. It's a destructive way to define breasts.

Ironically, for all the fuss about breast self-exam, most women don't do it—even women who are at high risk because they have a mother or sister with breast cancer.[1] Only about 30 percent of women do BSE with any regularity. If you talk to women about BSE, most of them say they don't do it because they're scared of what they'll find. Sometimes they have lumpy breasts (see Chapter 6), and they can't tell whether one of their little bumps is actually a lump. But even when they're not doing BSE, it dominates their thinking about their breasts. I keep coming across women in their 30s and 40s who are very fearful of breast cancer—out of proportion to the real risk they face. Some of this comes from the idea of breast self-exam and the "need" to search their bodies constantly for signs of betrayal.

The idea of breast self-exam originated with Cushman Haagensen, who was a breast surgeon at Columbia University in New York in the 1950s, before mammography. Haagensen and his colleagues had women coming in with huge lumps in their breasts, far too big to be removed surgically. This was also an era when women were taught that it was bad to touch themselves "down there"—anyplace below the chin. Haagensen hoped that BSE would encourage women to touch their breasts and find cancerous lumps earlier, when they were still operable.

There are a couple of problems with his thinking, well intentioned though it was. He assumed that most of these women didn't touch their breasts because they were ashamed to. But that may not have been the case. They may have touched their breasts and found their lumps long before they came to the doctor: shame and fear may have prevented them not from touching their breasts, but from admitting it to the doctor, or from going to a doctor about a problem in that "shameful" area.

Still, in its early days it might have been useful to some women who did indeed feel ashamed to touch themselves without a medical directive. But the idea of BSE soon grew into something more than a permissible way for women to touch their breasts. It became standardized into a technique to find a cancer early, with the implication that this would save lives. That assumption is really not true, as I'll discuss in Chapter 14.

This rigid, standardized technique has become ubiquitous and serves mostly to make women very anxious. They'll read a book or go to a lecture about breast self-examination, and come home and stand in front of a mirror and do the exam. Then they feel these little bumps, and if they've never felt their breasts before, they start to get scared. There are these lumps here, and then they feel the other breast and the bumps are there too, and they think the "cancer" had spread. This gets them so upset they avoid touching their breasts anymore. They feel guilty if they don't keep doing their BSE every month and scared if they do.

Many women will stop me at this point and tell me that they or their friend found their cancer themselves. This is undoubtedly true: 80 percent of cancers not found on mammography are found by the woman herself. But when I question such women I find that few actually did a formal breast self-exam, as seen on those shower cards you get from the American Cancer Society. More typically, the woman just rolled over in bed, or felt a lump while soaping up in the shower, or had it pointed out by a lover. This touching and knowing your body is what we are after, not the rigid routine of looking for cancer.

Breast self-exam as currently presented is not a good model. It's important to learn how your breasts feel, but not so you can go on a search-and-destroy mission once a month, cataloguing every grain-sized nodule you feel and deciding that this is the one that is going to kill you. It's important to help give you a good, integrated sense of your body.

This process should start in adolescence. Its side benefits are marvelous—it teaches the girl to be comfortable with her own body, and it can be a pleasing rite of passage, a confirmation and exploration of her womanhood. Every woman should continue to explore her breasts periodically for the rest of her life, noting and embracing each change that all the stages of life entail in her breasts, as in the rest of her body. There is a powerful feeling that comes from knowing and becoming comfortable with your body—a feeling and a power that is yours alone and that no one can take from you.

3

Variations in Development and Plastic Surgery

Breasts come in many different shapes and sizes. Medically speaking, a "normal" breast is one that is capable of producing milk, so there's nothing "abnormal" about large, small, or asymmetrical breasts, or about extra nipples.

There are a number of common variations in breast development. They fall into one of two categories: those that are obvious from birth and those that don't show themselves until puberty. The latter are far more common. (There are also variations due to accident or illness, the surgical remedies for which are essentially the same as those used for genetic variations.)

VARIATIONS APPARENT AT BIRTH

The most common variation to appear at birth is polymastia—an extra nipple or nipples. These can appear anywhere along the milk ridge (see Fig. 1-8). Usually the milk ridge—a throwback to the days when we were animals with many nipples—regresses before birth, but in some people it remains throughout life. Between 1 and 5 percent of extra nipples are on women whose mothers also had extra nipples. Usually they're below the breast, and often women don't even know they're there, since they look like moles. When I would point out an extra nipple to a patient, it was usually the first time she'd been aware of it.

Extra nipples cause no problems and usually don't appear cosmetically unattractive. One patient was actually fond of her extra nipple: she told me that her husband had one too, and that's how they knew they were meant for each other! Men sometimes have extra nipples, though as far as we know, less frequently than women do. This may be due to some biological factor we don't yet know about, or it may simply be that men and their doctors don't notice the nipples because they're covered by chest hair.

Extra nipples don't cause any problems, though they may lactate if you breast-feed. There's nothing wrong with this, unless it causes you discomfort.

A variation of the extra nipple is extra breast tissue without a nipple, most often under the armpit. It may feel like hard, cystlike lumps that swell and hurt the way your breasts do when you menstruate. Like extra nipples, this extra breast tissue is often unnoticed by doctor and patient. One of my patients found that she had swelling under both armpits during her second pregnancy. It was probably caused by extra breast tissue and it went down after she finished lactating. The extra tissue is subject to all the problems of normally situated tissue. I have had patients with cysts, fibroadenomas, or even cancers in such tissue.

Unless the extra nipple or breast tissue causes you extreme physical discomfort or psychological distress, there's no need to worry about it. If it does bother you, it's easy to get rid of surgically. The nipple can be removed under local anesthetic in your doctor's office, and the extra breast tissue can be removed under either local or general anesthetic.

A much rarer condition is amastia—being born with breast tissue but no nipple. It's usually associated with problems in the development of the chest bone and muscles, like scoliosis and rib deformities. Aside from whatever medical procedures you may need because of the associated problems, you might want to have a fake nipple created by a plastic surgeon, the same way a nipple is created during reconstruction after a mastectomy. The nipple can be tattooed on or a skin graft can be taken from tissue on the inner thigh. The skin becomes darker after it's grafted and, if it still doesn't match the color of your other nipple, it can be tattooed to a darker shade. Though this artificial nipple will look real, it won't feel completely like a real nipple. There is no erectile tissue, so it won't vary as your other nipple does. It's usually constructed midway between erect and flat. It will have no sensation because it has no nerves. Because it won't have ducts, it can't produce milk. Its advantages are wholly cosmetic.

Some women have practically no breasts at all. This condition is sometimes called Poland's syndrome, and it involves not just the breast but also the pectoralis muscle and the ribs, as well as, in some cases, abnormalities of the arm and side on one side of the body. A woman with Poland's syndrome may have a small but very deformed breast. A patient of mine in Los Angeles was doubly unlucky. She had been born with Poland's syndrome and had a very undeveloped breast on one side. When she developed breast cancer in the good breast, she was anxious to have a lumpectomy rather than a mastectomy. She very much wanted to preserve her only functional breast.

Some women have permanently inverted nipples (they grow in instead of out)—a congenital condition that usually won't manifest until puberty.

Various injuries can affect breast development. This may happen surgically or with trauma. If the nipple and breast bud are seriously injured before puberty, the potential adult breast is destroyed as well. Sometimes injuring the skin can limit future breast development. Most commonly this occurs as a result of a severe burn. The resulting scars are so tight that breast tissue cannot develop. In the past, some congenital conditions such as hemangiomas (birthmarks) were treated with radiation, which damaged the nipple and breast bud and prevented later growth. Any serious injury to the breast bud can cause such arrested development.

VARIATIONS APPEARING AT PUBERTY

Three basic variations appear when the breasts begin to develop: extremely large breasts, extremely small breasts, and asymmetrical breasts.

Very Large Breasts

Very large breasts can occur early in puberty—a condition known as "virginal hypertrophy." After the breasts begin to grow, the shutoff mechanism, whatever it is, forgets to do its job and the breasts keep on growing. The breasts become huge and greatly out of proportion to the rest of the body. Sometimes the condition runs in families. In very rare instances, virginal hypertrophy occurs in one breast and not the other. It's worth noting here that "large" is both subjective and variable. A five-foot-tall woman with a C cup is very large-breasted; a five-foot-eight woman with a C cup may not feel especially uncomfortable with her size. A five-foot-eight woman with a DD cup is likely to be very uncomfortable.

Large breasts have been a problem for a number of my patients. "I almost never wear a bathing suit," one patient told me, "because people stare at my breasts." Another, at 71, still "hunches over" when she walks to avoid having her breasts stared at.

Huge breasts can be very distressful to a teenage girl. She faces ridicule from her schoolmates, and—unlike the small-breasted girl—extreme physical discomfort as well. She may be unable to participate in sports, and she may have severe backache all the time. She usually needs a bra to hold the breasts in, but the bra, pulled down by the weight of the breasts, can dig painful ridges into her shoulders.

If the breasts cause this much discomfort, the girl might want to have reduction surgery done while she's still in her teens. (See later in this chapter.) In some cases, the nipple will have to be moved further up on the newly reduced breast, threatening the possiblity of breast-feeding. For this reason, some mothers refuse to let their daughters have reduction surgery, urging them to wait until they've had children. Both mother and daughter must weigh the physical and emotional damage the girl will go through first. If she decides to have children, pregnancy may worsen her problem. When the breasts become engorged with milk, they become even larger and, in a woman with huge breasts, more uncomfortable. Though it's unfortunate that someone so young is faced with a decision that affects her whole life, it's important to realize that not having the surgery will also affect her life. Many girls of 15 or 16 are mature enough to make their own decisions if all the facts are carefully explained to them, including the possibility of bottle-feeding. In any case, the losses and gains of either choice are the girl's, and she should be given the right and the time to decide for herself what to do. She should be encouraged to talk to doctors, mothers of young children, and very large-breasted women; to read all the material she can find about the pros and cons of the procedure and of breast-feeding; and to make her decision only when she feels she is fully informed.

Not all problems with huge breasts appear right after puberty. Some comfortably large-breasted women find that their breasts have expanded considerably after pregnancy; others become uncomfortable after their breast size has increased with an overall weight gain. Many surgeons are reluctant to operate in this latter case, preferring to wait till the woman has lost weight. Sometimes, however, this can backfire psychologically. I've known women who were so depressed by their huge breasts that they compensated by overeating, thus intensifying both problems. In such cases, the pleasing appearance of their breasts created by reduction surgery can be a spur to continue their self-improvement.

In any case, the decision must be made by the individual woman; she's the one who lives with the problem and she's the one who can best judge its impact on her life. Some women with very large breasts don't mind them. One patient, who admits they cause her discomfort, says that she nonetheless enjoys their size. "They feel feminine and sexy," she says.

Very Small Breasts

The opposite problem is extreme flat-chestedness. Like "large-breasted," the notion of "small-breasted" is subjective and relative, and culturally determined. Some women, however, have breasts so small that their chests look like men's. This causes no physical or medical problems but can make a woman feel unattractive and sexless. Plastic surgeons often, and inaccurately, call very small breasts a "disease," contributing further to the woman's lack of comfort with her anatomy.

Because very small breasts can feed babies and respond sexually, some women aren't bothered by them. Others are satisfied simply by wearing "falsies" or padded bras. Some want to have the breasts altered surgically. (I'll discuss silicone implants later in the chapter.)

Asymmetrical Breasts

In some women breasts develop unevenly, resulting in severe asymmetry. For a woman who is bothered by this, cosmetic surgery can help achieve a reasonable match. Either the larger breast can be reduced or the smaller one augmented—or a combination of both can be done. It's important for the surgeon to discuss these options. Often we assume a woman will want her small breast made larger and neglect to suggest the possibility of reducing the larger breast. What a woman decides will depend on the size of both breasts, the degree of asymmetry, and above all her own esthetic judgment.

It's fortunate that plastic surgery techniques exist for women who want them. But don't assume that because you have atypical-looking breasts you have to get them altered. Many women are quite pleased with how their breasts look. Some women with large breasts feel, as did the patient I mentioned earlier, that their breasts are "feminine and sexy." Small breasts too have their advantages. One of my patients liked her small breasts because "they're unobtrusive, and they worked well during nursing. Occasionally some male person will intimate that they're less than optimal. That's his problem, not mine." Another liked her tiny breasts ("they're really just enlarged nipples") because they didn't get in her way when she engaged in sports. A patient with asymmetrical breasts said she used to feel self-conscious but had "come to terms with them" since she nursed her child.

And another patient tells a wonderful story about a friend of hers who had inverted nipples. "When I was 12 and my cousin was 14, we stood before the bathroom mirror and compared breasts. I noticed how different her nipples were; they didn't protrude the way mine did. We had this big discussion about whose were 'normal.' I was convinced mine were, but she insisted hers were, and since she was older and, I thought, more knowledgeable, I decided she must be right.

"After she graduated from college and was studying in Paris, she became ill and had to be hospitalized. The doctor who was examining her asked if her nipples 'had always been like that.' That's how she learned that she had inverted nipples—and that mine were the normal ones!"

PLASTIC SURGERY

Some women, deeply unhappy with their atypical breasts, turn to plastic surgery. Interestingly, the first recorded breast surgery was done on a man with gynecomastia, in A.D. 625.[1] Mammoplasty was not performed on a woman until a thousand years later, in 1897—but we needn't feel too deprived. With the primitive state of surgery in the past, that poor man in the seventh century couldn't have had a comfortable time.

Good breast reduction techniques have now been with us for decades. Augmentation, as I mentioned earlier, is a much more recent procedure.

From a surgical standpoint the procedures are quite safe. They are often labeled "unnecessary surgery," and of course they *are* unnecessary in the sense that you won't die without them. But for many women the risk is well worth the chance of improved self-image and, in the case of large breasts, increased physical comfort.

Plastic surgery has always raised ethical concerns, especially for feminists. We have been told that we aren't right as we are, that we need to change our looks to please men, or a particular man. Cosmetic surgery is often seen as only a high-tech version of painful assaults on the body that women have experienced for centuries—like foot binding, corsets, genital mutilation. Rather than subjecting our bodies to procedures that carry the risk all surgery entails and may even cause other health problems, many activists in the women's health movement argue, we should change society's approach so that we don't feel the need to have "perfect" or "ideal" bodies.

While there is some merit to this concern, it doesn't seem reasonable to me. First, it takes a very paternalistic—or maternalistic—view of what's best for other people. Second, some women have practical needs for bodies that society defines as ideal—like the young women I used to meet in my Los Angeles practice who were trying to succeed as actresses and models. Third, even for women whose needs are emotional rather than practical, the feelings are deeply ingrained—they can't just decide not to feel that way. Years of fighting an uphill battle against internalized social expectations can be as devastating as physical illness. A nose job, a face-lift, or a breast enlargement can make a major difference in a woman's life—and whether that would or wouldn't be the case in an ideal world is beside the point.

Not everyone who wants to alter her body is a bimbo. Over the years, I've had a range of patients who wanted their breasts augmented. Among them was a married gynecologist, a well-educated professional, not terribly young, who had silicone implants and said they had made a tremendous difference in her life, and that she'd do it again if she had to make the choice today. Another had gotten her implants in 1980 at the age of 40. "For the first time in my life I was proud of my figure," she told me. "I felt like a new woman." Perhaps it's a pity that society has made these women feel that way, and we can work to change the way we're taught to view our bodies. But meanwhile, we all have irrational feelings that deeply affect our lives, and nobody needs to be a martyr.

Before we get into the various kinds of plastic surgery, there's a practical consideration you need to address: insurance. You'll need to check with your insurance company about what forms of plastic surgery it will or won't pay for. You'll also want to find out if the insurance company has a disclaimer or exclusion for coverage of future implant-related health problems (medical/surgical). You may have to shoulder the financial responsibility for the procedure yourself.

Breast Reduction

Most women come for this operation because they're embarrassed by their large breasts or because they have discomfort from neck and back pain. As with the other operations described in this chapter, a woman who is over 35 should have a mammogram to make sure there's no cancer.

On the patient's first visit, says my old colleague Dr. Goldwyn, "I show them photos of breasts that have had reduction surgery to make sure they know there will be scars." The doctor will explain what sizes are possible; most of Dr. Goldwyn's patients want to be a B, and some want to be a C. Dr. William Shaw, a plastic surgeon and one of my former colleagues at UCLA, points out that it is difficult to be sure that the patient and the surgeon both have the same idea of what a B or C cup is. He often asks patients to bring in pictures from magazines to be sure he knows what their expectations are. Then the operation is scheduled. It's not always possible to get exactly the size you want, but a good surgeon can approximate it. There are a number of variations of the breast reduction operation, but all start with the same basic procedure.

The operation is usually done under general anesthesia and takes place the day you're admitted to the hospital. It may last up to four hours. Your nipples can be either removed and grafted back, or left on breast tissue and transposed. Most doctors today prefer not to graft the nipples except in extremely large reductions, since they lose sensitivity if all the nerves are severed.

Most procedures involve some variation of the keyhole technique. The amount of tissue to be removed is determined and a pattern drawn on the breast (Fig. 3-1). The nipple is preserved on a small flap of tissue while the tissue to be removed is taken from below and from the sides. This allows the surgeon to elevate the nipple and bring the flaps of tissue together, giving both uplift and reduction. The resulting scars are below the breast in the inframammary fold and come right up the center to the nipple. In recent years, says Dr. Shaw, there is a preference for shorter incisions under the breast. In some cases only a circular scar around the nipple is used—the so-called doughnut, or concentric, reduction pattern.

Patients experience pain the first day after the operation, but very little after that. You can go home the next morning, wearing a bra or some form of support. The stitches are out in one to two weeks, and you can go back to work; in three to four weeks you can be playing tennis.

Side effects include infection, which can occur with any operation. There's a slight risk that you'll need blood transfusions, but it's very rare. If you're worried, however, give your own blood to the hospital two or three months in advance, and it will be there in case you need it. There's some danger of the operation interfering with the blood supply of the nipple and areola; if this happens the nipple and areola die and need to be artificially reconstructed. It's not a very great danger—it happens in less than 4 percent of operations. The larger your breasts are, the greater the danger. Reduction does not affect a woman's risk of cancer. Your ability to breast-feed will be decreased; studies show that about half of women who have had reductions can still nurse their babies.

Some of the erotic sensation in your nipples may be reduced, though for many women the increased relaxation actually makes sex more pleasurable after reduction surgery. Also, because the nerves in the nipple of the overlarge breast are so stretched out, the nipple is unlikely to have much sensitivity to begin with, and the loss of sensation—in terms of both sexual activity and breast-feeding—will proba-

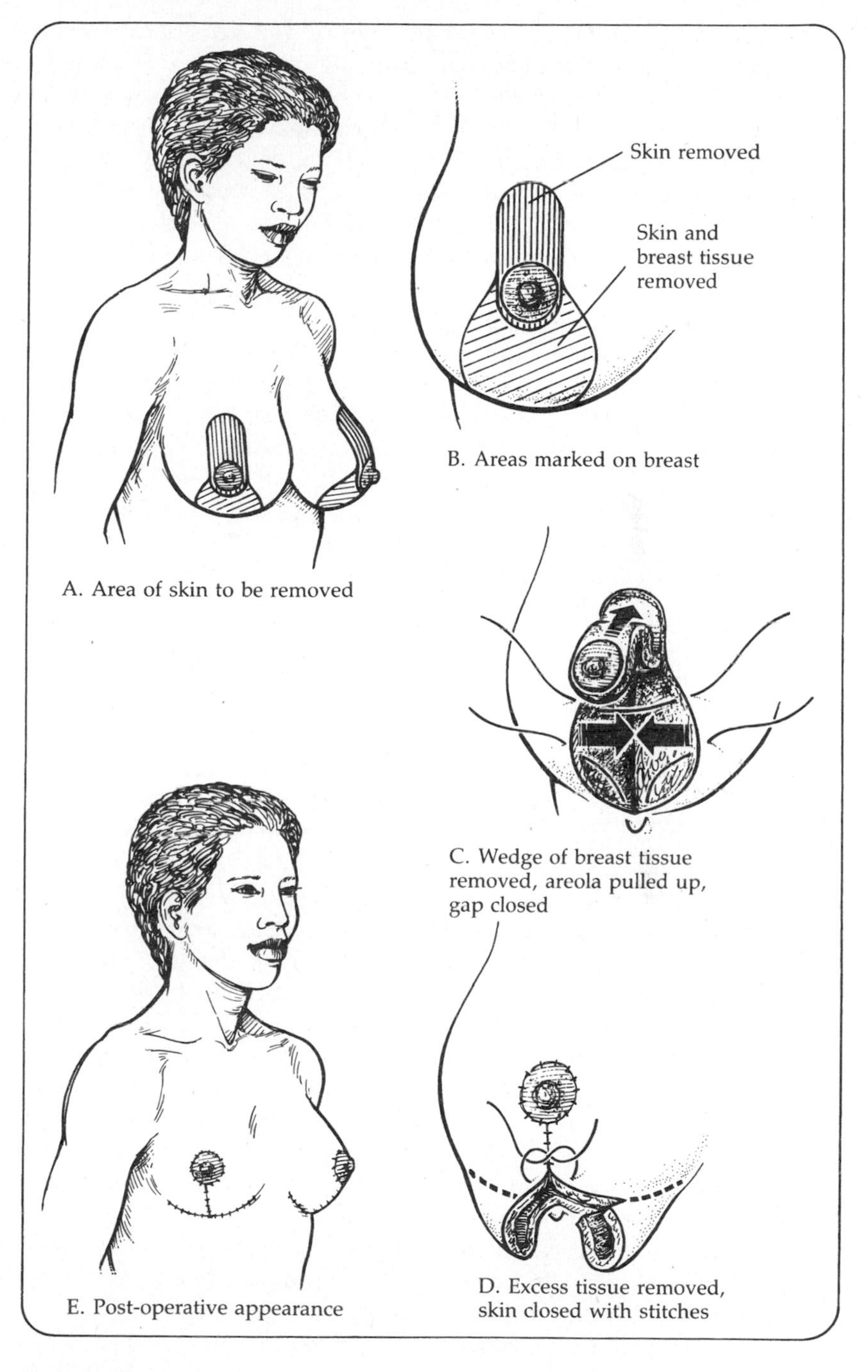

A. Area of skin to be removed

B. Areas marked on breast

C. Wedge of breast tissue removed, areola pulled up, gap closed

D. Excess tissue removed, skin closed with stitches

E. Post-operative appearance

FIGURE 3-1

bly go unnoticed. There's also a possibility of some reduction of sensitivity in the breast itself, although again this is minimal. There's no way to know in advance whether or not you'll experience reduced sensation, so you have to decide for yourself how important full sensation is, compared to whatever physical or emotional discomfort your large breasts create for you. In any case, you'll still retain most of your breast sensation.

If you do decide to have reduction surgery, be aware that if you later gain weight, your breasts will probably also gain weight, just as they would without the surgery. This has happened to a number of my patients. One woman had her size 36EE breasts reduced to a 36B, but they ended up a 36D. According to Dr. Goldwyn and Dr. Shaw, the more the patient sees the operation as reconstructive, the happier she'll be, while the more she sees it as cosmetic, the more critical she'll be about the result. When it's only cosmetic, she's more likely to focus on the scars; if it relieves pain and discomfort, she'll focus on how much better she feels.

Silicone Implants

Silicone implants have been the source of much controversy since the first edition of this book came out. I don't mean to dismiss women's concerns about silicone implants. The biggest concern of the activists, however, is one that remains unproven: the idea that the gel can cause an *autoimmune* disorder (a condition in which the immune system, once turned on, gets carried away and starts attacking the body and connective tissue). The most common of these are scleroderma, lupus, rheumatoid arthritis, dermatomyositis, and Sjorgen's syndrome. No studies have made any connections between the incidence of such diseases and silicone implants. A comprehensive review of over 15 epidemiological studies covering 4,000 women showed no increased risk of connective tissue diseases among women with breast implants.[2] So the fact that someone with implants gets such a disease doesn't mean there is a connection: they may simply be two unrelated facts in the woman's life.

One hypothesis is that some women are allergic to silicone, and that for those women a leak causes autoimmune disorders or other health problems, while women who aren't allergic to silicone have no negative reactions to it. We can't rule out this possibility until the proper studies have been done.

Another concern is whether silicone implants increase the risk of breast cancer. The best study was in Los Angeles County, where over 3,000 women who had silicone implants were studied for a number of years, and their breast cancer rates compared to the expected incidence of breast cancer in LA.[3] Not only was there no increase in breast cancer in women with implants, but there appeared to be a possible decrease. This was substantiated by a second study in Alberta, Canada, in which 13,577 women with breast cancer were studied and only 41 of them had implants.[4] The researchers concluded that there was a lower risk of breast cancer in these women. This may be because plastic surgeons are less likely to put implants into women who are high risk for breast cancer. Women with implants also tend to be thinner and thus at lower risk. Interestingly, there are data in animals showing that silicone may protect against breast cancer. We have no idea at this point why this may be so. It does not, of course, suggest that women should run out and get implants as a way to protect themselves from breast cancer. But it certainly does suggest that silicone implants aren't the grave danger many have portrayed them to be.

Implants do, however, interfere with how well mammograms can detect tumors in the breast. A study by Mel Silverstein and his colleagues showed that implants create shadows on mammograms, blocking areas from the picture and leading to a decrease in accuracy.[5] However, small breasts are hard to see through on mammograms, which are not always a surefire way to detect breast cancer. Still mammography remains the best tool we have for finding breast cancer before it spreads, and any process that interferes with its effectiveness should be entered into only with great forethought. Women who do have implants need to remember that a normal mammogram cannot be considered reassuring and that they need to take any abnormality seriously.

There are more common problems that can happen with implants, which, though less serious than breast cancer, need to be considered. Silicone isn't the wholly inert substance it was once thought to be, and it always creates some reaction around it. Minuscule amounts of silicone will always leak. The reaction may be something that you'd never notice or be bothered by—the sort of thing that only shows up if the breast is biopsied.

Contracture—which means the formation of a thick, spherical scar tissue that causes the breast to be overly firm (Fig. 3-2)—is a real possibility with most implants. It occurs in 1–18 percent of cases in which the implant is under the muscle, and in 18–50 percent of cases in which it's between the muscle and breast. This firmness can be unnoticeable or it can feel like solid wood—or anything in between. Contracture can be painful, and it can change the appearance of the breast. Contracture, warns Dr. Shaw, may happen to one implant and not the other, or may happen differently in the two implants, leaving one side higher than the other. Further, the incidence of contracture tends to increase over

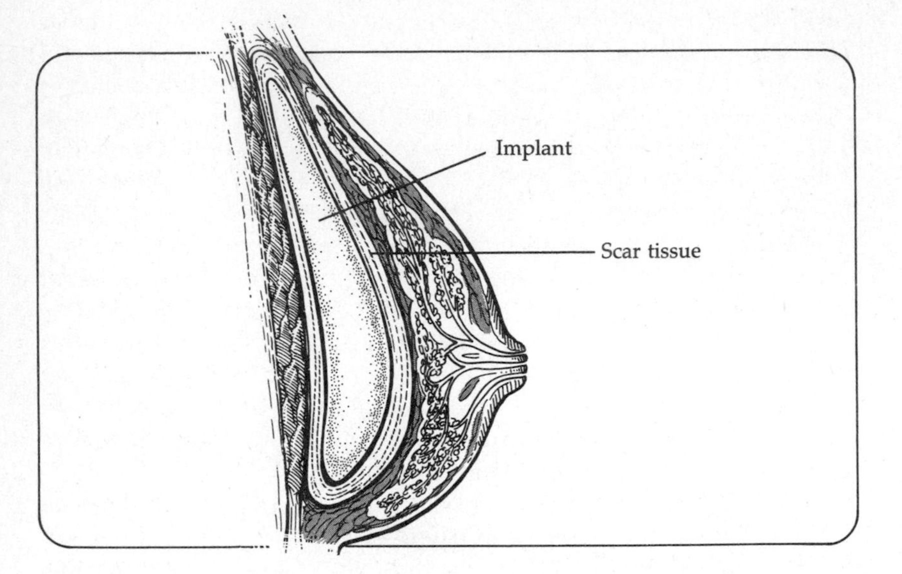

FIGURE 3-2

time. Thus results that look great five to 10 years after the procedure may develop progressive distortion and contracture by 15 or 20 years.

Failures of reconstruction or augmentation result mostly from surgical problems such as infection, poor healing, and recurrent capsule formation. Some silicone always escapes from the surface of an implant. When levels of silicon (which is found naturally in everyone's body) are measured in the blood of women with implants, they are significantly higher than in women without implants. In addition, silicone has been found in several other areas of the body, including the skin, pleura (sac surrounding the lungs), chest wall muscles, and lymph nodes. The actual incidence of silicone spread or rupture, however, is unknown. Most of the studies have been on women who were having their implants removed, which is usually done for a reason. This gives us an estimate of rupture in women who have symptoms but not in women in general. It does appear, however, that the longer an implant is in place, the higher the chance for rupture. Some reports suggest that the rate of rupture is as high as 55 percent 10 to 15 years after surgery.[6] As a result, some plastic surgeons recommend that implants be replaced every 10 years.

Rupture is usually diagnosed by seeing a change in the size, shape, or consistency of the implant. It can also be detected through mammography coupled with ultrasound. The most sensitive tool, however, is MRI, which can show very accurately whether there has been a rupture and where.

The idea of a rupture sounds ominous, but what does it really mean? For one thing, it can defeat the purpose of the implant by creating a cosmetically unappealing effect. It also requires surgery, as I discuss later. But the more serious question is whether it is dangerous. What does the body do when exposed to silicone? The immune system responds to the silicone by trying to clean it up with an inflammatory reaction. This response is what ultimately leads to fibrosis, or contracture formation. This varies in degree and in hardness around the implant. In some cases, it can be accompanied by local symptoms of pressure sensation and even pain. The leaked silicone has been known to travel to the vicinity of the brachial plexus and nerves of the arm, causing chronic irritation and pain. We don't know if that leakage is dangerous or not. No randomized study has ever been done on the long-term health of women who had silicone injections before they were banned: such a study might tell us if silicone in the breast and other parts of the body causes harm. Dr. Shaw has had a number of patients who had silicone injections years ago, and has seen cases in which hard lumps have formed in the breast, making early cancer detection more difficult, and other cases in which there was infection and dead tissue in the breast itself. This suggests that similar problems can occur with leakage from implants. The mystery is why capsules occur in some women and not in all. It may be, as we said, that some women are more sensitive to silicone than others.

The alternative is an implant filled with saline. This works similarly to silicone, except that saline—salt water—is inside the silicone shell instead of silicone gel. Saline implants are no more likely to leak than silicone, but when they do leak the saline becomes absorbed by the body fairly quickly, so that you realize suddenly that your breast has shrunk. When gel implants rupture or leak, the bulk of the material stays together inside the fibrous scar capsule. Therefore the outside appearance may not change for some time. Saline leakage won't cause any medical problems.

Saline has a somewhat less realistic feel than silicone. Dr. Shaw describes it as "less fleshy than silicone; it's more like a bag of water, particularly when the covering tissue is thin."

Patients with saline implants have complained about problems of capsular contracture, poor aesthetic results, asymmetry, a fluidlike feeling in the breasts, and "rippling" of the breast skin surface due to rippling of the implant shell and capsule. These, however, are all part of the standard issues related to the use of implants; imperfect results occur sometimes. There are no known, specific, documented problems with the saline material itself, in contrast to gel material.

Luckily for women who want implants, a number of studies are now being done. First, each implant (silicone gel or saline) put in the body is documented in a prospective manner. Surgeons are required to keep information about implants in a prospective study and to report problems periodically. Over many years, this will give us better information about the magnitude and nature of potential implant-related problems. Second, plastic surgeons and manufacturers are now studying alternative materials to be used as fillers in breast implants in place of silicone. While we might anticipate certain improvements, particularly in terms of mammogram, it is unlikely that future implants will be totally trouble-free. We don't know if these new materials could cause infection. Further, they would still be in a silicone pouch; in addition to the possible problems with the pouch itself, we still don't know if there would be reactions caused by the silicone rubber interacting with the filling material on the one side and the patient's body on the other. "In the best possibility, it's still a foreign implant," Dr. Shaw warns. "Not every patient will have a good result." Unfortunately there are no studies on possible substitutes for the silicone pouch, since no solid substance is less inert than silicone.

According to Dr. Shaw, after a patient has had implants for many years, there may be reasons to remove them surgically, for example, local problems with capsular contracture, poor results, or ruptures, or systemic conditions that may or may not have a direct link to the implants. Also, some patients, after many years, may not wish to have such large breasts anymore and do not want to live with possible future problems with implants. In all of these cases silicone breast implants may be removed surgically to improve the patient's sense of comfort and security. The problem is that the removal of silicone breast implants requires surgery that is often tedious. Another issue is that the reduction of the volume of the breasts may be a shock to a woman after so many years of having larger breasts. Finally, many breasts would become saggier and relatively deformed after implant removal. Dr. Shaw says he gets better results by doing an immediate *mastopexy,* or reshaping of the breasts, similar to breast reduction or *ptosis* (sagging breasts) correction. Many women are pleased with their resulting smaller but more shapely breasts. In most cases, immediate mastopexy can be performed at the same time as implant removal surgery.

Breast Augmentation

As noted earlier, women over 35 who are considering plastic surgery for their breasts should have a mammogram to rule out cancer. In addition, the surgeon should check for cysts that will require needle aspirations (see Chapter 6). As Dr. Goldwyn puts it, "You don't want to be sticking needles into the patient's breast when there's a silicone gel bag inside it." The plastic surgeon will also take a careful history.

The surgeon should show you pictures of breasts that have been augmented, including those that have left very visible scars, so you know both the best and the worst possible results of your operation. You and the surgeon should also discuss what size you want your new breasts to be, and you need to be realistic about that—you won't have enough breast tissue to turn tiny breasts into huge ones. Dr. Goldwyn tells of a petite woman who wanted to go from a size 34A to a size 34D. "Not only did she lack sufficient soft tissue to harbor such implants," he says, "but the results would have been poor, even bizarre." Dr. Shaw emphasizes that the augmentation should be appropriate for the size and build of the patient.

If you're married, some surgeons will want to make sure your husband feels okay about augmentation, since an angry husband might later try to sue the doctor. Dr. Shaw points out that it is not so important for medical or legal reasons, but may be important for the marital relationship. If you feel that it is your decision alone, let the surgeon know and try to work it out. Otherwise, find a surgeon willing to do what you want.

The operation can be done under either local or general anesthetic. Some patients, says Dr. Shaw, prefer to use general anesthetic because they fear pain, and some surgeons also prefer it.

The incision is made either through the armpit, underneath the breast, or around the areola (Fig. 3-3). All of these have their proponents. The implant can be placed under the breast tissue between the

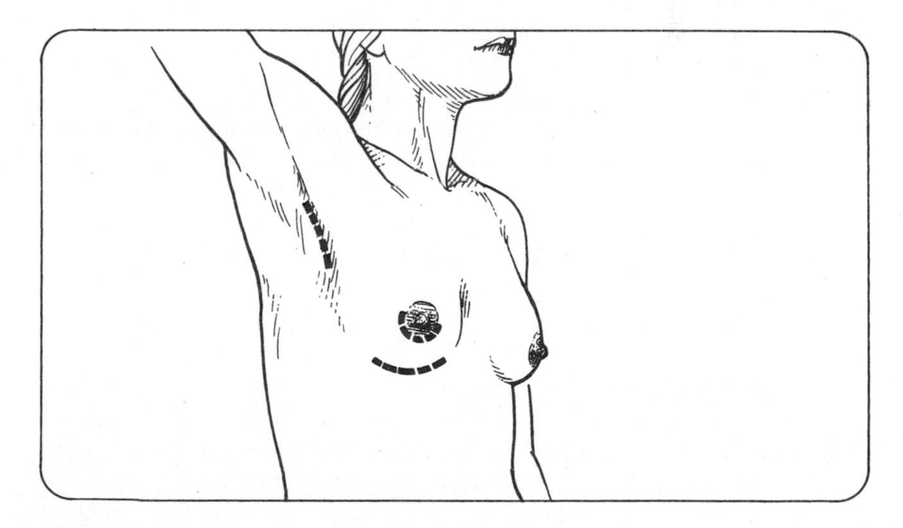

FIGURE 3-3

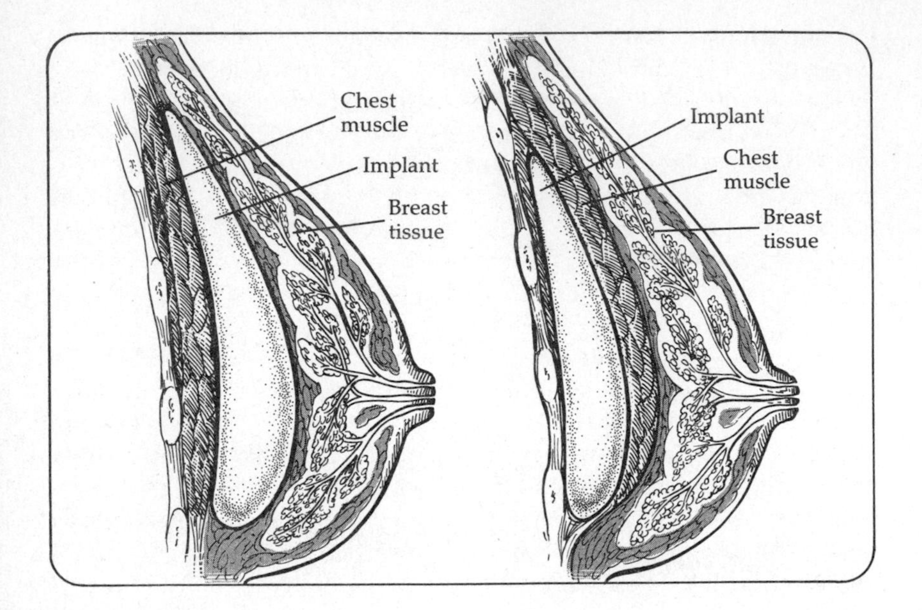

FIGURE 3-4

breast and the muscles or under the muscle itself (Fig. 3-4). According to Dr. Shaw, putting the implant under the muscles has two disadvantages: a tendency for a flatter breast and the possibility of movement of the breast with the muscle. But it has two advantages: it seems to carry less risk of contracture and, even more important, it's less likely to hide a future cancer.

The operation is usually done on an outpatient basis; it takes about two hours or more, depending on whether or not the surgeon puts the implant under the muscle, which takes more time. You go home after the operation. The stitches will be removed about 10 days later. You'll be out of work for about two to five days, and shouldn't drive a car for a week. In three weeks you'll be able to jog or play tennis.

Side effects can include infection, which occurs in less than 1 percent of cases, and bleeding, which is equally rare. There may be permanent altering of sensation in the nipple or areola, which occurs in less than 2 percent of cases, and there is also a slight possibility of reduced sensation in the breast. There's also the possibility of visible scarring and of contracture, both mentioned earlier. And there is some possibility that lactation can be affected, unless the surgeon makes sure the scar is not next to the areola and no ducts are severed.

Implant rupture, as noted earlier, is a possible serious complication, though not a common one. It can occur through strenuous physical force or just spontaneously. The implant needs to be removed immediately and the surgeon must try to take out all the silicone in a procedure known as *explantation.* This is difficult surgery because it involves trying to remove all of the silicone, so it requires a surgeon experienced in the procedure.

Unfortunately, for now at least, some form of implant is the best we can do for women wanting to have their breasts enlarged. There are operations using the body's own tissue that are done for breast reconstruction after mastectomy (see Chapter 22), but they really don't make much sense for less drastic cosmetic purposes, says Dr. Shaw. "It's a big operation, and you'd have large scars on the area the tissue is taken from, so you'd create an esthetic problem as great as the one you're trying to fix. Particularly for a very young woman, it wouldn't be worth it. For a middle-aged woman with very, very small breasts, whose tummy is probably pushing out a bit and whose cosmetic expectations may not be as great, it's a possibility, especially if she's had implants and now needs to have them removed." He warns also that insurance rarely pays for this kind of operation.

Surgery for Asymmetry

To correct major asymmetry, the doctor can use one of three procedures, and it's important for you as the patient to know which of the three you want. You can, as noted earlier, have an implant put in one, or you can have the other made smaller, or you can have a combination of both.

The procedures used to reconstruct a breast are also possible, but for the reasons noted above, probably aren't a good idea. If your asymmetry results from Poland's syndrome or an injury, appropriate breast reconstruction utilizing expanders, implants, or your own tissues will achieve a reasonable result. Unlike the situation of the woman with small but symmetrical breasts, the scars created in the area the tissue is taken from are likely to disturb you less than the asymmetry itself.

If you're thinking of implants for asymmetry, keep in mind that exact matching is unlikely. If there's a difference in nipple and areola size, the implant operation will stretch the nipple and areola on the smaller breast. And, since silicone has now been added under tight skin, the augmented breast will tend not to sag like a normal breast does as you age. Still, these differences are minor compared to the original asymmetry, and it's likely that you yourself will be the only one to notice. Remember, you may need to have your implant replaced at some point, so be sure you know what size it is.

The Breast Lift

As already mentioned, sagging breasts (known medically as ptosis) can be made firmer through an operation called a mastopexy, which Dr. Goldwyn describes as "a face-lift of the breasts." A mastopexy can give your breasts uplift, but Dr. Goldwyn warns that it will not make your breasts look like a 20-year-old's. And it will leave scars—sometimes bad ones, depending on how your body usually scars. Like a face-lift, it won't last forever. Remember, you've got gravity and time working against you.

As with the other procedures we've considered, your plastic surgeon will take a very thorough medical history, and you should get a mammogram before proceeding further, if you haven't had one recently. Be sure to get a full description of both the best and the worst possible results of a mastopexy.

This operation usually involves removing excess skin and fat and elevating the nipple (Fig. 3-5). If you're very large-breasted, you may want reduction surgery as well, especially since a mastopexy is less effective on very large breasts: gravity pulls them down. If you're very small-breasted, you may want an augmentation.

If your operation doesn't involve reduction or augmentation, it's a simpler procedure and can be done either in the hospital under general anesthetic or in the doctor's office with local anesthesia. Since insurance won't pay for it, most women prefer the latter. The operation lasts about two and a half hours; the stitches are removed in two weeks. By three weeks, you'll be able to participate in sports. You should wear a bra constantly for many weeks after surgery. Follow-up is minimal—three or four visits during the year after surgery.

You may experience some very slight loss of sensation in the nipple or areola. Other than that, there are no particular side effects to mastopexy.

Inverted Nipples

There is an operation that can reverse nipple inversion, but it doesn't always work and the inversion may recur. It's a simple procedure, usually done under local anesthetic with no intravenous medication, and you can go back to work the next day. The stitches come out in about two weeks.

Nipples are usually inverted because they are tethered down by scar or other tissue from birth. To reverse it, the surgeon will reach down and pull the nipple, stretch it, and make an incision, releasing the constricting tissue (Fig. 3-6). There are a number of procedures, and each

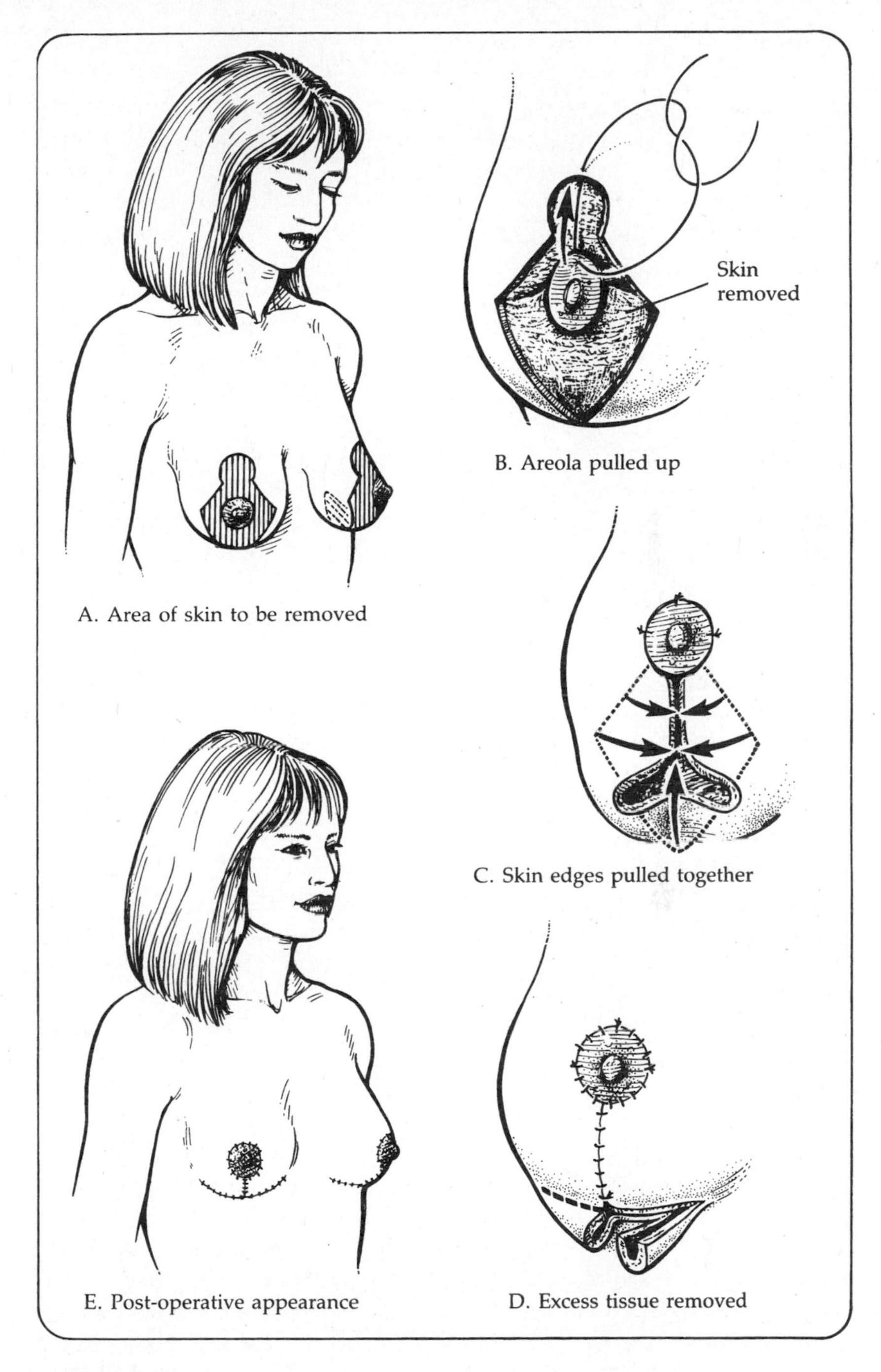

A. Area of skin to be removed

B. Areola pulled up

C. Skin edges pulled together

D. Excess tissue removed

E. Post-operative appearance

FIGURE 3-5

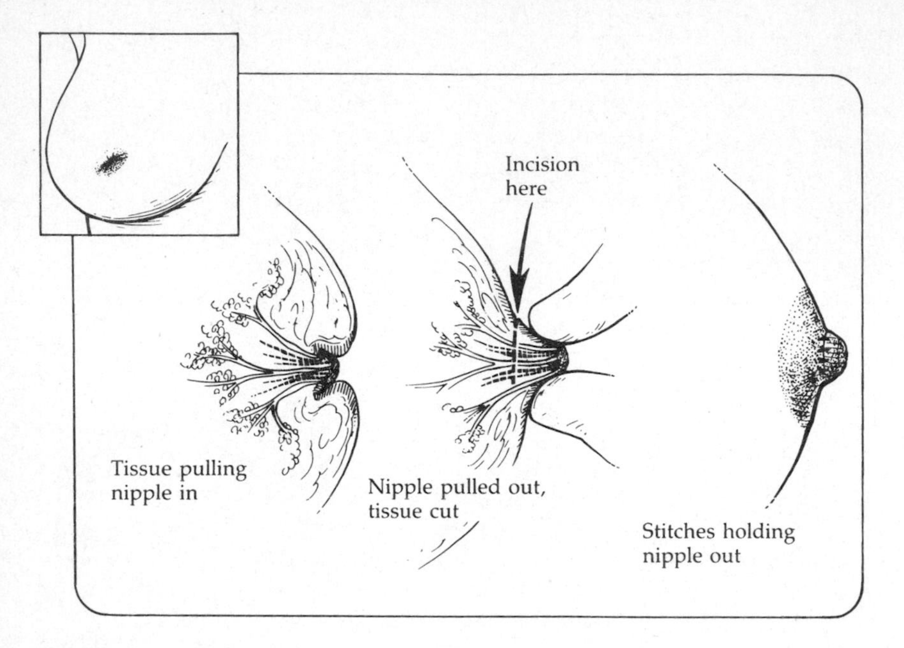

FIGURE 3-6

one has its advocates. If the inversion recurs, the operation can be redone.

This operation can make a psychological difference for teenagers, who often feel self-conscious about having inverted nipples. It definitely interferes with breast-feeding, but women with inverted nipples usually have difficulty with breast-feeding anyway.

THINKING ABOUT PLASTIC SURGERY

None of these operations is medically necessary. Still, we're lucky to live in an age when they're available. For a woman deeply unhappy with the way her breasts look, plastic surgery offers a solution that can make a major psychological difference in her life. No operation will make you look "perfect" (whatever that is), but all of these procedures will help you feel more normal and more comfortable in your body.

If you're thinking about plastic surgery, you should ask yourself a few questions. The first and probably most important is, Who wants the surgery? If you're content with your breasts, but your mother or boyfriend or someone else is pressuring you into surgery, you probably shouldn't do it. It's your body, not theirs.

The second question is, How realistic are your expectations, and how clear an idea do you have about the kind of breasts you want? Dr. John T. Heuston, a noted plastic surgeon, has written some wise words about reduction surgery that can apply to all forms of cosmetic surgery for the breasts.[7] "The concept of an ideal operation," he writes, "carries with it the concept of an ideal breast. The surgeon seeks the best means to construct the breast form—but for whom? For him or her, or for the patient, or both?" As Heuston notes, there is no objectively ideal breast; each of us has her own ideal. So you should have a clear sense of what size and shape breast you want, and what your own goals are. The surgeon can't make your breasts absolutely perfect, but if your goals are fairly reasonable, they can come close to being met. If you do decide on plastic surgery, make sure you know the range of possible results. Some plastic surgeons like to "sell" their operation—a practice Dr. Goldwyn abhors. "Too often doctors use pictures to seduce patients into surgery," he says. "I think it's a form of hucksterism. If you're shown pictures of a surgeon's best results, insist upon seeing pictures of the average and worst results as well." Dr. Shaw concurs. "Communication between plastic surgeon and patient can be very tricky," he says. "It requires a tremendous amount of honesty and self-restraint. Both the patient and the surgeon constantly need to separate wishes for perfection from the reality of what can be reasonably expected."

Once you know what you want, don't hesitate to shop around for the right plastic surgeon. You should choose someone you feel absolutely comfortable with and confident in. Above all, it should be someone who respects your ideal and doesn't seek to impose her or his ideal on you. The surgeon's "beautiful breast" and yours may be very dissimilar. Make sure you find someone who will construct *your* breast. And make sure you find someone who respects who you are, and why you're making your decision. If the surgeon you've approached acts insulting or condescending, go out and find someone with a more professional, more humane approach.

Of course, even if you have taken every precaution possible there's no guarantee that you'll be happy with your operation after it's done. But the odds are on your side. I've had very few patients who regretted having their breasts cosmetically altered, but I've had several who regretted not having it done. One of my Boston patients was an 80-year-old woman with huge, uncomfortable breasts. When she was younger, she went to a surgeon to try and get her breasts reduced. He told her she shouldn't have the operation. She took his advice—those were the days when doctors were gods; you didn't question them—and since then had been uncomfortable and unhappy with her breasts. After we talked she decided to have the surgery done. She was very happy with her small breasts—and very sad about all the years she could have been this comfortable.

Another of my patients was a sophisticated career woman in her early 30s. During our first visit I noticed that her breasts were extremely asymmetrical, and after a few visits I asked her if she'd ever thought about plastic surgery. Her face lit up. "Can I really do that?" she asked me. I assured her that she could, and gave her a list of plastic surgeons. She didn't even wait till she got out of the building to call them; she found a phone booth downstairs, made an appointment, and had her implant within the month. She was absolutely delighted with it—but she needed me to suggest it and to give her "permission" to seek help for her asymmetry. My coauthor, who had silicone injections for her asymmetry, has found that her breasts are no longer perfectly matched, and, as she grows older, the augmented breast sags much more than the natural one. But she is very happy about her decision and says she would make the same choice again today. She keeps in her closet an old V-necked sweater her mother gave her after she finished her injections—a symbol of a freedom she hadn't known before.

Because the news tends to focus on women who have trouble with their silicone implants, it's easy to forget that the vast majority of patients—those that don't get in the news—are happy with their decision to alter their breasts. Psychiatrist Sanford Gifford writes about a patient feeling she had "gained something lost in early puberty."[8] He observes that the degree of satisfaction is much greater among women who have had plastic surgery for their breasts than among those who have had face-lifts or nose jobs—they don't have the same unrealistic expectations. Often they're happier with their still-imperfect breasts than the surgeon thinks they should be. For some reason people don't go into this kind of plastic surgery with the same dreams of impossible perfection they bring to facial surgery.

If you are considering plastic surgery for your breasts, make sure you have all the information you need about risks, dangers, and reasonable expectations—and then do what you want. And don't let age deter you from the cosmetic surgery you want. My 80-year-old patient was delighted with her belated operation, and I've had many women in their 50s, 60s, and 70s who have had their breasts reduced or augmented. If your health is good enough to sustain surgery, it doesn't matter how old you are.

PART TWO

Common Problems

4

"Fibrocystic Disease" and Breast Pain

You're concerned about your breasts: they get swollen and hard just before your period. Or they're so painful you can't get any work done. Or there's discharge when you squeeze your nipple.

So you talk to a friend who says, "Oh, I know what that is! I had it a few years ago, and my doctor told me it was fibrocystic disease."

You decide, quite sensibly, to talk to your doctor. After all, if you've got a disease you want to know about it. Probably nowadays your doctor will tell you not to worry about "fibrocystic disease" and will then look at your specific symptom. But if your doctor is a bit more old-school, you may hear that you do indeed have fibrocystic disease.

Well, you don't have fibrocystic disease any more than you have a werewolf bite: there's no such thing. "Fibrocystic disease" is a meaningless umbrella term—a wastebasket into which doctors throw every breast problem that isn't cancerous. The symptoms it encompasses are so varied and so unrelated to each other that the term is wholly without meaning. To an examining doctor, "fibrocystic disease" can be swelling, pain, tenderness, lumpy breasts (a condition not to be confused with breast lumps—see Chapter 6), nipple discharge—any noncancerous thing that can happen in or on the breast. That's the clinical version of our mythical disease.

To a pathologist, fibrocystic disease is any one of about 15 micro-

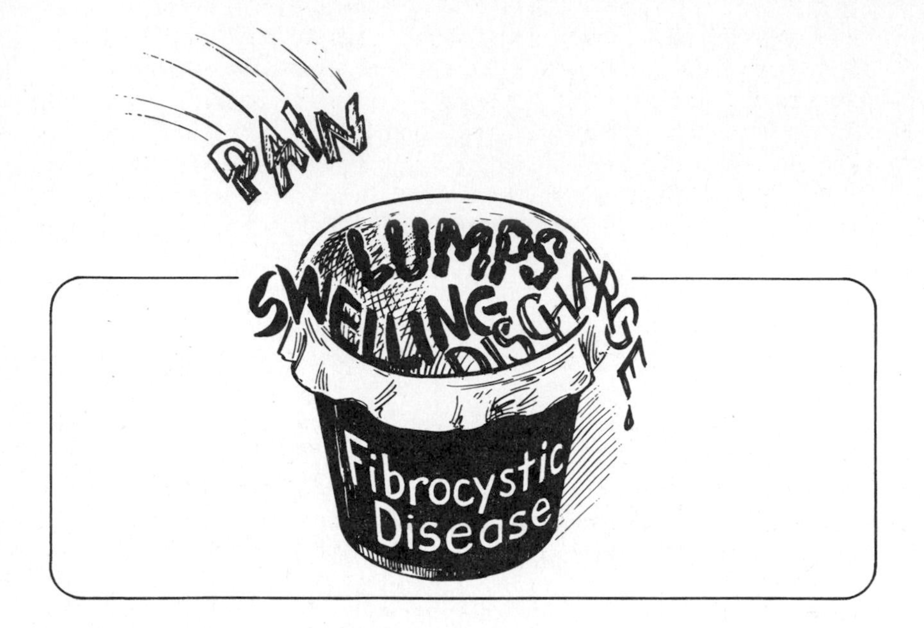

scopic findings that exist in virtually every woman's breasts and never reveal themselves except through a microscope. They cause no trouble, and they have no relation to cancer—or to anything else, except the body's natural aging process. They were found in the particular breast tissue that was biopsied only because it was biopsied, not because they had any relation to whatever symptom the examining doctor was concerned with. Only one of these microscopic findings is a danger sign: it's called atypical hyperplasia, and, combined with a family history of breast cancer, it can suggest an increased breast cancer risk (see Chapter 10).

The radiologists who read mammograms have another version of fibrocystic disease altogether—dense breasts. Dense breasts are normal in young women, as explained in Chapter 1. Breast tissue that is unusually dense for one's age is, however, related to hormonal stimulation of the breast, which has been implicated in the increased risk of breast cancer.[1]

So whatever problem you have with your breasts, it isn't fibrocystic disease. But the invention of this mythical disease has caused a number of problems. Insurance companies have refused to cover women diagnosed with the "disease" or have excluded coverage of breast problems. If such women do develop breast diseases, their medical bills can be devastating.

Women have also been subjected to a number of "treatments"—ranging from eliminating caffeine from their diets to getting prophylactic mastectomies. Finally, for a long time researchers didn't bother to study any of the conditions defined as fibrocystic disease, since they believed a diagnosis already existed. As a result, we haven't had the studies necessary to help us learn what does cause some of the real problems, such as breast pain, that women actually experience.

I'm proud of being a pioneer in debunking the myth of fibrocystic disease. After doing a lot of research into the studies claiming to define the "disease," I wrote about my findings in the *New England Journal of Medicine* in 1982. Although no doctor wrote to the journal to argue against my findings, the College of American Pathologists took four years to come out with a statement that fibrocystic disease doesn't increase the risk of cancer.[2]

In this chapter and the two following ones we'll consider the various kinds of benign breast conditions. One common breast symptom is pain—frequently called either "mastalgia" or "mastodynia" (one is Latin, the other Greek, and they both translate to "breast pain"). It can run the gamut of discomfort—from a minor irritation a couple of days a month through permanent, nearly disabling agony, and everything in between.

A clinic in Cardiff, Wales, documented three main categories of breast pain: cyclical (pain related to the menstrual cycle), noncyclical ("trigger zone" pain), and pain that does not originate in the breast. Of these the most common by far is cyclical.[3]

The best way to determine which kind of pain you have is to keep a breast pain chart—a calendar where you mark every day whether your pain is severe, mild, or gone.[4] In addition, you mark the days of your period. Looking at this, you can easily determine whether your pain is premenstrual or everyday (cyclical or noncyclical), or nonbreast in origin.

CYCLICAL PAIN

We know that cyclical mastalgia is related to hormonal variations. The breasts are sensitive right before menstruation, then less sensitive once the period begins. For some women, tenderness begins at the time of ovulation and continues until their period, leaving only a couple of pain-free weeks during their cycle. For some, it's barely noticeable; others are in such pain they can't wear a T-shirt, lie on their stomach, or tolerate a hug. Sometimes it's only in one breast, and other times it radiates into the armpit and even down to the elbows, causing its poor victim to think she's got cancer spreading to her lymph nodes.

Understanding precisely the part hormones play in cyclical mastalgia is clouded by the fact that women's hormonal cycles haven't been all that well researched. Although we know roughly how the levels of estrogen and progesterone go up and down during each cycle and that FSH and LH are the main pituitary hormones, we don't yet understand the fine-tuning of these hormones or how the hormones regulate and affect the different parts of the body. Just as we don't understand menstrual cramps and bloating and PMS, we don't understand breast pain. Recent data done in the United Kingdom has shown that tamoxifen gel rubbed on the breast has shown success in alleviating breast pain.

Hormones may also affect cyclical breast pain in a more subtle way—for example, as a result of stress. We know that stress can affect the menstrual cycle: you can miss your period or have a particularly heavy period or an early or late period when you're under great stress, positive or negative. Similarly, your breast pain can increase or change pattern with the hormone changes of stress. We also know that hormones vary at different points in your life and that the incidence of breast pain often follows these shifts. It's usually most intense in the teens and then again in the 40s—at both ends of the fertile years. It almost always ends with menopause, though in some rare cases it lasts beyond menopause—perhaps because of the continuing estrogen production of the ovaries and breast tissue (see Chapter 1). And of course, if a postmenopausal woman is taking hormones, her body thinks she's still premenopausal and she's as likely to get breast pain as she was before.[5] We also know it's common in pregnant women; indeed, unusual breast pain can be an early sign of pregnancy.

The relation to hormones doesn't appear to be absolute—there must be other factors, since most often the pain is more severe in one breast than in the other, and a purely hormonal symptom would have to affect both equally. It appears to be caused by a combination of the hormonal activity and something in the breast tissue that responds to that activity. More research needs to be done.

Breast pain is annoying, but it usually isn't unbearable—what can be unbearable is the fear that it's cancer. The best treatment, therefore, is reassurance. The study in Cardiff suggests that 85 percent of women with breast pain worry much more about the possibility of cancer than about the pain itself. Most of them, when reassured that their problem has no relation to cancer, are relieved and feel they can live with their pain. This study was repeated in Brazil to see if it was only Welsh women who responded to reassurance. Sure enough, Brazilian women also responded to reassurance with a success rate of 70.2 percent.[6] Only 10–15 percent of the women have pain that's incapacitating and needs treatment.

A wide variety of treatments have been proposed for cyclical breast pain. Some work and some don't. Many clinicians suggest stopping caffeine or taking vitamin E, despite studies showing that this approach does not work. Some physicians who believe the pain comes from water retention recommend diuretics (water pills). These give little relief. Others have tried everything from ginseng tea, vitamin A, vitamin B complex, and antibiotics, to just a firm support bra.

If you have breast pain, the first step is to get a good examination from a breast specialist or someone knowledgeable in the field who will take your symptoms and concerns seriously (this may take some searching). If you're over 35, have a mammogram. Once you know you don't have cancer you can decide whether you are able to live with your discomfort or want to further explore treatment. You may also want to look into Chinese herbs and acupuncture, which have been used for centuries in China. In some cases, herbs and acupuncture are used together; in others, the patient and/or practitioner prefer to use one or the other. They can also be used for noncylical pain (see page 65).

Another possibility is the use of meditation and visualization techniques, such as those discussed in Chapter 25. A number of studies have shown that these techniques can be effective in reducing pain, and they may well help relieve both cyclical and noncyclical breast pain.

If you are in your 20s, you may want to try the pill. Analgesics like aspirin, Tylenol, and ibuprofen can offer some relief, and wearing a firm bra will prevent bouncing breasts from increasing your discomfort.

A reasonable treatment plan for moderate to severe mastalgia has been proposed by the breast pain group in Wales. Although different women will respond better to different drugs, they ensure relief of pain in 70–80 percent of women when their regimen has been followed.[7] They recommend evening primrose oil (a natural form of gamolenic acid) as the first step for women with moderate pain and those who are taking oral contraceptives. It can be obtained in health food stores as tablets containing 500 mg of gamolenic acid. Six capsules should be taken twice a day. It has minor side effects, but the reaction to therapy can take a while so a trial of treatment should last at least four months and be monitored by keeping your pain chart. This treatment has been shown to benefit 44–58 percent of women. If pain has decreased, evening primrose oil is continued for one to two months more and then discontinued. Many women will have long-lasting effects after discontinuing therapy.[8] But don't take it if you're pregnant or trying to get pregnant as it can cause a miscarriage.

The next step for treatment in those women for whom evening primrose oil doesn't work is hormonal. Danocrine (Danazol) and bromocriptine have been shown to have some benefit. If you are taking oral contraceptives, you should not use either drug; only women who are not taking oral contraceptives and are using adequate mechanical contraception should use them. Danocrine is given at 200–300 mg per day and slowly reduced to 100 mg a day after relief of symptoms. Danocrine will relieve pain in 70–80 percent of women.[9] Side effects are common, including menstrual irregularities, leg cramps, weight gain, and decreased libido. The symptoms are related to the dose, and so the recommendation is to start with 200 mg a day for a month and, if the pain is diminished, to reduce it to 100 mg a day for the second month and then to stop. Few women need a longer course of therapy.

Bromocriptine inhibits the release of prolactin and has been shown to be effective in up to 65 percent of women treated for cyclical breast pain at doses of 5 mg a day. These results were demonstrated in a European multicenter randomized controlled trial.[10] Mild side effects such as nausea, dizziness, headaches, and irritability have been reported in 30 percent of women and 10 percent complained of severe side effects. Most of these effects can be avoided by gradually increasing the dose, taking the drug with meals, and using the smallest amount necessary to get an effect. (See Fig. 4-1 for an explanation of where the treatments described have their effects.) If bromocriptine is tried first and does not work, about 30 percent of women will respond to danocrine, and vice versa if danocrine is tried first. These two drugs are the only ones approved for the treatment of breast pain at this time. Other drugs have been shown to be effective but are not as yet approved for that purpose.

Tamoxifen is an estrogen blocker (see Chapter 28). According to an English study, it's very good at relieving mastalgia (80–90 percent).[11] Side effects include hot flashes and menstrual irregularities. Luckily, it was shown to be just as effective at 10 mg per day as at 20 mg, and three months of treatment were just as good as six. A group in Minnesota reports using 10 mg for two months with good results and only a 30 percent recurrence rate.[12] LH-RH analogs are drugs that put you into a reversible menopause. In one study they achieved an 81 percent response rate when given by injection.[13] Side effects include hot flashes, headaches, nausea, and irritability. Because these drugs decrease bone density (see Chapter 18), they should only be used for a short period of time.

A more benign remedy, a low-fat diet, has been studied and shown to have some effect on cyclical mastalgia and hormone levels.[14] W.R. Ghent and colleagues have theorized that the absence of dietary iodine may render duct lining cells more sensitive to estrogen stimulation.[15] As a result, they have been studying the use of molecular iodine as a treatment for breast pain with some success.

Eventually we will be able to invent something specifically for breast pain like the prostaglandin inhibitors (ibuprofen) that work so well with menstrual cramps, and women will no longer have to suffer from it.

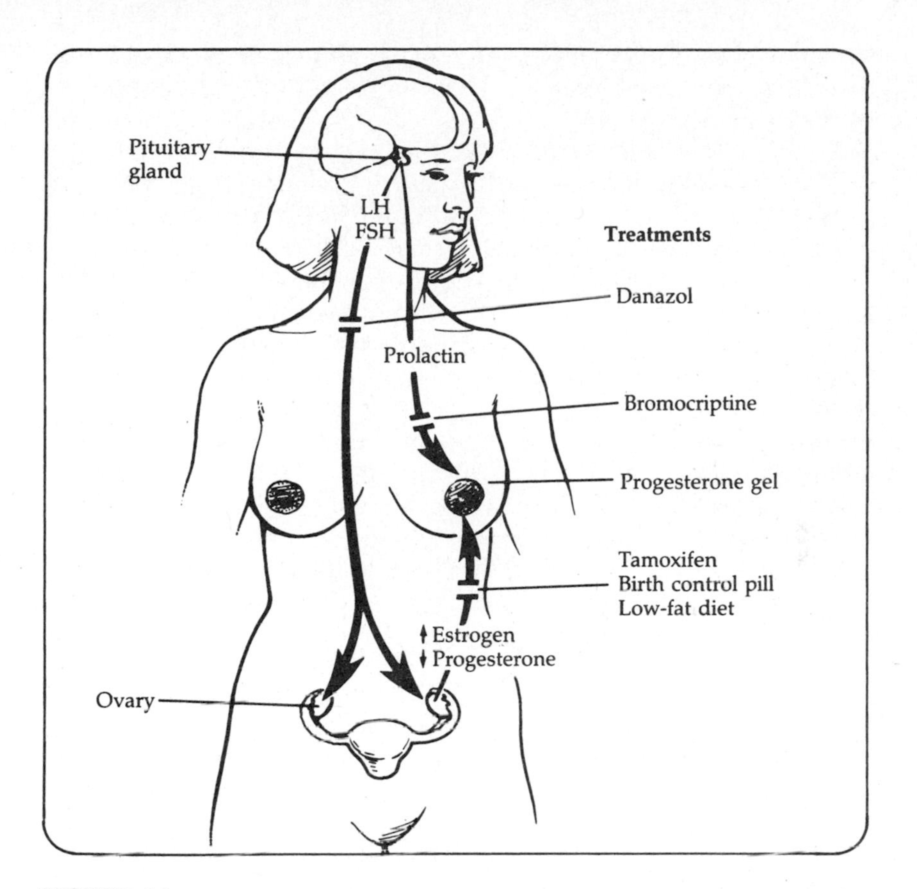

FIGURE 4-1

NONCYCLICAL PAIN

Noncyclical pain is far less common than cyclical pain. It also feels a lot different. To begin with, it doesn't vary with your menstrual cycle—it's there and it stays there. It's also known as trigger zone breast pain because it's almost always in one specific area: you can point exactly to where it hurts. It's anatomical rather than hormonal—something in the breast tissue is causing it (although we usually don't know what). Rarely, it can be a sign of cancer, so it's always worth checking out with your doctor, especially if you are over 30.

One cause of noncyclical breast pain is trauma—a blow to the breast will obviously cause it to hurt, and a breast biopsy is likely to leave some pain (see Chapter 8). Many women get slight shooting or stabbing pains up to two years or more after a biopsy. And you're never quite perfect after any surgery—just as after breaking a leg you can always tell when it will rain. This kind of pain is usually pretty obvious: it's on the spot where your scar is. It's unpleasant, but it's nothing to worry about.

Often we simply don't know what causes noncyclical breast pain; we'll operate and remove the area, have the tissue studied, and find nothing abnormal. Unfortunately we don't relieve the pain.

Treatment for this kind of breast pain is more difficult than for cyclical breast pain. Again, start with a good exam, and, if you're over 35, a mammogram. If there's an obvious abnormality it can then be taken care of. For example, sometimes a gross cyst (see Chapter 6) causing localized breast pain or tenderness can be cured by needle aspiration.

Since noncyclical pain is rarely caused by hormones, hormonal treatments are less likely to work. Some women, however, find relief with the kinds of treatments mentioned under cyclical breast pain.[16] You may want to try them. Sometimes, though not invariably, having a biopsy relieves the pain—though you will experience pain from the biopsy itself. A good test is for your doctor to inject some local anesthesia into the spot. If it gives relief then surgery may work well; if not, then it probably isn't worth it.

The best treatment is most likely a good exam and a negative mammogram with the reassurance that goes with it. This, of course, does nothing to relieve your pain, but it does relieve what's usually much worse than the pain—the fear that you have cancer.

NONBREAST-ORIGIN PAIN

This third category isn't really a form of breast pain, though that's what it feels like to the patient. It's usually in the middle of the chest and doesn't change with your period. Most frequently it's arthritic pain, in the place where the ribs and breastbone connect—an arthritis called costochondritis (Fig. 4-2).[17] When men get costochondritis they think it's a heart attack; when women get it, they think it's breast cancer. You can tell it's arthritis by pushing down on your breastbone where your ribs are—if it hurts a lot more, that's probably what you've got. Similarly, if you take a deep breath and the middle part of your breast hurts, it's probably arthritis. If you take aspirin or Motrin and it relieves the pain, it's probably arthritis, since they're anti-inflammatory agents and thus work especially effectively on conditions like arthritis. Having your doctor inject the spot with local anesthetic and 40 mg of methylprednisolone (steriods) will relieve 90 percent of chest wall pain.[18]

You can also get nonbreast-origin pain from arthritis in the neck (a pinched nerve).[19] This pain can radiate down into the breast the way

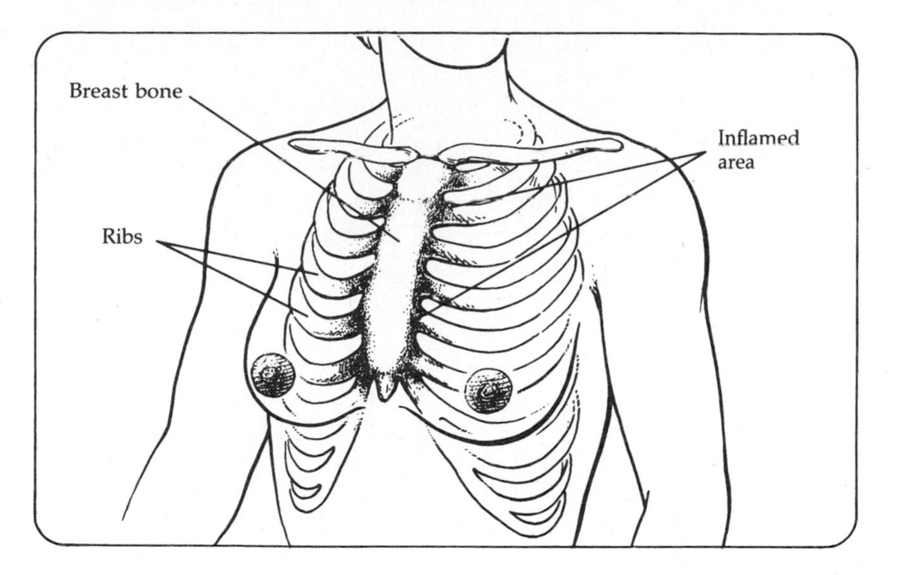

FIGURE 4-2

lower back arthritis goes into the legs. There's also a special kind of phlebitis (inflamed vein) that can occur in the breast, called Mondor's syndrome. It gives you a drawing sensation around the outer edge of your breast that extends down into your abdomen. Sometimes you can even feel a cord where it is most tender. None of these problems is serious. A nonbreast condition that appears in the breast area is treated as it would be in any other part of the body. That usually means, for the conditions just mentioned, aspirin or another anti-inflammatory agent. These pains are usually self-limited and will go away in time.

Cancer Concerns

How likely are any of these forms of breast pain to be cancer? Cyclical pain has no relation to cancer, so don't worry. Noncyclical pain is rarely a sign of cancer, but it can be, so it's worth checking out. One of my patients discovered while she was traveling in Europe that her breast hurt when she lay on her stomach; though she couldn't feel any lump she had it checked when she came home and discovered she did indeed have a tiny cancer on the spot. About 10 percent of all "target zone" breast pain is cancer. Nonbreast-origin pain, as already noted, is probably arthritis, and you can confirm this by the methods I suggested. If you're still in doubt, have it checked by your doctor.

5

Breast Infections and Nipple Problems

Breast infections and nipple discharge are fairly uncommon and usually are not much more than a nuisance. But they can cause great anxiety to the woman who experiences them. There are two major categories of breast infection: intrinsic and extrinsic. Intrinsic breast infections—those occurring only in the breast—break down into three categories: lactational mastitis, nonlactational mastitis, and chronic subareolar abscess.

BREAST INFECTIONS: INTRINSIC

Lactational Mastitis

Lactational mastitis is the most common of these infections.[1] It occurs, as its name suggests, when the woman is breast-feeding. The breast is filled with milk, a medium that encourages the growth of bacteria. You've got a baby biting and sucking on your breast on a regular basis, causing cracks in the skin and introducing bacteria—it's really amazing that more nursing mothers don't get infections.

Probably it happens as seldom as it does because milk is always flowing through and flushing the bacteria out. However, sometimes

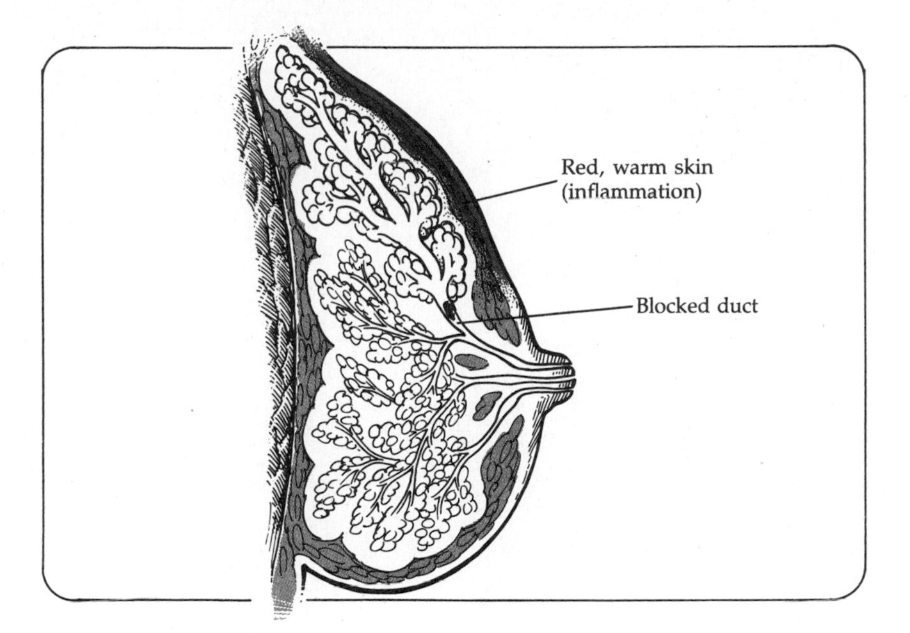

FIGURE 5-1

when you're breast-feeding a duct will get blocked up with thick milk that doesn't flow very well. Then bacteria become trapped in the breast, the milk helps them grow, and suddenly you've got a reddened, hot, and very painful breast (Fig. 5-1).

Your doctor will probably suggest that you try to unblock the duct with massage and warm soaks; sometimes a doctor suggests heat (which liquifies the milk for better flow, but unfortunately increases the blood flow to the breast tissue and thus accelerates the bacterial growth) or ice packs (which slow the bacteria's growth rate but unfortunately thicken the milk). If the infection persists, antibiotics are the next step. Usually that will take care of it. Don't worry about the antibiotics affecting your nursing child. Your obstetrician will know which antibiotics are safe for children to ingest. Nor will the bacteria hurt the child, since they will be killed by the baby's stomach acid. It's actually good for you if the child goes on nursing. The sucking helps keep the duct unblocked.

Antibiotics almost always get rid of infection, but in about 10 percent of cases an abscess forms, and antibiotics are useless in eliminating abscesses. An abscess, like a boil, is basically a collection of pus, and the doctor has to drain the pus. If it's a small abscess, the pus can be aspirated with a needle. If it's fairly big, the doctor will have to make an incision large enough to allow the pus to drain (Fig. 5-2). This

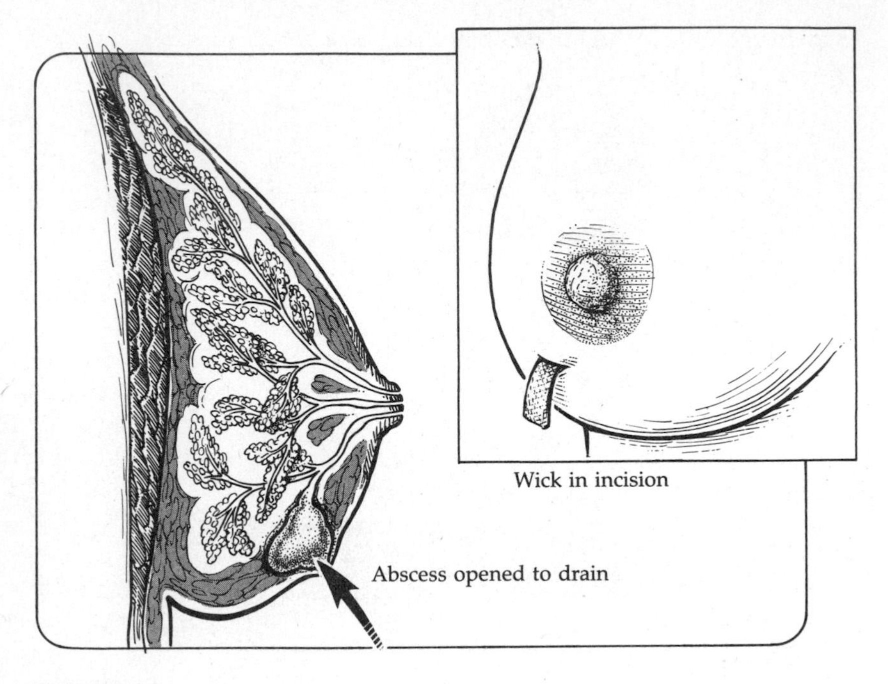

FIGURE 5-2

can be done under local anesthetic, but it's difficult because the inflamed tissue is highly sensitive and it's hard to inject an anesthetic that will really numb the area well. If my patient had an extremely small infected area, I'd tell her to bite the bullet, the pain would soon be over, and go with the local. But if it was a large area, I found it far more effective to put the patient to sleep. (See Chapter 21 for a discussion of general anesthetic.)

Once the cut is made, the pus drains out and the pain abates quickly. Surgeons never sew up a drained abscess; that would lock bacteria into the cavity and almost ensure the infection's return. I'd tell my patients to go home and rest, then, after 24 hours, begin taking daily showers; let the water run over the breast and wash away the bacteria. Then put a dressing over it to absorb oozing fluids from the incision. Some surgeons will put a wick, or drain, in the corner of the incision to keep it open; that way it heals from the inside out and closes within a week or two.

Some surgeons will tell you that if you need an operation you have to stop breast-feeding. Many women really want to breast-feed, and there's no reason they should give it up. It's messy, since not only are you oozing fluids, you're also oozing milk. But if you're willing to put up with the mess there's no reason not to breast-feed. It's usually just one breast, and just a segment of the breast at that; there's plenty of room for your baby to suckle.

Nonlactational Mastitis

Though the kind of mastitis described above is usually found only in lactating women, mastitis can also occur in nonlactating women, especially in particular circumstances. For example, it may occur in women who've had lumpectomies followed by radiation, in diabetics, or in women whose immune system is otherwise depressed: such women are prone to infections either because some of the lymph nodes, which help fight infection, have been removed, or because their immune systems are generally less strong than those of most people. This type of infection will usually be a cellulitis—an infection of the skin—red, hot, and swollen all over rather than in one spot. It's generally accompanied by high fever and headache, both characteristics of a strep infection (staph infections, by contrast, are usually local). Your doctor will treat it with antibiotics, usually penicillin, and you may be briefly hospitalized.

Skin boils (or staph infections) can form on the breast, as they can on other parts of the body. If you're a carrier of staph and prone to infection as well—as in the case of diabetics—this is more likely to occur than in noncarriers or people less infection prone. It's also possible to get an abscess in the breast when you're not lactating and don't have any of the other risk factors, although this is unusual. Both cellulitis and these abscesses can mask cancer (as we'll discuss below), so, though such cancer is rare, if you've got one of these conditions it's important to have it checked out by a doctor.

I had several patients with what has been called chronic mastitis. In each case the patient had an infection, which her doctor drained. Unlike lactational mastitis, discussed earlier, these infections are abscesses, and so the first treatment should be to drain them. If the abscess recurs or fails to heal completely the patients are sent to an infectious disease specialist who starts them on antibiotics. Some of the women I saw had been on these antibiotics for years, often given intravenously at home through a Hickman catheter (see Chapter 24). Most of the time I found that the problem could have been easily treated with a minor operation, a solution the infectious disease specialist, lacking experience in breast surgery, had overlooked. If you have a so-called chronic infection, make sure you see a breast surgeon early on. You may save yourself a lot of suffering and expense. Diseased tissue, like the chronic subareolar abscess which I discuss next, has to be removed surgically.

Chronic Subareolar Abscess

The second most common breast infection—and it's rather infrequent—is the chronic subareolar abscess, which we don't understand very well, though there is some evidence that it is more common in smokers. Two theories about its cause demonstrate the fact that we also don't really understand the anatomy of the breast ducts and the nipples (see Chapter 1). One theory states that this infection is caused by ducts that become blocked with keratin and then get infected.[2] But Dr. Bruce Derrick at Temple University and Dr. Otto Sartorius put forth a different view, which I find more compelling.[3, 4] As you'll recall from Chapter 1, there are little glands on the nipple, as well as ducts. These small, dead-ended glands can get infections, whether you're nursing or not. Bacteria from the skin or mouth of your child or lover gets into the gland; thickened secretions block it so it can't drain well, and it gets infected. This kind of infection is most common in women with inverted nipples, because their glands have narrower openings.

Whether the culprit in this condition is the ducts or the glands doesn't matter much to the patient. Either way, an abscess forms that can't drain through the usual exit and therefore tries to drain through the weakest part of the skin in the area—the border of the areola and the regular skin (Fig. 5-3). The abscess is a red, hot, sore area on part of the border of the areola—like a boil. It looks and feels fairly awful, and the frightened woman often thinks she's got breast cancer. She doesn't, and the infection doesn't affect her vulnerability to breast cancer.

If the infection is caught very early, before an abscess forms, it may be helped by antibiotics. But often it can't be and needs an incision and a draining. I think it's best to make the incision on the border of the areola, so that it doesn't show later. Once the pus is drained, it's okay—for the time being. The trouble is that this type of infection is apt to recur. The gland is a little blind passage with no internal opening, so it can reinfect itself and drain again at the same point. Eventually this leaves a permanent open tract.

We've had some luck reducing these recurrences by removing the entire gland or tract. To get the whole tract, the surgeon must excise a wedge of nipple. The method isn't perfect, but its success rate is a lot better than that of other methods.

Since the gland is small and the surgery relatively minor, I used to do it under local anesthetic. But it's hard to get a chronically infected area thoroughly numb, especially one as sensitive as the nipple—the same problem as in lactational mastitis, only more severe. So I found that, in my anxiousness to end my patient's discomfort, I sometimes didn't get the whole gland out and the infection recurred. Later I gave women short-acting drugs to complement the local. I passed a probe

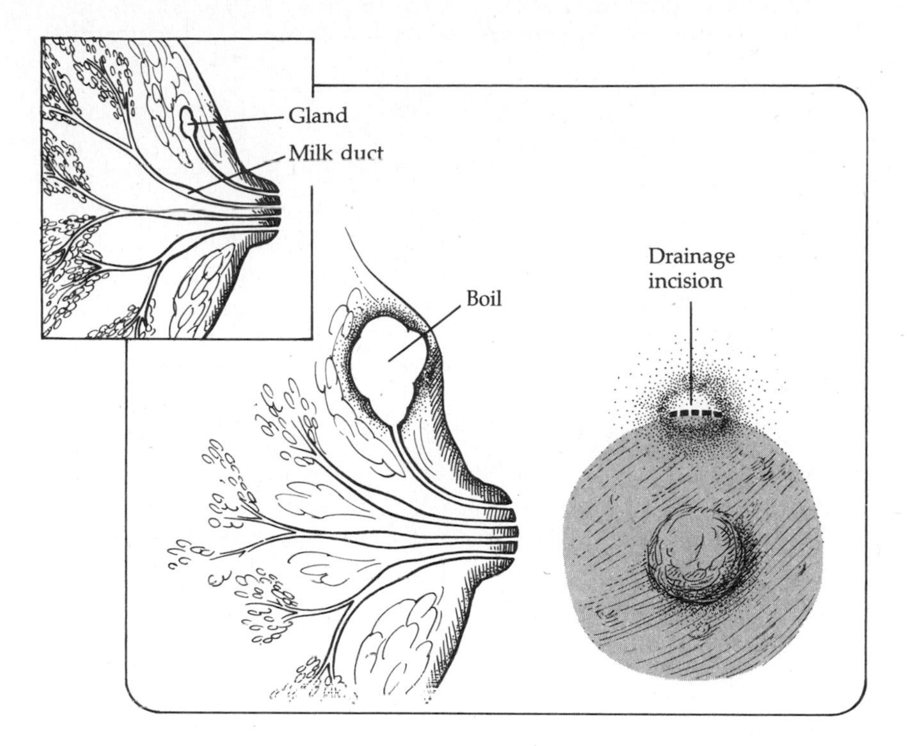

FIGURE 5-3

through the tract and then took out the wedge of nipple that contained the tract, including both openings (Fig. 5-4). I then closed the nipple and sewed it up.

There's some controversy about whether or not to close the incision: some doctors are afraid that if there are lots of bacteria to begin with there's a greater chance that the gland will reinfect itself if it's closed off; others are more concerned about the cosmetics of a nipple with a hole in it. I prefer to close it, but I always tell my patient the pros and cons, then do what she wants.

Unfortunately, even in the most skillfully done operations, the problem often recurs.[5] Perhaps the infection spreads from one gland to another, or perhaps there's still lining left from the old gland that the surgeon isn't aware of. So if you have a chronic subareolar abscess, it's well worth trying to have it taken care of. But understand that you might have to keep dealing with it. About 40 percent of these infections do recur, sometimes as often as every few months.

As so often happens, many doctors think disfiguring surgery on women's bodies is called for. One patient came to me after her doctor said he was fed up with these recurrences and wanted to remove both

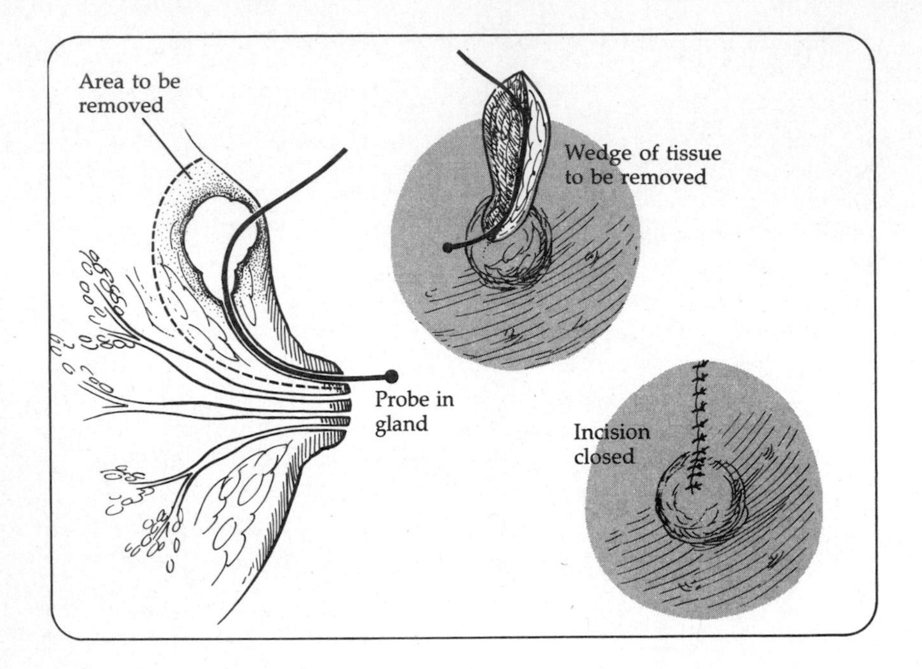

FIGURE 5-4

breasts. Fortunately she had the sense not to listen to him. A well-planned, nonmutilating operation solved her problem—but even if it hadn't, the most drastic procedure that would have made any sense at all would have been to remove the nipple alone—then at least a plastic surgeon could reconstruct a new nipple, leaving the breast intact (see Chapter 3).

But if you have this condition it's unlikely you'd want even that done. A chronic absess is unpleasant and a nuisance, but not life-threatening. It doesn't interfere with breast-feeding, nor should it restrict your sexual life, except that you're not likely to want your nipple touched while it's hurting.

BREAST INFECTIONS: EXTRINSIC

Extrinsic breast infections are those that involve the whole body but show first on the breast. These are extremely rare in this country, so I'll mention them only briefly. TB and syphilis have both been known to emerge first on the breast; such infections are treated the same way the diseases would be treated if they showed first anywhere else.

INFECTION AND CANCER

As I said earlier, breast infections never lead to breast cancer. However, some breast cancers lead to infections or look like infections (see Chapter 16). As the cancer cells grow, noncancer cells die off for lack of blood supply, and the necrotic (dead) tissue can get infected. So it's possible, though extremely unusual, for a breast cancer to show up first as a breast abscess.

A form of cancer called inflammatory breast cancer can be mistaken for infection (see Chapter 16). This starts with redness of the skin, warmth, and swelling. There usually is no lump. What distinguishes it from infection is that it doesn't get better with antibiotics. Anyone with a breast infection that persists after 10 days to two weeks of antibiotics should see a breast surgeon, who will probably want to do a biopsy.

If you get an infection, don't worry about it—but do see your doctor right away. The infection won't give you cancer, but it should be treated and gotten rid of, and you do want to make sure it is in fact an infection.

NIPPLE PROBLEMS

Discharge

The nipple is an especially sensitive area and subject to a number of problems, such as the subareolar abscess discussed earlier. The most common nipple problem—or rather concern, since it's not always a problem—is discharge. As I explained at length in Chapter 2, most women do have some amount of discharge or fluid when their breasts are squeezed, and it's perfectly normal (Fig. 5-5). In a study at Boston's Lying-in Hospital breast clinic women had little suction cups, like breast pumps, put on their nipples and gentle suction applied.[6] (See Chapter 13.) Eighty-three percent of these women—old, young, mothers, nonmothers, previously pregnant, never pregnant—had some amount of fluid. As I will explain in Chapter 13, this fluid can be analyzed for precancerous cells.

The ducts of the nipple are pipelines; they're made to carry milk to the nipple, so a little fluid in the pipes shouldn't be surprising. (It can come in a number of colors—gray, green, and brown, as well as white.)

Sometimes people confuse nipple discharge with other problems—weepy sores, infections, abscesses (see above). Inverted nipples (see Chapter 3) can sometimes get dirt and dried-up sweat trapped in them, and this can be confused with discharge.

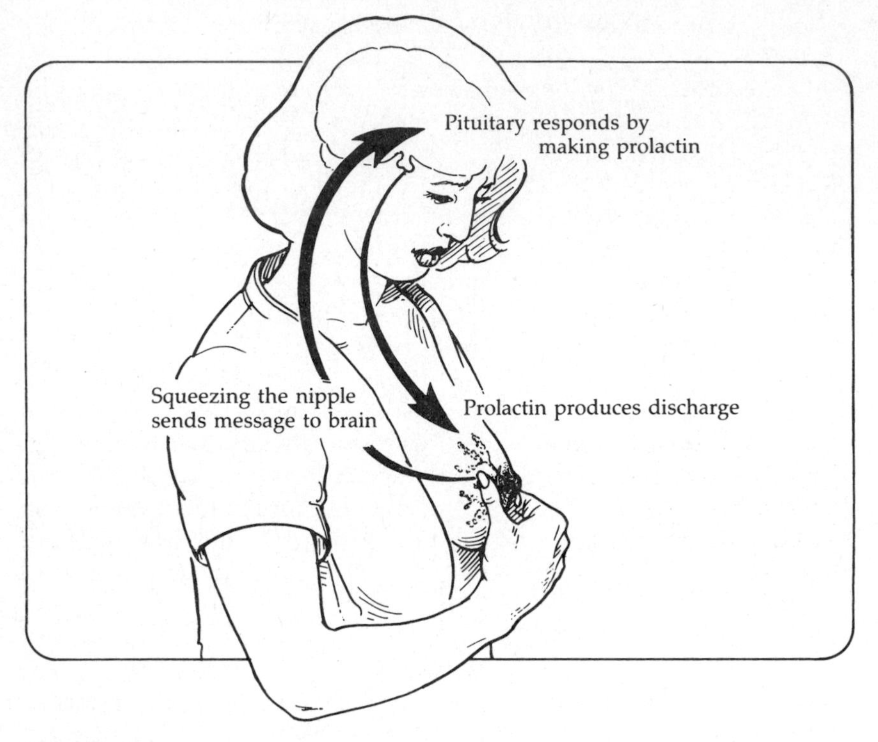

FIGURE 5-5

Some women are more prone to lots of discharge than others: women on birth control pills, antihypertensives such as Aldomet, or major tranquilizers such as thorazine tend to notice more discharge, because these medications increase prolactin levels. It may seem aesthetically displeasing, but beyond that there's nothing to worry about.

There are also different life periods when you're more likely to get discharge than others: there's more discharge at puberty and at menopause than in the years between. And there's the "witch's milk" that newborn babies get (see Chapter 1). This makes sense, since the discharge is a result of hormonal processes.

When Should You Worry?

The time to worry about nipple discharge is when it's spontaneous, persistent, and unilateral (only on one side). It comes out by itself without squeezing; it keeps on happening; and it's only from one nipple and usually one duct. It's either clear and sticky, like an egg white, or bloody. You should go to the doctor right away. There are several possible causes:

1. Intraductal papilloma. This is a little wartlike growth on the lining of the duct. It gets eroded and bleeds, creating a bloody discharge. It's benign; the surgeon removes it to make sure that's what it is.
2. Intraductal papillomatosis. Instead of one wart, you've got a lot of little warts.
3. Intraductal carcinoma in situ. This is a precancer that clogs up the duct like rust: it's discussed in detail in Chapter 12.
4. Cancer. Cancers are rarely the cause of discharge. Less than 10 percent of all spontaneous unilateral bloody discharges are cancerous. But it's important to have it checked.

Age is an important factor in predicting whether the discharge is related to cancer. Among patients with nipple discharges, only 3 percent who are younger than 40, and 10 percent who are between 40 and 60, will have cancer, but the number jumps to 32 percent of those over 60.[7]

Your clinician should first test for blood by taking a sample, putting it on a card, and adding a chemical (hemacult test). If it turns blue, there's blood (which may not be visible to the eye because of the color of the discharge). The doctor may do a Pap smear, very like the Pap smear you get to test for cervical cancer. Discharge is put on a glass slide and sent to the lab for the cells to be examined. A recent study from Vermont showed this to be quite accurate when done on women with abnormal discharge.[8] Next the doctor will try and figure out the "trigger zone" by going around the breast to find out which duct the discharge is coming from, though often the woman herself can give the doctor this information. If you're over 30 you'll be sent for a mammogram to see if there's a tumor underneath the duct.

You can then have your duct lavaged (see Chapter 13). If the cells are abnormal, this might give you another tipoff that there's a problem. Unfortunately, if the cells look normal, it doesn't guarantee that all is well. So you'll want to follow this procedure with a ductogram—a tool I find vital. The radiologist takes a very fine plastic catheter and, with a magnifying glass, threads it into the duct, squirts dye into it, and takes a picture (Fig. 5-6). This sounds fairly ghastly, but it really isn't that bad—the duct is an open tube already, and the discharge has dilated it. The ductogram provides a "map" for the surgeon who may do a biopsy and may also show the source of the discharge. Not every surgeon will order a ductogram or lavage, but I find them worthwhile. Two studies have documented that preoperative ductography increases the chance that if there is any abnormal tissue causing the pathology, it will be found.[9]

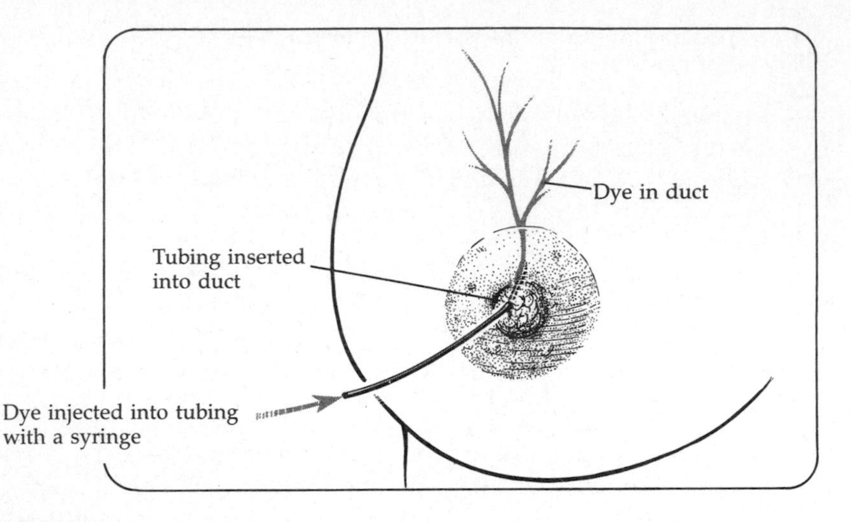

FIGURE 5-6

You may also have a simple biopsy, a specialized form of the regular breast biopsy (see Chapter 8). It can be done under local anesthetic on an outpatient basis. A tiny incision is made at the edge of the areola; the areola is flipped up, and the blood-filled duct located and removed (Fig. 5-7). Sometimes the radiologist will cut a fine suture and pass it into the duct to the point to be removed, or blue dye can be injected into the duct to help identify it. Both of these techniques will help pinpoint the right area. Sometimes if the ductogram has shown the lesion to be far from the nipple, the surgeon will localize the area with a wire, as described in Chapter 8. That way the duct won't get blocked, which interferes with breast-feeding, or numbed, which interferes with sexual pleasure.

Because the lesion can be far from the nipple itself, the old standard surgical practice of removing the ducts under the nipple has largely been abandoned nowadays. This is because though this procedure stops the discharge (by disconnecting the ducts from the nipple), it may or may not remove the tumor or other problem causing the discharge.

Some centers are using duct endoscopy to figure out what's causing the discharge. An endoscope is a thin scope put directly into the nipple duct, by which the surgeon can view the inside of the ducts on a video screen. They have reported success in seeing intraductal papillomas and other pathology and are devising intraductal techniques to treat them.[10]

Another form of problematic discharge is one that is spontaneous, bilateral (on both sides), and milky. If you're not breast-feeding and

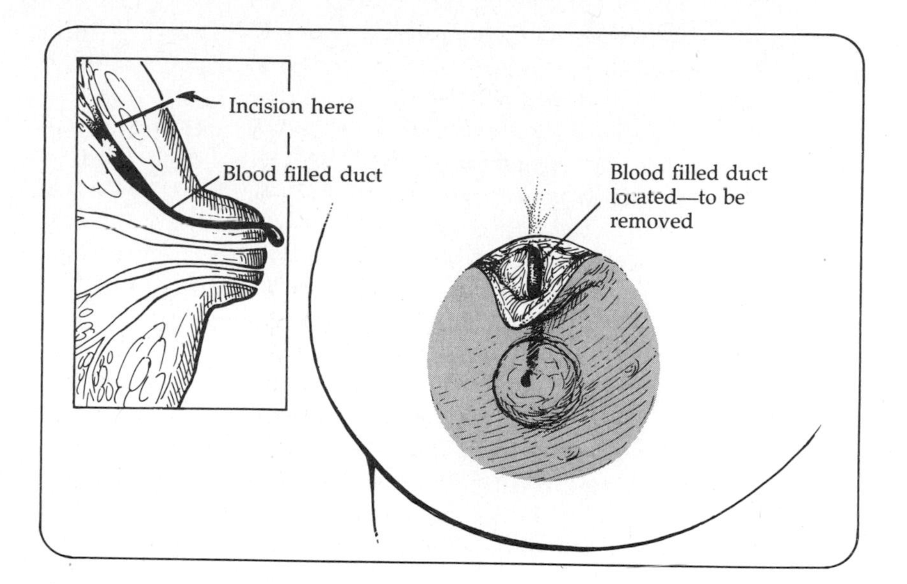

FIGURE 5-7

haven't been in the past year, this is probably a condition called galactorrhea—excessive or spontaneous milk flow. It occurs because something is increasing the prolactin levels—sometimes a small tumor in the brain. This may not be as alarming as it sounds: often it's a tiny tumor that may not require surgery. A neurosurgeon and an endocrinologist together need to check this out. You may be given bromocriptine to block the prolactin. Galactorrhea is often associated with amenorrhea—failure to get your period. It can also be caused by major tranquilizers, marijuana consumption, or high estrogen doses.

Galactorrhea is diagnosed only when the discharge is bilateral. Many doctors don't understand this, and send patients with any discharge for prolactin level tests. They shouldn't; the unilateral discharges are not associated with hormonal problems. Unilateral spontaneous discharge is anatomical, not hormonal, and the money spent on prolactin tests is wasted.

Other Nipple Problems

There are a few other problems women can have with their nipples. Some patients complain of itchy nipples. Usually this doesn't indicate anything dangerous, especially if both nipples itch. You can get dry skin on your nipples as elsewhere. You may be allergic to your bra or to the detergent it's washed in. Pubescent girls with growing breasts often experience itching as the skin stretches. Otherwise, we don't know what causes itchy nipples. If they bother you, you can use calamine lotion or other anti-itch medication.

There is a form of cancer known as Paget's disease that doctors and patients often confuse with eczema of the nipple. It looks like an open sore area and it itches. If it's on only one nipple and doesn't go away with standard eczema treatments, check it out. A biopsy can be performed on a small section of the nipple. (Paget's disease is discussed at length in Chapter 19.)

If the rash is on both nipples and you tend to get eczema anyway, don't worry. Anything that can happen to other parts of the skin can happen to the nipple.

Most of these infections and irritations are benign—they're more of a nuisance than anything else. If they appear, get them checked out, just to make sure they're what they appear to be and to get the relief available.

Finally, I should mention currently fashionable nipple piercings. In general they are not harmful, although, like any piercing, they can get infected. What is really worrisome is that such piercings might interfere with and even scar the openings of the milk ducts, affecting both later breast feeding and potential new avenues of treatment and prevention of breast cancer. (See Chapter 18.) For this reason I think it's wise to discourage it.

6

Lumps and Lumpiness

Lumpiness, as I explained in Chapter 1, isn't the same as having one dominant lump. It's a general pattern of many little lumps in both breasts, and it's perfectly normal. The distinction between "lumps" and "lumpiness" is important; confusing the two can cause a woman days and weeks of needless mental anguish.

Doctors who don't usually work with breast cancer—family practitioners and gynecologists—often get nervous about lumpy breasts and may fear they're malignant. So your doctor may send you to a specialist—a surgeon or a breast specialist—to make sure you don't have a cancerous lump. If you or your doctor are uncertain about whether you've got a lump or just lumpy breasts, it's probably not a bad idea to check it out further. But understanding more about what a lump really is might make the trip to the specialist unnecessary.

Ellen Mahoney, a fellow breast surgeon, tells her patients to visualize what their breasts may be like inside—from butter to gravel to bubble wrap—and if it's the same all over, it's just the way they're made. The only area to be concerned about is the one that is different from all the rest. The most important thing to know about dominant lumps—benign or malignant—is that they're almost never subtle. They're not like little BB pellets. They're usually at least a centimeter or two, almost an inch, or the size of a grape. The lump will stick out prominently in the midst of the smaller lumps that constitute normal lumpiness. You'll know it's something different. In fact, that's why most breast cancers are found by the woman herself—the lumps are so clearly distinct from the rest of her breast tissue.

The obvious question here is, How do I know the BB-size thing isn't an early cancer? The answer is that you usually don't feel a malignant lump when it's small. The cancer has to grow to a large enough size for the body to begin to create a reaction to it—a fibrous, scarlike tissue forms around the cancer, and this, combined with the cancer itself, makes up the palpable lump. The body won't create that reaction when the cancer is tiny, and you won't feel the cancerous lump until the reaction is formed.

At the same time, if it's much bigger than a walnut—if it feels like a quarter of the breast itself—you're probably still okay. You'll know by checking it through a couple of menstrual cycles, when you'll see that it changes through different parts of your cycle. A cancer lump that large would probably have been noticed earlier by even the most absentminded person. But if it doesn't go away or change significantly after two menstrual cycles, have it checked out. It's not likely to be a cancer, but it could be, and you don't want to take the chance. It will be easier for you to notice changes if you've become acquainted with your breasts, as I discussed in Chapter 2.

There are four types of dominant lumps, three of which—cysts, fibroadenomas, and pseudolumps—are virtually harmless. It's the fourth type—the malignant lump—that you're worrying about when you have your lump examined by a doctor. (I'll talk about cancerous lumps at length in Chapter 16.) Only 1 in 12 dominant lumps in premenopausal women is malignant. We don't know the cause of any of the noncancerous lumps, though we do know they're somehow related to hormonal variations (see Chapter 1). Two kinds of lumps—cysts and fibroadenomas—form during a woman's menstruating years but can show up years later, when breast tissue has shifted. Pseudolumps can occur in women of any age. It's interesting that two of the three kinds occur most often at opposite ends of a woman's fertile years: fibroadenomas occur when the woman is just starting to menstruate, and cysts when she's heading toward menopause.

CYSTS

Usually when you think of nonmalignant lumps you think of cysts, since doctors have a tendency to describe all nonmalignant lumps as cysts. They're not. A cyst is a particular, distinct kind of lump. Typically it occurs in women in their 30s, 40s, and early 50s, and is most common in women approaching menopause. It rarely occurs in a younger woman or in a woman who's past menopause. However, I've had patients in both categories—including a teenager and a woman who'd finished with her menopause long ago and wasn't on artificial hormones. (As I said earlier, a woman taking estrogen to combat menopausal symptoms fools her body into thinking it's still premenopausal.)

A gross cyst (gross meaning "large," not "disgusting") is a fluid-filled sac, like a large blister, which grows in breast tissue. It's smooth on the outside and "ballotable"—squishy—on the inside, so that if you push on it, you can feel that it's got fluid inside.

This, however, can be deceptive. Cysts *feel* like cysts only when they're close to the surface (Fig. 6-1). Cysts that are deeply embedded in breast tissue tend to distend that tissue and push it forward, so that what you're feeling is the hard breast tissue, not the soft cyst. In these cases the cyst feels like a hard lump.

The classical cyst story goes something like this. A woman in her 40s comes to a specialist and says, "I went to the gynecologist six weeks ago and everything was fine. I had a mammogram, and that was fine too. Then all of a sudden, in the shower last night, I found this lump in my breast, and I know it wasn't there before." So the doctor examines her and sure enough, there's a hard lump in her breast.

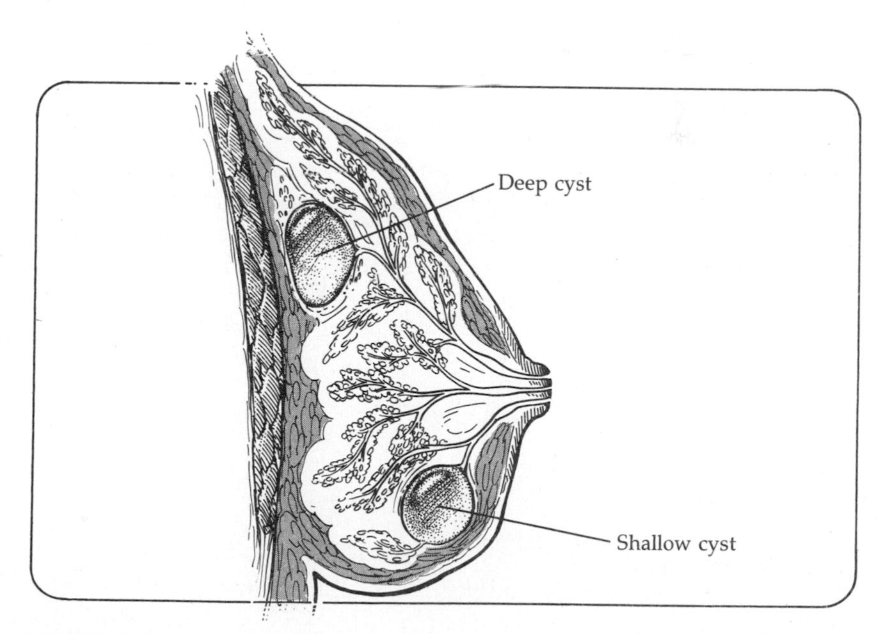

FIGURE 6-1

Because of its overnight appearance, the doctor is pretty sure it's a harmless cyst, but of course it's something the doctor—not to mention the patient—wants to be absolutely certain about: some cancers do seem to appear overnight. So the doctor tries to aspirate it.

To do this, the doctor takes a tiny needle, like the kind used for insulin injections, and anesthetizes the sensitive skin over the breast lump. Then a larger needle—like the kind used to draw blood—is attached to a syringe and stuck through the breast and into the cyst, where it draws out the fluid (Fig. 6-2). The cyst collapses like a punctured blister, and that's that.

Aspirating cysts was one of the medical procedures I most enjoyed doing. It's very easy, and as soon as it was done, my patient and I both knew she was okay. We were both delighted that she didn't have cancer, and she thought I was the greatest doctor in the world, having simultaneously diagnosed and cured her condition. It did wonders for my ego.

An added pleasure is that, though it sounds scary, it's usually almost painless. Most of the nerves in the breast are in the skin, and that's been anesthetized. Some women with greater sensitivity to pain or especially sensitive breasts do find it painful, but most don't. The only possible complications from aspirating a cyst are bruising or bleeding into the cyst, neither of which is more than slightly uncomfortable.

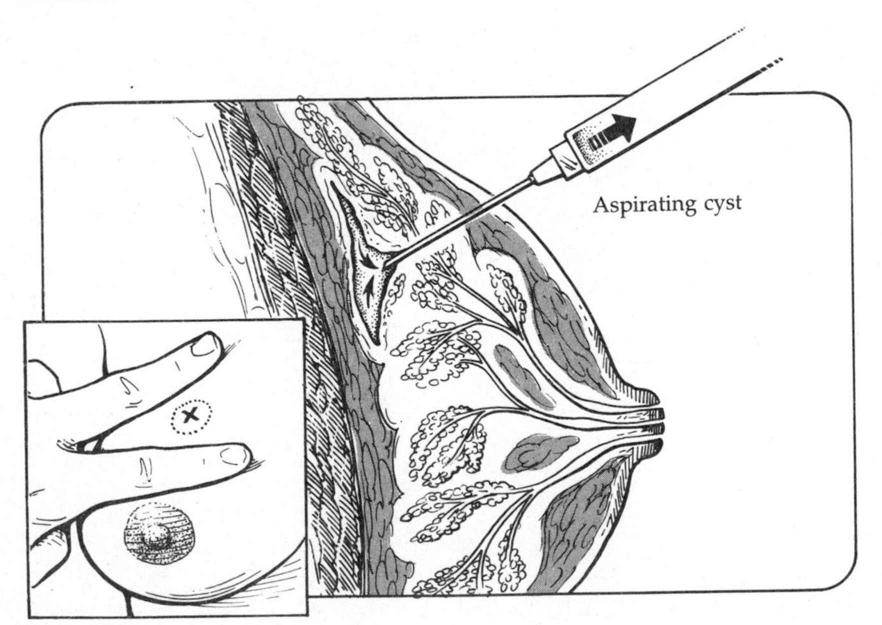

FIGURE 6-2

The fluid looks disgusting, but it's harmless. It can be almost any color, but usually it's green, brown, or yellow. Sometimes the fluid can even be milk—a breast-feeding woman can form a milk-filled cyst, called a galactocele, which is treated the way any other cyst is. There can be any amount of it—from a few drops to as much as a cup. One patient came to me with asymmetrical breasts; after I aspirated her cyst, her breasts were the same size.

Some doctors have the fluid analyzed in the lab, but I think it's pointless. The chances of getting a correct diagnosis from cyst fluid are very low, and false positives are common. The fluid's usually been around awhile and it's old, and its cells, though harmless, often seem weird when they're checked. The tests are virtually useless, and they're costly. Most specialists just throw the stuff down the sink.

Usually a woman will get only one or two cysts in her entire life. But some get many, and they get them often. If a patient had recurring multiple cysts, I would see her every three to six months, and aspirate as many as I could to keep the multiplication of cysts under control. If a malignant lump is forming, the cysts, harmless in themselves, can obscure it, and that, of course, is dangerous. When a woman has multiple cysts chances are she'll go on getting them until menopause—only rarely are they a one-time occurrence.

If cysts are harmless why do we bother to aspirate them? There are a number of reasons, but the most important one is that we need to be sure it is a cyst. You can't be sure a lump in the breast isn't cancer until you find out what it really is. Once we know it's a cyst, doctor and patient can both rest easy.

There are other ways of finding out you have a cyst—it may show up as an area of density on a routine mammogram, and then you can have an ultrasound test done to see whether it's a cyst or a solid lump. The ultrasound test works like radar. If you have a solid lump, the waves from the ultrasound will bounce back showing a brighter spot and there'll be a dark shadow behind it. If it is a cyst, however, the sound waves will go right through it and there won't be a shadow. (See Chapter 7 to read about mammograms and ultrasound techniques.)

If you've discovered a cyst through a mammogram and ultrasound and it doesn't worry you, don't bother having it aspirated—you already know it isn't cancer. Sometimes a cyst is painful, especially if it developed quickly. Aspirating the cyst will relieve the pain.

Cysts are almost never malignant. There's a 1 percent incidence of cancer in cysts, and it's a seldom dangerous cancer called intracystic papillary carcinoma (Fig. 6-3). It usually doesn't spread beyond the lining of the cyst, and unless there are specific signs that it might be present, it's not worth the risk of a biopsy. A biopsy is surgery, though minor, and it's better to avoid it when you can.

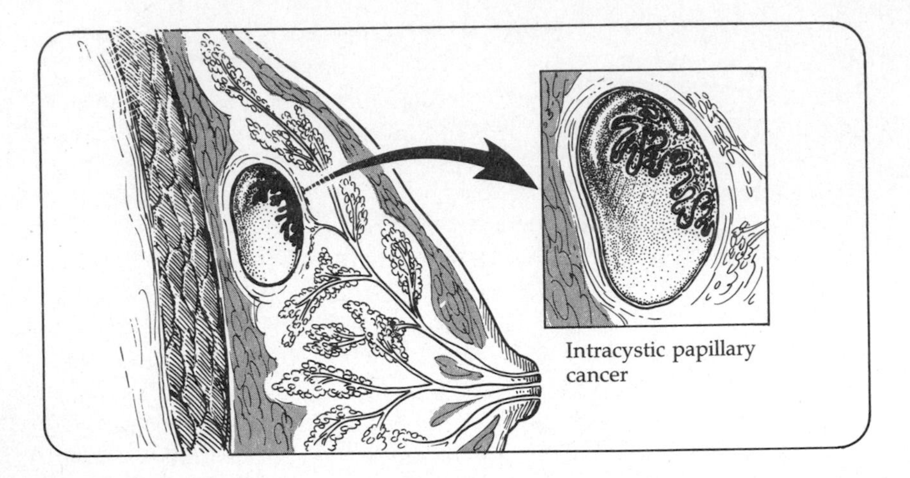

FIGURE 6-3

If there are signs that cancer might be present in the cyst, I'd operate on it—never otherwise, and only if the ultrasound looks suspicious.

Sometimes a doctor will aspirate a cyst and won't get any fluid. This isn't a cause for panic. It can happen for a number of reasons. The lump may not be a cyst after all, but a nonmalignant solid lump like those discussed below. Or the doctor may have missed the middle of the cyst. The doctor tries to get the cyst between her or his fingers and then puncture it, but it's easy to miss the middle, especially in a fairly small cyst. When this happened to me, I'd send the patient for ultrasound and let them aspirate it under direct vision. Operating on a cyst should only be a last resort.

Aspirating a cyst was once thought to be dangerous if someone had an unknown breast cancer, since the process of aspiration would spread the cancer over the needle's track. We now know that's completely untrue.[1] Any dominant lump should be aspirated before it's biopsied. It might be a cyst, and surgery can be avoided.

Cysts don't increase the risk of cancer. Only one study—by Dr. Cushman Haagensen of Columbia—suggests it does, and his evidence is slight.[2] Dr. David Page's research is a little better; he's found that there is a slight risk increase in women who have gross cysts and a first-degree relative—a mother or sister—with breast cancer. Most other research shows no relation between cysts and cancer.

The real risk is mental rather than physical. A woman with frequent cysts is likely to feel a lump and shrug it off as just another cyst—only to learn later that it was a malignant growth. Every lump should be checked out to be sure it isn't dangerous.

FIBROADENOMAS

Another common nonmalignant lump is the fibroadenoma. This is a smooth, round lump that feels the way most people think a cyst should feel—it's smooth and hard, like a marble dropped into the breast tissue (Fig. 6-4) where it can move around easily. It's often found near the nipple but can grow anywhere in the breast. It's also very distinct from the rest of the breast tissue. It can vary from a tiny 5 mm to a lemon-size 5 cm. The largest are called "giant fibroadenomas." A doctor can usually tell simply by feeling the lump that it's a fibroadenoma; if a needle aspiration is done and no fluid comes out, the doctor knows it isn't a cyst and is even more convinced it's a fibroadenoma. We can get a diagnosis by doing a core biopsy (see Chapter 8) and sending the tissue off to the lab just to make doubly sure. Fibroadenomas are usually distinct on a mammogram or ultrasound test (see Chapter 7). They are harmless in themselves and don't need to be removed as long as we're sure they're fibroadenomas. Most investigators believe that fibroadenomas usually grow over a 12-month period to a size of approximately 2–3 cm, after which they remain unchanged for several years.[3] Studies in which women were followed for up to 29 years found that the fibroadenoma shrunk or disappeared in 16–59 percent of all cases. They concluded that a fibroadenoma would probably disappear after five

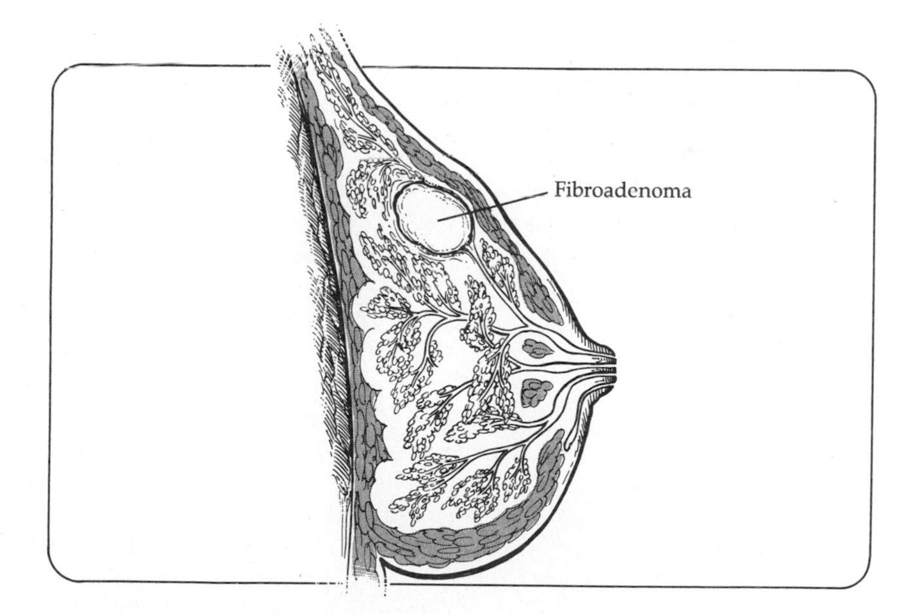

FIGURE 6-4

years in approximately 50 percent of cases and that in the others its lifetime is about 15 years.[4]

Since fibroadenomas develop at puberty, teenagers are more prone to have them and less likely to get breast cancer than are older women, so we might consider not removing fibroadenomas in teens. In older women we tend to remove all fibroadenomas to be sure they're not cancer.

Fibroadenomas are easy to remove, and the procedure can be done under local anesthetic. The surgeon simply makes a small incision, finds the lump, and takes it out (Fig. 6-5). (Some surgeons prefer to make a small incision around the nipple and then tunnel their way to the lump, to minimize scarring. I don't think this is a great idea, however; it's harder to find the lesion that way. If you cut over the fibroadenoma you're bound to get it, and the scarring doesn't usually remain noticeable in most patients.) If you feel nervous about your fibroadenomas, it's probably a good idea to get them removed for your own peace of mind; if there's no reason to get them removed and you don't want to, don't worry about it.

Since the last edition of this book, a third option has been developed, which should appeal to many women: a minimally invasive procedure in which the fibroadenoma is frozen in place under ultrasound guidance. It is almost painless because the cold is numbing, and it takes about a half hour in a doctor's office. Over about a year the fibroadenoma disappears.[5]

Gradually a woman has only one fibroadenoma; it's removed or treated, and she never gets any more. But some women get several over a lifetime—and a few women get many of them. One of my pa-

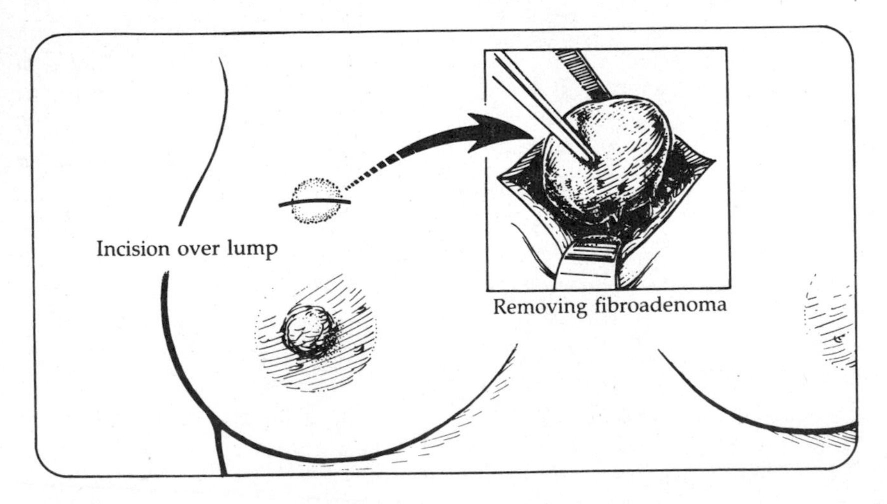

FIGURE 6-5

tients had a fibroadenoma in her left breast, and I removed it; she returned a couple of years later with another one on the exact same spot in her other breast—a kind of mirror image. Occasionally a woman will have multiple fibroadenomas at once. Once they are removed, more form. I had one woman with this problem and I must admit it is a difficult one. Obviously a surgeon can't keep removing them, but equally obviously a woman with this condition will be worried. One woman I talked to was told to have prophylactic mastectomies so the surgeon would not have to worry. This is pretty drastic for a benign condition that does not increase breast cancer risk. I'd generally recommend surgery only for the patient's needs, not for her doctor's peace of mind. A more sensible suggestion is to try danocrine (Danazol), a drug used for breast pain (see Chapter 4), which will put you into a reversible menopause. Stopping the hormonal stimulation of the breast should help control the fibroadenomas.

Fibroadenomas shouldn't be confused with fibroids, which by definition exist only in the uterus. There are similarities between the two conditions in that in both cases, one section of glandular tissue becomes autonomous, growing as a ball amid the rest of the tissue. But there's no other correlation—having one doesn't mean you're likely to get the other. In fact, they usually occur at different times in a woman's life: fibroids when you're heading toward menopause, fibroadenomas in your teens or early 20s.

However, fibroadenomas can occur at any age, up until menopause. As with cysts, you can get them after menopause if you're taking hormones that trick your body into thinking it's premenopausal. As we do more mammograms on "normal" women, we find more and more fibroadenomas in women in their 60s and 70s. Probably they've had them since their teens and simply, in those premammography days, didn't know about them. There are some very rare cancers that can look like fibroadenomas on a mammogram, so, in postmenopausal women, we usually do either a fine-needle aspiration, core biopsy, or, if those don't give us the information, an excisional biopsy (removal of the whole lump), just to make sure it is a fibroadenoma.

Ellen Mahoney, a breast surgeon friend of mine, says, "I tell people it has to come out if it bothers you, or if it grows—following this rule, I have never missed the occasional indolent cancer. One of my patients had three in the same quadrant. A baseline was done and repeated in six months—two had grown. All were removed and all were cancer. Following this rule too, I have diagnosed some of the 2–3 mm tumors sitting next to fibroadenomas and stimulating them. I think there are two types of fibroadenomas: hamartomas, which rarely grow larger than 2.5 cm (like the sponge toys in the gelatin capsules), and neoplasms, which may grow in response to a number of factors. I make sure I have a good measurement by ultrasound or by my little cloth tape measure, whichever is appropriate to the location."

There's also a rare cancer called cystosarcoma phylloides (see Chapter 19), which can occur in a fibroadenoma. It is found in about 1 percent of fibroadenomas, and those are usually giant fibroadenomas—lemon-size or larger. It's generally a relatively harmless cancer that doesn't tend to spread to other parts of the body. Some doctors will insist on removing all fibroadenomas on the theory that this cancer might be present. It's not a very sensible attitude, because of both the rarity and the lack of danger. Unless the lump is large, it's almost never going to be this cancer—and even if the cancer is present for a long time, it probably isn't going to kill you. When it's discovered, the surgeon simply has to remove the lump and it's gone.

Finally, fibroadenomas do not turn into cancer. Rarely a cancer will arise in a fibroadenoma, but it won't be missed as long as you check the size at diagnosis and at six months. If all is stable, size doesn't have to be checked again until there is a suspicion of change.

PSEUDOLUMPS

Studies have shown that pseudolumps are the most confusing to surgeons. If you line up patients with fibroadenomas, with cysts, and with breast cancers, and have surgeons who haven't been told which patient has which kind of lump examine them, usually the surgeons will agree in their diagnoses. Give them patients with pseudolumps, however, and you'll get all kinds of different diagnoses. These innocent areas of breast tissue cause no physical problems but all kinds of confusion.

"Pseudolump" is a descriptive term for an area of breast tissue that feels more prominent and persistent than usual. The surgeon checks it out and just can't be sure that it isn't another kind of lump.

If I thought a patient had a pseudolump, I'd usually see her at least twice, several months apart and at different parts of her cycle, just to make sure it wasn't normal lumpiness. Deciding what is or isn't a lump in these cases can be very subjective. Now that we have easier ways to make a diagnosis with a core biopsy, I would recommend that any lump which remains questionable be biopsied. (See Chapter 8.)

A pseudolump, then, is usually just exaggerated lumpiness. It's distinct and persistent enough, however, that we have to check to be certain that's all it is. It's usually what's meant when doctors say you have fibrocystic disease (see Chapter 4). Or a pseudolump can be caused by a rib pushing against breast tissue and causing it to feel hard and lumpy (Fig. 6-6). Sometimes women who had silicone injections years

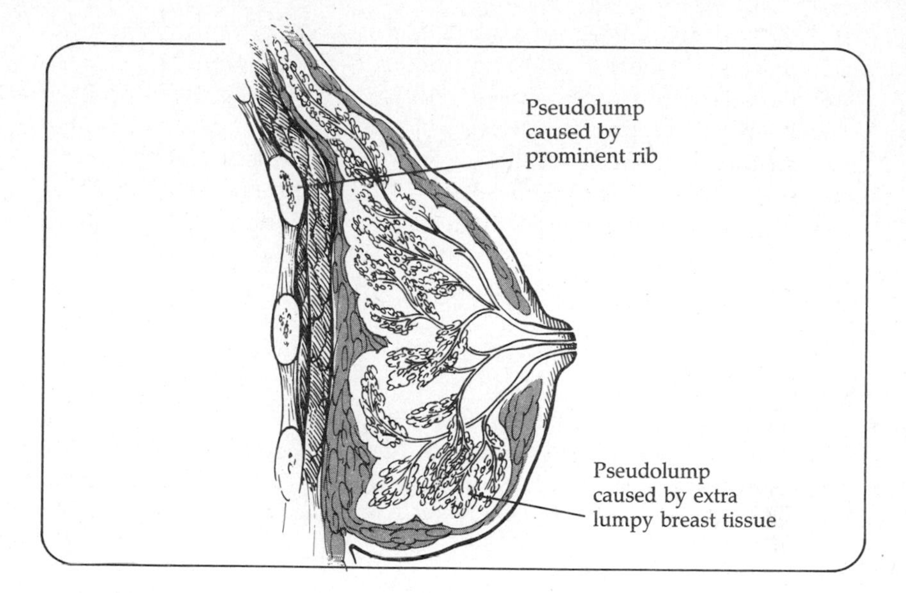

FIGURE 6-6

ago to enlarge one or both breasts (see Chapter 3) will get lumps that turn out to be hardened chunks of silicone. If you've had injections and get a lump, check with either a breast surgeon or a plastic surgeon (preferably one who's old enough to have worked with silicone injections when they were legal). Surgery on the breast can cause pseudolumps through hardened scar tissue. A pseudolump can also be caused by fat necrosis—dead fat—resulting from trauma due to a lumpectomy and radiation in the removal of an earlier, cancerous lump (see Chapter 23), or to breast reconstruction surgery (see Chapter 22). But in all these cases the best judge will be a breast surgeon who's done all the procedures.

CANCER

The fear of cancer is, of course, the main reason we worry about any of these lumps. When you get a cyst aspirated or a fibroadenoma or pseudolump biopsied, it's chiefly to make sure there is no cancer.

It's reasonable to be afraid of getting breast cancer and to check out any suspicious lump. But remember that a dominant lump doesn't mean you have cancer. In premenopausal women there are 12 benign lumps for every malignant one. The statistics change dramatically in postmenopausal women who aren't taking hormones, not because they get that much more cancer but because they no longer get the lumps that come with hormonal changes, cysts, and fibroadenomas. Yet even for postmenopausal women it's only a 50–50 chance that a lump is cancer. We'll consider malignant lumps in Chapter 16. The main thing to remember is to be cautious but not frantic. If you've got a lump, it may be cancer but it probably isn't. Get it checked out right away. If it's cancer, you can start working on it; if it isn't, you can stop worrying.

WHAT TO DO IF YOU THINK YOU HAVE A LUMP

If you have something that feels like it might be a lump, the first thing to do, obviously, is go to your doctor. Chances are that the doctor will check it out, tell you it's not a lump, and send you home. But a doctor who's a general practitioner or a gynecologist and hasn't spent years working on breasts might not be sure, and may send you to a breast surgeon for further examination. Often when you hear the word "surgeon" you get scared—sure that the doctor knows you've got something awful and that you will have to undergo major surgery.

Probably you won't. The doctor is simply, and sensibly, taking no chances, and sending you on to someone who has more experience with breast lumps and is thus better able to determine whether or not it's a true dominant lump. But sometimes even the surgeon can't be sure. In this case, depending on your age, the surgeon will probably send you for a mammogram and ultrasound to get additional information. The mammogram might show evidence of a real lump or a pseudolump. If it doesn't—if even the combination of an examination and a mammogram doesn't give the surgeon the necessary clarification—it's wise to do a biopsy to find out what it is. In the past we were afraid of unnecessary surgery and didn't want to biopsy these "gray area" lumps. Now with the minimally invasive core biopsy we can easily get an answer without surgery.

It's important to stress one thing: if you're certain that something is wrong with your breast, get it biopsied, whatever the doctor's diagnosis. Often a woman is sure she has a lump, the doctor is sure she doesn't, and a year or two later a lump shows up on her mammogram. She believes the doctor was careless. Usually that's not the case. A cancer that shows on a mammogram probably wasn't a lump two years earlier, or it would be a huge lump at that point. It's likely that the patient—who, after all, experiences her breast from both inside and outside, while the doctor can only experience the patient's breast from outside—has sensed something wrong and interpreted that in terms of the concept most familiar to her, a lump. I'm convinced that this is the basis of many of the malpractice suits that arise when a doctor "fails" to detect what later proves to be cancer. If you really feel something is wrong in your breast, insist on a biopsy. If you're wrong, you'll put your mind at rest—and if you're right, you may just save your own life. It's a minor procedure with low risks and potentially high gains.

PART THREE

Diagnosis of Breast Problems

7

Diagnostic Imaging: Mammography, Ultrasound, MRI, and Other Techniques

Although mammography is most commonly thought of in relation to cancer, it's actually a diagnostic tool for a variety of breast problems. It shares this capacity with a number of other imaging techniques. ("Imaging" means ways of seeing body tissue.) For example, a woman with localized breast pain might have a mammogram to see if she has a cyst. A woman with an abscess might need an ultrasound to delineate its extent. A woman with nipple discharge might have a ductogram (type of mammogram; see Chapter 5) to find the lesion and plan surgery. Both magnetic resonance imaging (MRI) and ultrasound are being used to determine whether silicone implants have leaked.

In this chapter we'll look at diagnostic mammography and other commonly used diagnostic tools. Later, in Chapter 14, we will talk about the use of mammography as a method of screening for breast cancer. (The same equipment is used for screening and diagnostic mammography, but different types of pictures may be taken.)

A mammogram is an X ray of the breast—"mammo" means breast and "gram" means picture. It isn't the same as a chest X ray, which looks through the breast and photographs the lungs. Mammograms look at the breast itself and take pictures of the soft tissue, allowing the radiologist to see anything unusual or suspicious. Mammography can pick up very small lesions—about 0.5 cm (or 0.2 inch), whereas you usually can't feel a lump until it's at least a centimeter (0.4 inch). These lesions can be benign or malignant. In addition, mammograms can sometimes pick up precancers (see Chapter 12).

Mammography has its limits, though. The mammogram can take a picture of only the part of the breast that sticks out—the plates are put underneath the breast or on the sides of the breast—so it's easier to get an accurate picture of a large breast than of a small one. The periphery of the breast does not get into the picture at all (Fig. 7-1). In addition, if your breasts are dense, the lump may not be visible through the tissue. So a mammogram isn't perfect. Physical exams and mammograms complement each other. You can see some lumps on a mammogram that you can't feel, and you can feel some lumps (palpation) that you can't see on an X ray.

You get a diagnostic mammogram when you find a lump or have another breast complaint and your doctor wants to get a better sense of what the problem is. If, for example, you have lumpy breasts and there's one area that may be a dominant lump, your doctor may send you for a mammogram. If a lump looks jagged, not smooth, on the mammogram, it's a sign that further investigation may be called for. If you've got a lump your doctor thinks may be cancerous, a mammogram can help determine if there are other lumps that should be biopsied at the same time; it can also document the location of the lump.

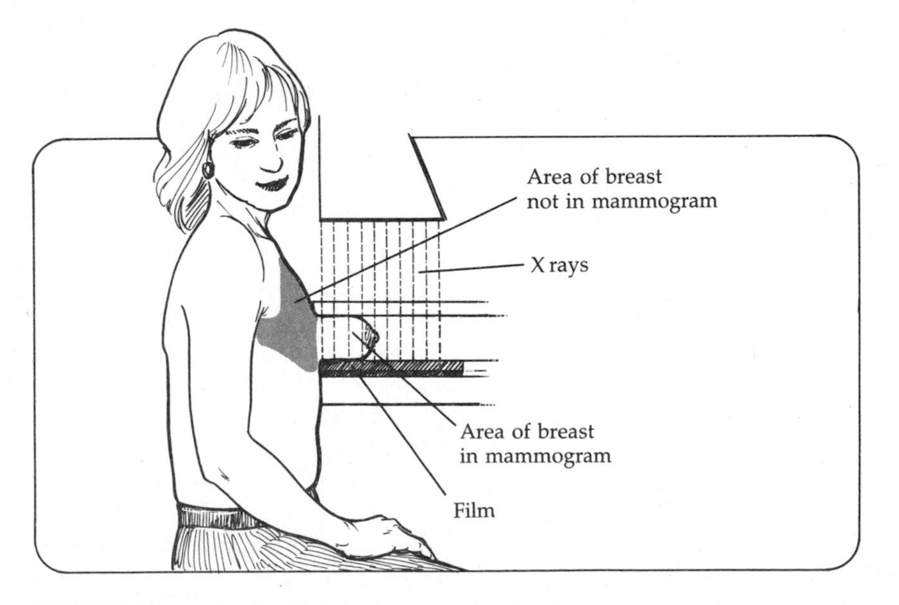

FIGURE 7-1

MAMMOGRAMS

What Mammograms Show

A mammogram, like any other X ray, presents a two-dimensional view of a three-dimensional structure. Denser areas appear brighter. Breast tissue, for example, is very dense, and shows up white on the mammogram. Fat, which is not very dense at all, shows up gray (see photographs on pages 100–101).

As you'll recall from the discussion in Chapter 1, when you're young—in your teens and early 20s—your breasts are made up mostly of breast tissue and are very dense. As you grow older, the breast ages, much as your skin does, and there's less breast tissue and more fat. When you're in your 30s and 40s, it's about half and half. (This varies with your weight; if you're very heavy it's more likely there'll be a lot more fat; if you're thinner, there'll be more breast tissue.) Once you're in menopause, the breast tissue will often go away, leaving behind only a few strands. However, women vary in the proportion of breast tissue remaining after menopause. And if they take hormone replacement therapy (see Chapter 9), their tissue may remain as dense as it was or even become more dense.

How does this affect the reading of a mammogram? Cancer and benign lumps are the same density as breast tissue. So if you've got a white lump in the middle of an area of dense tissue, it won't show up on the mammogram—the tissue will hide it. It's like looking for a polar bear in the snow. But if the same lump is sitting in the middle of fat, it'll be very obvious—a white spot in the midst of gray: a polar bear in the sea. So mammography is more accurate in older women, who have more fat, than in younger women, who have more breast tissue. Sometimes I'd get a patient who'd had a mammogram and was told that her breasts were so dense that mammography wasn't useful to her. That's ridiculous—what it means is that mammography wasn't as useful to her now as it would have been if she had fatty breasts. Typically this happened with women around 30—when breasts should be dense. There's a 9 to 20 percent chance that something could be missed—but there's also an 80 to 90 percent chance of picking up something.This isn't to say I'm recommending screening mammograms for women at 30, but that a diagnostic mammogram may have some value if there is a breast problem that needs to be explored.

When mammograms show something round and smooth, it's likely to be a cyst or a fibroadenoma (see Chapter 6). The mammogram can't distinguish between these; you'd follow up with an ultrasound (discussed later in this chapter) to see if it's a cyst. If a mammogram shows jagged, distinct, radiating strands pulling inward, it's more likely to be

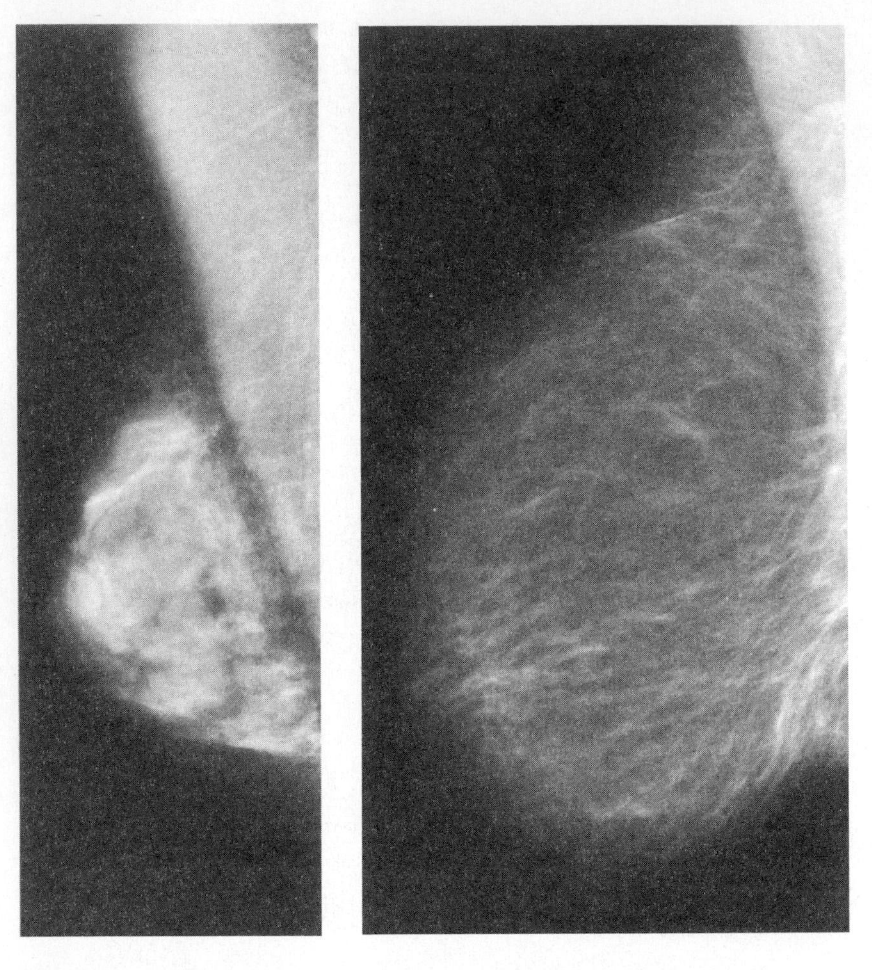

Dense breast in young woman

Fatty breast in older woman

cancer. But until it is biopsied, we can't tell for sure. Several benign conditions can mimic cancer on a mammogram. Scarring or fat necrosis (dead fat) will look very suspicious. A noncancerous entity called a *radial scar* is caused by an increase in local fibrous tissue (see Chapter 1) trapping some of the glands in a way that can look suspicious. It can be confusing even under the microscope and often requires an expert breast pathologist to be sure it is not cancer.

A mammogram may also show intramammary (in the breast) lymph nodes. In fact, until the mammogram came along, we didn't know that lymph nodes are found in the breast. We now know that 5.4 percent of women have them. Sometimes you'll hear about a "normal"

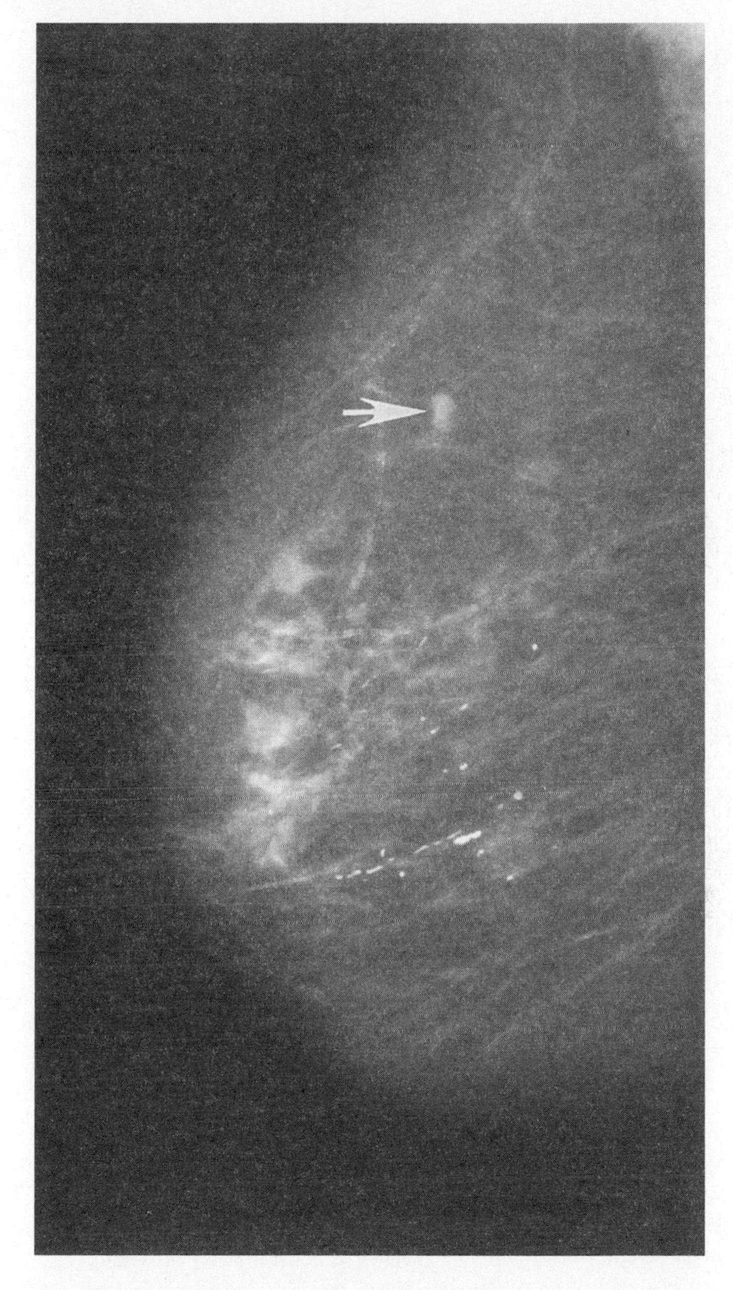

Small cancer in fatty breast (*arrow*) and benign calcifications

mammogram. But there's really no one pattern you can call normal, since there's no "normal" breast.

In mammography reports, some radiologists use words loosely—as if they can see what the pathology is when they're looking at the shadows on the mammogram. So they'll tell you you've got "cystic changes," which is a variation of our old nemesis fibrocystic disease. All that means is that you've got dense breast tissue. Or they'll tell you you've got "mammary dysplasia," which sounds very serious and means you've got abnormal cells en route to cancer. But the cells aren't visible on the mammogram—only a biopsy can show cells. What they really mean is, once again, you've got dense tissue in your breasts. All a radiologist can tell you is how much breast tissue there is and how much fat tissue, and whether there are abnormal areas of density. It is for these reasons that a standardized reporting system for mammography was developed and is now used by most radiologists who interpret mammograms. This is called the breast imaging reporting and data system (BI-RADS; see Table 7.1). It is important that the radiologist who interprets your mammogram uses BI-RADS for the report so your doctor won't be confused by the report findings.

Just as 20 percent of women have some degree of variation in the size of their breasts, breasts vary on the inside as well. It will appear on the report as "asymmetry," and it probably doesn't mean anything. Rarely an asymmetry can be caused by cancer, so you might want to get a second mammogram several months later, just to make sure: if it's cancer, it's likely to have changed somewhat during that time. In some cases the radiologist may recommend additional views or an ultrasound. One of the most absurd cases I've come across is that of a patient who'd had a mastectomy on one side, with a reconstruction. She came to me because the report on the mammogram said it showed "marked asymmetry." Of course it did! The breasts were completely different in their composition; they were meant to look the same on the outside, not the inside.

Types of Mammograms

Though early mammography in the 1950s produced a fair amount of radiation, over the years X ray techniques have been refined so that now very little radiation is actually used. It's commonly said that a mammogram exposes you to the same amount of radiation you'd get in a plane flying over Denver. One radiologist I used to work with in Boston explained it in more colorful terms: the amount of radiation of one mammogram is equal to the amount of radiation you would get by walking on the beach nude for 10 minutes or until you got caught.[1]

Table 7-1. Breast Imaging-Reporting and Data System (BI-RADS)

Category	*Assessment*	*Description, Recommendation*
1	Negative	There is nothing to comment on: routine screening
2	Benign	A definite benign finding
3	Probably benign	Findings that have a high probability of being benign (<2%)
4	Suspicious abnormality	Not characteristic of breast cancer but has a reasonable probability of being malignant
5	Highly suggestive of malignancy	Lesion that has a high probability of being malignant (95%)
6	Known biopsy proven malignancy	Lesions known to be malignant that are being imaged prior to definitive therapy

Film-screen mammography, the conventional type of mammography, gives a precise definition of what the tissue looks like. It can be a bit uncomfortable because the breasts have to be squeezed between the plates to get an accurate picture. The slight discomfort is well worth the increased accuracy and low radiation. A 1993 study tried letting women control the compression themselves. Not surprisingly, they ended up with the same amount of compression, equally good quality films, and fewer complaints.[2]

A relatively new technique is the digital mammogram. Like a digital camera, digital mammography is a way of computerizing the image so it can be viewed on a computer monitor screen and can also be printed out like conventional mammograms. Because it's a computerized rather than a photographic technique, the radiologist can magnify different areas to focus on what she or he wants to see. Just as you can play with digital photos on your computer and remove Uncle Jack, on a digital mammogram all the fat can be blocked out so only breast tissue shows up, or it could erase the breast tissue so that only fat shows up. A recent study has shown that it does this successfully. In a paired comparison of digital and regular screen-film mammograms the same number of cancers were found. But with the digital technique, fewer additional films were needed to sort out an abnormal shadow before a biopsy was recommended. The technique allowed the radiologists to manipulate the images and figure out if what they were seeing was real, whereas the screen-film had to be repeated in a different view to accomplish the same thing.[3,4] Though the hope has been that this technique will be more sensitive and accurate than film-screen mammograms, so far this has not happened; however, a very large multicenter prospective study comparing the two techniques is due out in 2005 and it should help answer the question definitively.

Another highly touted promise for digital mammography was computerized reading of mammograms (computer-aided-detection or CAD). A computer pre-screens mammograms and points out the worrisome areas so that the mammographers can examine them more carefully. It was hoped that this would make reading more accurate, as computers don't get easily distracted or blink at the wrong moment. In one study it did help find more cancers; unfortunately, this benefit did not seem to translate to the real world when tested in a large clinical practice.[5,6]

At this point, we've gotten almost as far as we can with mammography. Each advance is incremental. We can hope for other imaging techniques to be developed in the future.

Calcifications

One of the more important discoveries from the study of mammograms is that cancer is often associated with some very fine specks of calcium that appear on the picture—they look a bit like tiny pieces of dust on a film.

We discovered that these microcalcifications, as we called them, were sometimes an indication of cancer or precancer (see Chapter 12). So the radiologist will always mention in a report any microcalcifications that show up. But it's nothing to panic about—80 percent of microcalcifications have nothing to do with cancer; they're probably just the result of normal wear and tear on your breast.[7] Ironically, when you age, calcium leaves your bones, where it's needed, and shows up in other places, where it's not. It can show up in arteries, causing them to harden, and in joints, causing arthritis. The microcalcifications in your breast won't cause any problems if they're not indications of cancer or precancer. (The appearance of this calcium in your body has no relation to how much calcium you eat or drink, by the way.)

How can we tell which are the bad and which are the harmless kinds of calcifications? We look at the shape, the size, and how many there are. If they're tiny and tightly clustered, and there aren't a whole lot of them, they're more likely to be precancer. If they're all over the place they're more likely to be benign.

Precancer occurs in the duct, which is very small. For the calcifications to fit in a duct, they have to be very tightly clustered and very small. The big chunks of calcium we see on the mammogram couldn't possibly fit in the ductal system, so we know they're benign. They're usually old fibroadenomas that you had as a teenager, which have faded and become soft and less dense and now are calcifying. Sometimes they're calcifications in a blood vessel that's getting older and harder.

There's a middle group of calcifications that are less easy to characterize. They may be new, but there are just one or two of them. In that situation, we'll usually repeat the mammogram in six months.[8] If it's precancer, we might see more calcifications, or a change in the shape or size, whereas if there's no change, it's more likely to be benign. Patients get nervous about that; if it's cancer and we wait six months, won't it grow and kill you? But in fact, if we wait six months it's probably because we don't think it's cancer. And even in the worst-case scenario, it's precancer, not cancer, and precancer takes 10 years to develop into cancer. So six months won't make any difference, and the wait prevents needless biopsies.

It's true that some precancerous calcifications don't grow or change, so they don't get picked up on the second mammogram. But that's because they aren't growing and thus aren't becoming cancer.

Any time doctors are worried about calcifications they can of course proceed to a biopsy. This can be a core biopsy or an open biopsy, depending on the available facilities (see Chapter 8).

Mammographic Workup

Screening is for asymptomatic women. In contrast, diagnostic mammography involves the workup of a lump felt by a woman or her doctor or of an abnormal finding on a screening mammogram.

One way to do this workup is to do a compression spot view. We do this when there is a dense area on the original mammogram that we're unsure of. It's an extra view on the mammogram; the radiologic technologist uses a small plate to press right over the abnormal area and takes a picture of that area. Since a mammogram is a two-dimensional picture of a three-dimensional structure, we see overlapping shapes. (It's as if you had a transparent balloon with different pictures on each side. If you took a photo from the front, it would look like one complex image. If you looked at each picture on the balloon from a different direction you'd see them as separate.) The technologist may also press on your breast at an angle and change it so that things aren't perfectly juxtaposed.

If there is an abnormal density on mammogram or a lump that can be felt but isn't visible on a mammogram, you may be sent to get an ultrasound.

If you have a palpable lump, the technologist should put a marker on your breast to be sure that the lump is on the film. If it is at the periphery of the breast it may be necessary to take special mammographic views to get it in the picture—like changing the angle of your camera to make sure Aunt Mabel's head doesn't get cut off in the photo. This is especially important for lumps that are near the armpit or in the lower fold of the breast.

If calcifications are present, we often do a magnification view, which is a mammogram that magnifies the area of the breast with the calcifications, so we can see them and characterize them better. So, for the most part, if you're told that the calcifications on your mammogram are worrisome, you should make sure they do a magnified view to see if the calcifications still look bad and how many there are. This is sometimes not necessary with digital mammograms. Sometimes mammographers will want to skip this step and send you for a biopsy. Don't let them. Why subject yourself to surgery if it may not be necessary?

Problems can arise when radiologists don't have enough experience reading mammograms (see quality of mammograms section below). How familiar your radiologist is with the procedure may determine how well the X ray is read. A more experienced mammographer may be willing to state the opinion that something is almost certainly benign. A radiologist anxious about missing something will be more likely to say, "I don't think it's cancer, but it could be, and a biopsy is recommended to be absolutely sure." As a result of these kinds of readings, we're doing more biopsies than ever on benign lumps.

For this reason it's very important, if you're told you need a biopsy for an abnormal mammogram, that you get a second opinion. Take your mammogram to another center—preferably a place that specializes in mammography—and have them review it. Studies show that 60 to 70 percent of biopsies done for abnormal mammograms could be avoided if the mammogram were reviewed by an expert.

A mammogram can't tell for certain what you have. But there are some situations in which the view from the mammogram shows signs that clearly suggest a diagnosis. It's a bit like seeing someone from the back. You don't know for sure that it's your friend Mary until she turns around and faces you, but if it's Mary's shade of red hair, arranged in the kind of ponytail Mary always wears, and she walks like Mary does and carries the kind of large briefcase Mary likes to carry, you can make a pretty good guess that it's Mary. How often you are right will of course depend on how well you know Mary. An experienced mammographer is better able to diagnose breast problems than an inexperienced one.

A typical story in my practice was that of a patient in her early 60s who came to my office after her first mammogram and told me they had found something strange. I looked at the X rays and saw a little asymmetry, so I sent her back for a compression spot mammogram—and the asymmetry completely disappeared. Because the radiologist didn't take it the next step, the patient had been needlessly scared.

In another common scenario a woman would tell me something strange had appeared on her mammogram. I would look at the X rays and see a small and smooth lump, like a fibroadenoma, but it would be new. The radiologist had written, "possible fibroadenoma; cancer can't be ruled out." I could have done one of two things. I could have waited six months and checked it out again; if it was cancer, it probably would have grown. If she was really anxious, I could have done a core biopsy under X ray or ultrasound guidance. If it wasn't cancer, that was fine; if it was, we could plan for the cancer surgery. If a diagnosis couldn't be made this way, we could do a wire localization biopsy. (We'll examine these forms of biopsy further in Chapter 8.)

QUALITY OF MAMMOGRAMS

Today all mammography units must be accredited by an FDA-approved body (certified by the FDA as meeting the standards) and must prominently display the certificate issued by the agency. The initial quality standards for mammography facilities to meet FDA certification went into effect in December 1994. They include the following: radiologic technologists who perform mammography, physicians who interpret mammograms, and medical physicists who survey equipment must all have adequate training and experience; each facility must have a system for following up on mammograms that reveal problems and for obtaining biopsy results. In 1996 the FDA along with the National Mammography Quality Assurance Advisory Committee developed additional and more comprehensive final standards, including (1) a consumer complaint mechanism to provide women with a process for addressing their concerns about mammography facilities; (2) special techniques and personnel qualifications related to mammography of women with breast implants; (3) communication of mammography results to referring physicians and *all examinees (that means you)* in writing; and (4) additional clinical image review and examinee notification requirements when a facility's images are determined to be substandard. In addition, there is standardized reading of mammograms, the BI-RADS system (mentioned above), whereby all mammograms are classified according to six categories (see Table 7-1).

Mammography now is the one place where we really do have quality control—something we have little of in the rest of breast care, and indeed in much of medicine.

Procedure

What actually happens on the day you have a mammogram? Preparations start before you leave the house. Don't use talcum powder or deodorant (except for those without aluminum, such as Tom's) the day you're scheduled for a mammogram—flecks of talcum can show up as calcifications on the mammogram. Avoid lotions that can make the breast slippery. Some instructions will tell you not to consume caffeine for two weeks before the X ray; unless you have experienced some problem with caffeine, ignore them.

The atmosphere you face when you get there will vary from one mammography facility to another. Some are cold and clinical; others provide a warm ambience and reassuring, friendly personnel. But the actual procedure is pretty standard. You have to undress from the waist up, and you're usually given some kind of hospital gown. You'll probably be x-rayed standing up. The technologist—usually, but not always, a woman—will have you lean over a metal plate and help you place your breast on the plate. It can be cold and a bit uncomfortable, and when the plates press your breast together, it can be somewhat unpleasant. Two pictures of each breast are usually taken, one from the side, the other vertical. But 20 percent of the time it will be necessary to take additional views or do special magnification or spot pictures. This isn't a sign that you have cancer—it just means that the mammography technologists and radiologists are being painstakingly careful to get accurate pictures. In addition, the way the technologist takes the X rays is important. The tighter your breasts are squeezed, the more accurate the picture is.

The process really isn't all that painful. One researcher did a multicenter study interviewing people right after their mammograms, asking how painful the process was and what point they were at in their menstrual cycle.[9] He was pleased that 88 percent of the women reported no pain or discomfort, and was surprised to learn that their cycle didn't seem to have any effect on their comfort level.

There's a small percentage of women whose breasts are unusually sensitive, and for them a mammogram can be painful. In this study none of the women who reported that the procedure was painful felt that it would stop them from having another mammogram exam. It's unfortunate that it's not painless, but I think it's well worth the slight—and brief—discomfort. At UCLA we actually timed the technologists, and we found that compression lasted at most 10 seconds. It doesn't leave bruises or tender spots when it's over.

Women with disabilities may have difficulty getting a clear mammogram, particularly if they're unable to stand up. Fortunately a good technologist can do a mammogram allowing a woman to sit for the procedure.

The whole process lasts only a few minutes; when it's done, you have to wait for a while till the pictures are developed, so you might want to bring along a book or an iPod. A digital mammogram is faster, since films do not have to be developed and the technologist can check the mammograms on a computer screen a few seconds after they are taken. The radiologist (an M.D., not the technologist) who looks at the pictures will sometimes see something on the periphery that isn't completely clear and will want to take another picture, focusing on that area. Or she or he will want a magnification view. If you are having a diagnostic mammogram the radiologist will usually discuss the results with you immediately following the examination. In some places, the radiologist will also come out and tell you what the *screening* mammogram shows. In other high-volume settings the radiologists will read the screening mammograms later in the day when they can focus and not be interrupted. Then the results are sent by mail and you have to wait several days to a week to get them. Since studies have shown that centers which do a high volume of mammograms and read them later often have more accurate interpretations, this is not unreasonable.

Please don't ask your technologist to interpret the mammogram for you. Technologists aren't doctors: their job is taking the pictures, not reading them.

Although, as I have often been quoted as saying, mammography must have been invented by a man (and there should be an equally fun test for men), it is the best tool we currently have. We have to be careful, regarding the risks and benefits of screening (see Chapter 14), not to throw the baby out with the bath water. It's an imperfect tool but, particularly for women with confusing breast problems, it's an important one.

Limitations of Mammography

Frustration with the limitations of mammography has led to a search for other ways of looking at the breast. Mammography uses radiation, which is potentially dangerous, and it is limited in its ability to see through dense breast tissue and determine clearly whether a lump is benign or malignant. These issues are especially important for young, high-risk women. Some of the techniques we've looked at are old, and some are new. The amount of promise varies significantly with each technique. So far none of these techniques promises to do away with mammography. Most are being proposed as an adjunct to mammography either to help figure out which suspicious lesions on mammogram are really worrisome to image-dense breasts or to determine which young woman might benefit from a mammogram.

ULTRASOUND

In the ultrasound method, high-frequency sound waves are sent off in little pulses, like radar, toward the breast. A gel is put on the breast to make it slippery, and a small transducer (a device that picks up sound waves) is slid along the skin, sending waves through it. If something gets in the way of the waves, they bounce back again, and if nothing gets in the way, they pass through the breast. It never picks out the small details, as an X ray can, but it can show other characteristics of a lump. Ultrasound is appealing because it doesn't use radiation. It is most effective in the dense breast, where mammography is limited. But ultrasound is limited in the fatty breast, where mammography is very effective.

This technique is used mostly for looking at a specific area; if we know a lump is there, we can use ultrasound to get more information about it. It can help determine whether a lump is fluid-filled or solid—if it's fluid-filled, like a cyst, the sound waves go through it, and if it's solid, like a fibroadenoma, pseudolump, or cancerous lump, the sound waves will bounce back. So if a lump shows up on a mammogram that we can't feel in a physical examination, and we want to determine whether it's a cyst or a solid lump, ultrasound can give us the answer.

Ultrasound can also be quite useful in helping us interpret a mammogram. If the doctor feels a lump and the mammogram shows just dense breast tissue, the ultrasound can sometimes see if there's a lump within the dense breast tissue. Mammography will only show overlapping areas of brightness, but ultrasound can sometimes distinguish differences in the density of the tissues causing the shadows. Remember the image of the transparent balloon mentioned earlier? Now imagine that the balloon has a few colored balls inside it. An ultrasound can distinguish the balls inside, which are different from the balloon itself. Ultrasound adds another dimension to the imaging possible with mammography. Most cancer centers, therefore, if there is a suspicious area on a mammogram, will also do an ultrasound.

Because, as far as we know, sound waves are harmless, ultrasound is often the best tool for studying benign problems at length, particularly in women under 35. So if a doctor has a younger patient who has a lump and wants to determine if it's likely to be a fibroadenoma or just dense breast tissue, ultrasound in that area can differentiate between a distinct lesion with edges or a mixed area without any definite lumps.

A limitation of ultrasound is that it depends, more than mammography does, on the experience of the person operating the equipment. Unlike mammography, which shows the whole breast on each picture, each ultrasound picture shows only a small section of the breast.

Therefore the technologist or physician who operates the ultrasound equipment must be able to first find the abnormality and then demonstrate it well on the pictures he or she takes. The technologist or physician holds the transducer directly over the suspicious area, and the angle at which it is held changes the image. Looking at the photograph of the image at another time can be difficult. The technologist or physician needs to be standing at the patient's side looking at the screen while performing the examination and taking the pictures. It may be hard for the physician to pick up an ultrasound picture after the fact and then interpret it accurately.

Since ultrasound produces no radiation and has the capacity to tell a cyst from solid tissue, why don't we just use it and not mammography? In a recent study of whole breast ultrasound, 37 additional cancers were found with ultrasound in 13,547 women with dense breasts and normal mammograms. Before you get too excited, consider that in women with dense breasts ultrasound found something not found on mammogram 0.27 percent of the time.[10,11] One problem is that it is not easy to ultrasound the whole breast accurately. There are a few ultrasonographers who are doing it, but it takes a lot of time, patience, and experience. It shows so many changes in contour and density that it becomes very difficult to differentiate normal breast tissue from abnormalities. Also, microcalcifications or other signs visible on a mammogram may not be identifiable on an ultrasound. In order to find out whether it is worthwhile, a large multicenter trial has been launched looking at the supplemental benefit that ultrasound combined with mammography might have in high-risk women with dense breasts. It will be interesting to see what they find, but the real question will be how it compares to mammography. The best use of ultrasound is for investigating one lump or area that has already been detected by physical exam or mammography.

We can also use ultrasound in much the same way we use mammograms to guide needle biopsies (see Chapter 8).[12] Sometimes ultrasound is a more effective tool for guiding us into the lump than mammography. Physicians experienced in breast ultrasound can approach the lump from different directions, which can make it easier to biopsy hard-to-reach areas in the breast, and many find the ultrasound method faster and more comfortable for the patient.

Ultrasound has also been used to look at women with silicone implants to decide whether the implant has ruptured or leaked. With a highly skilled technologist and radiologist, it's very accurate for that purpose.[13]

Just as digital mammography is attempting to make mammography clearer, there are many scientists working on improving the resolution of ultrasound. Three-dimensional ultrasound with even better resolution will be more useful in the diagnosis of breast problems, especially in young women with dense breasts. Color Doppler ultrasound and power Doppler ultrasound are used to show the increased blood vessels associated with a mass. Cancers often have an increase in blood supply, but so do some benign lesions. One study compared the color Doppler images with later examinations of the tumors under the microscope. They found that increased blood flow shown on the color Doppler ultrasound correlated with the size of the tumor and the number of involved lymph nodes but did not correlate with the tiny new blood vessels in the tumor (microvessel density). In other words, color Doppler ultrasound is better at picking up bigger blood vessels than at showing the very new ones that we think are important at predicting the behavior of tumors.[14]

Whether these new and improved ultrasound technologies will finally prove to be useful for detecting more abnormalities or in making diagnostic decisions will depend on clinical research studies. Meanwhile, ultrasound continues to be an important diagnostic tool for breast cancer diagnosis.

MRI

Magnetic resonance imaging (MRI) takes advantage of the electromagnetic qualities of the hydrogen nucleus. Hydrogen is part of water, and water is part of our bodies. MRI is a huge magnet. You are put in the middle of the magnet, and the hydrogen nucleus lines up with the magnetic field. Then the MRI technologist turns on a radio frequency wave to tip the hydrogen nucleus off the new magnetic axis. When the radio frequency wave is turned off, the hydrogen realigns with the strong magnetic field. The way the hydrogen realigns with the field allows the MRI machine to make an image of the tissues.

This test was initially used in the brain, and has been very accurate in diagnosing brain tumors. It's finally taking its place in breast diagnosis. It is now recognized as the most sensitive and specific way to evaluate whether a silicone breast implant has leaked. It is also gaining acceptance as a technique that can identify breast cancer and further define abnormalities identified on mammography or ultrasound.

A silicone-specific technique has been developed to differentiate rupture of the capsule from other benign breast problems. This has been accurate in experienced hands. Detection of invasive breast cancer is not quite as good.

Most of the studies on MRI and breast cancer are done with contrast material (a dye) that is injected into the woman's veins. This material is picked up rapidly by areas with lots of blood vessels and therefore by cancers. Unfortunately a few cancers are slow growing and do not have increased blood vessels, and a large number of benign conditions also have an increased number of blood vessels. MRI also does not pick up many precancers that show up on mammograms as calcifications. Results that appear to be cancers but are actually benign are called false positives, while the cancers that are missed are false negatives. MRI's problem is many false positives. It is sometimes used preoperatively to determine the extent of a tumor and the advisability of breast conservation techniques. As I mentioned in Chapter 6, this may not be wise since it often leads to extra biopsies and sometimes even mastectomies for benign disease. Its best potential use seems to be as an additional screening test in women who carry mutations in BRCA 1 or BRCA 2 (see Chapter 10). Studies on these high-risk women have shown that MRI can find cancers missed by mammography and ultrasound.[15] Since the chance of cancer is high for a woman who has a mutation in BRCA1/2, this makes sense. If we used MRI in addition to mammography on all women, aside from the expense, we would be doing many unnecessary biopsies and finding few cancers.

The MRI exam is done with the patient lying face down on a table with her breasts hanging into the machine. To get good results, the woman should have an injection of contrast material that is picked up by lesions and not by normal tissue. We do this by injecting a dye called gadolinium intravenously before the procedure. Though this improves the accuracy of the MRI, it is not foolproof; it often lights up with a fibroadenoma and other benign conditions, and it misses some cancers.

MRI is not going to replace mammography, at least at this stage. It's not as good a screening test—it's too expensive; it's too hard to do; and it is not yet accurate enough. Nonetheless much research is going on to determine the exact role MRI can have in the detection and diagnosis of breast cancer. I predict we will see more of it in the future.

PET SCANNING

Positron emission tomography (PET) is another technique that has received a lot of press. Other techniques create pictures, but PET is a completely different way of imaging breast tissue. We don't look at the structure itself, but at the activity going on in it. All tissues need glucose as fuel to survive. Cancers are rapidly growing and turning over, so they use more glucose than normal tissue. PET scanning looks at how much and how fast glucose is being used by a tissue. Like MRI, PET was first developed to study the brain, and it has been very useful for that.

To do this scan we give the patient a radioactively labeled glucose molecule, which is taken up and metabolized by the tissue. The scanner can demonstrate how much and how fast glucose is taken up by the tissues. When imaging the brain with the PET scan, we can have the patient do a number of things that use different parts of the brain. If the patient talks, the scan lights up in the area of the brain that connects for talking; if the patient reads, it lights up another area. So it's very useful in mapping the brain and seeing where different problems lie.

Potentially PET scanning could be the answer to detecting virtually any cancer, since it can examine the whole body. Cancers are faster growing and use more glucose than normal tissues, so they should light up better. PET scans have been able to demonstrate areas of metastatic disease that cannot be seen by other imaging techniques. The major question is how small a cancer it can pick up—how sensitive it really is. If it could pick up micrometastatic disease, it would be very helpful. At this stage in its development, it does not show the area involved very clearly and therefore is not good for finding a cancer and helping us know where to biopsy. As with MRI, we are still in the process of determining its usefulness. It may have a role in distinguishing benign lumps from malignant ones based on how much glucose they use.

Another thing we're looking at with PET scanning is whether it can be used to find the spread of breast cancer in women with locally advanced disease (see Chapter 27).[16] One of the biggest drawbacks to the PET scan is that it is very expensive and can be found only in selected centers. Researchers are trying to develop a PET scanner that would work only on the breast and therefore would be easier to buy and operate as well as be less expensive.

MIBI SCAN

MIBI scan (Sesta MIBI scan) is a nuclear medicine scan. MIBI stands for 2-Methoxy IsoButyl Isonitral. It can be useful in determining the difference between benign lumps and cancer. The radioactive particle Tc–99m Sestamibi is injected intravenously (through the foot), and a scanner, much like a bone scan machine, takes a picture and shows whether the radioactive particle is taken up by the breast lump more than by the rest of the tissue. Since cancer is likely to pick up more of the particles, it will often light up. It was hoped that the MIBI scan would help determine the difference between benign lumps and cancer. Review of several studies suggests that this technique in women with palpable lesions has a high sensitivity (84–94 percent) and specificity (72–94 percent).[17] *Sensitivity* is the ability to find cancers; that is, it has a 6–16 percent chance of missing them. *Specificity* is the ability to correctly diagnose them as cancer; that is, it has a 6–28 percent chance of being wrong. It is not as good in diagnosing lumps that are nonpalpable or were not seen on a mammogram, with a reported sensitivity as low as 50 percent. It is therefore best for palpable lumps that are hard to interpret on mammogram. This might be especially helpful for a young woman with dense breasts who feels a lump that her doctor can't find. A negative MIBI scan is not 100 percent accurate but should put her mind at rest. It's not particularly good for screening because it requires an injection of radioactive material, and also because it doesn't localize things very well. It's very fuzzy and far less distinct than a mammogram.

CT SCANNING

Another type of test, CT scanning (the CAT scan), also uses radiation—far more than mammography does. It works by imaging cross-sectional slices of the body. It's very good for detecting brain tumors and cancer in the belly and the lungs, because of the composition of those organs. But the amount of radiation needed to make slices close enough to pick up a 5 millimeter lump in the breast is simply too high for safety, and you're wiser to stick with mammograms. One recent study used contrast to enhance the CAT scan in women who had been diagnosed with cancer.[18] The contrast-enhanced CT was good at detecting the extent of disease and therefore in planning surgery. But MRI, which does not involve radiation, is also good at this.

THERMOGRAPHY

Thermography is based on the premise that cancer gives off more heat than normal tissue. It doesn't involve radiation or putting anything else into the body. A sensor is put on the breast, and heat coming from different parts of it is measured. From this a map is constructed, making beautiful colored pictures in which blue shows cold areas and red shows hot areas. The hot areas are supposed to be the cancerous ones.

Unfortunately this technique hasn't proved accurate—there are too many false positives and false negatives. Not all cancers give off heat, and of those that do, some are too deep or are located under wedges of fat and the heat doesn't register on the device. An Australian company has developed what is said to be a more accurate thermography machine. It has yet to be tested in the United States. A Scottish group has developed an interesting device called the Chronobra—a bra fitted with heat sensors and an electronic memory chip that can record the level of heat in the breast.[19] According to its developer, Dr. Hugh Simpson, women who are high risk tend to reach their peak breast temperature a day or two earlier in the menstrual cycle than their low-risk counterparts. Another new approach is termed dynamic thermography. Here the pattern of change in heat becomes an important factor in the analysis. One type of dynamic thermography involves lowering the temperature of the breast by blowing cool air on it and then mapping its return to normal temperature. Although the test is safe, its accuracy has not been demonstrated.

OTHER TECHNIQUES

Transillumination is an old technique used long before mammography appeared on the scene. Its purpose was to help determine whether a lump was a cyst or solid. It functioned like a flashlight; if the light shone through the lump, it was assumed to be a cyst; if it didn't, the lump was solid and potentially dangerous. That technique became more sophisticated, and equipment was developed that could monitor the exact amount of light in transmission.This advanced form of transillumination is called *diaphanography.* Since it doesn't use radiation, there was great hope that diaphanography would replace mammography, but it hasn't proved to be a great screening test. I have known some practitioners who have found it useful in conjunction with mammography.

Electrical impedance scanning uses the measure of current (no radiation) to detect changes in the breast. It has been used in one study to determine which women under 40 would benefit from further study.[20] Its sensitivity is only 50 percent at this point and so a negative scan would not mean that you were home free but a positive scan might indicate more imaging. At this point it needs more study to see whether it has clinical utility.

THE FUTURE

All of these are attempts to find ways other than mammography to diagnose breast lesions. What we really need is a diagnostic test that does not involve radiation and can determine the difference between dense breast tissue and benign lumps and cancer.

One possibility is combining biology and imaging. New techniques are exploiting the fact that cancers need a new blood supply if they are going to grow and spread. New MRI techniques are trying to use this to make the imaging more sensitive. Other work in animals combines antibodies to certain tumor genes with tags which can be seen on imaging. The future of breast cancer imaging will certainly be a long way from the rather crude tools that are available today.

Researchers are also exploring whether there are diagnostic tests that are different from imaging, like a blood test that could determine whether or not a lump is malignant or if there is malignancy in the body. As you'll see in Chapter 13, we now also have a way to analyze nipple duct fluid that may point the way to the future direction of screening.

8

Biopsy

When the doctor says you need a biopsy, you'll want to find out what kind. There are two types of biopsies that are done with needles and two "open" biopsies that require surgical cutting (Fig. 8-1). A fine-needle (like the kind used to draw blood) biopsy takes only a few cells out of the lump; a larger-needle biopsy, called a core, cuts a small piece out of the lump. An incisional biopsy takes out a much larger piece of the lump, while in an excisional biopsy the entire lump is removed (Fig. 8-2).

If you aren't clear about what kind of biopsy the surgeon or radiologist is planning, you may be assuming only a little piece will be removed whereas the surgeon really means to remove the whole thing. Then you'll end up angry because you've had an operation, and the surgeon will end up defensive because you were told you were getting a biopsy done.

The term *biopsy,* by the way, refers to the operation itself, not the process of studying the lump in the laboratory, which the pathologist does later. Anything that we cut out of the body is always sent to the pathologist for analysis, and the connection between the two procedures causes people to confuse them with each other. If you're having a biopsy performed, it's useful for you to know the precise meaning of the term.

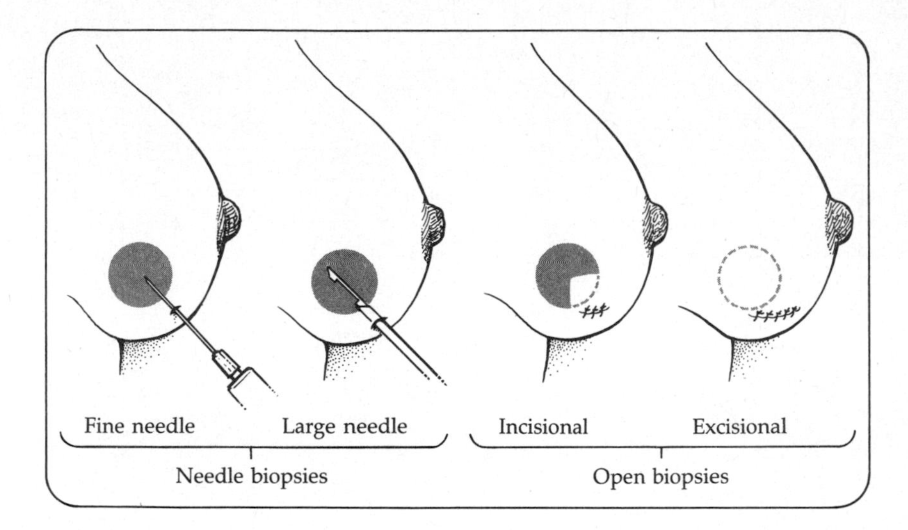

FIGURE 8-1

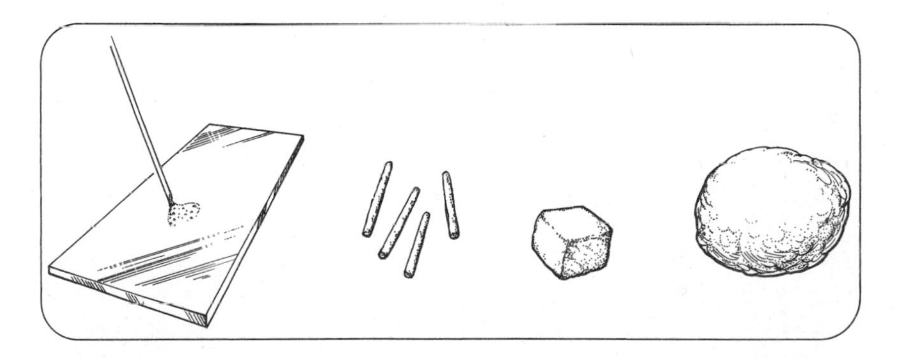

FIGURE 8-2

FINE-NEEDLE BIOPSY

If you have a palpable lump, the surgeon will anesthetize your breast with a small amount of lidocaine and then use a needle and syringe to try to get a few cells (Fig. 8-3). The material is squirted onto a slide, which is examined under a microscope. This can often show whether it is benign or cancerous.[1] However, since there's no tissue to look at, just individual cells, the procedure requires a good cytologist—a specialist in the field of looking at cells rather than tissue—who can identify cells out of context.

Fine-needle biopsies can also be done on lesions that can be seen

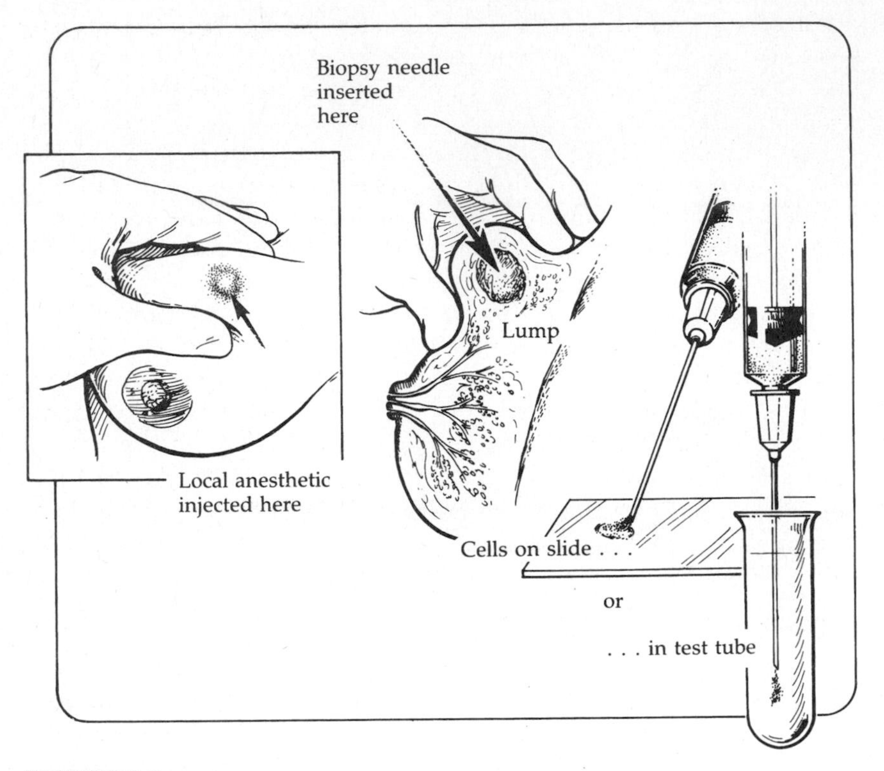

FIGURE 8-3

only on mammogram, although generally we use a core biopsy in that setting.

The rule of thumb with needle aspiration is that three elements should be consistent to determine that the lesion is benign.[2] If I think on examination that it's a fibroadenoma, if it looks like one on the mammogram, and if it also looks like one under the microscope after a needle aspiration, then I feel certain that's what it is. But if one of those elements is different—if it seems like it's not a fibroadenoma to me, even though the mammogram and needle aspiration suggest it is, or if I think it is but either the mammogram or the needle aspiration biopsy suggests something different—then we go on to a larger biopsy.

CORE BIOPSY

A core biopsy is similar to a fine-needle biopsy. The major difference is that we use a larger needle. We always did needle biopsies on palpable lumps. But with the increased use of mammography, doctors were finding more and more lesions that couldn't be felt. There's always a good chance that such lesions are harmless, but of course there's no way to be certain of that. So we faced the question of what to do about them.

One way we tried was with wire localization, a form of biopsy described later in this chapter. But it always made some of us uncomfortable. Here was a lesion we couldn't even feel, and yet we were doing surgery—always invasive and always with some risk. So a procedure was developed called *stereotactic core biopsy.*

When these biopsies are done on lesions that can be seen only on mammogram, we use a device called the stereotactic biopsy machine (Fig. 8-4). This procedure is now widely used. Sometimes it's done by a radiologist, sometimes by a surgeon; it doesn't matter which, as long as the individual is competent.

In some cases stereotactic core biopsies shouldn't be done. Large, diffuse areas of calcification are better surgically removed with a wide excision because a core biopsies only part of the lesion, which may not be representative. Radial scars (see Chapter 7), which can be confused with cancer, are better taken out entirely because the doctor may have difficulty diagnosing a small piece. In addition, there are other reasons that stereotactic biopsies may not work. People who weigh over 300 pounds won't fit on the machine. The patient has to remain immobile in a prone position for as long as 45 minutes. This eliminates anyone with significant anxiety (unless the anxiety is being controlled successfully with medication), with arthritis in the neck or back, with chronic cough, with severe kyphosis (a condition that causes the person to hunch over), or anything else that prevents absolute immobility for 45 minutes. It's also a problem if the lesion is very superficial because the needle will poke through the skin. The needle is 3 centimeters long, so if the breast, when compressed, is less than 3 centimeters, it won't work. Often this happens in very elderly women. Although their breasts may appear fairly large when they hang down, there actually isn't much breast tissue for the machine to grasp.

Luckily, core biopsies can also be done with ultrasound, which utilizes a handheld device that can accommodate these situations. It will also work better with a lesion that's palpable but can't be seen on a mammogram. Even if the lesion is not palpable but can be visualized on ultrasound, a core biopsy can be done this way.

The ultrasound approach is becoming more popular because it does not require equipment such as X ray machines and does not expose the woman to radiation. Surgeons may have an ultrasound machine in their offices but will rarely have the X ray equipment necessary for a stereotactic core. Why don't we do all core biopsies that way? Because not all lesions are visible on ultrasound. Microcalcifications, for example, are too small for an ultrasound machine to detect and require a stereotactic core.

No doctor should ever do a core biopsy in place of a 6-month follow-up mammogram; rather, it is done in place of surgical biopsy. So when a doctor is first examining a lesion, the question is always, Should we do a biopsy? If the answer is no, we should repeat the mammogram.

When should core biopsies be done? Different surgeons have different ideas on this. Many, like me, feel that when a biopsy is needed, it should be a core rather than a surgical biopsy whenever possible. This gives the surgeon the information, and after that the surgeon and patient can sit down and talk about what comes next. If the core biopsy shows cancer, you can then have the surgery you need, and you've had only one surgical procedure, rather than the two that you might have with a surgical biopsy.

If the lesion appears likely to be malignant, some surgeons would rather do a wire localization biopsy (see below), diagnosing the lesion and then removing it. Core biopsy is ideal if you're likely to want a mastectomy, since it entails only one surgery. People with multiple lesions do better with core biopsies because multiple surgical biopsies can leave your breast looking like Swiss cheese, and multiple core biopsies are far less disfiguring. If it's very likely that the lesion is a fibroadenoma (see Chapter 6), a core is also ideal because it will assure you and your surgeon that it is indeed a harmless lump. But if you know it's going to worry you and you want the lump removed whatever it is, then you may as well have that done right away and not bother with the core.

Medical device manufacturers have been mobilized by the success of core biopsies and are trying to come up with machines that will allow a surgeon to do an entire lumpectomy this way. Their theory is that surgery could be altogether avoided if there were a needle bigger than that used for core—enlarged a centimeter or two—that could take out an entire lesion. There are several devices out there and all have their pros and cons. What is important is that the surgeon or radiologist using the biopsy device is experienced with it and comfortable with the results.

Doing a lumpectomy with a device rather than doing an open, surgical one always entails the difficulty of ensuring that the doctor gets clean margins. When there's a small lesion that the doctor feels is probably benign but the patient wants removed, margins won't matter. In the rare case where the lesion turns out to be cancerous, a surgical re-excision can be done. This kind of lumpectomy also works well if the patient is in her 60s or older, has fairly fatty breasts, and has a small, well-circumscribed cancerous lesion. In this case the doctor should be able to remove the lesion and still get good margins.

The Procedure

Core biopsy differs mainly in whether it is being done under X ray guidance or ultrasound. When X ray is used (stereotactic), the patient lies down on the table with her breast suspended below her between two X ray plates (Fig. 8-4). The patient is given local anesthesia. A small incision is made over the site where the biopsy needle will go in. After exactly localizing the area with mammograms and a computer, the biopsy device enters the breast rapidly and drills a core of tissue. Although this sounds scary, it is similar to having your ears pierced with the device used in jewelry outlets. Usually several passes are taken to make sure the lesion is well sampled. The size of the incision depends on how big the core biopsy needle is; with some of the devices, it will have to be sutured closed when the procedure is finished. If only a small core (about 1 cm long and 1 mm wide) is taken out, a little, bandage-like covering called a steri strip is adequate to close it. Usually five cores are taken out for lumps; for microcalcifications it may be 10 or more. After the biopsy the breast is x-rayed to see the line of air in the middle of the lump, to prove that the doctor actually took out what she was going after. (The inventor of these things was clearly a man: they were first called biopsy guns. Only a man would think of aiming a gun at women's breasts! In the UCLA breast center, I got them

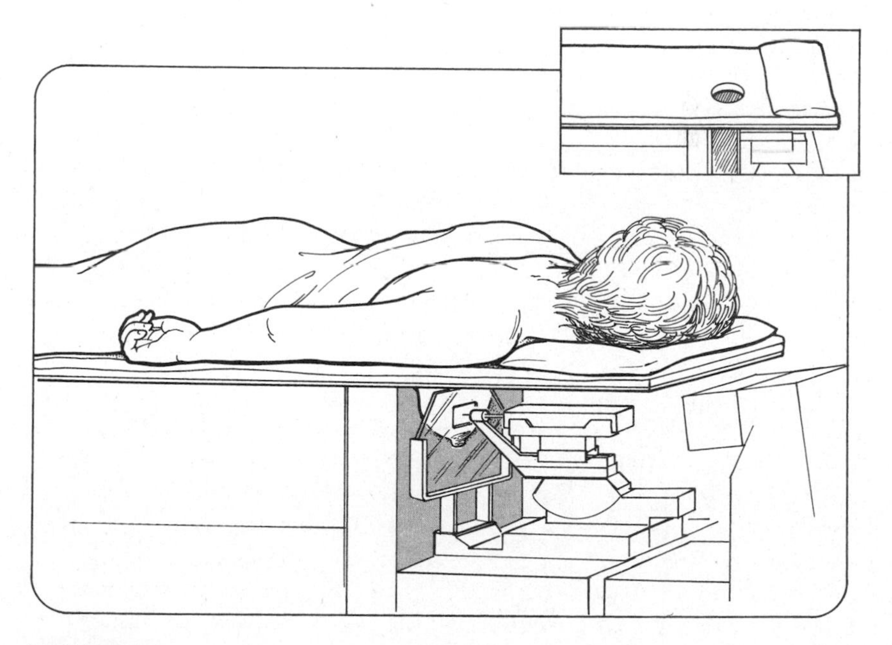

FIGURE 8-4

to use the less lethal-sounding "biopsy device.") Afterward a metal clip is used to permanently mark the site of the biopsy; then pressure is applied to the breast for a few minutes, until it stops bleeding. If swelling is a concern, it may be covered with an ice pack.

When the procedure is done by ultrasound, the woman lies on her back on a table and the radiologist or surgeon identifies the lesion using a handheld ultrasound device. Once the lesion is identified, the doctor proceeds with the biopsy, watching the core needle enter the lesion on the ultrasound monitor. The core biopsy is done by the physician with a handheld device.

There are few complications, whether done under X ray or ultrasound. The doctor might miss the lesion, but this rarely happens. There may be infection or hematoma (blood collection), but these occur in only about 1 percent of patients. You may have some minor bruising.

SURGICAL BIOPSY

What is an incisional or excisional biopsy like? You may have your biopsy performed in your doctor's office or, more frequently, in the hospital's minor operating room. If you had a biopsy several years ago, you might find this confusing. In the past, most surgery was performed in what we now call the main operating room, and the surgical rituals may differ from those you recall.

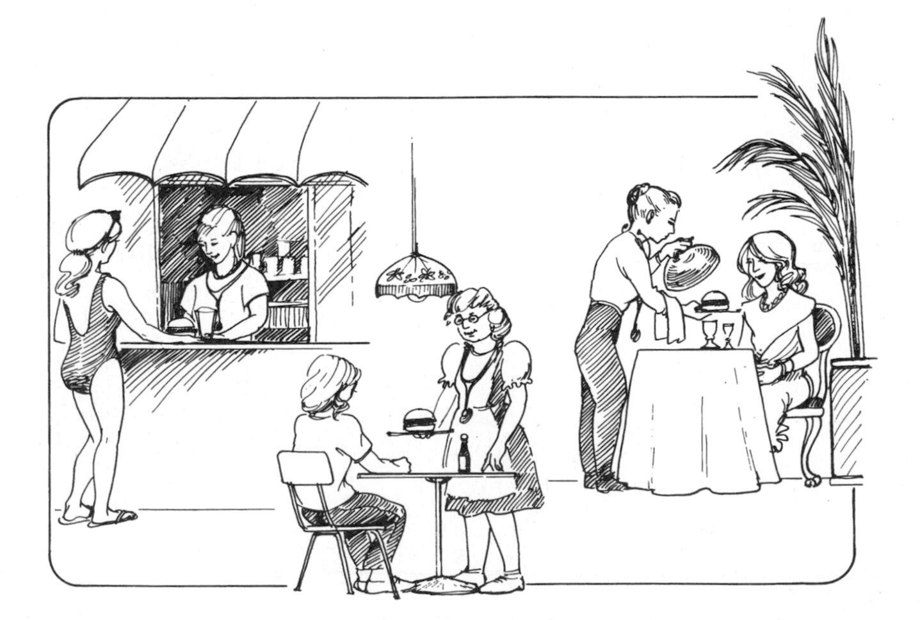

Biopsies may be done in two or three kinds of operating rooms. I like to compare them to types of restaurants that serve basically the same food but in somewhat different venues. The minor operating room can be in the doctor's office or a hospital and is like a snack bar—you can go in barefoot, dressed in your bathing suit, and order your hamburger, and it's cheap and it tastes good. The ambulatory surgery room is located in a surgicenter or hospital and is more like a coffee shop; you have to be fully dressed, but it's okay to wear jeans, and you sit at a table and are waited on.There's a larger menu, which still includes your hamburger. And finally there's the main operating room only found in the hospital, which is like the formal dining room—you've got to dress up, there's a fancier menu, and the waiter grinds pepper onto your salad. Again, you can still get your hamburger, though it will cost you more. In each place, the hamburger is the same, but the context different.

Similarly, you can have your biopsy in any of the three operating rooms, though the ambulatory and main rooms are equipped with a larger "menu" that includes more complex operations as well. The difference is in the ritual. The rituals are always defined by the room they're performed in, not the particular operation.

There's nothing wrong with rituals—every profession has them, and they're useful. But if you don't know what the rituals are or even that they are rituals, they can be intimidating.

Most surgical rituals are holdovers from the turn of the century, when they served a practical purpose. Little was known about germs and the danger of spreading them through unsanitary practices. The

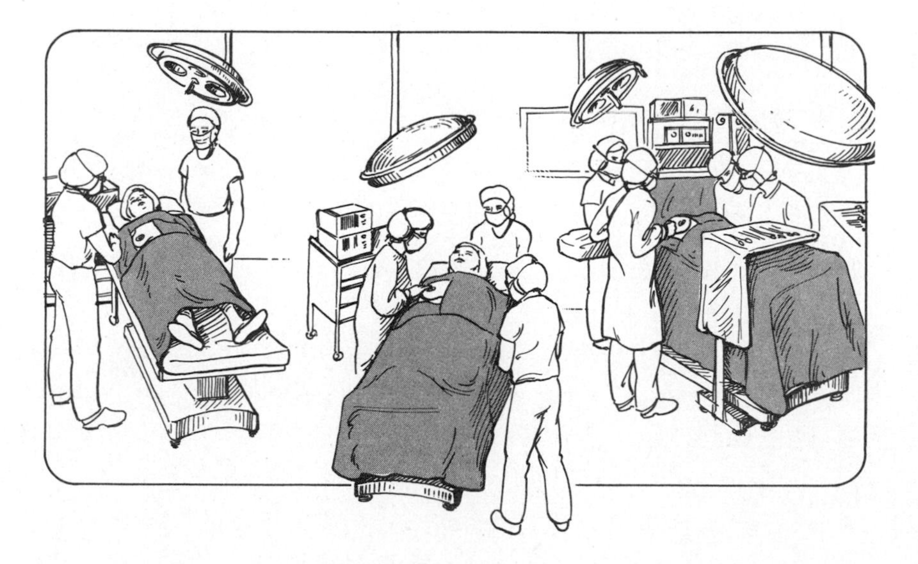

majority of the rituals began then—the frequent hand washing, the surgical gowns and masks, and so on—but nowadays, when people shower every day and wash their hands a lot and we have antibiotics to combat infections, the extreme degree of attention to sterile cleanliness is less necessary and, as I said, partially ritualistic. Predictably, the fancier the operating room, the fancier its attendant ritual.

Today breast surgery is mostly done in either outpatient, freestanding ambulatory clinics or the minor operating room. It's much cheaper than the same surgery performed in the main operating room. In the latter, you're paying for all that specialized equipment used for complicated procedures like open-heart surgery. Neither patients nor their insurance companies want that, so the "snack bar" facilities are being increasingly used. (The ambulatory room is a bit more sophisticated than the minor operating room, but far less so than the main.) Often the ambulatory and minor operating rooms are used interchangeably. Keep in mind, however, that all this varies from hospital to hospital, and region to region.

If you had a biopsy 30 years ago in the "formal dining room," you may be expecting all the formal ritual and may find its absence disturbing. Don't worry. The operation and the care you're receiving are the same, and they are what matters.

If a patient has other medical problems—a heart or a respiratory condition, for example—then it's probably wiser to perform the operation in the main operating room, in case complications arise that need more sophisticated equipment. If you're concerned about possible complications and how they'll be handled, talk with your doctor beforehand about which room will be used and what you're likely to need.

Wire Localization

If your lesion cannot be felt and a needle biopsy is not possible, we may use a wire localization biopsy. Performing a biopsy on something that can only be seen on an X ray is difficult. In this procedure we use a thin wire to show the surgeon where the lesion is. It's usually done in the X ray department. The radiologist will give you a local anesthetic and put a small needle into your breast under X ray guidance, pointing toward the lesion (Fig. 8-5). She will then pass a wire with a hook on the end through the needle, and then position the hook so the end of the wire is on the site of the calcifications or density. The wire is left in the breast and you're taken to the operating room. The biopsy procedure that follows is very similar to the procedure used to take a lump out, except that we use the wire to direct where we'll remove the tissue. The surgeon gives you more local anesthetic, makes an incision, follows the wire, and then takes out the area of tissue around it, hoping it's the right

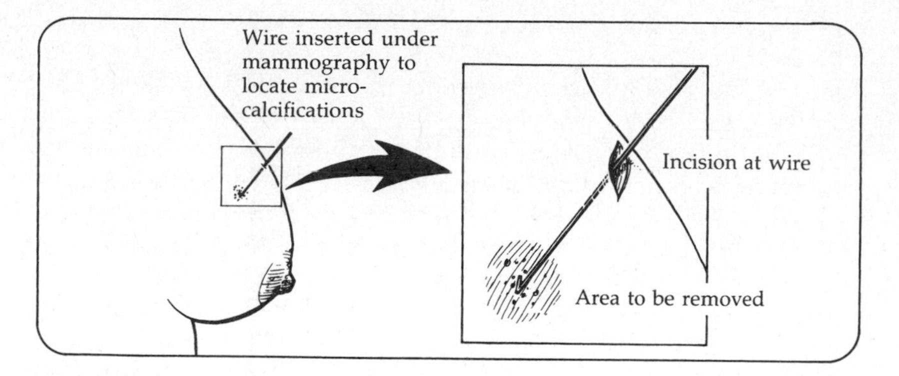

FIGURE 8-5

place. The tissue is then sent to the radiology department. There they x-ray it to make sure it's from the area with the calcifications or lesion and then send it to the pathology department where they make slides and look at it under the microscope. Meanwhile the surgeon sews you up.

The X ray of the specimen will tell you if the surgeon got the calcifications or area that was seen on the mammogram. Since the surgeon can't see or feel calcifications, it is also possible to miss them with the surgery. In this case the X ray of the specimen will not show calcifications and you may need to get another biopsy.

The specimen won't, however, tell you if the surgeon got all the calcifications in your entire breast. If the area is benign this won't matter, but you will want to know whether there are still some benign calcifications inside. So it's important that you get another mammogram three to six months later to show how you look after the surgery.

Biopsy Procedures

Whether a wire, local, or regular biopsy, the procedure can be done under either local or general anesthetic, but most doctors and patients prefer local. Some doctors like to give their patients a tranquilizer; I prefer to help them stay calm through reassuring conversation. A device called a pulse oximeter fits over your finger (like the pulse monitors often used by fitness enthusiasts) and monitors both your pulse and the amount of oxygen in your blood. It is an important safeguard whenever sedation is used. In some cases "local/standby" is used. This means the operation is done under local anesthesia, but an anesthesiologist or nurse-anesthetist is standing by in case you need mild drugs that will make you indifferent to the procedure. The anesthesiologist can also put you to sleep if general anesthesia becomes necessary. There are now drugs that are very fast acting and don't last long. They put you into a kind of twilight sleep, in which you don't care about what happens and won't remember it, but you're not totally unconscious. These are often used in conjunction with a local anesthetic. This is known as monitored anesthesia (MAC). If MAC is used, we need to do the same preoperative preparation we use for general anesthesia. When local anesthesia alone is used, you arrive, have your procedure, and go home. So it's a trade-off between being relatively more comfortable with a longer procedure or having more discomfort but getting in and out more quickly.

Which anesthetic people prefer is a very personal choice. Some people don't want to know what's going on, and they're willing to put up with the extra inconvenience. Others hate being out of control and want to know what's happening. You should discuss with your doctor which way makes more sense for you. Some drugs allow the patient to be awake but leave her with no memory of the experience afterward. If a woman wants to remember what happens during surgery, she needs to tell the anesthesiologist or anesthetist so that a drug such as Versed, for example, is not given to her.

If the biopsy takes place in the minor operating room or the doctor's office, the patient usually changes from the waist up; in the main operating room, where the dress code is more formal, the patient has to change into a hospital johnny and the surgeon wears a scrub suit. Depending on whether you are being operated on under local anesthesia or MAC, you may be more or less aware of what happens next.

Often the surgeon uses a machine called an electrocautery to seal off the small blood vessels and prevent bleeding. Since there's a slight risk of a short circuit, which would give you an electric shock, a plastic pad is put on your leg, back, or abdomen to ground the current and prevent electric shock. It is filled with a cool gel, and initially it feels freezing cold.

Next, the surgeon washes her hands, puts on surgical gloves, and then paints you with an antiseptic solution. Usually this is done two or three times—no particular reason, but three is a nice ritualistic number, so why not? Then sterilized towels (paper or cloth, depending on which room you're in) are framed around the area that's going to be operated on (Fig. 8-6).

With a sterile felt-tip pen, the surgeon marks the spot over the lump and then injects the local anesthetic through a small needle. (We usually use lidocaine, not Novocaine, these days, but "Novocaine" is still the popular term—like calling any facial tissues "Kleenex.") When the needle first goes in, you may feel a little pain or a burning sensation.

Don't be misled by the lidocaine—it's not exactly like the anesthetic you get at the dentist's. For one thing, it hurts a lot less. The dentist has to poke around your mouth looking for a nerve and then deaden it,

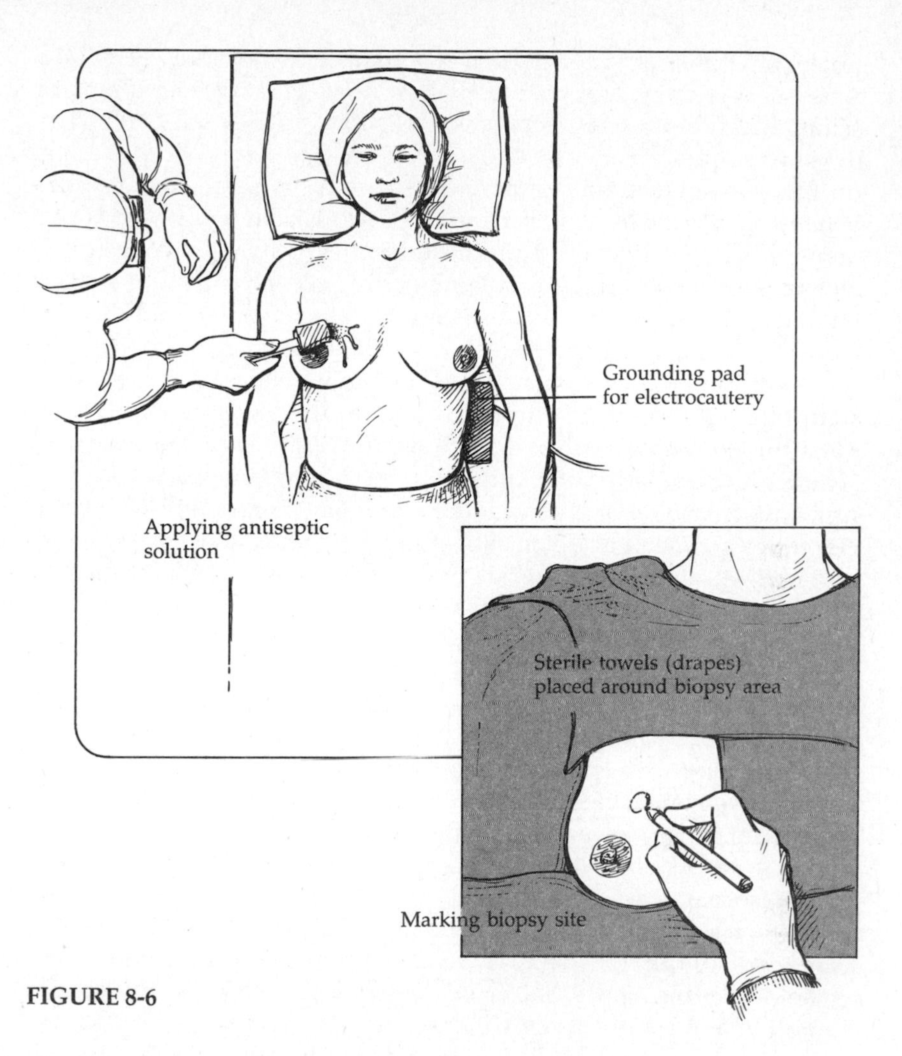

FIGURE 8-6

and you have to wait till it takes effect, and then your whole mouth goes numb and you end up chewing the inside of your cheek. It's not the dentist's fault: dental work requires a nerve block, since drilling into a tooth is felt all through the jaw.

In the biopsy we're cutting only into soft tissue, and consequently we can use "local infiltration," which numbs just the area where it's put, not the whole breast. And it works immediately. (This confuses some alert patients, who get scared when the surgeon starts to work right after injecting the anesthetic.) It's possible that you will feel some pain, even with the local anesthetic we give you for the biopsy. Some people are especially pain sensitive. This is not bad, nor are you being weak. Everyone's pain sensitivity is different and can change, depending on a number of factors, including medications you may be taking, stress, and prior experience. You can always ask for more anesthetic or sedation. Don't try to be "polite" or a "good girl"—there's no reason for you to suffer.

Now the surgeon makes the incision, going through skin, fat, and tissue to get to the lump. Most of the process isn't actually cutting; it's just spreading tissue apart until the lump is reached. There's little bleeding because there aren't many blood vessels here, and the cautery takes care of the few there are. The lump is cut away from the surrounding tissue and removed (Fig. 8-7).

The incision is then sewn up, usually in layers—tissue, then fat, then skin. This prevents a dent from forming in the breast when it heals. Most surgeons use dissolvable stitches that tend to leave less scarring.

After the operation the surgeon bandages the incision and will probably tell you when you can take the bandage off and when you can shower. I usually had the patient remove the bandage the next day and shower as soon as she wanted to. We used to think that you shouldn't shower until the stitches came out, but we've found that water doesn't hurt stitches at all.

The more you bounce, the sorer you'll be, so whether or not you usually wear a bra, it's a good idea to wear one for a couple of days after the surgery—a good firm, sensible bra, not a lacy, flimsy one. You'll probably want to keep it on all night as well. Some women, though, find the bra so uncomfortable in bed that they prefer the soreness. If the incision is near the bra line, the bra may cause more discomfort than it's worth. Use your own judgment; the point is to make you as comfortable as possible.

The anesthetic wears off more quickly than the dentist's does. Just as it goes to work right away, it wears off right away, generally within an hour after the biopsy. You're usually not in much pain after the operation; many patients only need Tylenol. Do not, however, take aspirin or a nonsteroidal pain medication such as Motrin, Nuprin, or Aleve. They increase the chance of postoperative bleeding or bruising. By the next day you can usually go back to work and resume your normal activities. (Be sensible, of course; if your normal activities include weight lifting, give it another couple of days.)

There will be some scarring, though usually very little. You should talk with your surgeon about it before you have the procedure done. You and your surgeon may have different ideas about what makes an acceptable scar. For example, surgeons have often learned in training that the most cosmetic scar results if they make the incision right around the areola and then tunnel up to the lesion, so that the scar is camouflaged by the color change between the areola and the rest of the breast. If that's done well, it can indeed give you a very unobtrusive

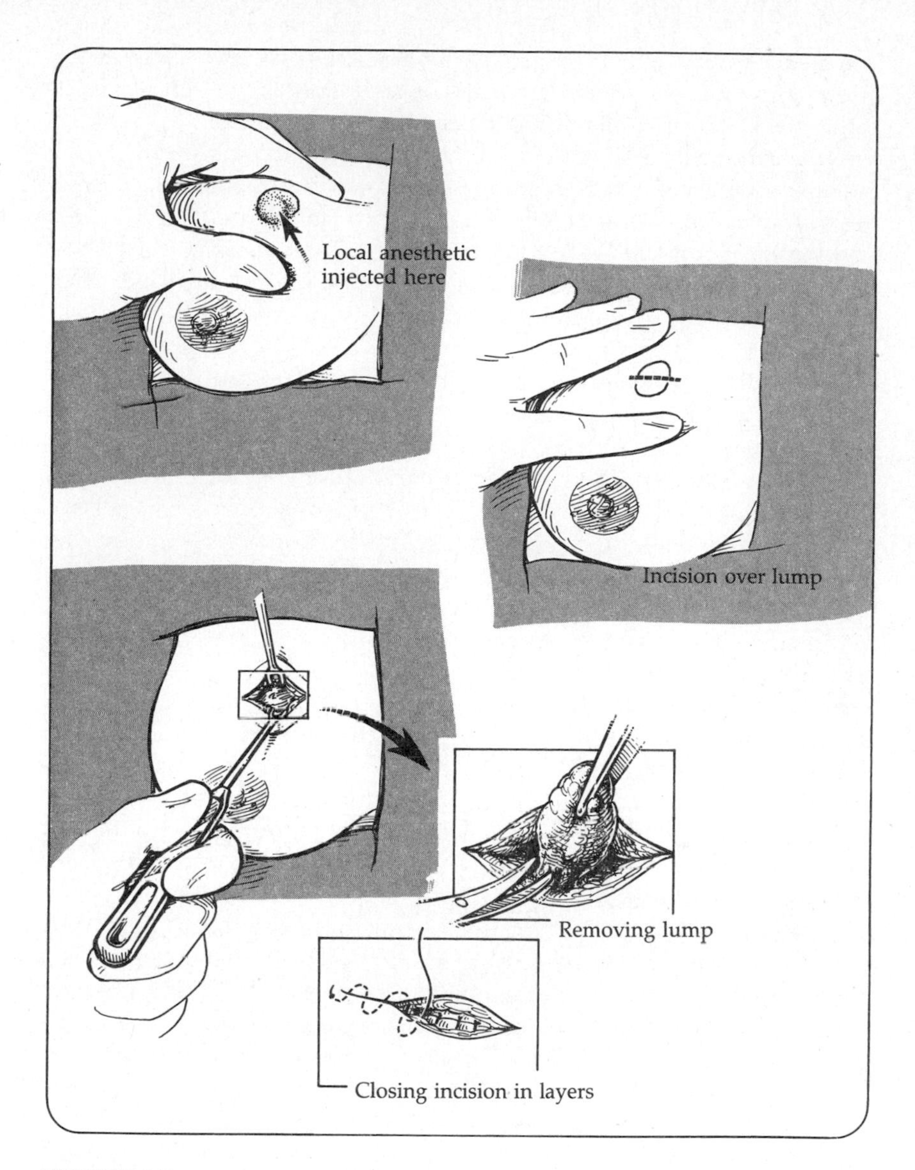

FIGURE 8-7

scar. Sometimes, however, depending on the length of the scar or the amount of tissue that's removed, it can decrease the sexual sensation in your nipple, or create other changes in your nipple and areola such as numbness or puckering. Also, the scarring might cause difficulties in breast feeding. Further, the tunneling increases the chance that you'll have bleeding complications and a hematoma (see below).

The alternative I favor is to make the incision directly over the lesion and just take out the lump. It's usually a smaller incision that way, and there's less chance of damaging the nipple.

Unless you discuss your preferences with your surgeon, he will make assumptions about your wishes that may or may not be accurate. Most surgeons are sensitive to patients' concerns and will try to give you the incision you want. If you feel the surgeon is being flippant or not taking your concerns seriously, find another one. At the same time, be aware that some people have bodies that make big keloid (thick) scars, and the best surgeon in the world can't prevent that. You probably know if you're one of these people from your own experience, although there's always the chance that, if you've never had a major cut before, you won't know till after the surgery.

With wire localization biopsies, it's important to know how much tissue the surgeon plans to remove. Some surgeons make their incision where the wire enters the skin and take out the tissue surrounding the whole length of the wire. This usually creates more deformity than making the incision over the place where the end of the wire is—going in directly and taking out only the lesion. With the increasing use of the core biopsy and the stereotactic needle aspiration, doctors can diagnose these things before the surgery and don't have to remove as much tissue. So find out exactly how much tissue the surgeon plans to remove and ask questions if you think it will be too much.

While you're resting up from the operation and resuming your regular activities, the lump is being analyzed by a pathologist. Sometimes the pathologist will do a "frozen section," which is a quick but crude method of testing the lump. The lump is cut in half; a piece is quick frozen to make it solid, then thinly sliced, placed on a slide, and stained right away. Sometimes this will give you the answer, but it's not 100 percent accurate. In the old days, when we did an immediate mastectomy if the lump was malignant, this method was always used to allow the surgeon to proceed with the operation immediately. Nowadays, however, we usually do it in two steps—the biopsy is performed; the results are discussed with the patient; if further surgery is called for it's done later (see Chapter 21). So we don't often do a frozen section anymore.

Far more reliable is the "permanent section." Here the tissue is removed and cut into small pieces. It goes through several stages. First it's dehydrated in different strengths of alcohol, then embedded in a block of paraffin wax. This is put on a microtome, a knife that cuts it into very thin slices. Each slice is then put on a slide, the wax melted away, and the tissue stained with different colors. This whole process takes between 24 and 36 hours.

When the slides are ready, the pathologist looks at them and makes a diagnosis; this takes a few hours. The pathologist then dictates a report that is sent to the doctor, who will probably have it in a week. Some doctors wait till the report comes in, but others prefer to call the pathologist the day after the operation. This is what I used to do because I liked to let my patients know what was happening as soon as possible, and because for all patients the waiting and uncertainty can be terrifying. Whatever your doctor's practice, you'll know in a week or so what the biopsy has shown.

As with any surgical procedure, in a breast biopsy there are sometimes complications. The two most common are hematoma and infection. If a hematoma occurs it will usually be within a day or two of the procedure. It's caused by bleeding inside the area where the surgery was done, causing a blood blister to form (Fig. 8-8). It turns blue and forms a lump right under the skin. The body usually simply absorbs and recycles it, as it does with any bruise. But sometimes, before the body can do that, you'll bump into something or someone will bump into you, and it will burst open, causing dark blood to come out. It looks gross and disgusting and you'll think you're dying, but don't worry—you're not. It's old blood; you're not bleeding now. What you need to do is go home, clean up the mess, and take a shower. If you're worried about it, call your doctor.

If an infection occurs, it will show up a week or two after surgery—there'll be redness and swelling and fever, and the doctor will treat it with antibiotics. Again, it's more of a nuisance than anything else.

Sometimes you'll get a combination of infection and hematoma—the blood mixes with pus, like an abscess or a boil, and needs to be drained by the doctor. Sometimes when stitches are removed after breast surgery—either biopsies or cosmetic procedures—a small nondissolvable stitch is overlooked and remains in the breast, which will then get infected, as was the case with one of my patients (no, I

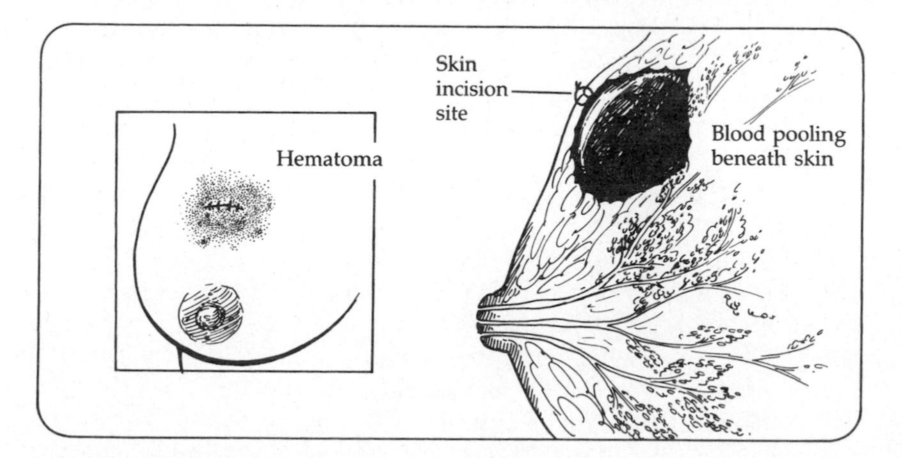

FIGURE 8-8

wasn't the surgeon who removed the stitches). It's easy to treat with antibiotics and removal of the stitch.

And, yes, the worst patient nightmares do occasionally occur. I had one patient who had a persistent infection after a biopsy, and a follow-up operation revealed that her surgeon had left a sponge inside her. I'm not quite sure how a surgeon could manage to do that, but this one did. Fortunately it's very, very rare—and she is fine now.

These complications occur in about 10 percent of breast biopsies, but they're not life threatening and they don't have any long-term effects.

One special situation is when you are pregnant or breast-feeding. If you do find a suspicious lump, get it checked out. Should a biopsy be called for, neither pregnancy nor breast-feeding need prevent it. When you're pregnant, it's best to have a biopsy done under a local anesthetic to avoid exposing the fetus to general anesthesia. And a core biopsy may well be easier for both mother and child than an open one.

A nursing mother can have either a general or a local anesthetic. I preferred to operate right after a woman had fed her baby or expressed the milk. I used the lowest percentage of local anesthetic possible, usually lidocaine, since the child could swallow some of it later. I would also advise the mother not to feed the baby from that breast for 12 hours after the surgery, since a gulp of the lidocaine might be harmful and it should be given time to disperse throughout the breast. Swallowing a tiny bit of anesthetic, however, should not harm the child.

It's messy to perform surgery on a lactating woman. The operation can create a milk cyst or leakage, but it's no great tragedy if it does. It can temporarily make the milk messy too, since blood from the operation can mix with it. Blood won't hurt your baby, so the problem is mostly esthetic.

Some surgeons tell a lactating woman she has to stop breast-feeding if she needs a biopsy. She doesn't. If your surgeon tells you this at a time when you're thinking of stopping breast-feeding anyway, it's probably a good time to stop. Otherwise, find another surgeon who will operate while you're lactating.

HOW TO READ YOUR BIOPSY REPORT

There are three possible biopsy findings—benign, cancerous, or not certain. The latter happens because the doctor often gets only a piece of the lesion. It's possible that the pathologist will find atypical hyperplasia, which often exists with cancer (see Chapter 12). If that's the case, the doctor is obligated to go back in and take more tissue out, to be certain that there are no cancer cells as well. According to a research article by Dr. Helen Pass, about 50 percent of atypical hyperplasia diagnosed from a core biopsy on a mammographic lesion turn out to be accompanied by cancer.[3] As with needle aspirations, three elements should be consistent to determine that it is benign.[4] The physical exam, mammogram, and pathology have to match. But if one of those elements is different—if it seems to the doctor that it's not a fibroadenoma, even though the mammogram and needle aspiration suggest it is; or if the doctor thinks it is but either the mammogram or biopsy suggests something different—then it's important to go on to a larger biopsy.

Even when the doctor tells you that the lump was benign, it's important to find out exactly what it was. "Benign" isn't enough. You should ask to see a copy of your pathology report.

The report will have two parts. The first is the "gross description." It describes what the surgeon gave the pathologist and the pathologist could see just by looking at it—a slide with some cells on it, or a core, or a piece of tissue measuring 3 by 5 centimeters. Then it will often describe cutting the tissue and what it looked like. It will say whether the surgeon saw a distinct mass or whether the lump just looked like breast tissue. If a fibroadenoma was removed, it will often be described as a distinct mass that's round and smooth and measures such and such number of centimeters. If it's a pseudolump and it's just breast tissue, it may be described as a piece of fibro-fatty tissue that contains no obvious lesions. If it's microcalcifications, the pathologist won't see these with the naked eye, and so they won't be described.

The second part describes what the lump looks like under the microscope. Some reports will give you a detailed description—what the cells look like, what the surrounding tissue is like, and so on. Others cut to the chase and give just the final diagnosis. So it might read, "1.fibroadenoma." It almost always adds, "2. fibrocystic disease" or "fibrocystic change." That's because, as I said in Chapter 6, the "fibrocystic change" is the background that we see normally in breast tissue, so it's always there. The report may say "fibrocystic change" alone if it's just breast tissue. That's not an adequate diagnosis. If your report says that, you should ask for a more specific diagnosis, even if it means making the pathologist go back, look at the slides again, and describe exactly what's there. Under the rubric of "fibrocystic disease" there is one entity that does increase your risk of subsequent breast cancer: atypical hyperplasia, which I describe in Chapter 12. You want to know if that's what you have. Usually if it says fibrocystic disease (or change) alone, you don't have atypical hyperplasia. Today most pathologists are aware of its importance and are likely to mention if it's there. But they might not. I wouldn't risk assuming they would have mentioned it and done nothing. Often you'll have hyperplasia that isn't atypical—extra cells in the lining of the duct that are normal. So if it says "hyperplasia of the usual kind," that's fine.

In addition, if you had a biopsy that was done for calcifications, you want to be sure that the pathologist saw calcifications under the microscope, so you can be sure that he's looking at the right tissue. Sometimes, if you have a very small area of calcifications and a big piece of tissue taken out, when they make the slides they don't get the area where the calcifications are. Then they can look at the tissue and say "totally benign." That has happened to me: I took out calcifications and the report came back benign. I asked if they'd seen the calcifications and they said no, but they'd put all the tissue through. I said, "You need to see the calcifications." So they took the blocks of paraffin, x-rayed them, found which ones had the calcifications, and made additional slides. Then they found the calcifications and indeed there was precancer, which they would have missed. So it's important to make sure the pathologists have seen what they were supposed to see. You may think it's your doctor's job to take care of all that, and you're right. But you can't assume that's happening, and you need to double-check.

Then you should get a copy of the report and save it. It may become relevant at some later time and it's important for you to have it in your records. One of the things we're starting to realize is that some of the changes in the basic molecular biology of the breast tissue (see Chapter 10) can be identified in earlier biopsy tissue. For example, suppose you have a family history of breast cancer and you have a biopsy for what turns out to be a fibroadenoma. In the past we thought that was all you needed to know. But, as I explained in Chapter 6, we've recently discovered that one kind of fibroadenoma can, when you have a family history of breast cancer, markedly increase your risk. It is important for you to be able to have the pathologist go back and look at the slides and determine what kind of fibroadenoma you actually had. Probably they won't keep the tissue, but if you at least keep a record of your biopsy, with the date and the hospital, you can go back and find the slides. That can be very important.

In fact, however, you may be able to save extra tissue from the biopsy in a tissue bank. As we do more and more research on benign and malignant breast problems, there's an enormous need to have tissue to test. Some of that needs to be saved fresh, and some can be saved in paraffin blocks. It's to your advantage to have the tissue saved because as new discoveries come along we can go back and test them out on this tissue. One of the things we're trying to do on a political level is create a regional network of tissue banks, so that everybody will be able to have some tissue saved from surgery.

It's really important, if you've had your biopsy because of a lesion seen on mammogram, to have a new baseline mammogram a month or two after the procedure. If the doctor doesn't suggest it, you should.

Sometimes even when we take out calcifications, we may not get all of them. If it's benign, that doesn't matter. But it's good to have it documented so that a year from now if you have a mammogram, it won't seem like there are new calcifications.

Similarly, if you have something taken out, your breast is going to look different: there will be scarring. A year later that might look like something new and alarming, unless there's a baseline fairly soon after the surgery for comparison.

PART FOUR

Prediction, Prevention, and Screening

9

Risk Factors: Nongenetic

When we talk about the risk of breast cancer, we look at two different types of risk factors: genetic and the range of nongenetic factors that include hormones, diet, alcohol consumption, environmental carcinogens, and radiation. We'll examine genetic risk factors in the next section, and the connection between the two kinds of risk factors in Chapter 11.

Nearly every day you turn on the television or open a newspaper and learn about "a new study" showing that this food increases the risk of getting breast cancer or that activity prevents that condition. The next week another new study appears to show that the activity doesn't work after all or the food causes a new and unforeseen problem. And you're confused—as well you may be.

The problem is that neither the media nor much of the public distinguishes between kinds of studies. Different studies have different degrees of significance, and to understand what a particular study means, you need information about the study itself.

There are many ways to conduct studies of diseases and of possible ways to control, treat, or prevent them. Unfortunately, a completely accurate, comprehensive study is impossible to achieve. There are too many variables in even the simplest area of study. But some studies are better than others. To understand how accurate a study is, you need to look at how it was designed. It may be weak in one area, strong in another, and excellent in a third. Different aspects of a study will make it more or less believable.

Few people understand study design. Doctors are as predisposed to self-deception as anyone else: we all tend to believe the studies that feed our biases rather than the ones that don't. This same tendency is reflected by the media. Reporters often don't understand the nuances of a study, and their quick-story reports usually fail to address limitations in the study's design. In addition, they often exaggerate the study's implications. Data that are only one brick in the complex design of a wall are presented as if they were the cornerstone. It's no wonder the layperson is confused about what a study's results might mean in real life.

OBSERVATIONAL STUDIES

There are two basic categories of study; each has its own values and limitations. One category is the *observational study,* which observes, without intervention, people doing what they would normally do. The other category is the *clinical trial,* or *intervention study,* in which a certain treatment is tested on a group of people who are assigned to use it in certain ways over a certain period of time. We will examine this category later. Here we will review the studies more relevant to risk and prevention.

Observational studies are great for generating a hypothesis. They observe a phenomenon and then try to think of an explanation. They do not, however, prove cause and effect. For example, a study done in Boston observed that women with breast cancer were more likely to get their clothing dry-cleaned, have exterminators come to their homes, and use lawn treatments. The hypothesis was that these poisons might lead to breast cancer. This is an interesting possibility, but it's far from proven. The next step might be to do an animal study and see if dry cleaning fluid increases cancers. We could also study women who work at dry cleaners to see if they had more cancer. If these studies still seemed to show a relationship, we could then go on to a controlled study in which women were randomized to use dry cleaners or not and then see how many developed breast cancer. This last study, of course, would be difficult to do, but it would be the one to give us the final proof. Many of the studies we hear about in the news are observational, but they are presented as if they demonstrate cause and effect. This does not mean they are useless. They are great at telling us what to study. They may even function as a warning sign for possible temporary actions: you might decide to wait and see about making a change until the definitive study is done.

UNDERSTANDING RISK

Every woman wants to know what her risk of getting breast cancer is and what she can do about it. Before discussing the figures, however, we need to be clear about where they come from, since they're often used in confusing and misleading ways. For example, an advertisement calling milk "99 percent fat-free" might suggest that it has 1 percent as much fat as whole milk. Actually, it means that 1 percent of the milk is made up of fat. Since only 3.6 percent of whole milk is made up of fat, whole milk could be called "96.4 percent fat-free." Thus, a more helpful ad would say, "less than one-third the fat of whole milk." Likewise, when media headlines say that three alcoholic drinks a week increase breast cancer risk by 50 percent they don't mean you have a 50–50 chance of getting breast cancer, but rather that these drinks increase the relative risk by 50 percent and your lifetime risk is now about 5 percent rather than 3.3 percent. Thus, it is important that we examine the common statistics used about breast cancer and review exactly what they mean. There are three kinds of risk commonly referred to in discussing breast cancer: absolute risk, relative risk, and attributable risk (Fig. 9-1).

Absolute risk is the rate at which cancer or mortality from cancer occurs in a general population. It can be expressed either as the number of cases per a specified population (e.g., 50 cases per 100,000 annually) or as a cumulative risk up to a particular age. This cumulative risk is the source of the familiar 1 in 8 for non-Hispanic white women. (Other racial and ethnic groups may actually have a lower risk; see Table 9-1.)

Future risk at any one time also depends to a great extent on your age. At age 20 the risk over the next 10 years is 1 in 2,152 (0.05 percent), while the risk over the next 10 years for a 50-year-old is 1 in 36 (2.78 percent) (see Table 9-2).

The second kind of risk we talk about determining is *relative risk.* This is the comparison of the incidence of breast cancer or deaths from breast cancer among people with a particular risk factor to that of people without that factor, or a "reference population." This type of measurement is more useful to an individual woman because she can determine her risk factors and thus calculate how they will affect her chances of getting the disease. Even here you have to be very careful. For comparison, you can't use the 1 in 8, or 12 percent, generated in the absolute risk equation (see above) because that is based on all women regardless of risk factors. Rather, you need a number that will reflect the risk of a woman without the factors being considered. For a woman with no clear risk factors at all (no previous cancers, no family history, menarche after 11, menopause before 52, first pregnancy before 30) this is 1 in 30, or 3.3 percent, significantly lower than the "average" risk of 12 percent.[1]

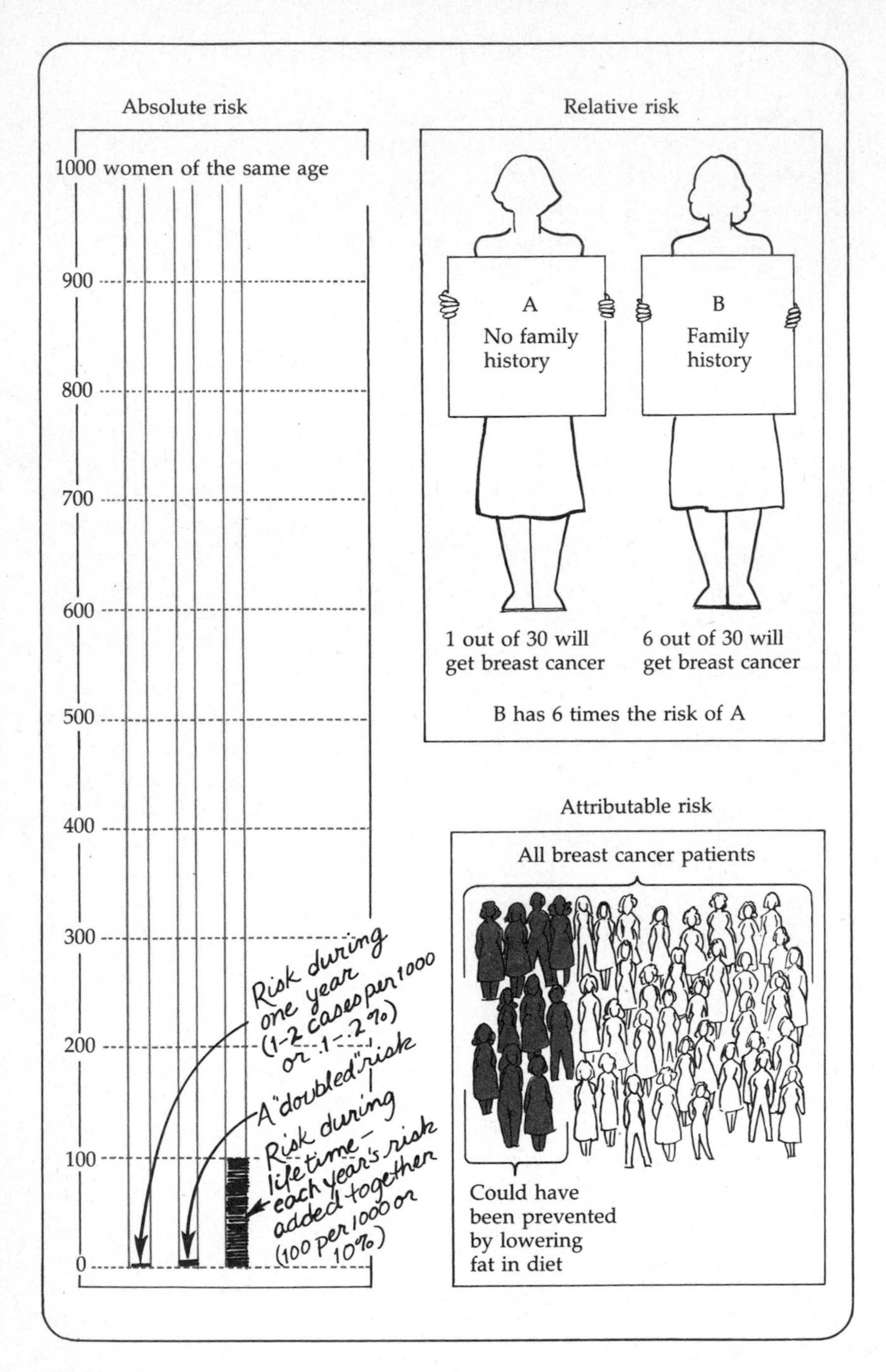

Absolute risk
1000 women of the same age
900
800
700
600
500
400
300
200
100
0
Risk during one year (1-2 cases per 1000 or .1-.2%)
A "doubled" risk
Risk during lifetime—each year's risk added together (100 per 1000 or 10%)
Relative risk
A
No family history
B
Family history
1 out of 30 will get breast cancer
6 out of 30 will get breast cancer
B has 6 times the risk of A
Attributable risk
All breast cancer patients
Could have been prevented by lowering fat in diet

FIGURE 9-1

Table 9-1. Breast Cancer Incidence in Different Racial/Ethnic Groups

	Age-adjusted Cases/ 100,000 women/year	*Lifetime risk percent*	*Lifetime risk*
Caucasian	141	14.1%	1 in 7
African American	122	10.2%	1 in 10
Asian/Pacific Islanders	97		
Hispanics	90		
American Indians/ Alaskan Natives	58		

Source: A. Ghafoor, A. Samuels, A. Jemal. *Breast Cancer Facts and Figures 2003–2004.* American Cancer Society, pg 3. Accessed online on 4/17/05 at www.cancer.org

Table 9-2. Age Specific Probabilities of Developing Breast Cancer

If current age is:	*Then probability of developing breast cancer in the next 10 years is:*	*Or 1 in:*
20	0.05%	2,152
30	0.40%	251
40	1.45%	69
50	2.78%	36
60	3.81%	26
70	4.31%	23

Source: American Cancer Society Surveillance Research 2003

If you call the risk of the woman without any particular risk factors 1.0, you can report the risk of those *with* a particular risk factor in relation to this. This is how relative risk is derived. A woman whose mother had breast cancer in both breasts before the age of 40, for example, has a relative risk of 2.7 over her lifetime—that is, 2.7 times that of the woman with no family history, not, as it might appear, 2.7 times the 12 percent mentioned above (see Table 9-3).

How an increase in relative risk will affect your absolute risk also depends on your age at the time. For example, a threefold relative risk (compared to that of the general population) at a young age will increase your absolute risk by about 20 percent, while by age 50, the woman with the threefold increased relative risk has a lifetime risk of about 14 percent. One-third of the breast cancers occur before age 50

Table 9-3. Factors That Increase the Relative Risk for Breast Cancer in Women

Relative Risk	*Factor*
Relative Risk >4.0	• Age (65+ vs. <65 years, although risk increases across all ages until age 80)
	• Certain inherited genetic mutations for breast cancer (BRCA 1 and/or BRCA 2)
	• Two or more first-degree relatives with breast cancer diagnosed at an early age
	• Personal history of breast cancer
	• Postmenopausal breast density
Relative Risk 2.1-4.0	• One first-degree relative with breast cancer
	• Biopsy-confirmed atypical hyperplasia
	• High-dose radiation to chest
	• High bone density (postmenopausal)
Relative Risk 1.1-2.0	
Reproductive factors	• Late age at first full-term pregnancy (>30 years)
	• Early menarche (<12 years)
	• Late menopause (>55 years)
	• No full-term pregnancies
	• Never breast fed a child
Factors that affect circulating hormones	• Recent oral contraceptive use
	• Recent and long term use of hormone-replacement therapy
	• Obesity (postmenopausal)
Other factors	• Personal history of cancer of endometrium, ovary or colon
	• Alcohol consumption
	• Tall
	• High socioeconomic status
	• Jewish heritage

Source: A. Ghafoor, A. Samuels, A. Jemal. *Breast Cancer Facts and Figures 2003-2004.* American Cancer Society, pg 3. Accessed online on 4/17/05 at www.cancer.org

and so her risk is only two-thirds of that. She has about a 4.5 percent chance of developing breast cancer over the next 10 years and about 10.5 percent in the next 20 years, compared with the average risks of 1.5 and 3.5 percent, respectively.[2]

When you read a study or see one reported in the media, it is important to check the basis for the relative risk numbers. Most authors compare women with a specific risk factor to women without it. They assume that all the other risk factors are equal in both groups, so that only their risk in terms of the risk factor of interest is being compared. It's like the fat in the milk: the numbers can be very misleading if you don't take the time to put them in context.

Finally, we must consider the *attributable risk*. This concept relates more to public policy. It looks at the amount of disease in the population that could be prevented by alteration of risk factors. For example, a risk factor could convey a very large relative risk but be restricted to a few individuals, so changing it would only benefit these individuals. Dr. Anthony B. Miller has hypothesized that if every woman in the world were to have a baby before 25, 17 percent of the world's breast cancer would be eliminated.[3] If you were looking at this from a public health policy perspective, you'd have to weigh the possible advantages of pushing early pregnancy against the problems of young and possibly immature parents, and possible increased population growth (Table 9-3).

What do we mean by risk factors and how are they determined? "Risk factor" is a term referring to identifiable factors that make some people more susceptible than others to a particular disease; that is, smoking is a risk factor in lung cancer, and high cholesterol is a risk factor in heart disease. Medical researchers attempt to define risk factors in order to discover who is most likely to get a particular disease, and also to get clues as to the disease's cause and thus to the possible prevention and/or cure. A risk factor is usually determined by an observational study.

Sometimes, as in the case of lung cancer and smoking, risk factors are dramatic and can make a clear difference in the individual's likelihood of getting the disease. Unfortunately, it usually doesn't work this way. In breast cancer, we have come up with some risk factors—such as family history—which we'll look at in this chapter. But so far, there is nothing comparable to the connections found between cholesterol and heart disease or between smoking and lung cancer. With breast cancer, the sad reality is that we can't say, as with lung cancer, "You're fairly safe because you're not in this particular population." In fact, 70 percent of breast cancer patients have none of the classical risk factors in their background.[4] It's important to understand this, for two reasons. Overestimating the importance of risk factors can cause needless mental anguish if you have one of them in your background. On the other hand, you may harbor a false sense of security if you don't have them. I can't count the number of times patients have come to me with a suspicious lump that turns out to be malignant and, stunned, say, "I don't know how this happened! No one in my family ever had breast cancer!" I tell them they're in good company—most breast cancer patients don't have a family history of breast cancer. By virtue of being women, we are at risk for breast cancer.

Risk factors don't necessarily increase in a simple arithmetical fashion: if one risk factor gives you a 20 percent risk of getting breast cancer and another gives you a 10 percent chance, it doesn't always mean that now you're up to 30 percent. The interaction of risk factors is a tricky and complicated process. One interesting example is studies on alcohol and breast cancer (which we'll consider later) showing that women with other risk factors who also drank liquor didn't increase their risk very much, while women with no other risk factors who drank raised their risk dramatically.[5]

If only we could say, "This causes breast cancer so don't do it!" But breast cancer is a "multifactorial disease"—it has many causes that interact with one another in ways we don't understand yet. So why do we even bother with all these risk factors if they don't really help determine the risk to the individual woman? We do it because it will give us hints as to the cause of the disease—and thus more tools for its prevention and cure. So read on, not to calculate your exact risk or that of your daughter or even to learn how to live your life risk free, but to explore the mystery that is breast cancer.

As I noted earlier, the older you are, the higher are your chances of getting breast cancer. The publicity about breast cancer, which has increased rapidly in recent years, gives the impression that the disease is hitting younger and younger women. That's partially true. The *percentage* of young women getting breast cancer is the same as it's always been. It's the *number* of younger women in the country that has risen in recent years, because the baby boomers are in their 40s and 50s. If you take 10 percent of 40, you get 4; if you take 10 percent of 400, you get 40. There are more 40-something women with breast cancer because there are more 40-something women around. (There's no breast cancer rise among postboomers, by the way. There are fewer of them than boomers, and breast cancer in really young women—teens and 20s—has always been unusual.)

Most breast cancer still occurs in women over 50—about 80 percent of cases. Your risk at age 30 of getting breast cancer in the next 10 years (see Table 9-2) is 1 in 251. By age 40, it's 1 in 69 in the next 10 years.[6] So the risk of getting breast cancer before you're 50 is very small. The median age for breast cancer diagnosis is 64, which means that half of women who get breast cancer will get it before age 64 and half will get it after.

So whenever you look at risk factors, you need to correct for age. Other risk factors (e.g., family history, hormonal factors) will most likely cause breast cancer only in combination with rising age.

Another factor we need to look at is the variation among ethnic groups. Almost all the data you read are based on non-Hispanic Caucasian women. Table 9-1 demonstrates that the risk for African American and Asian women is lower than for white women. But this is deceptive. At age 30 the 10-year risk for an African American woman is 0.5 percent, while it is 0.4 percent for a Caucasian woman, 0.3 percent for a Hispanic woman, and 0.4 percent for an Asian/Pacific Islander. The disparity between white and black women exists because African American women have rates similar to those of white women premenopausally, but lower than those of whites postmenopausally. That won't necessarily be comforting news to African American women, however, since, though it's less common in that group, it's often more deadly (see Chapter 19). When Rowan Chlebowski looked at the postmenopausal women who participated in the large Women's Health Initiative study, he found that most of the differences in incidence attributed to race and ethnicity could be explained by known risk factors except for those in African Americans.[7]

Interestingly, there's also a class variation—white women of higher socioeconomic status get more breast cancer than poorer white women.[8] Black women of higher socioeconomic status also have a higher risk than poorer black women. Breast cancer seems to "discriminate" opposite to the way our society discriminates.

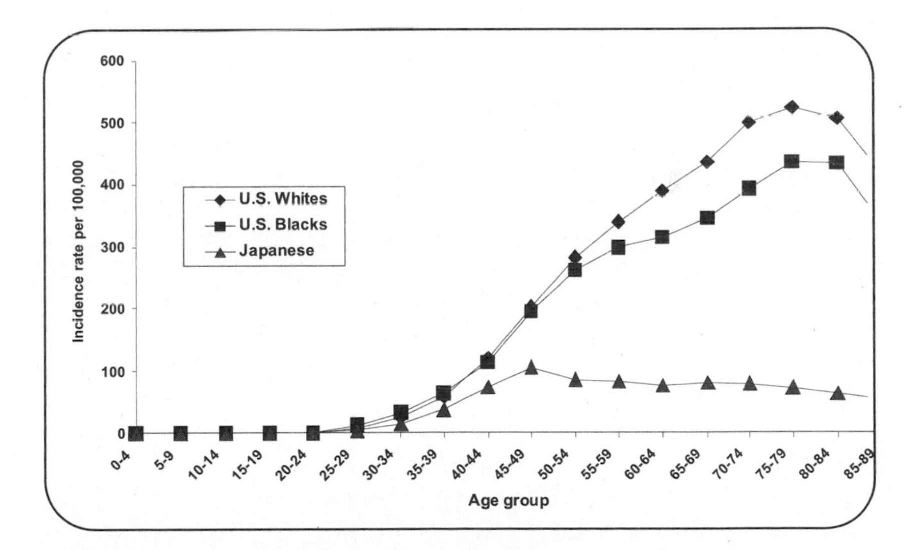

FIGURE 9-2. Age-Specific Breast Cancer Incidence Rates

Source: W.C. Willett, B. Rockhill, S.E. Hankinson, D. Hunter, G.A. Colditz, "Nongenetic factors in the causation of breast cancer," Chapter 16 in Harris JR, Lippman ME, Morrow M, Osborne CK, eds. *Diseases of the Breast*, 3rd ed. Philadelphia: J.B. Lippincott, Williams & Wilkins, 2004, p. 225.

The difference in vulnerability to breast cancer works on an international level as well. Third World countries have less breast cancer than highly industrialized countries do.

The only likely possibility that we've come up with so far is one I'll discuss in a later chapter. These days many white middle- and upper-class women tend to have their first child later in life, and a small subset of these women choose to have no children at all. In addition, they are more likely to take hormones. This trend doesn't follow in non-Caucasian women or women of lower socioeconomic groups in the United States, nor in women of Third World countries. But that's not enough to explain the whole difference.

Risk in Lesbians

In 1993 there was a lot of publicity about the possibility that lesbians are at higher risk of breast cancer—1 in 3 instead of 1 in 8. This was based on research done by Suzanne Haynes from the National Cancer Institute.[9] She had looked at studies done on lesbians who frequented gay bars in the 1950s and had filled out questionnaires about their lifestyle. Then she took the characteristics identified in those studies and matched them with known breast cancer risk factors. She hypothesized that there should be a larger amount of breast cancer in lesbians than in heterosexual women. The factors she was looking at were not directly related to their sexual preference, but to the lifestyle common to the lesbians who had been studied. Since they spent a lot of time at bars, they tended to drink a lot of alcohol and many were obese. Most had not been pregnant. These are in themselves risk factors for breast cancer. Haynes did not necessarily believe lesbians had a greater risk of breast cancer than heterosexual women. But there hadn't been any studies on lesbians and breast cancer, and she was trying to show the research establishment that it was a population that needed to be studied. As a result of her work, studies are now being done. The Women's Health Initiative, which is researching estrogen, diet, and other aspects of women's health, includes a question about sexual preference so that we can begin to get information that will tell us whether lesbians are indeed at higher risk, or have particular risks.

In 1998, the *Journal of the Gay and Lesbian Medical Association* published a study by Stephanie Roberts, done for the Lyon Martins Women's Health Services. Roberts looked at a group of women 35 and older, half of whom were lesbians and half not. She asked them a number of questions. Interestingly, though the lesbians didn't seem to have a greater incidence of breast cancer than the straight women, they did have more breast biopsies. This finding was a bit surprising and she is researching it further. They also had a higher body mass (possibly because they were less concerned with looking thin, which is perceived in our culture as necessary to "catch a man"). The heterosexual women had higher rates of smoking and—less confusingly—of birth control pill use, pregnancy, and miscarriage.

HORMONAL RISK FACTORS

Aside from genetic risk factors, which we will examine in the next chapter, the other obvious group of risk factors is hormonal. We know that hormones play a large part in breast cancer because it is common in women and rare in men, and, as noted in Chapter 1, women's breasts undergo a complex hormonal evolution that men's don't. We don't yet understand what the hormonal risk factors are, but we have some interesting clues.

Early Influences

Some of the most intriguing data since the third edition of this book suggest that prenatal influences may affect breast cancer risk. Data are pretty consistent that birth weight (which gives us clues as to what in

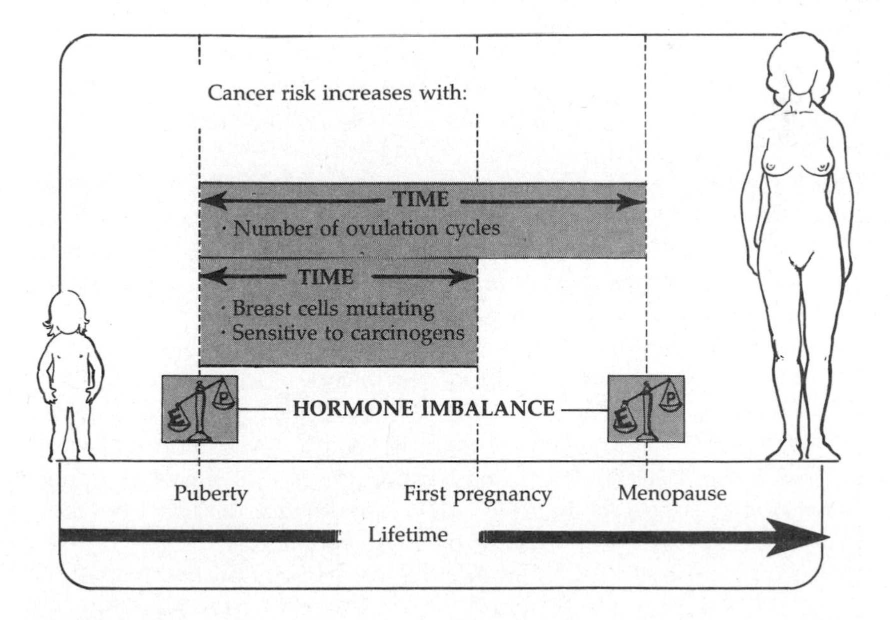

FIGURE 9-3

utero estrogen levels were) correlates with later breast cancer risk.[10] On the other hand, preeclampsia, a condition associated with low estrogen levels, decreases the subsequent breast cancer risk of the child.[11,12] Other factors that indicate good nutrition during childhood also correlate with breast cancer risk. The hypothesis is that early stimulants for growth also increase the number of breast stem cells that are available to undergo mutations later in life.[13] The mutations can be inherited or acquired by exposure to carcinogens.

As we will see in Chapter 28, breast cancer is not just based on abnormal cells with mutations but also on the local environment they find themselves in. The hormones we are exposed to during our lives (our own or those we take) probably influence this aspect of cancer development.

For example, the younger a woman is at her first period and the older she is when she goes into menopause, the more likely she is to get breast cancer (Table 9-3). The longer a woman has reproductive levels of hormones, the more prone she is to breast cancer. If she menstruates for more than 40 years, she seems to have a particularly high risk. If your ovaries are removed early and no hormone replacement is given, your risk of breast cancer is greatly reduced.[14] It's not exactly a cure-all, however, since it would also greatly increase your danger of osteoporosis. If you've had a hysterectomy, it may or may not influence your vulnerability to breast cancer, depending upon whether your ovaries were removed. If you still have ovaries, your body is still going through hormonal cycles, even though you have no periods.

Pregnancy also appears to affect breast cancer risk in two ways. During a pregnancy and for the ten years following it, a woman has a greater risk of developing breast cancer, presumably because the hormones of pregnancy cause more cell division.[15,16] However, women who have never been pregnant seem to be more at risk than women who have a child before 35. The hormones of a pregnancy carried to term will mature the breast tissue, making it less susceptible to carcinogens. Women who have their first pregnancies after 35 have a greater risk than women who have never been pregnant at all. Although it had been hypothesized that therapeutic abortion or miscarriage might increase breast cancer risk, large studies have shown no association.[17,18,19] Breast-feeding is protective against breast cancer, the relative risk decreasing 4.3 percent for every 12 months, in addition to a decrease of 7 percent for each birth. This in part explains some of the discrepancy between more developed and less developed countries, as there tends to be more and longer breast feeding in poorer countries.[20]

After menopause, high blood levels of estrogen and testosterone, which often reflect earlier reproductive and menstrual factors, lend themselves to an increased risk of breast cancer.[21,22]

Breast Density

One marker for hormonal effects on the breast appears to be mammographic density. You will recall from Chapter 7 that breast tissue, which is dense, shows up white on the mammogram, while fat tissue shows up gray. Women whose mammograms show very dense tissue are at significantly higher risk of breast cancer. Although some researchers have attributed this to an increase in breast cells, I think the evidence suggests it is the stroma, or local environment, that is being affected. For example, one of the dangers of hormone therapy is that a third of women taking it show increased breast density on mammogram, which starts right away. As noted in Chapter 7, there are some epidemiological data showing that this is a problem for two reasons. One is that dense tissue makes it more difficult to see lumps on the mammogram. The other is that the stroma in the breast tissue is being stimulated. When I was first told this, I thought it was foolish—the dense breast tissue that shows on the mammogram isn't what gets cancer; the cells within the ducts get cancer. But now we're learning that there is constant "cross talk" between cells and their neighbors, and it isn't quite so easy to dismiss. Further, observational studies have suggested that progestin added to estrogen increases the density, resulting in risk more than estrogen alone.[23] One interesting but not yet proven hypothesis is that if you begin hormone therapy and your mammograms start to get a lot denser, it *might* be a sign that you're one of the people who shouldn't be taking hormones. On the other hand, if your mammograms don't show more density, *maybe* you could feel better about taking them.

There are increasing data to support this theory, though they're not yet conclusive. As we'll see in Chapter 11, Malcolm Pike from the University of Southern California has developed a pill for breast cancer prevention that essentially puts a woman into a state of reversible menopause. It blocks all hormones (see Chapter 18). After six months in a small study, the volunteers' mammograms were much less dense. Tamoxifen also reduces breast density almost immediately.

Along with the hormones our bodies produce, there are all the hormones we willingly ingest over our lives. As we might expect, studies show that such hormones also have effects on the breast.

Birth Control Pills

The birth control pill, originally seen as the magic solution to unwanted pregnancy, was vilified when its negative side effects became apparent. As is often the case, the reality of the pill is more complex.

Especially in its early forms, the pill seemed to contribute to a number of illnesses, including stroke (especially in combination with cigarette smoking in women over 30). Later studies, however, have suggested that it may also be useful in protecting against certain diseases such as ovarian cancer. It stops ovulation, and the more you ovulate the more chance you have of getting ovarian cancer. So if you take the birth control pill and decrease the total number of ovulations, you can decrease your risk. It has consistently been shown to reduce endometrial cancer as well.[24,25]

Part of the problem in discussing "the pill" as though it were a single entity is that it, like some other inventions, has gone through many permutations. The earlier pills used much more estrogen and progestin than current pills do; we've changed both the amounts and the proportions of those hormones. So early findings aren't necessarily applicable to the pill used today. A study that says it's looking at women who have been on the pill for 10 or 20 years is actually likely to be looking at women who have been on a number of different pills at different times—which explains in part why we seem to get so many contradictory results with studies on the relationship between breast cancer and the pill. A 2002 study looked at 9,257 women between 35 and 64 (old enough to have taken oral contraceptives early in their reproductive years). It found no increased risk of breast cancer in either current or former users of the pill.[26] This may not be true for all women, however, since at least one study suggests that women who carry the BRCA 1 gene for breast cancer had a 3 percent to 40 percent increase in breast cancer compared to gene carriers who did not take the pill.[27]

I am more concerned with the use of the birth control pill to treat the symptoms of perimenopause. Here we are dealing with women who are closer to the age of menopause and increased breast cancer risk. It is becoming common for gynecologists to use birth control pills to treat hot flashes and perimenopausal symptoms in women who are still menstruating. It makes sense that the pill could help hot flashes by balancing out hormone shifts, although I have been unable to find any studies on this approach. (Smokers and women with high blood pressure, however, should not take the pill because of the possible increased risk of stroke.) An analysis of the effect of birth control pills on the risk of breast cancer by age found no increased risk among women age 24 to 39, but did find a risk for women under 24 and over 39 who were currently taking the pill. Specifically, women between 46 and 54 had just about double the risk of breast cancer. Among those who stopped taking the pill, the additional risk disappeared after three years. This would suggest that women should approach this therapy with the same caution as they would menopausal estrogen therapy.

DES

Another external hormone women have taken is the estrogen DES. It was used in the 1940s through 1960s to increase fertility and prevent miscarriage. A 1984 study showed a slight increase—1.4—in breast cancer among women who took DES while pregnant.[28] Since there's a lot of estrogen going through your body anyway when you're pregnant, it's not clear why an increased external dosage would be harmful, but it appears to have been, at least for some women. One theory is that exposure to estrogen during the period of rapid growth of breast tissue during pregnancy may increase risk.[29] We don't know yet what effects DES had on the breast cancer rate among daughters of women who'd taken it, since the daughters are only now approaching the age when breast cancer is most common. There has been an increase in vaginal cancer among this population, but it's not as aggressive as we once thought it was.

Postmenopausal Hormone Therapy

Over the past several decades we have shifted from considering menopause as a natural part of life to thinking about it as a disease that needs to be treated. It is hard sometimes to determine how much of that approach is thinly veiled marketing for the panoply of drugs offered to us as we age. Menopause is a natural part of life, just as fertility is. Our bodies need high levels of hormones to reproduce, and they need the downshift to a more reasonable level postmenopausally (see Chapter 1). Those who favor hormone therapy argue that we're not "supposed" to live long enough to go into menopause in the first place; in the old days people died in their 30s and 40s. But in fact people *didn't* all die in their 30s and 40s. The "average life expectancy" was low—as low as 32 in 1640. But that average was drawn from all deaths and did not represent a "typical age of death." Until modern medicine came along, there were large numbers of deaths at all ages, and especially in childhood. It was no more usual to die at 35 than at 65. Men were considered fit for military service until they were 60, and a fair number of people of both genders lived into their 90s.[30,31,32] So that argument makes no sense.

We once believed that the ovaries stopped functioning at menopause. Recent studies have shown that to be a fallacy—most women's ovaries don't stop functioning. But until recently, there was no test available that could detect lower levels of estrogen, and so it was assumed that there weren't any such levels. Actually most women continue to produce hormones well into their 80s—testosterone, androstenedione (both "male" hormones), and even some estrogen.

And we are starting to understand the symptoms of menopause better as well. The traditional belief is that the symptoms of perimenopause come from low levels of hormones, but recent studies have shown that what's really at the core of symptoms is the *fluctuation* of hormones as the body rebalances at a new level. The transition typically takes between three and six years, and then the body settles into its new situation.

Although menopause is a normal passage of life, it has been redefined as a disease called "estrogen deficiency." And since it's a disease, the assumption is that it should be treated. In reality if "estrogen deficiency" is a disease, then all men are sick. Imagine how they could decrease their risk of heart disease, prostate cancer, and osteoporosis if they took the "miracle drug" menopausal women are so often prescribed! Notice we even call the treatment "hormone replacement therapy," which implies we are missing something that needs to be replaced. A far better term is "hormone therapy," which implies rightly that these are drugs being given to treat or prevent disease—if and when they're needed.

It's important, when discussing hormone therapy, to differentiate between the two very distinct reasons women might want to use it: symptom control and disease prevention. Hormone therapy helps reduce hot flashes, vaginal dryness, insomnia, night sweats—the vast range of uncomfortable, usually short-term symptoms many women experience during their perimenopausal years. In natural menopause, these symptoms are usually transient—they last about three to five years. After that, your body readjusts itself and you're fine. The use of hormones short-term (three to five years) for women who do not have breast cancer or clotting disorders is probably safe. At the end of the period they should taper off the hormones over six to nine months in order to ensure that the abrupt change doesn't bring back their symptoms. In women who have had breast cancer it is better to explore alternative methods to decrease symptoms, which we discuss at length in Chapter 26.

The third edition of this book had a long explanation of my concerns about the safety of taking hormone replacement therapy (HRT or estrogen and progestin) for prevention of the diseases of aging. For this edition I actually have some data. The Women's Health Initiative is a large randomized study of menopausal women. It has several components: HRT versus placebo, estrogen replacement therapy (ERT) versus placebo, low-fat diet, calcium and vitamin D, and an observational study. In 2002 the study made headlines when the estrogen and progestin arm was stopped prematurely after finding an alarming increase in breast cancer risk of 24 percent. It concluded that "relatively short-term combined estrogen plus progestin use increases incident breast cancers, which are diagnosed at a more advanced stage compared with placebo use and also substantially increases the percentage of women with abnormal mammograms. These results suggest estrogen plus progestin may stimulate breast cancer growth and hinder breast cancer diagnosis."[33] Some critics suggested that the effect on mammography and cancer was too fast for it to have been caused by the HRT. However, the effect may have been on the stroma rather than the epithelial cells. This would also correlate with an increase in mammographic density. The study also showed an increase in stroke, heart disease, and dementia.

Although the data surprised many, they confirmed numerous observational studies that had gone before.[34] In these studies the women who were currently taking HRT and had taken it for the longest time showed the greatest risk for breast cancer. As with birth control pills, stopping the drugs causes the risk to go away over time.

The estrogen-alone study was continued, but it also was stopped prematurely in 2004.[35] Here the findings were even more surprising: there was no increase in breast cancer risk or benefit to heart disease. This latter is highly significant, as the supposed capacity to prevent heart disease was one of the big selling points of estrogen therapy. As with HRT, there was an increase in stroke and a decrease in fracture rate. Again, this was consistent with earlier observational studies, which had shown that the risk of estrogen alone was significantly less than that of estrogen plus progestin (1 percent versus 8 percent/year).[36] And estrogen alone has less effect on mammographic density than estrogen plus a progestin.[37] In addition, studies that have looked at the *duration* of estrogen use show the biggest risk. Bruce Ettinger of Kaiser Permanente looked at a series of women who had used estrogen for at least seventeen years. The study found a doubling of the risk of breast cancer.[38] (It may seem odd that the study was called Reduced Mortality, but the decreases in cardiovascular disease that it also found appeared to counteract the effects of the increased breast cancer.)

Criticisms of the Women's Health Initiative include the fact that it studied conjugated estrogen (Premarin) and medroxyprogesterone acetate (Provera), synthetic hormones, rather than the newer "bioidentical" hormones that are closer to what our bodies make. (See Chapter 27.) The implication is that natural progesterone and estradiol will be safer for the breast. Perhaps—but we have no data to support that hypothesis. In fact, in the PEPI study progesterone increased mammographic density to almost the same degree as medroxyprogesterone acetate (Provera) did, suggesting that its effect on the breast is the same.[39] Other studies have looked at bioidential hormones, especially ones done in Europe, where conjugated estrogen (Premarin) was not as widely used, and they also show an increased risk.[40]

In October 1997, the Collaborative Group on Hormonal Factors in Breast Cancer brought together and reanalyzed about 90 percent of the worldwide epidemiological evidence on the relation between the risk of breast cancer and the use of hormone replacement therapy of all types. Individual data from 51 studies in 21 countries were collected, checked, and analyzed centrally. They included 52,050 women with breast cancer and 108,411 women without the disease. The analysis found a 35 percent increased breast cancer risk after five years of use, escalating to 53 percent increase after more than five years. Five years after stopping hormones, this increased risk completely disappeared.[41] The Million Women Study from the United Kingdom was an unselected prospective study of a million postmenopausal women initially identified when they had their first mammogram. In the women who used hormone therapy, after 2.5 years they found a 66 percent increase in the incidence of breast cancer, with a 22 percent increased chance of dying of breast cancer within four years. Again the estrogen plus progestin showed the biggest increase. Interestingly they looked at more than just conjugated estrogen (Premarin) and medroxyprogesterone acetate (Provera)—they also included estradiol as well as several different types of progesterone and found very little difference between them.[42] To me the conclusion is clear: there's an increased risk of breast cancer for women who take conjugated estrogen, with or without medroxyprogesterone acetate, postmenopausally for five or more years. It is not a huge increase, however. In the WHI study there were eight more cases of invasive cancer per 10,000 women per year. After five years this would be 4 out of 1,000 women. After 30 years it would be 24 women out of 1,000. And the risk was across all groups of women, not just those with a family history of breast cancer. In fact, the big surprise to me from the WHI is that the risk is not higher. Nonetheless, this risk does give pause. When HRT was believed to decrease heart disease, that was reasonably considered more important. Now the studies are showing no benefit in heart disease but an increase in dementia and stroke; the only thing HRT seems to prevent is osteoporosis. And there are better things you can do for that condition.

One crucial question being being looked at is whether cancers caused by postmenopausal hormone therapy are the same as cancers that occur on their own. At least four recent studies have shown an increase in lobular cancers in women on HRT.[43,44,45,46] This makes some sense, since lobular cancers are almost always sensitive to estrogen. However, they are harder to feel or see on a mammogram and are often diagnosed at a later stage.

Alcohol consumption may also play a role. A couple of studies have shown that the estrogen levels of a woman on hormone therapy are

300 percent higher after she's had a drink. This is particularly true when the medication used is conjugated estrogen (Premarin), which is metabolized by the liver. The liver, as you know, is strongly affected by alcohol. This suggests that if you want to use hormone therapy, you should probably have fewer than three alcoholic drinks a week—maybe save your drinks for very special occasions. (Remember, as I explain elsewhere in this chapter, drinking already increases your breast cancer risk.)

Finally I take a cautionary stance on using testosterone. There is an increasing call for the use of testosterone to treat decreased libido in postmenopausal women. However, there are no long-term safety data on this drug. As we have learned, just because you had more of it when you were premenopausal doesn't mean it is safe to take it when you are postmenopausal. We noted earlier in this chapter that women who have higher levels of testosterone have higher levels of breast cancer. Even the over-the-counter supplement DHEA is suspect. You need to be careful about what you put in your body and demand long-term safety data. At the very least, ask yourself if the risk is worth what you believe the gain to be, before taking such medications for the long-term.

FERTILITY DRUGS

Fertility drugs are being used a lot these days as the baby boomers who postponed childbearing are now trying to get pregnant. We don't know how safe fertility drugs are or how they interact with breast cancer. Some data suggest that use of clomiphene citrate (Clomid), which makes your ovaries work harder, will increase ovarian cancer since the more you ovulate the stronger your chance is of getting ovarian cancer, and the drugs make you hyperovulate.[47] Then there are drugs like Human Menopausal Gonadotropin (Perganol), which, like conjugated estrogen (Premarin), comes from the urine of pregnant mares, and which also causes you to hyperovulate. These all stimulate the ovaries. There's also HCG, human chorionic gonadotropin—the hormone that actually goes up in pregnancy. By the time you're taking fertility drugs you're probably over 30 and haven't had a child yet—a combination that already increases your risk of breast cancer. The drugs and hormones might also add a promoter effect. It's very important for women to realize that we don't know the relationship of these drugs to breast cancer, but they're likely to have some effect, since DES and the other hormones do.

Some of the differences in effects between our own levels of hormones and those we take may be from our ability to metabolize them. One interesting study suggests that the risk of breast cancer with oral contraceptives may be related to the way they are broken down by the body and that this may be different in different women.[48] This may explain why postmenopausal hormones don't increase breast cancer risk more. The other factor may be the breast itself. We now know that the breast is capable of making estrogen locally, at least in some women, and that the tissue around a tumor has higher estrogen levels than the tissue far from it.[49] The problem may be less the hormones we take than the ones found locally in the breast. That research is just beginning to be done, so stay tuned.

PESTICIDES AND OTHER ENVIRONMENTAL HAZARDS

Sources of estrogen in the environment are organochlorines (DDT) and PCBs, persistent environmental contaminants known as estrogen mimics that have been identified throughout the global ecosystem in, for example, fish, wildlife, and human tissue, including blood and breast milk.

One reason many people believe that DDT and PCBs are related to breast cancer is that a lot of them are broken down in the body to weak forms of estrogen, which, it's thought, can stimulate and cause breast cancer just as estrogen can.

But this isn't always the case with weak estrogens. Phytoestrogens like soy and the weak estrogen of tamoxifen have very different effects, as we'll see in Chapters 11 and 26. Weak estrogens are not necessarily linked to the effects of estrogen. The biology of estrogen, estrogen

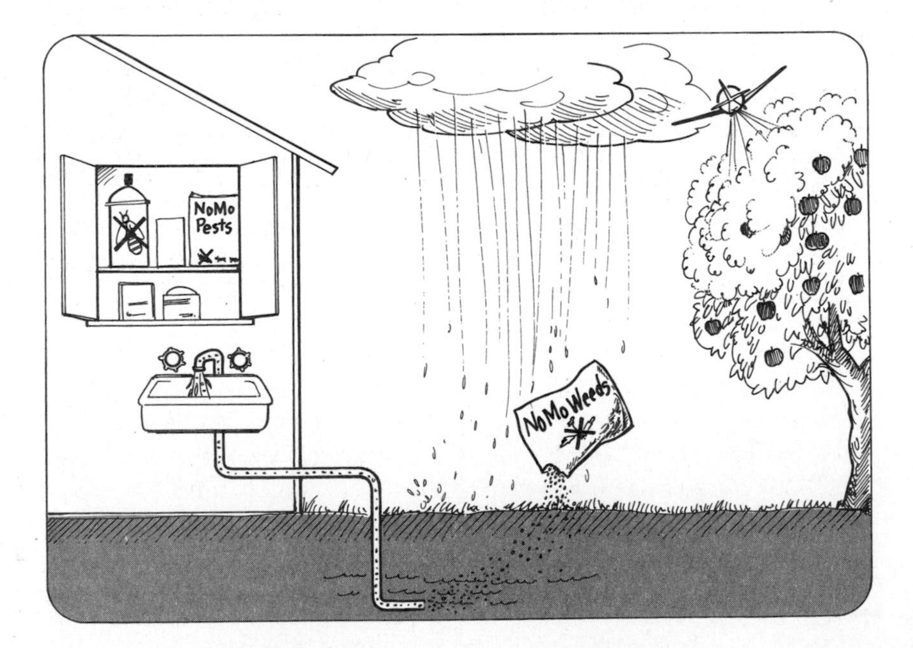

receptors, and the selective estrogen receptor modulators is very complex.

Several observational studies have been done and have failed to demonstrate a relationship between occupational exposure to pesticides and breast cancer. For example, the Nurses Health Study, a European study, and one from Mexico, where levels are especially high, have all found no relationship between blood levels of DDE and PCBs and breast cancer.[50,51,52] At the same time, observational studies can miss connections. Many of the studies that initially showed a relationship found it disappeared with further follow-up.[53]

Breast cancer activists on Cape Cod and Long Island (where there is very high risk of breast cancer) were responsible for some of the studies done in the early 1990s. They demanded that the Centers for Disease Control (CDC) investigate the high incidence of breast cancer in their areas. Though the studies have shown no relation between breast cancer and pesticides, it opened the way to breast cancer activism and raised some questions that remain unanswered.[54] Why were these populations getting more breast cancer?

I think that the issue is complex and must take into consideration time of exposure and other associated risk factors. There still may be an environmental relationship, but it is probably small. Nonetheless, this lack of definitive answers is no excuse for not cleaning up the environment. There are enough known health problems from environmental pollution to convince us that it needs to be seriously curtailed. This is a fairly new area of scientific study. Who knows what we'll find in the next 5 or 10 years?

Equally important are nonhormonal external factors that can create a breast cancer–causing mutation or accelerate the growth of breast cancer or, for that matter, prevent the growth of breast cancer. Diet, alcohol, and certain medications carry risks over which we have some control. The amount of fat and liquor you consume may play a role in increasing your susceptibility to breast cancer. Radiation has always been known to increase cancer risk, and may or may not be something over which you have control.

DIET

The idea that dietary fat can contribute to breast cancer has been around for a long time. It began with the observation that breast cancer is lower in Japan than in the United States, and that the incidence increases when women move from Japan to the United States. As proponents of this theory note, one of the many cultural differences in the immigrant group is diet. Charts of fat intake in different countries

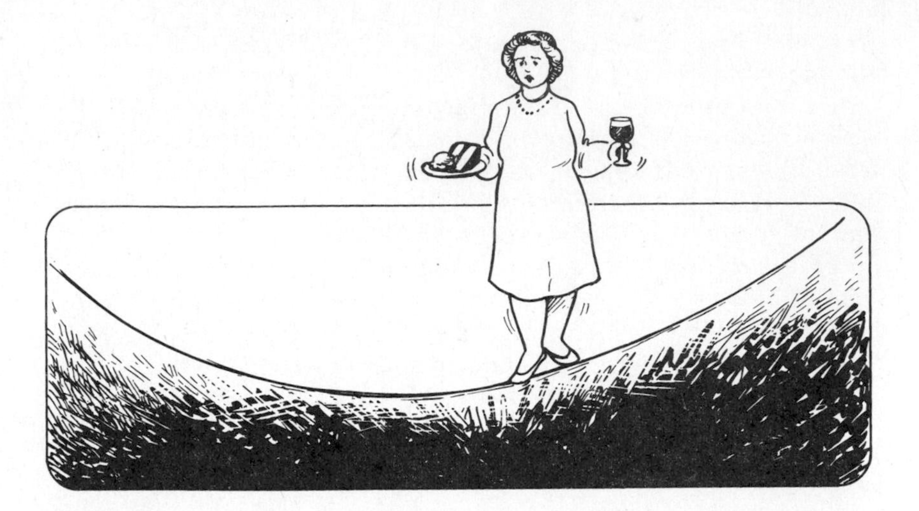

overlaid on charts of breast cancer incidence appear to confirm the association.

But, as I've mentioned a number of times, this kind of parallel doesn't necessarily mean cause and effect. Northern European countries tend to have both a high-fat diet and an increase in breast cancer. But they also have a high-calorie diet. Further, they tend to have the same genetic background, which has been passed on to most of us in the New World. These, or other factors, might be equally or even solely significant.

The high-fat breast cancer hypothesis was put to the test in rats, and it was found that the total calorie count seems to be more important than the amount of fat. Further tests on human subjects suggest that this is true in women as well.

Some researchers feel that the type of fat may be important, but a recent analysis of the Nurses' Health Study failed to find an association between any type of fat and breast cancer.[55] Although the large numbers of women in this study increase its power to demonstrate a relationship, it is an observational study and thus not as conclusive as we'd like. The Women's Health Initiative, which is randomized and prospective, has the best chance of answering the fat and breast cancer question.

It won't, however, be the definitive study by any means. Postmenopausal women are more likely than younger ones to get breast cancer, but the factors that give them the cancer may, as noted earlier, begin during adolescence. So if it turns out that changing her diet at age 55 doesn't affect a woman's chance of getting breast cancer, that doesn't necessarily mean fat has no role in the disease. We need another study, one that starts in adolescence and monitors the young woman's diet throughout her life.

Designing such a study seems difficult at this point. My teenager doesn't welcome advice about what to eat. Still, we must figure out a way to create such a study. We desperately need research to not only identify the culprits in our Western high-fat diet but pinpoint when they do their dirty work. If it's during adolescence, then it's pointless for us to encourage 50-year-old women to change their diets as a method of lessening breast cancer risk.

Of course, the fact that fat intake probably doesn't cause breast cancer doesn't mean you should scarf down a pound cake and a wheel of Brie every day. Fat still plays a large role in heart disease and other illnesses.

Indeed, some studies suggest that the amount of fat we eat may be an indirect cause of breast cancer for just this reason. Being high in calories, fat creates greater weight. Some data show that the taller and fatter a postmenopausal woman is, the more susceptible she is to breast cancer.

Thus it's quite possible that the problem isn't fat but overall nutrition: people who eat more may be more vulnerable to breast cancer. Overnutrition might also have a connection with other risk factors: girls with lower food consumption stay thinner and often begin menstruating later than more heavily nourished girls. People who eat more also tend to be those who can afford to—those with an overall higher standard of living, who appear to be at greater risk for breast cancer.

If fat intake in itself does indeed increase the risk of breast cancer, what makes it happen? There are a number of theories. Some researchers think it changes the metabolism of estrogen. According to one study, people with a high-fat diet tend to have more estrogen in their blood and low urinary excretion of estrogen; vegetarians who eat dairy foods excrete more estrogen, leaving less in the blood, and people on macrobiotic diets, which include a very low amount of fat, have even lower levels of estrogen in their blood and secrete less in their urine.[56] As I noted in Chapter 1, your fat cells can make estrogen, so it is also possible that if you're obese you have an oversupply of estrogen, which could increase your vulnerability to cancer. Studies attempting to confirm this hypothesis have been inconsistent.

It's also possible that cancer cells grow better in an environment with a lot of overnourished cells, and the fatter you are the more such cells there are for the cancer cells to grow with. There's also some evidence that among women with breast cancer those on low-fat diets have a better prognosis than those on high-fat diets.

It may be that fiber, rather than fat, is the important element. Usually diets very high in fiber are very low in fat. It may be that with a low-fat diet it's the fiber or the high-complex carbohydrates or the vegetables you're replacing the fat with that are helping you.

The other possibility is that it isn't the food at all that contributes to breast cancer but the carcinogens and hormones that are in the food. Beef in this country, for example, still has artificial hormones. Unfortunately meat isn't the only problem. Fish are heavily contaminated, since most of our fresh and coastal waters are polluted. Among other things, there is a lot of mercury in the fish we eat. Even vegetables aren't completely safe, since they're sprayed with pesticides.

Overall, the various studies suggest that weight and calorie intake affect your vulnerability to breast cancer. While there isn't nearly the solid proof that there is with smoking and lung cancer, the data are strong enough to make it worthwhile to seriously consider cutting back the calories and animal fat in your diet—especially when you consider that animal fat has proved to be a factor in many other illnesses, and nothing good has ever been shown about high animal fat consumption, except perhaps its nice taste. If you're the parent of a teen or preteen daughter, consider encouraging her to eat a healthy diet, since the evidence suggests that much of the damage may be done early in life. You may want to encourage your kids to spend less time at MacDonald's and eat a bit more low-fat, nutritional food. Don't, however, expect miracles. Even if changing your diet does have an effect, it is likely to be a small one. (See also Chapter 11.)

ALCOHOL CONSUMPTION

Alcohol, the other major dietary substance that has been associated with breast cancer, has received less attention—which is ironic, since the data are more solid. A number of studies suggest that drinking alcoholic beverages, even in moderate amounts, may increase your risk of breast cancer. An analysis of six prospective studies found an increasing risk of breast cancer as larger amounts of alcohol are drunk.[57] Beer, wine, and hard liquor all contribute to breast cancer risk, and as your consumption rises, so does your risk. Another large study asked whether it is what you drink now or what you drank in your wild and crazy youth that makes the difference. Don't worry. You may have made an ass of yourself, but you probably didn't give yourself breast cancer. While recent consumption of three or more drinks per day was associated with a doubling of risk, what you drank between 16 and 29 had little effect.[58]

There is even a reasonable explanation for this effect, since consumption of approximately two alcoholic drinks per day increased levels of estrogen in the blood of premenopausal women, while single doses of alcohol acutely increased them in postmenopausal women.[59,60] Fortunately, good eating habits can help. Several large studies show high intake of folic acid, found in spinach, broccoli, corn, legumes, and multivitamins, appeared to mitigate completely the excess risk of breast cancer due to alcohol.[61,62,63] Since one to two drinks a day have been shown to decrease heart disease, this gives those of you who enjoy your cocktail or glass of wine an out: increase your green leafy vegetables and take a multivitamin. I can just picture it—a spinach martini, with a multivitamin instead of an olive. Actually, one of my friends who dislikes vegetables bought a juicer and invented a broccoli–apple concoction she swears is palatable. Personally, I haven't tried this, but it works for her.

Seriously, whether to stop drinking or not is one of the many decisions we all must make on inadequate information. The risk increase isn't great, but it definitely exists. You alone know how much pleasure you get from your glass of wine or beer, and how alarmed you are at the thought of breast cancer. If it's not all that important to you to drink, you might want to reduce your alcohol consumption to a glass of champagne on New Year's Eve and major celebrations. Although it may be wise for any number of reasons to discourage your daughters from drinking, this is an area, like many in parenting, where you may not have a lot of control.

RADIATION

One of the known risk factors for breast cancer, as well as a variety of other cancers, is radiation. At least three major studies have confirmed that there is indeed a link between radiation and increased risk of breast cancer.

The first study came out of one of the major tragedies of the twentieth century—the bombings of Hiroshima and Nagasaki at the end of World War II. The people in the immediate area of the bombings died instantly, or shortly after the bombs were dropped. But it has become evident that those within a 10-kilometer radius of the bomb sites developed far more cancer than others in comparable populations, and scientists began studying these survivors to learn more about the dangers of radiation. They measured the amount of radiation these people had been exposed to and then followed them over the years to see what cancers they developed.[64]

The best analysis of this sample reports that women exposed to the bomb have a relative risk of developing breast cancer that is much higher if it happened before they were 20 than when they were older.[65] The effects were greatest among women in their teens and early 20s, and nearly nonexistent in women in their 50s and 60s. Reports have indicated an increased risk in the women who were less than 10 years old at the time of the exposure. The effect took longer to be revealed because it didn't appear until the women had reached the age at which breast cancer normally occurs. This supports other findings about the particular vulnerability of the developing breast to carcinogenic agents.

An interesting finding among the A-bomb survivors is that those who had early full-term pregnancies were at significantly lower risk than those who hadn't. Remarkably, this protection occurred among women who were exposed as children, as well as among those exposed as adults. Here is confirmation that the maturation of breast tissue that occurs during a full-term pregnancy drastically reduces the ability of a cell to progress to cancer, even if it has received earlier damage that would predispose it to cancer.[66] This provides us with even more evidence that it often takes more than one factor to cause a breast cancer.

Other studies of radiation exposure support the atom bomb data. The first is a Canadian study that looked at women treated for tuberculosis with fluoroscopy.[67] This was a common treatment in the 1930s and 1940s before we knew of the dangers of radiation and saw it as a magic cure-all. The typical treatment for TB was to collapse the infected lung to rest it and then check it with X rays every day to see how it was doing. When the women were studied in the 1970s, they were found to have an increased incidence of breast cancer. I came across a similar case in my own practice. A 58-year-old patient I diagnosed with breast cancer had TB in her early 20s. She lived in France and was treated with intensive radiation in a sanitarium. Her two best friends at the sanitarium, treated with the same radiation therapy she was given, also developed breast cancer.

Another study examined a group of 606 women in Rochester, New York, who had suffered postpartum mastitis—painfully inflamed breasts (Chapter 5)—and had been given radiation averaging between 50 and 450 rads for both breasts to alleviate their pain.[68] They too had a rate of breast cancer higher than that of the general population. And the risk was dose related. This study is interesting for a second reason. The radiation was given after the first pregnancy, which should have been protective. But nonetheless it was during lactation, a time of high activity in the breast.

There are other studies confirming the existence of radiation-induced breast cancer. One showed an increase in the disease among women with scoliosis who had a lot of X rays to monitor their backs during puberty.[69] Another showed an increase among a group of women who had radiation therapy to their chests for acne—also during puberty.[70] Still another study found an increase in women who had their thymuses radiated in infancy or early childhood to shrink them. (The thymus, a normal gland in the middle of the chest, shrinks with age. At one time before we realized that it shrank normally, radiation therapy was used to shrink it.)[71]

All these studies show that the danger is from exposure to moderate doses of radiation (10–500 rads), and the last two show that the danger is only to the area of the body at which the radiation has been aimed. Thus people exposed to radiation for cancer of the cervix did not show an increased rate of breast cancer.[72] Nagasaki and Hiroshima survivors had their whole bodies exposed to radiation, and they have suffered increased vulnerability to virtually all kinds of cancer. Another interesting finding in all these studies is the long latency period. The excess risk does not appear until the age at which breast cancer commonly occurs. This suggests that radiation is only part of the early picture and that other moderating influences come later and affect the development of breast cancer. The duration of the increased risk from radiation is also not known, but in the atomic bomb survivors, fluoroscopy patients, and mastitis patients, it appears to have lasted at least 35 years from the time of exposure.

This exposure differs from the kind you get with diagnostic chest X rays and mammograms. Many people are legitimately concerned about such X rays, but it's a mistake to throw out a highly useful diagnostic tool. Remember that the danger comes with a total cumulative dose of radiation. If you had a chest X ray every week for two years, you probably would increase your risk of getting breast cancer. But the danger of leaving pneumonia undetected, if you have reason to believe it may exist, is far greater than any danger from infrequent chest X rays. Similarly, the level of radiation in up-to-date mammograms (1/4 of a rad) won't increase your risk of breast cancer, except if you carry a very rare gene that makes you more sensitive to radiation.

Radiation used to treat cancer falls at the other end of the spectrum: very high levels of radiation are used, on the order of 8,000 rads. In these cases, however, the risk from radiation is far outweighed by the risk from cancer. For example, radiation is used to treat Hodgkin's disease, a cancer of the lymph nodes. By itself and in conjunction with chemotherapy it has been responsible for many cures. However, some women who had this treatment years ago are now showing up with breast cancer. We suspect that the radiation to their chests, which saved their lives, is responsible for the second cancer.[73] In a study examining second cancers in those treated for childhood Hodgkin's disease, breast cancer was reported as the most common solid tumor detected. Women in the group studied had 75 times greater risk of developing breast cancer than did women in the general public, and the cancers almost all developed in the radiated area. The younger a woman was when she was radiated, the higher her risk. A second study showed the relative risk of breast cancer after 15 years of follow-up was 11.4 for women who had been under 30 when they were treated and 41.9 for women who had been under 20 when they were treated. When you consider that most risk factors are 0.3, this increase is considerable.

Women who have received radiation exposure to their breasts, especially at a young age, might consider some of the current prevention practices such as taking tamoxifen for five years or even getting prophylactic mastectomy. If those approaches seem too drastic, they should certainly get regular breast exams and mammography beginning 10 years following their radiation.

The type of cancer that occurs after radiation therapy for Hodgkin's disease is similar to the type found in the general population, with 81 percent of lesions detectable by mammography. It usually occurs about 15 years after treatment. While it is for the most part unilateral, it occasionally will occur in both breasts. Treatment is usually a mastectomy because the woman has already had radiation to the chest and cannot get radiation there again.

It won't be surprising if some of the children treated today for cancer with radiation in the chest region will eventually have an increase in breast cancers.[74] This is unfortunate, but since radiation is probably responsible for their living long enough to get a second cancer, few of those patients are likely to have regrets.

OCCUPATIONAL EXPOSURES

You're probably unaware of many breast cancer risks. I used to ask all my patients if they had any environmental or occupational exposures to carcinogens. Almost to a woman, they'd say no. Then I'd ask what they did for a living. Very often they did in fact have exposures. For example, one of my patients worked as a manicurist for 15 years, inhaling fumes from nail polish remover and nail polishes in a close area. Could that be a carcinogen? Another woman was an artist who used oil paints. She was exposed to the solvents used to clean the oil paint as well as the cadmium in the paint, which some studies indicate is a very strong carcinogen.

There are probably a lot of environmental exposures that don't occur to us because we're not used to thinking about life that way. In 1993 the National Cancer Institute held the first conference on occupational risks of cancer in women. (Until then, the assumption seemed to be that women didn't have occupations.) Women who work at home are exposed to many different cleaning solvents and insecticides, which may be among the factors that lead to breast cancer.

Occupational exposure to radiation has been linked to an increased risk of breast cancer in a sample of medical diagnostic X ray workers in China, female employees at a nuclear plant, female and male Finnish

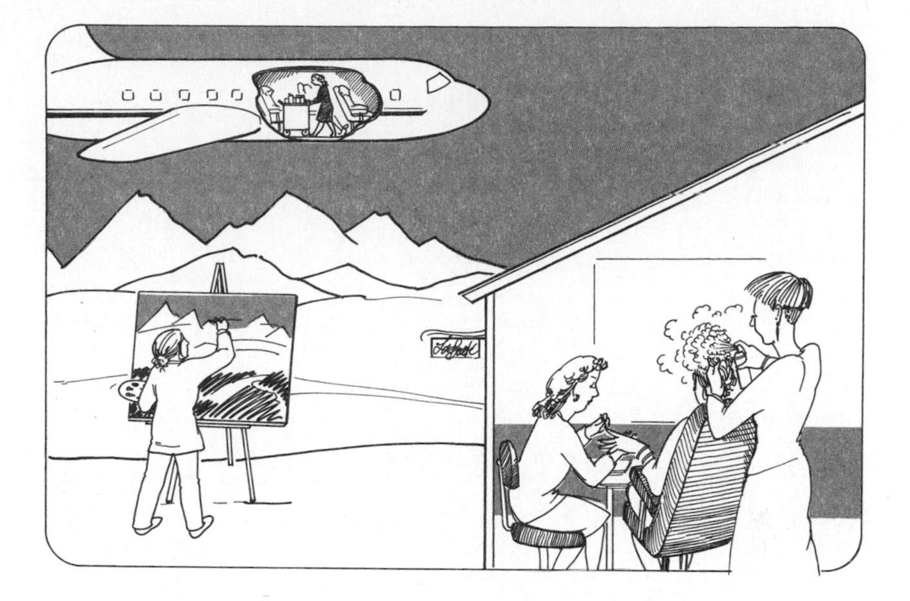

airline cabin attendants, and radiologic technologists in the United States.[75,76,77,78] As opposed to carcinogenic exposures that simply promote cancer, radiation is known to cause mutations in the breast cells. In addition, mutations known as radiosensitizers enhance the effects of radiation. At present at least 21 of these cancer-predisposing genes (see Chapter 10) have been isolated and cloned (9 tumor suppressor genes, 11 DNA repair genes, and 1 proto-oncogene). Also, at least eight other tumor suppressor genes and a gene involved in ataxia telangectasia (AT), a neurological disease, have been found on a specific chromosome. These genes are involved in the control of cellular proliferation, programmed cell death (apoptosis), and DNA repair pathways. Several are examples of radiosensitizers.[79]

ELECTROMAGNETIC FIELD (EMF) EXPOSURE

Another subject that hasn't been well studied is electromagnetic fields. Electric and magnetic fields arise from the motion of electric charges. They are characterized as *nonionizing radiation* when they lack sufficient energy to remove electrons from atoms, as opposed to *ionizing* radiation such as X rays and gamma rays. EMFs are emitted from devices that produce, transmit, or use electric power such as power lines, transmitters, and common household items like electric clocks, shavers, and blankets, computers, televisions, heated waterbeds, and microwave ovens.

There is concern that EMF exposure may increase the incidence of cancers, especially brain tumors and childhood leukemia, although studies have had inconsistent findings.

Artificial light is another source of EMFs. An interesting study done in Seattle on men with breast cancer showed that those who spent many hours in artificial light had a higher rate of breast cancer than men who didn't.[80] (Men were chosen because, since breast cancer is so rare in men, it's easier to find something in common than in the much larger female population. A similar study on women is now under way.) There are several possible theories to explain this. For example, the vitamin D in sunlight may work as a form of breast cancer prevention, whereas artificial light obviously doesn't contain vitamin D.

The researchers in Seattle favor an explanation involving the little organ under the brain called the pineal gland, which is involved in helping you distinguish day and night. It produces a hormone, melatonin, that is excreted in a strong daily rhythm that peaks at night and decreases during the day. It appears that melatonin can be protective of the breast. Electric power produces light at night (electric lighting) and a range of nonionizing electric and magnetic fields. According to a hypothesis developed by Richard Stevens, both light at night and low-level EMF may lower melatonin levels, which may in turn increase breast cancer risk.[81]

The effect of melatonin on breast cancer is based on studies in rats given a carcinogen.[82] The control group developed cancer, but the rats given melatonin didn't. The mechanism for this effect is unclear, but it may be through an increase in estrogen and prolactin, which stimulate breast tissue and/or prevent the growth and spread of cancer cells.

As promising as this hypothesis is, it's only a hypothesis, accompanied by a lot of circumstantial evidence. One problem is the perennial limitation of animal studies: we are not rats. Further, there are vast differences between how light suppresses melatonin, nighttime melatonin levels, and patterns of melatonin release. And while there have been interesting laboratory studies, findings in the laboratory may not reproduce what happens in life. Charles Graham described his findings from double-blind studies in a human research laboratory, which found no effect of overnight exposure to EMF on melatonin levels.[83] But real-world research on garment, utility, railway, and video display terminal workers indicated suppressed levels of melatonin. The different results may be due to differences between laboratory settings and the real world—laboratory research is over a short period of time, while chronic exposure may have more of an effect. Further, laboratory exposures are consistent, while real-world exposure may be relatively low over time with infrequent high exposures that occur in microseconds. These short-term high-energy peaks also occur in the home from utility operation and, unlike low-level EMF, may have enough power to alter cells. An ongoing study is investigating this possibility.[84] We know that women who work on telephone lines have a higher incidence of breast cancer.[85,86] A study of women who were completely blind (and therefore might have high melatonin levels) showed that they had less breast cancer than did the sighted women in the control group. Several other studies have been launched to investigate the potential association between EMFs and breast cancer. A study is in progress at Fred Hutchinson Cancer Center and another at the University Medical Center at Stony Brook in New York as part of the National Cancer Institute's Long Island Cancer Study. Both studies will measure in-home magnetic field exposures and proximity to power lines as possible risk factors. A project at the Brigham and Women's Hospital in Boston is evaluating whether electric blankets are associated with breast cancer in a group of 121,700 nurses who have been studied since 1976.

While we await the results of these studies, you might want to consider some lifestyle modifications. Try to put more space between yourself and devices that emit magnetic fields. Avoid being too close to computers, microwave ovens, and televisions. Turn off electric devices when you aren't using them (this also saves on your electric bill and energy waste). Avoid electric blankets and don't keep electric alarm clocks close to your bed. Discourage children from playing below power lines. Avoid prolonged use of cell phones. And sleep in a dark room.

How much you want to change your lifestyle to avoid a possible risk increase depends on you. My coauthor, for example, can't sleep in a completely dark room. Many people's livelihoods depend on heavy use of computers and cell phones. As with any risk question, there's always a compromise between your needs and your efforts to avoid risk.

10

Risk Factors: Genetic

We divide breast cancer occurrences into three groupings. The first, and largest, is the sporadic—women with breast cancer who have no known family history of the disease. The second is genetic—one dominant cancer gene is passed on to succeeding generations. The third group, the polygenic, is much larger than the second group. It occurs when there is a family history of breast cancer that isn't directly passed on through each generation in one dominant gene—some members of the family get it and others don't. Women in this category are at greater risk for cancer than the general public, though less so than women with hereditary cancer.

When I wrote the previous editions of this book, there was no test to identify which women were at risk, and so doctors developed an elaborate system of guesswork based on what knowledge existed. It was like searching for a criminal before the discovery of fingerprints or DNA, but with a fairly good description. If the suspect was a tall, blond man with glasses, many men matching that description might get rounded up, but only one would be the criminal.

So it was with determining cancer risk. A woman who (1) had a mother or sister with bilateral breast cancer, (2) was diagnosed with breast cancer at an early age, or (3) had more than two relatives with breast cancer was considered at risk. But we later learned that a woman who had the risk factors didn't necessarily have the one element that put her at genetic risk—a mutation in the BRCA 1 or BRCA 2 gene. Now that we have a way to test for these mutations, the old rules are much less relevant.

Some women have a family history of breast cancer but not an inherited gene. About 20 percent of breast cancers fall into this category. This doesn't mean the cancer is pure coincidence. These people may have inherited a mutation in a gene that has not yet been discovered or a gene for something that makes them more prone to breast cancer. What could make you more prone to breast cancer? You may inherit a gene that causes you to begin menstruating at an early age or a gene that makes you particularly susceptible to estrogen—which means other family members are also more likely to get breast cancer.

Another possibility is exposure to similar external risk factors. I have a friend who is one of five sisters who got breast cancer. The sisters were all tested for BRCA 1 and 2, and were shocked to discover they didn't have it. When all the cancer is in one generation, as in my friend's case, it's possible that they were all exposed to an environmental factor that caused the cancer. Of course it could still be genetic, but it would not be a mutation we can currently test for.

The Collaborative Group on Hormonal Factors in Breast Cancer reanalyzed the data from 52 studies, including 58,209 with breast cancer and 101,986 without. It determined that eight out of nine women who develop breast cancer do not have an affected mother, sister, or daughter. Although women with first-degree relatives who have a history of breast cancer are at increased risk of the disease, most will never develop breast cancer and most who do will be over 50 when their cancer is diagnosed. In countries where breast cancer is common, the lifetime excess incidence of breast cancer is 5.5 percent for women with one affected first-degree relative and 13.3 percent for women with two.[1] This should be reassuring for the majority of women.

BRCA 1 AND 2

In 1990 the BRCA 1 gene, which is a tumor suppressor gene linked to genetic breast cancer, was discovered; in 1991 the gene was shown to be linked with genetic ovarian cancer. Families who have mutations in this gene tend to have a high incidence of breast cancer, often at a young age, in both breasts, as well as ovarian cancer.

In 1994 the BRCA 1 gene was cloned. In that same year, a second gene was discovered, BRCA 2. It is less common than BRCA 1 and can also affect men. The risk of ovarian cancer carried by BRCA 2 is lower than that carried by BRCA 1.

The risk for women who have mutations in BRCA 1 or BRCA 2 is anywhere from 50 to 80 percent. At first the researchers believed that anyone with the BRCA 1 gene had an 80 percent lifetime risk of getting breast cancer, based on studies of families with a lot of breast and ovarian cancer.[2] Additional studies were then done on women who, though they had the gene, came from less clear situations—they had perhaps one or two relatives with breast cancer. The studies found, predictably, that the risk was commensurately lower in this group—more like a 37 to 60 percent chance.[3] Just as we were getting comfortable with that range, Dr. Mary-Claire King and her colleagues did a large study in New York on women of Ashkenazi Jewish descent (more about that later) and found that the lifetime risk was 82 percent and seemed to be increasing in time: the risk by age 50 among mutation carriers born before 1940 was 24 percent, but the risk for women born after 1940 was 67 percent. Lifetime risk of ovarian cancer was 54 percent for BRCA 1 and 23 percent for BRCA 2 mutation carriers.[4]

Male carriers of mutations in BRCA 1 or BRCA 2 are also susceptible to cancer; however, their risks remain poorly understood. Male BRCA 1 carriers are at increased risk for cancer of the prostate and breast. In women BRCA 1 mutations carry the greatest risk; in men it is BRCA 2. The relative risk to male BRCA 2 mutation carriers is high before age 65, mostly due to breast, prostate, and pancreatic cancer. And of course they can pass the gene on to their children.[5]

But why weren't all the carriers getting breast cancer and why was the risk increasing over the years? The word we use to describe this variability is *penetrance.* Whether or not the mutation in the breast cancer gene results in cancer depends on whether the mutation in the gene has an effect. We don't know what causes this difference in penetrance, but some of these people probably need an additional genetic alteration before the gene turns cancerous. Or they may have inherited other genes that protect them. Several mutations in sequence are probably needed to cause breast cancer (Fig. 10-1). For example, initially you'd be susceptible to a mutation caused by hormones; the second mutation would be caused by diet. The person with genetic breast cancer passes the gene on to her daughter, so the girl is born with her first mutation and only needs the second to get breast cancer. If the second mutation was for something that could be altered (e.g., diet, which we'll consider in Chapter 11), it would be possible that changing the situation (e.g., by switching to a different diet) could prevent her from getting breast cancer. For example, in Dr. King's study, physical activity and lack of obesity in adolescence were associated with significantly delayed breast cancer onset.

There are over 700 mutations in each of the genes, just as the same word can be mistyped in a number of different ways. Interestingly

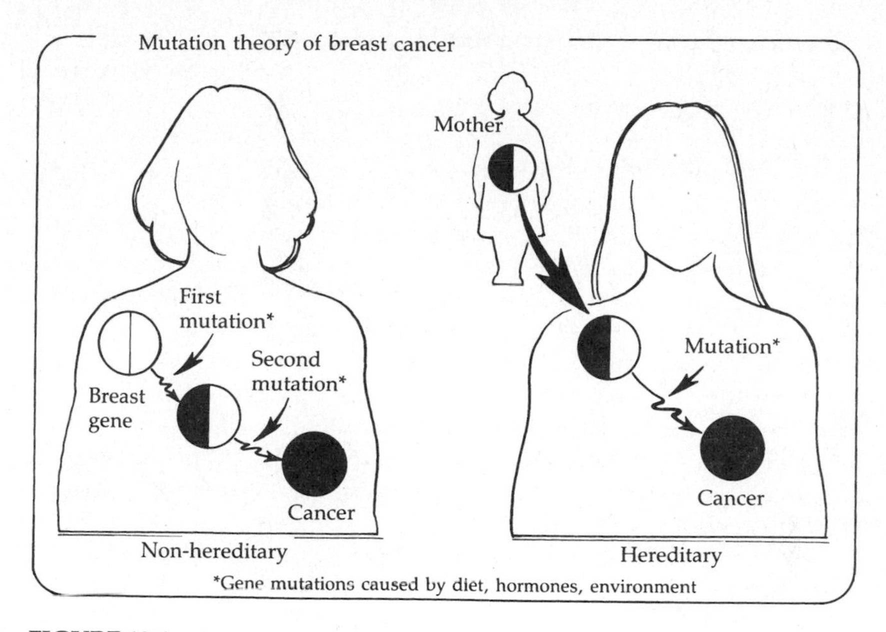

FIGURE 10-1

three of these mutations were found consistently in women of Ashkenazi descent, like a word always mistyped in one of the same three ways. These mutations were 185delAG, 538InsC, and 614delIT. These are often called founder's mutations and are caused by the founder effect because they're more common in populations with a lot of intermarriage. The founder is the first person who got the gene, inadvertently "founding" it and then passing it down to her or his descendants. Intermarriage perpetuates the gene through many generations. Since one of the three founder mutations is present in 2 percent of Ashkenazi Jews, this group has been studied extensively. Much of our knowledge about penetrance and the natural history of hereditary breast cancer has come from this relatively small group.

Such an effect isn't exclusive to Ashkenazi Jews. When researchers started looking at other populations, they found similar situations. In Iceland, where there's a lot of intermarriage, there is also a predominant mutation of BRCA 2.[6] (Only 9 percent of people in Iceland with the BRCA gene have BRCA 1, while 54 percent have BRCA 2. This is the reverse of the case in most other countries, in which BRCA 1 is far more common than BRCA 2.) In Norway it's even more specific. Though Norwegians get both BRCA genes, which mutation a person gets depends on which fjord she lives on.[7] One fjord has one mutation, while another has one of the others.

Returning to the typo metaphor, there are 700 to 1,000 possible typos with the BRCA 1 or BRCA 2 genes. It's as though all Ashkenazi Jews used the same typewriter, with an *e* that didn't work. All the Icelanders used a different typewriter, on which the *t* didn't work.

All of this is important when it comes to testing. If you're from an Ashkenazi family and have breast or ovarian cancer, instead of looking for any of the 700 to 1,000 possible mutations, doctors focus on the three common mutations—and the gene is much easier to test for. If doctors have to study the whole paragraph to find the typo, it's more time-consuming, and thus more expensive, to test.

In some cases, there are mutations whose effects, if any, we haven't yet determined. Even among the known mutations of BRCA 1, we can't be sure. Suppose the mutation is one that is ultimately found to be a harmless—you still test positive for BRCA 1. Again, as research continues, we'll know more and more about this, but we don't have all the answers now.

Penetrance varies from country to country, and the reasons may be unrelated to genetics. For example, use of oral contraceptives, age of first childbirth and oophorectomy may all influence the risks of ovarian and breast cancer.[8]

The risk also differs depending on whether the mutations are in BRCA 1 or BRCA 2. Although both BRCA 1 and 2 mutations seem to have penetrance values of up to 80 percent for breast cancer, the risk for ovarian cancer is about 40 percent for BRCA 1 mutations and about 20 percent for BRCA 2. And BRCA 2 carriers develop ovarian cancer at an older age.[9] The risk of breast cancer in BRCA 1 or 2 carriers increases significantly after age 30 but appears to taper off after menopause in BRCA 1 carriers, while it appears to continue to increase after menopause in BRCA 2 carriers. The risk of ovarian cancer rises steeply after age 40 in both BRCA 1 and 2 carriers, with an average age of 51.2 years at diagnosis.[10]

What do these genes do? Why does a mutation in BRCA 1, which exists in every cell of your body, cause breast and ovarian cancer and not, say, kidney cancer? BRCA 1 and 2 are thought to be involved in checkpoint or quality control of the DNA. Before a cell can divide and replicate, its DNA has to be checked out to make sure there are no mutations. Since BRCA 1 and 2 are involved in quality control, it is not surprising that they are also involved in tagging badly damaged DNA for degradation (this is called, impressively, ubiquitylation). Both BRCA 1 and 2 are also involved in DNA repair. When a carcinogen like radiation causes a mutation in the DNA, these genes repair it (see Fig. 10-2). When the genes themselves are mutated, they cannot do the repair and the damaged gene persists. But this still does not explain why the cancers occur in the breast and ovary specifically. One theory is

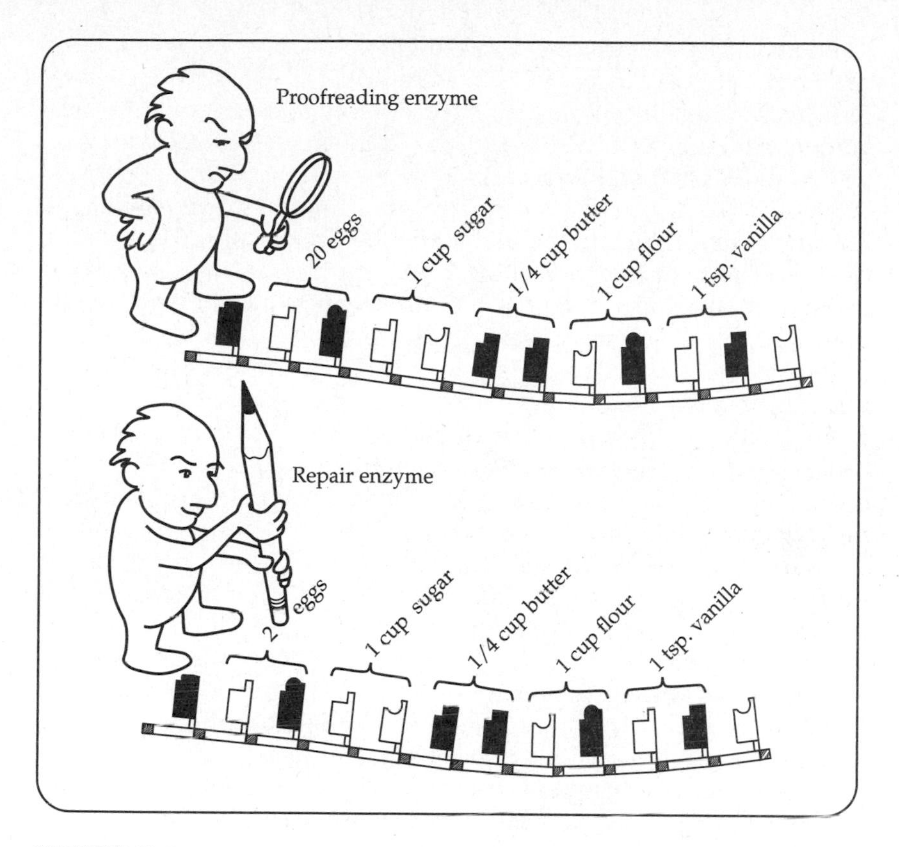

FIGURE 10-2

that absence of functioning BRCA 1 and 2 can exacerbate the action of tissue-specific carcinogens like estrogen and progestin. As I was researching this chapter, I thought for a minute about this theory and then said, "Hmm. I thought BRCA 1 caused cancers that are not sensitive to estrogen. Why would BRCA care about estrogen?" This sent me back to the books, only to find a new hypothesis: the breast cancer stem cells that seem to develop into BRCA 1 cancers are indeed estrogen receptor negative breast cancers. But the cells right next door are not.[11] Could it be that these surrounding cells might respond to estrogen and send pro-survival signals to the estrogen receptor negative cancer stem cells? I'll discuss this later when I review the options for mutation carriers. For now, I simply want to note that most of the treatments that reduce estrogen also reduce the estrogen receptor negative tumors of BRCA 1. Obviously we have a far way to go to understand how these mutations work, but research is moving rapidly and I am sure the answers are not far off.

TESTING

Now that we have a simple blood test that can detect many of the mutations that occur in BRCA 1 or BRCA 2, the questions become, Who should undergo it? and What does it mean?

We are using the test clinically at the same time we are researching it. We aren't yet clear who should be tested, when they should be tested, or why they should be tested. If you test positive, we don't know how much of a risk that gives you. If you test negative, it doesn't mean you don't have *any* breast cancer gene, it just means you don't have BRCA 1 or BRCA 2. You could have an as-yet undiscovered BRCA 3 or BRCA 4.

All we can do is look for "typos" in these two different paragraphs. If you happen to have a typo in another paragraph and that mutation causes breast cancer, we won't know it. Or if you have a typo that doesn't change the meaning of the sentence, you might test positive and not get breast cancer. With each new bit of discovery, the answers to those questions can change.

If you want to be tested, it makes sense to find out if there is a breast cancer gene in your family by having a relative with breast cancer tested first. If your mother has breast cancer, is tested, and discovers that she doesn't have a genetic alteration, there's no need for you to get tested. If we find that she has a mutation in the BRCA 1 gene and you don't, then we know you didn't inherit that gene. Again, that's no guarantee you won't get breast cancer, but the risk is much reduced and is the same as that of anyone whose mother did not have breast cancer.

In an interesting article for the *Annals of Surgery*, J.D. Igelhart looks into the responses of women who were considering getting tested for BRCA genes and sought counseling at the testing center.[12] Even after they had talked it over with counselors who explained the tests' limitations, most women still believed that if they tested negative they wouldn't ever get breast cancer. When you desperately want something to be true, you often mentally edit what you hear to transform it into what you want it to be.

Whatever the limits of counseling, however, it's far more frightening when women go into testing without it. And for the most part, they do. Says Dr. Iglehart, "Physicians without genetic training are more likely to provide testing and least likely to provide counseling."[13] And in fact few doctors have genetic training.

In the Iglehart study, women likely to be positive were asked before testing to estimate their risk of having the gene. The patients far overestimated their risk, thinking they had a 100 percent risk. The doctors, meanwhile, thought most patients had zero risk. They thought a few had a 10 percent risk, and a few had a 20 percent risk.

Interestingly, women with doctors who do have expertise—the ones who work in clinics where counseling is part of the process—are much less likely after the counseling to get tested. When they recognize the limits of what the test can do, they reconsider. Women who go to their local doctors and receive no counseling are more likely to have it done.

Some people have asked why the test for the breast cancer gene is being offered only to women at high risk for the disease. Why isn't it being suggested for all women with breast cancer, or even all women in the country? Part of the reason is that the chance of having the gene is so low for most people that it wouldn't be worth it. A study by Beth Newman, reported in the *Journal of the American Medical Association,* looked at a general group of women between 20 and 74 with breast cancer to see how many had the mutation.[14] Only 3 percent had the BRCA 1 gene.

J. Peto and his group did a study in the United Kingdom in the summer of 1999, looking at women with hereditary breast cancer.[15] They divided them into age-groups and looked at the correlation between hereditary cancer and the BRCA genes. In the group most likely to have the gene, women who had gotten cancer before they were 36, only 3.5 percent had BRCA 1 and 2.4 percent had BRCA 2. In women between 36 and 45, 1.9 percent had BRCA 1 and 2.2 percent had BRCA 2. So it's a very small percentage, even among young women.

The Risks of Getting Tested

What precisely are the risks? One is financial. The testing is expensive—typically $2,750 in the United States—and insurance companies don't necessarily pay for it. If a particular mutation is identified, then other family members can get tested for around $400. That's because the really hard work is searching for the specific mutation. It's like proofreading an entire manuscript to find the typo; once you know where it is, finding it in other copies is fairly easy.

Initially there was fear that insurance companies would discriminate against women who had been tested. So far this has not been the case. Still, it would be smart to check the laws in your state and the policy of your insurance company before proceeding.

Further, it isn't only you who will need to deal with the consequences of your decision. It becomes a family issue. If I get tested and I'm positive, this will have implications for my sisters—who may or may not want to get tested. It also has implications for my daughter. If you choose to be tested and learn you have the gene, you will then need to decide what to do with the information.

You should have the testing done at a research center. Don't go to your gynecologist or primary care doctor or even the medical school in the next town. Even if it means flying to the closest research center, do it. You'll only do this once, and it will affect the rest of your life, so do it well. A research center will include counseling and will perform the tests appropriately, giving you the most accurate information available at this time. To find such a center, you can check with a nearby medical school. You can also call 1-800-FOR CANCER. There is a website that lists genetic counselors for cancer geographically throughout the United States: http://cancer.gov/search/geneticsservices.

When you already have breast cancer, the emotional conflict over gene testing intensifies. You tend to think that you're unlucky and you must have the bad gene. Further, your own psychological issues get mixed into your perceptions. Were you mean to your mother when she had breast cancer, so now you're being punished by inheriting a killer gene? The most sophisticated of us are to some extent trapped by our own unconscious expectations.

There are, of course, rational reasons for women with breast cancer to consider getting tested. They may want to know if others in their family are likely to get it. Or they may be thinking about having children, and the possibility of passing on a breast cancer gene could play a role in their decision. Women with cancer in one breast are more likely to get it in the other, and they may want to consider having a double mastectomy if they know they have the gene. In women without the gene, the risk of a second primary is between 0.5 and 1 percent a year, and 15 to 25 percent over their lifetime. For someone with the gene, it's probably between 1 and 2 percent a year, 30–50 percent over their lifetime. Similarly, a woman with BRCA 1 or BRCA 2 may want to have her ovaries removed. People with the BRCA 1 gene also have a slightly higher risk of getting colon cancer. If you know you have the gene, regular colonoscopies are a must. Some studies indicate that prostate cancer may also be more common among men with the gene.

It doesn't make sense for every woman with breast cancer to be tested, since hereditary breast cancer is so rare. Still, there are some profiles showing your likelihood of carrying a genetic alteration. If you are a Jewish woman younger than 40 with breast cancer, there is about a 33 percent chance that you are a carrier. If you are not Jewish and have breast cancer before 30, you have a 12 percent chance of having a mutation. If you develop bilateral breast cancer between age 40 and 50 and have a first- or second-degree relative with breast or ovarian cancer before 50, there is a 42 percent chance that you carry a mutation. If you got breast cancer after 50 there is a lower risk that it is hereditary;

in fact, having more than two breast cancers in first- or second-degree relatives after 50 only gives you a risk of about 2 percent of having a mutation.[16,17]

And if you don't have breast cancer, should you get tested? The general recommendation is that someone with a 10 percent or greater risk of getting breast cancer should be seen by a genetic counselor and consider testing. This would include:

Family member with a known mutation in a breast cancer susceptibility gene

Two or more first-degree relatives or two or more first- and second-degree relatives on the same side of the family with

1. Breast cancer diagnosed before 50
2. Breast cancer diagnosed before 50 in one or more relatives and ovarian cancer diagnosed at any age in one or more relatives
3. Breast cancer in a family member, at least one of whom also had ovarian cancer diagnosed at any age
4. Ovarian cancer diagnosed at any age
5. Breast cancer diagnosed at any age and Ashkenazi Jewish ancestry
6. Male breast cancer and a female diagnosed with breast cancer less than age 50, or ovarian cancer at any age on the same side of the family

If you decide to be tested, there are several possible results. Most satisfying are the true positives and true negatives. In a true positive, the test is positive for a known mutation. In a true negative it is negative for a mutation that has been identified in the woman's family. In this case she knows she did not inherit the family gene. More complex is the situation where no known mutation is found. Then you do not know whether there is a gene but it is not one of the ones we know how to look for, or if there is no genetic alteration. Also, genetic alterations of unknown clinical significance can be found that are abnormal but have not been linked to breast cancer. In both of these situations the woman is left with as many questions as answers.

And what should you do with the information? Luckily in the past year we have identified several prevention strategies from prophylactic oophorectomies to chemoprevention. These will be discussed further in Chapter 11.

The question of testing depends on you, your family, and your values. The answer will be different for each person. If you are considering it, by all means get counseling for up-to-date information on the risks and benefits to you and your family.

What Kind of Cancer?

One of the important unanswered questions in our study of the BRCA genes is about prognosis. Does the woman with a cancer gene have a different *kind* of cancer than the one who doesn't have the gene? There is some evidence that BRCA 2 cancers are more likely to be estrogen receptor positive, while BRCA 1 cancers tend to be estrogen receptor negative. In fact, there is some preliminary information suggesting that BRCA 1 tumors are more likely to be what is being called basal type—estrogen receptor negative, Her-2/neu negative and often epidermal growth factor positive. This is a mixed blessing. They are more likely to be aggressive but also more likely to be sensitive to chemotherapy.

There is some indication that medullary carcinomas (see Chapter 16), which tend to look very aggressive but do not always act that way, are more common in women with BRCA 1. If that turns out to be true, it might partially explain the mortality rates.

CHOICES

If you test positive for the BRCA 1 or BRCA 2 gene, what next? First, getting a positive test result is not an emergency. It just confirms what you undoubtedly suspected: that you are at high risk for breast cancer. The question is, What are you comfortable doing about it? The choices range from ignoring it (probably not too wise) to close monitoring through chemoprevention or surgical prevention.

Again, you want to be seen by a clinic that specializes in high-risk women or women with genetic risk. They will review your options with you and consider your particular situation. Many factors have to be taken into consideration, from whether you still want to conceive your own children (which would preclude having your ovaries removed) to whether you are claustrophobic and cannot tolerate an MRI. All these need to be discussed and digested before you launch into a plan that will work for you and your life.

Surveillance

Monitoring for mutation carriers has been evolving. Usually it involves having an exam every six months beginning around age 25–35, as well as a yearly mammography. The latter is controversial because, as mentioned in Chapter 7, mammography doesn't work as well in young women with dense breasts. In fact it detects less than half of the breast cancers in mutation carriers.[18,19,20] Still, it can find microcalcifications and sometimes a cancer. Ultrasound is often added to the mammography, especially if there are palpable lumps. More recently we have been testing MRI in this setting. As you may recall from Chapter 7, one of the problems with MRI is that it is too sensitive, meaning it is positive for lots of things that are not cancer. But if you are at high risk, you want a very sensitive test and are probably willing to trade off unnecessary biopsies for the chance of finding a tumor early. In a Dutch study 1,909 women with a risk of over 15 percent were screened, including 358 carriers of germ-line mutations.[21] The study used mammography and MRI and in a period of 2.9 years detected 51 tumors. MRI was the most sensitive—79.5 percent versus 33 percent for mammography. Not surprisingly, they found that the breast cancer detection rate overall increased with the risk: there were 26.5 cancers per 1,000 carriers of BRCA 1 or BRCA 2 mutations. MRI was not as good at detecting DCIS, but luckily DCIS is not a prominent feature in most cancers associated with BRCA 1. At the current time, MRI with mammography and ultrasound starting around age 30 seem to be the best approach to surveillance. But you must make sure you are getting the best breast MRI available, in a high-risk or genetic clinic. Images are only as good as the person taking and then reading the pictures.

There may also be a place for ductal lavage (see Chapter 13) surveillance in this high-risk group, and many ongoing studies are attempting to validate the usefulness of analyzing the breast duct fluid for precancer cells, genetic mutations, or specific protein patterns.

Of course, the risk is not limited to the breast. You also need to monitor for ovarian cancer; the fact that this tends to occur after 40 allows for better detection with mammography. In many ways, as I noted earlier, ovarian cancer is more frightening than breast cancer, although it's also much less common. Breast cancer may or may not prove fatal; ovarian cancer almost always does. Unfortunately it is also a very sneaky cancer: there are no symptoms until it's far developed. Pelvic exams rarely show signs of ovarian cancer. A blood test called CA125 is good for monitoring metastatic ovarian cancer, but it works only about 50 percent of the time when the cancer is in an early stage. It's particularly tricky in premenopausal women. There are a lot of false positives, leaving the patient terrified that she has an incurable disease and leading to unnecessary surgery. Transvaginal ultrasound is a more recent technique. An ultrasound tool is placed in the vagina and the technician can look around the ovarian area. The process has a very high resolution, but most of what it finds is benign. It may be a good idea for very high-risk women, but even then out of 1,000 women screened they'd find suspicious signs in 50 women, all of whom would undergo major surgery and only one of whom would turn out to have cancer.

There are currently reports on a blood test for ovarian cancer based on protein patterns that is being tested.[22] This would be a wonderful addition to surveillance for mutation carriers.

Prevention in BRCA 1 and 2 Carriers

What kind of prevention can you try if you have the BRCA 1 gene? Beyond surveillance there are lifestyle changes that may have some impact. Remember Mary-Claire King's study showing that adolescents who participated in physical activity and were not obese had less penetrance of the mutations? Other ways to modulate estrogen also appear to be relevant; for example, pregnancy and oral contraceptives appear to increase breast cancer, probably because of their higher hormone levels.[23] This certainly doesn't give you many choices. It is also unfortunate because the pill decreases ovarian cancer. If you do give birth, however, breast-feeding will reduce your risk.[24]

On the surgical prevention front there are more positive data. Having your ovaries removed before age 50 reduces the risk of ovarian cancer by 96 percent and decreases the risk of breast cancer by 47–61 percent.[25] You may be wondering why it doesn't reduce the risk of ovarian cancer 100 percent, since there are only two ovaries and they are much easier to remove than breasts are. The reason is that there can be specks of ovarian tissue in the peritoneal lining of the abdomen (this is the smooth glistening lining of the inside of your belly, something like the inside of your mouth) that can still become cancerous. In a large follow-up study of women at high risk for ovarian cancer at the Gilda Radner Familial Ovarian Cancer Registry, 6 of the 324 women (2 percent) who underwent prophylactic oophorectomy developed peritoneal carcinomas.[26]

The more surprising finding was that having your ovaries out helped prevent breast cancer as well. In a large follow-up study over 8 years, women who had their ovaries out before age 35 had no cases of ovarian cancer and a 61 percent reduction in breast cancer risk. If they had the surgery between 35 and 50, there was a 97 percent reduction in the risk for ovarian and a 51 percent reduction in breast cancer. And finally over 50 the risk reduction was 89 percent for ovarian cancer and 48 percent for breast cancer. Earlier is definitely better, though not that much better.[27] Interestingly in at least one study HRT did not seem to affect this lowered risk, probably because the hormones are given at a lower dose than that which one would expect premenopausal women to have naturally. It is not clear how much additional benefit bilateral mastectomies would contribute.[28] Probably more relevant is whether adding tamoxifen to oophorectomy in mutation carriers is worth it. An

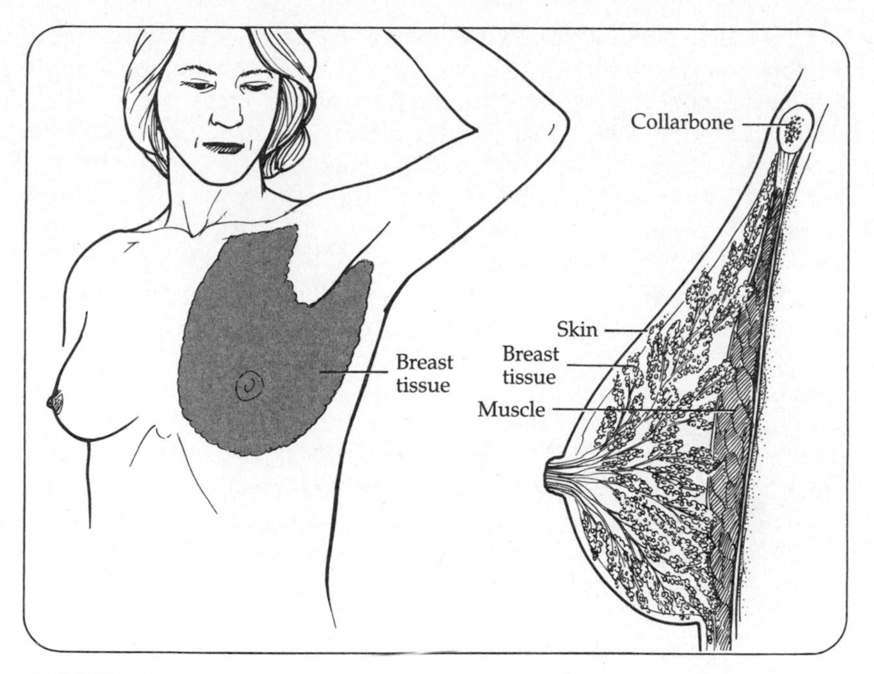

FIGURE 10-3

epidemiological study suggests that the protective effects of tamoxifen and oophorectomy may be independent and additive.[29]

Most people assume that the foolproof way to prevent breast cancer is to remove the breasts. If you don't have breasts, the reasoning goes, you won't get breast cancer. It's a drastic solution. Most women like their breasts for esthetic and erotic reasons, even if they're not planning to use them for breast-feeding. Yet some women are so terrified of the possibility of breast cancer that preventive mastectomy seems to be a good idea.

This procedure doesn't completely eliminate the risk of breast cancer. No mastectomy can be guaranteed to get out all the breast tissue, which extends from the collarbone to below the rib cage, from the breastbone around to the back. Further, it doesn't separate itself out from the surrounding tissue in any obvious way (Fig. 10-3). The most brilliant surgeon in the world couldn't be certain of digging all the breast tissue out of your body. When we do a mastectomy we do our best to get out as much as possibe.[30] The million-dollar question is, Does removing most of the tissue get rid of most of the risk? This was a big question when I wrote the first edition of this book. We now have data from nonrandomized studies that suggest that the answer is yes.

First there were data following up women who had undergone prophylactic mastectomies in the 1950s at Mayo Clinic. Using a complicated process, the researchers tried to compare the breast cancer risk in these women to that in their sisters. Overall seven women still got breast cancer after the prophylactic mastectomy, and two died of it.[31] Instead of 20 deaths from breast cancer, there were two.

Since then there has been one prospective study showing no cancers in 76 women with mutations in BRCA 1 or BRCA 2 in three years following prophylactic mastectomy.[32] This is a short but encouraging follow-up. Two other small studies in mutation carriers observed significant reductions in risk in women undergoing the surgery.[33,34]

What we really want, though, is a prospective, randomized control study—to have identical twins living in the same place all their lives who have BRCA 1. We'd give one a prophylactic mastectomy and see what happened to both. Since such a study is unlikely to happen, the two studies we do have give us a good clue. They tell us there's probably 90–95 percent reduction of breast cancer risk among mutation carriers who have prophylactic mastectomy.

PUTTING IT TOGETHER

A decision analysis model concluded that there is survival benefit to most prevention strategies, but the benefit is age dependent. Indeed the model predicts that BRCA 1 or BRCA 2 mutation carriers who take tamoxifen after oophorectomy or undergo mastectomy and oophorectomy by age 30 have an overall survival similar to that of women in the general population with no mutations.[35]

A review of the more common situation of women with breast cancer who elect to have their opposite breast removed suggested that there may even be a decrease in the chance of dying of breast cancer. Of women with cancer in one breast there was a 2.7 percent chance of developing breast cancer in the other breast; double mastectomy reduced this to 0.5 percent.[36] Although there appeared to be a reduction in mortality from breast cancer in this series, with a median follow-up of five years, it was small; 8.1 percent of women who had the prophylactic mastectomy died of breast cancer while 11.7 percent of the group that did not have the extra surgery died.

An editorial discussing the Mayo Clinic study summarized it well: "In the end, what the study demonstrated most dramatically is the cost of prophylactic mastectomy. Even in the cases with an unprecedented 80 percent reduction of breast cancer and deaths from breast cancer, the fact remains that 639 women, because of the fear of breast cancer, underwent a disfiguring and potentially psychologically damaging operation. As a result, instead of the 20 deaths related to breast cancer that were expected during this period of observation, there were only two. The saving of those 18 lives was clearly important. But the 621 women who probably would have survived without prophylactic mastectomy paid a price that will probably be considered unacceptable in the future."[37]

If you are diagnosed with breast cancer, should you be tested for the gene? Should you have both breasts removed? What about your ovaries? If you come from a family with a lot of breast and/or ovarian cancer on either parent's side, you should consider being tested. (This can be done at any time, even years later.) If the prognosis of the first cancer is good and you test positive for a mutation, you may want to consider oophorectomy, mastectomy, or both. If your prognosis is poor, it does not make sense to have surgery for prevention. Better to get on with treatment ASAP. Ask to talk to a genetics counselor, as most oncologists and breast surgeons are not well educated in genetics and will not be able to advise you as well. I sometimes hear of women who are being pressured to have gene testing prior to their cancer surgery so that they can decide between bilateral and unilateral mastectomies. While getting everything done at once has its appeal, there are many women who need more time to think about all the options. In that situation I usually advise that they go ahead with the appropriate treatment for the first cancer and then when the dust settles have the counseling and gene testing if indicated to see if they are mutation carriers. If they are, they can then explore their options for prevention and make a careful decision about what is the best choice for them.

Whether you have breast cancer or a genetic mutation, it is important to remember that this type of a decision is not an emergency and you have time to explore what it will mean to your life. Also, there are many studies going on that may make prophylactic surgery obsolete. We remove healthy body parts preventatively only when we don't know what else to do. Local therapy down the ducts, for example, may work as well (as it has done in rodents) and prevent breast cancer, precluding the need for surgery (see Chapter 13). On the other side, a sensitive blood test could predict ovarian cancer early enough to make oophorectomy unnecessary. This chapter has been expanded with data since the last edition and studies are ongoing. The hopes for true prevention have never been better.

11

Prevention

Each edition of this book has included more information on strategies of prevention. In this fourth edition I cover new studies on chemoprevention as well as new data on lifestyle changes. In Chapter 13 on the intraductal approach I will talk about a novel approach to prevention I have been working on that has been demonstrated in rodents and is being tested in women. To me this is the most exciting part of the book.

According to Canadian epidemiologist Anthony Miller, the major factors that seem amenable to change and therefore have potential for prevention are controlled diet, reduction in obesity, reduction in the use of estrogens at menopause, and—more controversially—a shift back to women having their first babies at an earlier age.[1]

Table 11-1 lists Miller's attributable risks for some of these environmental and lifestyle risk factors. Remember, attributable risk is the amount of breast cancer that can be attributed to a certain risk factor (or eliminated if that factor is changed). The degree of certainty varies for each risk factor. These are all very interesting from a public health standpoint, but may or may not be applicable to any one individual woman, and I don't advise using them as the sole influence in decision making. For example, I had my first child at 40 and do not regret it. The advantages to me far outweighed the slight potentially increased risk for breast cancer. Would I have been wiser to have had a child in

Table 11-1. Attributable Risks for Breast Cancer (Percentage of Breast Cancer Cases That Can Be Attributed to Each Factor)

	Attributable Risk (%)
Age 25 or older with first birth	17
Estrogen replacement therapy	8
High-fat diet	26
Obesity	12

Source: A.B. Miller, "Epidemiology and Prevention," in J.R. Harris, S. Hellman, I.C. Henderson, and D.W. Kinne, eds., *Breast Diseases* (Philadelphia: Lippincott, 1987).

my 20s, when I wasn't ready for it? Or, since having no children is actually less of a risk than having a first child later in life, should I have deprived myself of the joy Katie has brought me? For me, there was no question. On the other hand, I do eat a good diet high in fruits and vegetables and low in animal fat. The occasional twinge I feel at the sight of a juicy hamburger or wedge of Brie is a reasonable price to pay for the possibility that I may be decreasing my breast cancer risk and improving my overall health. These are very personal decisions.

DIET

As you'll recall from the discussion in Chapter 9, the possibilities that a low-fat diet may decrease breast cancer are looking less promising, but the final answer should come from the Women's Health Initiative. The question about dietary fruits and vegetables as a means of preventing breast cancer was given a blow when the report came out in 2005 from the European Prospective Investigation into Cancer and Nutrition (EPIC). An amazing 285,526 women between the ages of 25 and 70 completed a dietary questionnaire and then were followed prospectively for a median of 5.4 years. Although a reported 3,659 breast cancers were diagnosed, there was no association between consumption of fruits and vegetables and risk of developing breast cancer.[2] However, this does not answer the question as to whether certain fruits or vegetables, consumed at certain times in a woman's life, may have an effect. A case control study from the United States suggested that fruits and vegetables were beneficial in postmenopausal but not premenopausal women. This study indicated that high intake of carotenoids and particularly lycopene (tomatoes) could reduce the risk of breast cancer.[3]

Further, the question is complicated by the fact that weight gain is a risk factor for breast cancer, as noted in Chapter 9. Since a diet high in fruits and vegetables is often low in fatty foods, any apparent connection may be incidental. It's not the apples and carrots you are eating but the hamburgers and cheesecake you *aren't* eating that make the difference. The WINS study, which shows that women with breast cancer who eat a low-fat diet have a decrease in recurrence, adds evidence to this premise (see Chapter 27).

Soy

Studies in Western populations have shown no association between high soy intake and breast cancer prevention. However, even the most avid soy eater in the West has a pretty low intake. On the other hand some case control studies in Asia, where soy is eaten in larger amounts, have suggested that soy intake, particularly during adolescence, was associated with lower breast cancer risk.[4]

Vitamins and Minerals

Vitamin A studies have been equivocal, with some suggesting a benefit and some not.[5] However, in studies that measure vitamin A compounds in the blood, low levels correlated with an increased risk of breast cancer.[6,7] Recent reviews of epidemiological data suggest that vitamin E in foods may provide some protection against breast cancer while vitamin E supplements do not.[8] Finally, increases in Vitamin D and calcium intake were associated with decreases in breast density on mammogram (see Chapter 7) and therefore could help prevent breast cancer. Again, the Women's Health Initiative will answer this because it has an ongoing randomized study of vitamin D and calcium.

Overall the data are not strong enough to talk about a "breast cancer prevention diet," but in general a diet low in animal fat and high in whole grains and fruits and vegetables is most likely to be healthy and help you maintain your weight. It also makes sense to drink alcohol only in moderation, since, as discussed in Chapter 9, regular consumption of alcohol may affect your vulnerability to breast cancer, in addition to all of its other effects, though folic acid has been shown to mitigate the risks.

EXERCISE

Exercise is important for cardiovascular health and for preventing osteoporosis and heart disease, and probably breast cancer. A study by

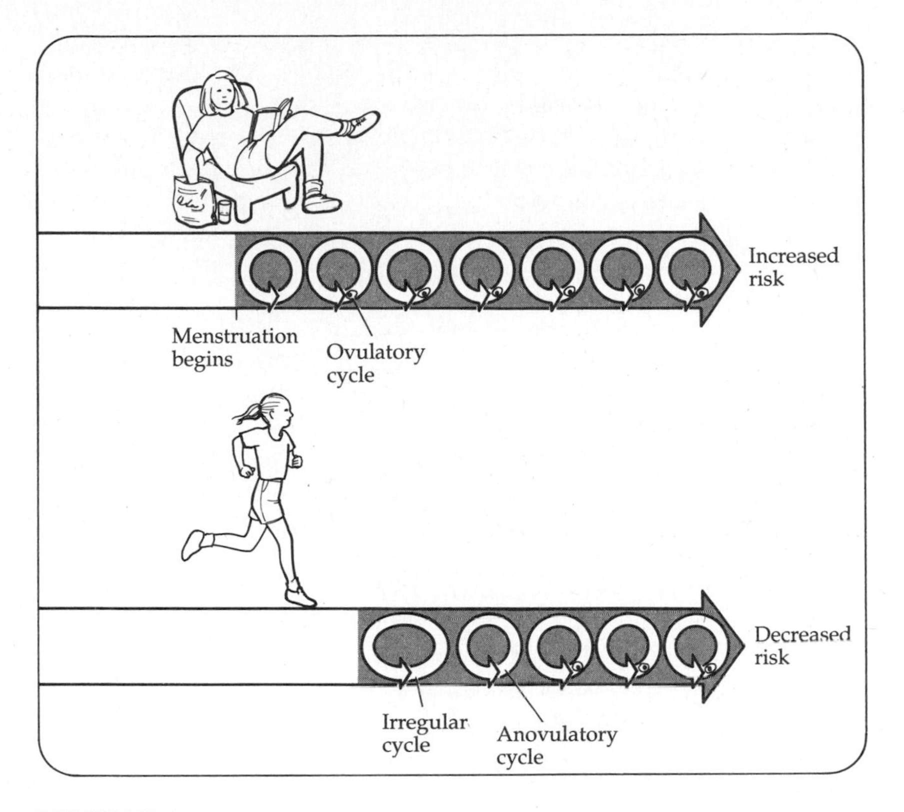

FIGURE 11-1

Leslie Bernstein at the University of Southern California came out in the fall of 1994 demonstrating that women who participated in four or more hours of exercise a week during their reproductive years have a 58 percent decrease in breast cancer risk.[9] This was very exciting because it is one of the first lifestyle changes shown to decrease risk. The mechanism is thought to be hormonal. Also, in young girls moderate exercise and associated alterations in menstrual cycle patterns and ovulatory frequency are correlated with lower risk.[10] Since late onset of menstruation works against breast cancer, this is significant (Fig. 11-1). A prospective cohort study of Norwegian women age 20–24 found that consistently active women had 37 percent less breast cancer than consistently sedentary women.[11]

A long-term prevention approach would be to get girls into the habit of exercising. Rose Frisch of Harvard Medical School and Harvard School of Public Health has shown that women who were involved in athletics during high school and college have a decreased risk of breast cancer.[12]

As a result, a delightful proposal has been put forth: increased funding to high school athletics for girls. Expanded participation in athletics would likely decrease breast cancer, strengthen bones, and prevent future osteoporosis; it would also help prevent heart disease. One caution in all this. There has been a near epidemic of eating disorders among teenage girls desperate to conform to our culture's "thin is beautiful" image. "Low fat" doesn't translate to "no food," and to be beneficial, exercise requires a well-nourished body. Breast cancer will not be an issue if a girl has so badly damaged her body with starvation that she doesn't live long enough to worry about it.

Exercise in adult women is valuable for a number of health concerns, although its effectiveness in terms of breast cancer is less clear. Besides, when you exercise every day you get to feel morally superior.

HORMONES

A more drastic approach to breast cancer prevention is to put women into temporary menopause, as mentioned in Chapter 9. Hormones are heavily implicated in the development of breast cancer. The earlier your first period and the later your menopause—the more menstruating years—the higher your risk of breast cancer. And the younger you are when you have your first child, the lower your risk. So there has been some thought that we might have an effect on breast cancer risk by coming up with a way to induce a hormonal "pregnancy," in which a teenager would be given the hormones of pregnancy for nine months to mature the breast tissue. To my knowledge, this has been tried only in rats so far, but it's an interesting possibility.

Because estrogen appears to have a central role in the development of breast cancer, it makes sense to reduce or block estrogen to prevent breast cancer. In Chapter 10 I talked about the use of bilateral oophorectomy (removal of the ovaries) as one approach to preventing breast cancer in women who carry mutations in BRCA 1 or 2. Although this is quite effective, it is not without side effects and probably not a reasonable alternative to women who are not mutation carriers at risk of both breast and ovarian cancer.

A related idea, which is actually being tried at USC by Dr. Malcolm Pike and Dr. Darcy Spicer, is devising a contraceptive that protects against breast cancer, based on the fact that reproductive hormone levels lead to an increased risk.[13] The women in the study are given GnRH inhibitors, which are drugs that inhibit the pituitary gland from stimulating the ovary (see Chapter 1). This puts them into a reversible menopause (Fig. 11–2). Staying indefinitely in this state would put young women at risk for osteoporosis, so they are given a low dose of

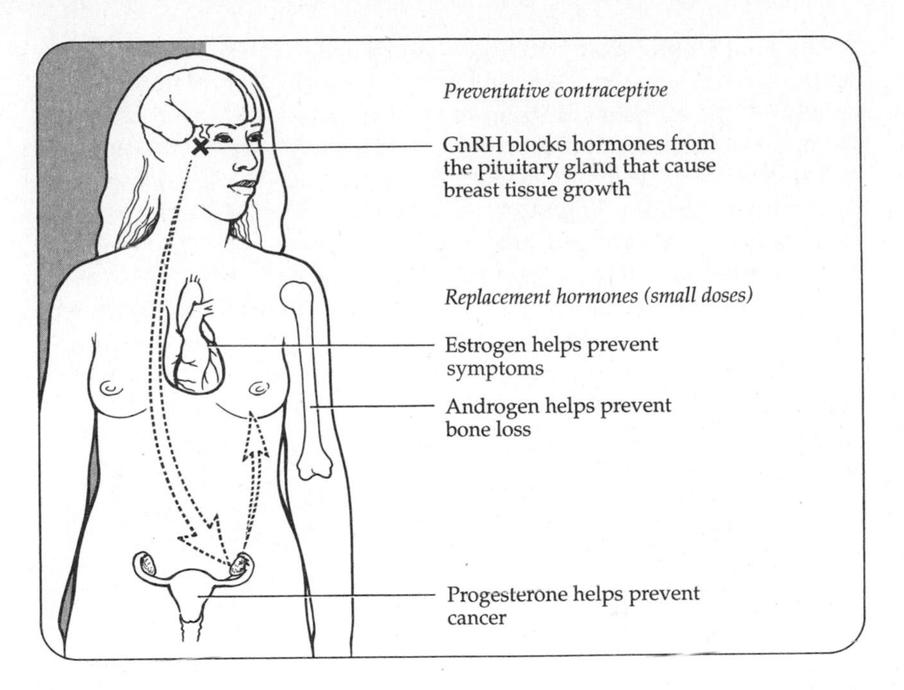

FIGURE 11-2

estrogen, enough to help prevent hot flashes but less than they'd have if they were regularly menstruating. Because taking estrogen alone would put them at risk for endometrial cancer, every two or three months they receive a small amount of progesterone. Careful monitoring (including regular mammograms) revealed after the first six to nine months of the study that they had an increase in bone loss, so a bit of androgen has been added.

This particular "cocktail" will, in theory, reduce breast, ovarian, and uterine cancer, while acting as a contraceptive. An interesting effect in the first 20 women to be studied on this new contraceptive was a change in their mammograms.[14] After a year on the study the density of breast tissue was reduced. We don't as yet know whether this means that the contraceptive is successfully preventing breast cancer or whether it will just make a cancer easier to detect. The study is provocative, however, and lends credence to Pike and Spicer's approach. This contraceptive is complicated and wouldn't be used by everyone. But it may be good for a woman whose family has hereditary breast cancer and who has a gene that makes it more likely that she'll get the disease. Again, I'm not too crazy about using medicine to prevent disease, but this could be right for a certain population of young women.

Finally it would make sense to try and prevent breast cancer in postmenopausal women by giving them a drug to block aromatase, the enzyme that makes estrogen from testosterone and androstenedione. In the one randomized controlled trial of anastrozole in the treatment of breast cancer, there was a reduction in second cancers similar to that seen with tamoxifen. This suggests that these drugs may prevent new cancers in women at high risk. Prevention trials using the new aromatase inhibitor drugs are going on. The drugs may, however, increase the risk of fractures and cognitive difficulties. In addition, some who take aromatase inhibitors experience vaginal dryness, hot flashes, fatigue, and joint aches and pains. For these reasons I do not recommend you trying an aromatase inhibitor for prevention outside of a clinical trial.

TAMOXIFEN AND OTHER SERMS

If eliminating estrogen production is one approach, the other is blocking the estrogen receptor so that it can't have its usual effect. This is the theory behind efforts to prevent breast cancer by giving women tamoxifen.

Tamoxifen didn't begin its life as a cancer treatment. It was actually-developed in 1967 as a fertility drug. (It is now being used for this purpose in breast cancer survivors, with the idea that it is safer than the usual ovulation-inducing cocktails.) But then the researchers realized estrogen's action in the breasts and decided to try tamoxifen in treating breast cancer.

There was initially some concern that tamoxifin would lead to more heart disease, since it blocks estrogen. I voiced that concern in the first edition of this book. As it turns out, however, not only does tamoxifen block estrogen in the breast but it also acts as a weak estrogen in the liver, resulting in a beneficial effect on LDL, one of the "bad" cholesterol derivatives. It doesn't, however, raise the helpful HDL, and in some women may increase triglycerides, which is also a risk factor for heart disease. It neither lessens nor increases osteoporosis; it increases bone density slightly but doesn't affect the number of fractures.

The real surprise was that it seems to increase the risk of uterine cancer. Why, we wondered, would something that blocked estrogen increase uterine cancer, which is *caused* by estrogen? It soon became apparent that tamoxifen acted like estrogen in some organs even as it blocked estrogen in other organs.

With this discovery, a new term was coined—selected estrogen receptor modulator, or SERM. Many like to think that we had set out to make the SERMs (also known as "designer estrogens") and, after much research, finally succeeded. But the reality is quite different: we stumbled on the phenomenon and then gave it a name. Still, if we weren't clever enough to figure out how useful SERMs were until we stumbled onto them, we learned quickly, and many drug companies set out to capitalize on the discovery. Soon raloxifene was on the market, followed by several others.

Even before the marvels of tamoxifen as a breast cancer prevention tool had given it a fancy new category, researchers who had used it to treat existing cancers had realized something: when women with breast cancer took tamoxifen, not only did they have fewer recurrences of the original cancer, but they also had 30–50 percent fewer cancers in the opposite breast. A woman who usually had a 10 percent risk of cancer in the other breast now had a 5 to 7 percent risk. If the drug could prevent new cancers in women who already had the disease, thought the researchers, perhaps it could further reduce the susceptibility of women who were at high risk. A study, the National Surgical Adjuvant Breast and Bowel Project (NSABP), was devised to examine that possibility.[15] It was a huge study—13,388 women. First researchers used the Gail model, a statistical combination of risk factors,to calculate who was at increased risk.[16] These factors included a woman's age at her first period, age at her first pregnancy, whether or not she'd ever had a breast biopsy, family history, and whether she had atypical hyperplasia or LCIS (see Chapter 12).

Since age is a risk factor for breast cancer (a 60–69-year-old woman has twice the risk of someone 40–49 and almost 10 times the risk of someone 30–39), they considered anyone 60 and over high risk. If a woman under 60 had risk factors that added up to those of a 60-year-old, she could take part in the study. Thus, a woman over 60 in the study might have only one risk factor, for example, she had her first child at a late age. But a 30-year-old would have to have three family members with breast cancer. (Limitations to the Gail model are discussed later in this chapter.)

Having picked the subjects for their study group, they then randomized them, giving half the group tamoxifen and half a placebo. Among these women, some had lobular carcinoma in situ and some had atypical ductal hyperplasia (see Chapter 12). Although the study included women with a five-year risk of 1.6 percent or more, most women in the study had a higher risk—and half of them had more than a 3 percent risk.

Overall, the study showed that taking tamoxifen decreased by 49 percent the danger of getting invasive cancer. This means that there were fewer cases of breast cancer among the women who took tamoxifen than among those who didn't. But the numbers aren't huge: 89 women in the tamoxifen group got cancer, while 175 women in the placebo group did. In an overall group of more than 13,000 women, those aren't very large figures.

The benefit persisted in all age-groups, though the numbers were small. In certain groups the difference was more dramatic. For example, women with previously diagnosed atypical hyperplasia had an 86 percent decreased risk. This was based on a small number of cases—3 in the tamoxifen group and 23 in the placebo group. Interestingly, all the cancers the placebo group got and the tamoxifen group didn't were estrogen receptor positive. This makes sense, since tamoxifen is an estrogen blocker. But it also shows the limitations of tamoxifen, since it does not affect tumors that are not sensitive to estrogen.

In addition, we know that women with estrogen receptor positive tumors have a better prognosis, although some do die of breast cancer. This raises a big question: is taking tamoxifen really worth it? If we prevent only cancers that we could cure if we caught them early on mammography, is it worthwhile? Prevention is certainly better than finding and not curing, but we can't be sure if it's better than finding and curing. Do we want long-term use or short-term use?

This study lasted only four years, and that is a serious limitation. It couldn't look at death from breast cancer because cancer takes time to develop, be detected, and kill. So there's no way of knowing if the tamoxifen prevented cancer deaths or only prevented the appearance of cancers that wouldn't have been fatal anyway.

Confusing the issue even more is the fact that the current study includes the prevention of DCIS. But only a third of DCIS becomes invasive cancer. So we can't say that preventing DCIS means preventing invasive cancer, let alone fatal cancer.

Another issue is that a lot of the prevention happened immediately, within the first year or two. So we need to question whether it is really preventing cancer or is treating a cancer that isn't yet detectable; remember that cancers are around for years before we're able to detect them. Or maybe, as discussed in Chapter 27, it is affecting the stroma around the cells and so any dormant cancer cells in the breast can flourish.

Not all studies show a reduction in risk of breast cancer with tamoxifen, and we have no data to indicate that tamoxifen saves lives. In one study, the International Breast Intervention Study I (IBIS-I), 7,152 women age 35 to 70 and at a high risk for breast cancer were randomized to take tamoxifen or a placebo for five years.[17] There was a significant decrease in survival, even though there was a 32 percent decrease in risk of breast cancer. Consequently tamoxifen should not be given to average risk women.

This type of study has some obvious problems. How do we define high risk for a prevention study? In the United States we have accepted the Gail model developed by Mitchell Gail from the National

Table 11-2. Risks and Benefits of Tamoxifen for Prevention

	Placebo	*Tamoxifen*
Breast cancer cases	175	89
Breast cancer deaths	6	3
Hip fracture	22	12
Endometrial cancer	15	36
Stroke	24	38
Pulmonary emboli	0	3
Deep vein thrombosis	22	35
Cataracts	507	574
Other fractures	54	37

Source: M. Gail, J.P. Costantino, J. Bryant et al., "Weighing the Risks and Benefits of Tamoxifen Treatment for Preventing Breast Cancer," *Journal of the National Cancer Institute* 91 (1999): 1829–1846. Used by permission of M. Gail.

Cancer Institute. It is based on age at menopause, age at first live birth, number of previous biopsies, presence of atypical hyperplasia, and number of first-degree relatives with breast cancer.[18] Although these are indeed risk factors, there are many that the Gail model doesn't address that may be equally important. For example, it doesn't ask if the woman is on hormones or whether she was exposed to radiation. The biggest problem, though, is family history. The model deals only with breast cancer in a subject's mother, sister, or daughter, not with cousins, grandparents, or aunts. But hereditary breast cancer can be passed down through either the father's or the mother's line. If your paternal grandmother and paternal aunts all had breast cancer, you would appear to be at low risk in the Gail model, but you could have inherited BRCA 1 or 2.

These new tools are interesting, but so far they are only tools. Their chief value is in setting standards for prevention trials.

Risks and Benefits of Tamoxifen for Prevention

Like all drugs, tamoxifen has some risks. In the study just mentioned, for some conditions there are more deaths among the placebo group (see Table 11-2). For others, though, there are more in the tamoxifen group. (Remember, there were the same number of women in both groups.)[19]

Most worrisome are the clotting problems leading to phlebitis, pulmonary embolism, and strokes, as well as the uterine cancers. These are probably risks worth taking to cure cancer. But prevention is a

Table 11-3. Potential Risks and Benefits of Tamoxifen for Prevention

Type of Event	*Expected Number of Cases per 10,000 Untreated Women*	*Expected Effect Among 10,000 Women Who Were Treated with Tamoxifen for Five Years*
		Potential Benefit
Invasive breast cancer	200	97 cases may be prevented
In situ breast cancer	106	53 cases may be prevented
Hip fracture	2	1 case may be prevented
		Potential Risk
Endometrial cancer	10	16 more cases may be caused
Stroke	22	13 more cases may be caused
Pulmonary embolism	7	15 more cases may be caused
Deep vein thrombosis	24	15 more cases may be caused

Source: M. Gail, J.P. Costantino, J. Bryant et al., "Weighing the Risks and Benefits of Tamoxifen Treatment for Preventing Breast Cancer," *Journal of the National Cancer Institute* 91 (1999): 1829–1846. Used by permission of M. Gail.

thornier question. You may well die from a pulmonary embolism you got trying to prevent a cancer you may never have had in the first place. The absolute risks of endometrial cancer, stroke, pulmonary embolism, and deep vein thrombosis increase with age. Most of the risk was in the women over 50. There were 75 percent more strokes and heart attacks among these women. Tamoxifen is also most beneficial for the women at highest risk of breast cancer. This leads to the conclusion that tamoxifen has the greatest benefit and fewest side effects in young, high-risk Caucasian women. Caucasian women under 50 have a very low chance of developing blood clots, strokes, or heart attacks. African American women have higher risks for these problems and consequently need a higher risk for breast cancer than Caucasian women to warrant the potential side effects from tamoxifen.

Dr. M. H. Gail, who created the Gail index, has developed a complex model to determine the risks and benefits according to the age and race of the woman. For example, a 40-year-old white woman with a uterus and a risk of breast cancer of 2 percent who took tamoxifen for five years may look at a chart like Table 11-3.

The good news is that the greatest risk of uterine cancer appears to occur in women who have previously taken estrogen therapy (without Provera) for menopause. For a woman who has not been on ERT the risks may be lower (see Chapter 9). There were also fewer severe problems—hot flashes and vaginal dryness.

Overall the best use of tamoxifen is in women for whom it has been shown to have the biggest benefit—those with atypical hyperplasia or lobular carcinoma in situ (see Chapter 12).

Raloxifene

The accidental discovery of tamoxifen's potential effect on breast cancer was followed by a furious search for drugs with similar capabilities. Raloxifene (Evista) is the first such drug—the first true designer SERM. Marketed in 1999, it was created to have the positive effect of estrogen on the body with none of its negative effects—in particular, uterine cancer. The biggest study to date, MORE (Multiple Outcomes of Raloxifene Evaluations), has been done by the pharmaceutical company Lilly. It's part of a study Lilly has been doing to see if raloxifene can affect the bones.[20]

The two-year study looks at women in their 60s who have low enough bone density to be diagnosed as having osteoporosis. It shows that raloxifene improves bone density by 3–4 percent—not as well as either alendronate (Fosamax) or estrogen (which improves bone density by 8 percent), but better than a placebo.

As part of the overall study, Lilly also tried to discover whether raloxifene could prevent breast cancer. It found that in postmenopausal women with low to average risk, invasive breast cancer decreased by 72 percent during three years of treatment. (Remember that women with low bone density have less risk of breast cancer, and women with low risk of breast cancer have a higher risk of osteoporosis.) In order to further study this benefit, the women from the MORE trial were continued for four more years in the CORE study. After eight years of treatment there was a 66 percent reduction in invasive breast cancer. As with tamoxifen, raloxifene affected only estrogen receptor positive tumors (see Chapter 16). It also shared tamoxifen's increase in pulmonary emboli. It did not, however, increase the incidence of uterine cancer. It's also the same as tamoxifen in terms of causing hot flashes, so it's probably going to intensify these symptoms only in women who have them already.

It might appear that a 76 percent reduction of breast cancer trumps tamoxifen's 49 percent decrease, but the data aren't comparable. To begin with, while the tamoxifen study looked at high-risk women, the raloxifene study looked at older women at low to average risk for breast cancer. Overall if you already have mild bone loss (osteopenia), raloxifene may help prevent severe bone loss (osteoporosis) and breast cancer. Further, postmenopausal women with measurable blood levels of estradiol (a type of estrogen) are most likely to benefit from raloxifene.

Whether raloxifene is equivalent to tamoxifen in high-risk postmenopausal women is the subject of the STAR (study on tamoxifen and raloxifene). In this study high-risk postmenopausal women are randomized to take one of the two drugs for five years. All the women needed for the study have been enrolled and the results are expected in 2007.

Other interesting data that have come out of the raloxifene studies have demonstrated that women with higher levels of estrogen in their blood are more likely to benefit. Maybe some day soon we will be able to have our hormone levels checked and only the women whose levels are high will consider taking this drug.

OTHER POTENTIAL CHEMOPREVENTION STRATEGIES

Other classes of drugs being tested include vitamin A derivatives[21,22] and anti-inflammatory drugs including aspirin and Cox-2 selective inhibitors such as celecoxib.[23] A provocative study presented at the American Society of Clinical Oncology in May 2005 suggested that the statins taken to reduce cholesterol may also prevent breast cancer. This would be an interesting side benefit of a widely used class of drugs, but it could also be that the type of woman who takes statins also exercises and eats a low-fat diet.[24]

PREVENTIVE SURGERY

Preventive surgery, both oophorectomy and prophylactic mastectomy, have been shown to decrease breast cancer risk (see Chapter 10) but are usually reserved for women who are gene carriers or already have had one breast cancer.

THE FUTURE

I think the next step in prevention will capitalize on the intraductal approach. Not only will we use it to identify which women are truly at risk, but we'll find it helpful for prevention (see Chapter 13).

The true answer to prevention probably is local, not systemic. We need to find ways to either block the carcinogens or reverse the damage to genes.

So, once again, what can most women do? There are some steps that the average woman can take to reduce her risk.

1. Take a multivitamin and make sure it includes adequate folic acid.
2. Exercise for at least 30 minutes a day, 5 days a week (enough to break a sweat).
3. Maintain a normal weight, especially if you are postmenopausal.
4. Have your children before 35 if you have a choice.
5. Breast-feed your children.
6. Avoid unnecessary X rays.
7. Drink alcohol in moderation and make sure you take folic acid when you do drink.
8. Avoid taking hormones (HRT, fertility drugs) unless necessary.
9. Evaluate any breast symptoms or changes that develop.
10. Have a mammogram when appropriate (see Chapter 7 on screening).
11. Consider raloxifene if you need to take a drug to prevent bone loss postmenopausally.
12. Join Love's Army (online at www.drsusanloveresearchfoundation.org) to participate in studies on the normal breast and the intraductal approach.

If you have a family history of breast cancer or think you are at risk, you can be evaluated at a high-risk center to see where you stand. Those who are at increased risk may well consider taking tamoxifen for five years. If you fit the criteria for genetic testing (see Chapter 10), you should see a genetic counselor to consider your options. Those who are mutation carriers will want to consider prophylactic surgery and close surveillance.

Finally, you can get involved in political action. It's vital that we continue the pressure to fund research into prevention. We can't just do one study and then wait for it to be over, and then another and wait for that to be over. That takes too long. We need to have several studies going on at once. And we have to demand that prevention become a priority.

12

Precancerous Conditions

The precancers that we will consider in this chapter are not to be confused with the symptoms misnamed "fibrocyctic disease." As explained in Chapter 4, virtually none of those symptoms is related to breast cancer. There are, however, certain microscopic findings in breast tissue that can lead to cancer.

The breast, as I've said, is a kind of milk factory. It has two parts—lobules that make the milk and ducts like hollow branches that carry it to the nipples (Fig. 12-1). Over the years, you can get a few extra cells lining the branch—sort of like a fungus. This is called *intraductal hyperplasia,* which simply translates to "too many cells in the duct." In itself, this is not a problem. Sometimes the cells become a bit strange looking, and this condition is called intraductal hyperplasia with atypia (also known as atypical hyperplasia, or ADH). If they keep on looking odd and multiply within the duct, clogging it up, they're known as ductal carcinoma in situ (meaning "in place") or intraductal carcinoma or DCIS (Fig. 12-2). These three steps are all reversible, and we suspect that this ability has something to do with hormones. Finally, if cells break out of the ducts and into the surrounding fat, they are called invasive ductal cancer. This same progression can take place in the lobules, leading to a sequence of lobular hyperplasia, atypical lobular hyperplasia (ALH), and lobular carcinoma in situ (LCIS). Since the very

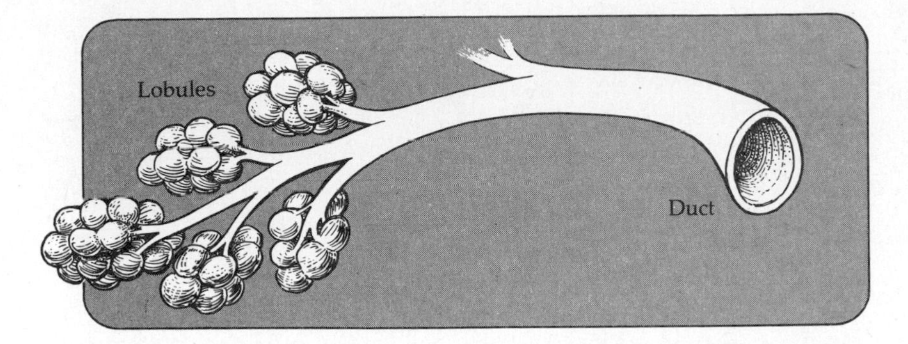

FIGURE 12-1

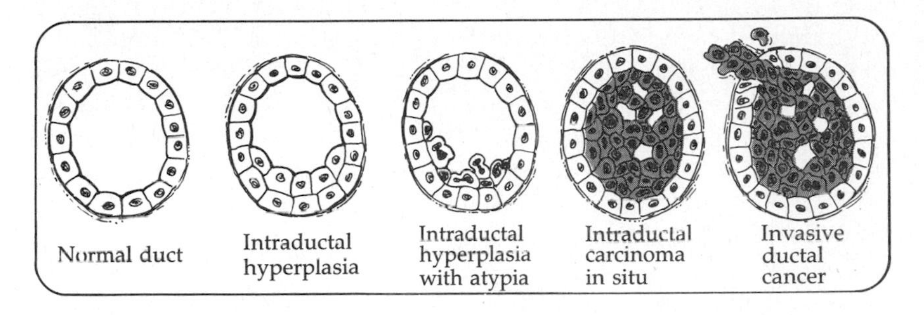

FIGURE 12-2

first changes that lead to cancer are thought to start at the junction of the duct and the lobule, it is interesting to consider what might cause it to go one way or the other.

The first two levels (hyperplasia and atypia) take place inside the duct or lobule, so you can't feel them by examining your breast. In the past they were only found incidentally (2–4 percent of the time) during a surgical biopsy, not in the lump itself but next to the lump in the rim of apparently "normal" tissue, and the pathologist came across them by accident.[1] Now with mammographic screening we are finding that some (12–17 percent) of the microcalcifications that are biopsied are associated with ALH or ADH.[2] If you look at autopsy studies of women who've died of causes other than breast cancer, you'll see that 30 percent or so had some degree of either hyperplasia or atypical hyperplasia.[3] So probably a lot of us are walking around with these conditions, and we don't know it because we have no reason to have biopsies and they don't show on mammograms.

The fact that we are finding more atypical ductal hyperplasia has led to several studies about what it means.[4,5,6] In general there is a progression of increased risk with each of these entities.[7] The women in these studies with ductal hyperplasia and no atypia had a slightly increased relative risk (barely significant), which was worse when compounded with family history (1.6–1.9 and 2.4–2.7, respectively). Finally, and most significantly, the women with atypical ductal hyperplasia had an increased relative risk of 4.1–4.3, and if they had a family history in a first-degree relative this rose to 4.7–8.4 over 15 years. This sounds high, until you realize that of the 10,000 benign biopsies studied in review, only 3 percent had atypical ductal hyperplasia.

Another factor that seems to affect risk is the age of the woman. Premenopausal women had a higher risk of getting cancer than postmenopausal women. Surprisingly hormone replacement therapy did not seem to affect the risk. Until recently no one had reported specifically on the significance of atypical lobular hyperplasia. Dr. David Page remedied the situation with a study of the 252 women in his records with atypical lobular hyperplasia that had been diagnosed on a surgical biopsy.[8] He found that 50 of them went on to develop invasive cancers, giving them a relative risk of 3.1. The cancers were on the same side as the ALH 75 percent of the time and took on average 14.8 years to show up. Obviously these lesions don't progress rapidly and often don't progress at all.

There are still many questions. For the woman diagnosed with atypical ductal or lobular hyperplasia, the most vital question is, What does it mean? The first step is to look at how it was diagnosed. If atypical hyperplasia is found on a core biopsy (see Chapter 8), there is a consensus that an open surgical biopsy is indicated. This is because of a 20–25 percent risk that the hyperplasia is the tip of the iceberg—that next to it there may be an in situ or invasive cancer.[9]

On the other hand, if it was found during a larger surgical biopsy, you can be more confident that the whole area has been removed. Most surgeons would agree that the best program is close follow-up, so that any in situ carcinoma or invasive cancer is found. This would include a physical exam by a doctor every six months and yearly mammograms.

For women who want a treatment, studies using tamoxifen for prevention have given us another option. The women with ADH who took tamoxifen for five years had 86 percent greater decrease in subsequent breast cancers than those who had no treatment.[10] It is certainly worth considering the risks and benefits of this approach (see Chapter 11). Some women may even consider a more drastic approach and have preventive mastectomies.

If we consider atypical hyperplasia as "pre-precancer," in situ cancer, the next step along the path can be considered precancer. Some doctors prefer to call it "noninvasive cancer"—a term I find misleading, since in most people's minds cancer is by definition an invasive disease. I prefer the term "precancer" because the lack of invasion means that these lesions can't metastasize, and therefore can't kill you. They have the potential to develop into an invasive cancer over time. I have had many battles over this nomenclature with colleagues who say cancer is cancer, whether it is invasive or not.

Precancers in the breast, like atypical hyperplasia, rarely cause lumps, pain, or any other symptoms and are also usually found incidentally. Unlike atypical hyperplasia, however, they can sometimes show up on mammograms, and the increased use of mammography for screening has shown us that they're actually far more common than we'd thought. The process of learning about and treating breast precancers is similar to that of cervical precancers, which were rarely seen until the routine use of Pap smears showed them to be fairly frequent.

There are two kinds of precancer of the breast: ductal carcinoma in situ and lobular carcinoma in situ (LCIS). As its name suggests, the latter occurs in the lobules.

LOBULAR CANCER IN SITU

Under the microscope, LCIS appears as small, round cells stuffing the lobules, which normally have no cells inside them (Fig. 12-3). If there are only a few cells and they're not too odd looking, you have lobular hyperplasia, while if they fill the whole lobule and look very atypical (odd), you have LCIS. Such lobules have been termed "multicentric" because they can be scattered throughout both breasts. However, no one has tried to tie them to one ductal system the way they have with DCIS.

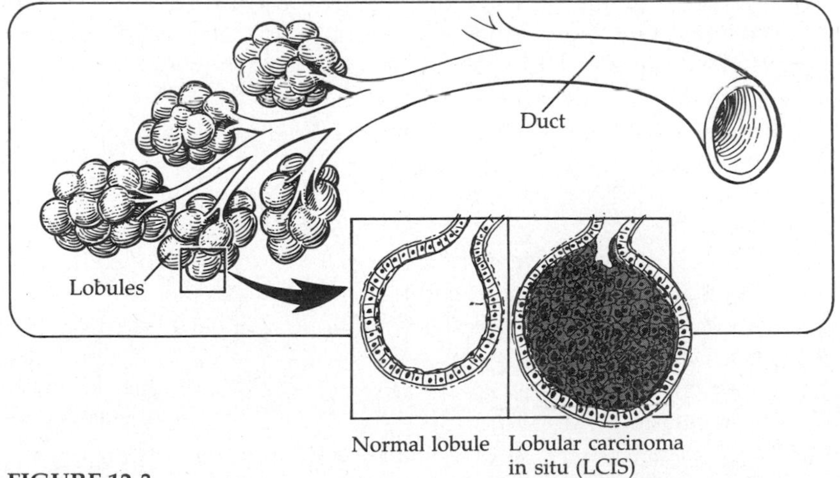

FIGURE 12-3

Since the lobules are at the periphery of each ductal branch, they could appear scattered while actually being part of the same branch of ducts.

We thought we knew the natural history of LCIS based on studies by Cushman Haagensen in 1978, but recent work has challenged our previous ideas. The old theory was that LCIS doesn't grow into cancer but signals a possible danger—the way, for example, an overcast day warns you it may rain. Because of this, many experts believed that lobular carcinoma in situ wasn't, in fact, a true precancer. Recent data suggest that this may not be the case. The first piece of evidence that LCIS can actually progress to invasive lobular cancer came from an analysis of 180 woman who had participated in a study of the National Surgical Breast and Bowel Project (NSABP).[11] Overall it found after 12 years of follow-up that nine (5 percent) invasive breast cancers developed in the same breast as the original lesions, eight (89 percent) of which were invasive lobular cancers—in the same area as the original LCIS. The risk of developing an invasive recurrence in the same breast was about the same within the first five years and after five years of follow-up. In addition, 10 invasive cancers developed in the opposite breast and six of the eight the study was able to review turned out to be invasive lobular cancers. These took longer to develop; most of them occurred after five years. Crucial for those diagnosed with LCIS, of the 180 women only 2 patients (1.1 percent) died of breast cancer: one who had a previous invasive breast cancer and one with a contralateral (on the other side of the breast) cancer.

A second piece of evidence was a study of women who had both LCIS and invasive lobular cancer in the same breast. The pattern of mutations in the involved cells was very similar, suggesting that one had indeed evolved from the other.[12]

Three other studies have been published since 1996, including one of 214 women with LCIS, which suggest a continuous risk of about 1 percent per year.[13,14,15] This risk can be compounded by other risk factors for breast cancer (see Table 12-1).

What can you do if you have lobular carcinoma in situ? Basically this is a prevention situation: you want to prevent yourself from getting breast cancer. There are a number of options; the most drastic is bilateral prophylactic mastectomy. Why bilateral (both breasts)? Because the risk occurs in both breasts. In the NSABP study mentioned above, there was a 5 percent chance of getting an invasive cancer in the same breast and a 5.6 percent chance of getting an invasive cancer in the opposite one.

Some women choose this because they want to know they've done everything possible. That way if they get breast cancer, they feel that at least it isn't their fault. If they hadn't done anything surgically and then developed the disease, they'd always wonder if they could have

Table 12-1. Benign Breast Disease and Risk of Breast Cancer[a]

	Relative Risk (%)
Previous biopsy[b]	1.8
Gross cysts	1.3
with first-degree family history	2.7
Atypical hyperplasia	4.4
with first-degree family history	8.9
with calcifications on mammogram	6.5
with first birth after 20	4.5
Lobular carcinoma *in situ*	7.2
Ductal carcinoma *in situ*	11.0

[a]Adapted from W.D. Dupont and D.L. Page, "Breast Cancer Risk with Proliferative Disease, Age at First Birth, and a Family History of Breast Cancer," *American Journal of Epidemiology* 125 (1987): 769.

[b]S.M. Love, R.S. Gelman, and W.S. Silen, "'Fibrocystsic Disease': A Non-disease?," *New England Journal of Medicine* 307 (1982): 1010.

prevented it. In the mid-1980s a patient told me, "I knew instantly what my decision should be. I was astounded to see how greedy for life I was." This woman was in a high-risk group because of her family history; she had relatives with breast cancer and was determined to do all she could to avoid suffering with it herself. She was uncomfortable with the studies about monitoring, which she thought were too recent, while mastectomy had been around a long time. She had reconstruction through one of the flap procedures discussed in Chapter 22. Others have silicone implants.

The alternative to surgery is to take the appearance of LCIS as a warning that you need to be closely watched. This means follow-up exams every six months, with a yearly mammogram. That way if a cancer does develop you're likely to catch it as soon as possible and can decide then if you want to have a mastectomy, or a lumpectomy and radiation (see Chapter 23). If a cancer doesn't develop, you've been spared the ordeal of major and disfiguring surgery. This is the consensus of surgeons, including myself, and one supported by the NSABP group. Most of my patients have opted for this course.

More controversial is the practice of taking tamoxifen for five years to prevent the subsequent development of breast cancer. This estrogen-blocking drug has been shown to decrease the chance of getting breast cancer by 56 percent in women with LCIS. Remember this means that the risk becomes 56 percent of the original risk— about 0.5 percent a year as opposed to 1 percent per year. Although there is some question as to whether its effect will last beyond five years, we have reason to believe it may. Other drugs are being developed that may have a similar benefit. As of yet none of them, including aromatase inhibitors (see Chapter 11) and raloxifene (or evista), have been tried in women with LCIS. All of the drugs have side effects that must be taken into consideration (see Chapter 24). In addition, they are not safe to take if you are trying to get pregnant. This is a decision that, like so many, depends very much on how you personally weigh the pros and cons.

Give yourself time to figure out what you want to do. LCIS doesn't call for an immediate decision. A woman called me recently in a panic because she had been diagnosed with LCIS and told by her oncologist that she should start on tamoxifen immediately. She was uncomfortable with this choice and worried about what to do. Remember that LCIS is a risk factor for subsequent cancer, not cancer itself. The risk of developing cancer is 1 percent per year, so there is no rush to begin a treatment. I suggested to this woman that she take the follow-up route initially, and see how she felt about it in six months or a year. If she was comfortable living with it, then she could continue this course for the rest of her life, or until a cancer occurred. You can always decide on tamoxifen or mastectomy later, but you can't undo a double mastectomy, and you may not be able to undo some of tamoxifen's side effects. However, if a woman finds herself living in a constant state of anxiety, waking up every morning thinking, "This is it—this is the day I'll find the lump," then maybe a bilateral mastectomy is best for her.

Radiation and chemotherapy are not necessary treatments for LCIS because it's not really cancer. As we reconsider the data on its ability to progress to cancer, we are also rethinking our treatment. Should we, or even could we, remove it all? Most of the time LCIS is scattered throughout an area of the breast. (Remember that the lobules are like the leaves on a tree.) Wide excision is probably not realistic and therefore not worth attempting.

Sometimes when a patient has a lump that turns out to be cancer, the pathologist will find LCIS in the adjacent tissue. What does this mean? In essence it suggests that the patient was at a higher risk of getting breast cancer and sure enough got it. A number of studies show that women with LCIS associated with their invasive cancer who undergo breast conservation have the same risk of local recurrence and contralateral breast cancer as those without LCIS.[16,17,18,19]

DUCTAL CARCINOMA IN SITU

DCIS is more common than LCIS. It's also more than a marker that cancer may appear in the breast: it's a lesion that can grow into an invasive cancer. DCIS rarely forms lumps but sometimes forms a soft

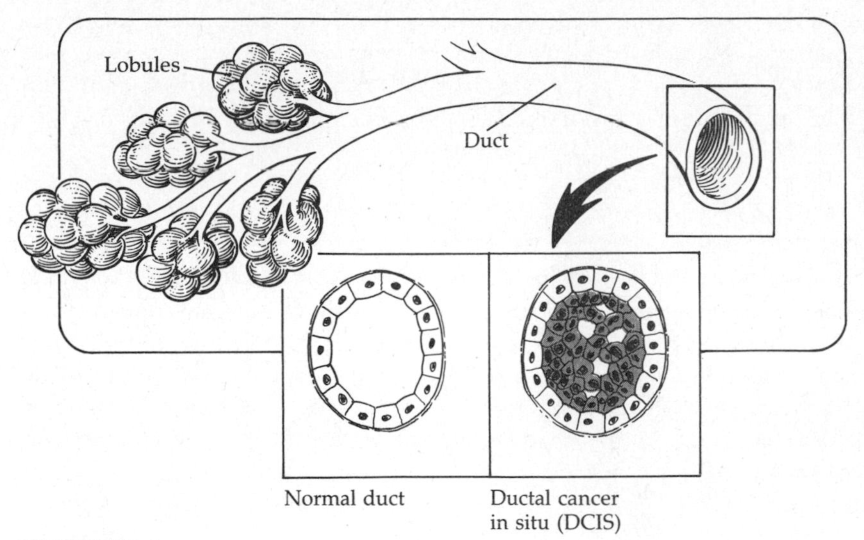

FIGURE 12-4

thickening (caused by the pliable ducts becoming less pliable because they're filled with cells; see Fig. 12-4). DCIS is now found far more frequently because of mammograms, where it appears with microcalcifications. A full 20 percent of malignancies detected by screening mammography are DCIS. In fact, it's probably very common. Autopsies done on women who died from all kinds of causes show that between 6 and 16 percent had DCIS.[20,21] This suggests that many of us have it unknowingly; it is probably not, as we used to believe, a rare condition.

In the past, standard treatment was a mastectomy of the breast with the lesion. That worked most of the time but might not have been necessary; since the breasts had been removed, we had no way of studying what happened when a breast that had DCIS *wasn't* removed.

A few small studies, however, have given us a clue. Two studies followed people who were biopsied and thought to have something benign. These studies have led us to believe that about 20–25 percent of women with untreated low-grade DCIS will go on to get invasive cancer up to 25 years after the initial biopsy, and in the same area of the breast in which that biopsy was done.[22,23] Since the studies together add up to only 78 patients, they may not be representative. Furthermore, their lesions were on the border between atypical hyperplasia and DCIS or they would have been diagnosed initially; the studies don't address the situation of women with obvious DCIS. What is clear from these studies, however, is that untreated DCIS can go on to invasive breast cancer but in the majority of women it does not seem to do so.

Unfortunately, we don't know how to tell which ones will become cancer and which won't. There's a lot of research going on in molecular biology seeking a marker that clearly shows which lesions are on their way to becoming cancer, and which will never become cancer.

DCIS and Invasion

We've always thought that invasive cancer cells are DCIS cells that have learned a new skill that allows them mobility, so they can break outside the ducts—sort of the way a tadpole grows into a frog. Perhaps a mutation gives them that ability, and from there they take off, make blood vessels, and become invasive cancer.

To determine this, researchers looked at DCIS cells and cancer cells, examining them for the molecular markers (such as p53, apoptosis, Her-2/neu; see Chapter 27) that are signs of cancer. They expected to find some of the markers in DCIS and many more in invasive cancers.

What they found, however, was that there were the same markers in both. We have yet to find anything that shows a difference between DCIS and invasive cells—something that would allow us to examine a lesion and say, "Okay, now it's not invasive, but if it develops X, we'll know it's crossed over that line." With such knowledge, we could probably catch invasive cancer at an extremely early stage by examining the DCIS.

We may still find it. Another hypothesis researchers are beginning to look at is the possibility that there may not be any difference in the cells—that in both situations, they're the same cancer cells. In that case, what would cause DCIS to stay within the duct would be not its inability to get out but the action of some other force keeping it in. They're not acting, say the researchers; they're being acted on.

If the second theory is correct, something is holding the DCIS inside the duct. Dr. Sanford Barsky, a breast pathologist who was at UCLA, has done some very interesting work looking at the myoepithelial cells that form a rim around the outside of the duct.[24] The cells are just sitting there in the background and no one has paid much attention to them till now. Barsky's studies have found that they produce an enzyme that actively blocks invasion. In order for cancer cells to invade, they have to be able to eat away proteins and get through the cells, and the enzyme stops them from doing this. Some hormones act differently on the myoepithelial cells. Think of these cells as a line of prison guards standing there and not letting anyone through. Then someone gives the guards whiskey, and they get mellow and laid back and decide to let everyone pass. On the other hand, tell them the boss is watching them and they get even tougher. Estrogen is the whiskey;

prednisone, another hormone, is the snoopy boss. Tamoxifen also tends to make the the myoepithelial cells tougher—which may be one of the ways it works.

Another component may be the local cellular neighborhood—there is "cross talk" between the cancer cells and the cells around them (see Chapter 28). Some of the tissues that these surrounding cells make up may also be involved in preventing invasion.

This is all preliminary, and probably it's only one factor. It shows up in the lab, and that's a revealing sign. But putting cells in a petri dish, dripping estrogen on them, and watching the myoepithelial cells get weaker doesn't tell us what happens in a human body. Still, it's promising. I'd love for it to work out because if it does, we may discover that even invasive cancer can be reversible. If we knew the elements needed to confine the cells, we could give patients whatever those elements were and send the cells back into confinement.

There are other important things to consider. In some women with DCIS, the ducts containing the abnormal cells are surrounded by microscopic extra blood vessels and also *stroma desmoplasia,* a hardening of the surrounding tissue. Both are reactions to something being secreted by the cancer cells. How can cancer cells trapped inside the duct get messages ordering the creation of new blood cells *outside* the duct? So far, we don't know. Maybe they're stimulating the myoepithelial cells to do it (the prison guards are getting messages to the gang outside). This ability to induce new blood vessels to grow (angiogenesis) and to increase the hardness of the surrounding tissue is shared with invasive cancer cells and may be an early indicator of which cells are likely to become invasive. These changes can sometimes be identified with an MRI, and they may be a clue to the more significant DCIS lesions.

Another significant change in the way we perceive DCIS is that we no longer necessarily see it as a simple progression from atypical hyperplasia to low-grade DCIS to high-grade DCIS and then to invasion. It now appears that low-grade DCIS becomes low-grade cancer, and high-grade DCIS becomes high-grade cancer.[25] This lends credence to the idea that the cells aren't changing. Their "personality" will stay the same, whether they're high-grade or low-grade, and there's something external making them behave differently.

If the high-grade DCIS cells recur or become invasive, they do so more quickly, which makes sense. They're more aggressive to begin with. Low-grade tumors appear to grow or invade much more slowly: the recurrences that David Page found 15 to 20 years after the diagnosis were all low-grade DCIS. This is very important to realize when we're doing studies: if a DCIS study follows its subjects for only five years, it will look as though only high-grade DCIS recurs or becomes invasive. We need longer studies following subjects with DCIS, and we also need to address additional questions. What were those cells doing for 20 years?

Without a thorough understanding of the natural history of DCIS, which we do not yet have, it's hard to devise a logical treatment. However, there is increasing interest in treatments for DCIS that are less drastic than mastectomy—chiefly wide excision. This is the same principle as the lumpectomy in breast cancer (see Chapter 21), except that there's usually no lump involved, so the surgeon tries to remove the entire area that has the DCIS, along with a rim of normal breast tissue.

Some experts argue against this, claiming that DCIS, like LCIS, is multicentric.[26] Their idea is that all ductal tissue is marching toward cancer, and is precancerous to a greater or lesser degree; this tissue has just gotten a little further on. So, says this theory, we must take off the whole breast or even both breasts, because just taking off part of one isn't going to solve the problem.

This unfortunate idea evolved from a number of studies in which breasts removed for DCIS were analyzed. The breasts were cut into four quadrants and then examined under the microscope. If they found DCIS in more than one quadrant, the researchers designated it as multicentric, implying that it was sprouting up in several ducts at once.[27]

This, however, presupposes that ducts are arranged in quadrants. They aren't. The breast isn't like an orange, with each duct in its nicely defined section. In fact, the ductal system isn't structured in quadrants at all. It's more like an arbor: it comes from the nipple, branches out, and fills up a certain amount of space. There are between five and nine separate ductal systems in each breast; they intertwine but they don't connect.[28] Thus one system may take up the whole upper part of the breast. If the breast is cut into quadrants, we could easily find DCIS in both quadrants even though it's all part of one ductal system.

This was demonstrated in a study done by Rolland Holland in Nijmegan, the Netherlands.[29] He took breasts that had been removed and cut them into four quadrants, and he too found that there was disease in several of the quadrants. But he went a step further. He very carefully mapped out the DCIS and found that in 80 of the 81 cases, even though it was in more than one quadrant, it was in the same duct, which branched into several parts of the breast.

The idea that DCIS is multicentric has been given less credence recently, especially since it was discovered to be *monoclonal*.[30] A clone, remember, is an exact replica of the original cell. This means that all of the molecular markers would be exactly the same. If you could be cloned, for example, your clones would be far more like you than an identical twin would. Everything, down to the tiny mole on your left buttock, would be the same. The monoclonal model suggests that one cell keeps replicating and all the cells up and down the duct look exactly the same.

This is important not only in terms of our scientific understanding of DCIS but in an immediate way for patients diagnosed with the disease. If it were multicentric, it would lend itself to the argument that you may as well have mastectomies in both breasts because it is only a matter of time until the second breast gets cancer. But if DCIS is actually unicentric and monoclonal, the wiser treatment would be to remove the one affected section of the breast.

Unfortunately, when pathologists look at DCIS on a slide and see several duct profiles filled with cells, they also use the terms "multicentric" or "multifocal." The clinician interprets that as meaning there's DCIS all over the breast. But the pathologist just means that there are several different ducts (or sections of the same duct) seen in cross-section that have DCIS in them (Fig. 12-5). Pathologists don't have a whole breast under the microscope, just one little piece. All they can say is whether there is DCIS all over that piece. This means if a doctor says you have multicentric DCIS and need a mastectomy, you need to probe further what is meant. If necessary, see if you can talk directly to the pathologist and ask what exactly was under the microscope. This will give you a better perspective on the problem.

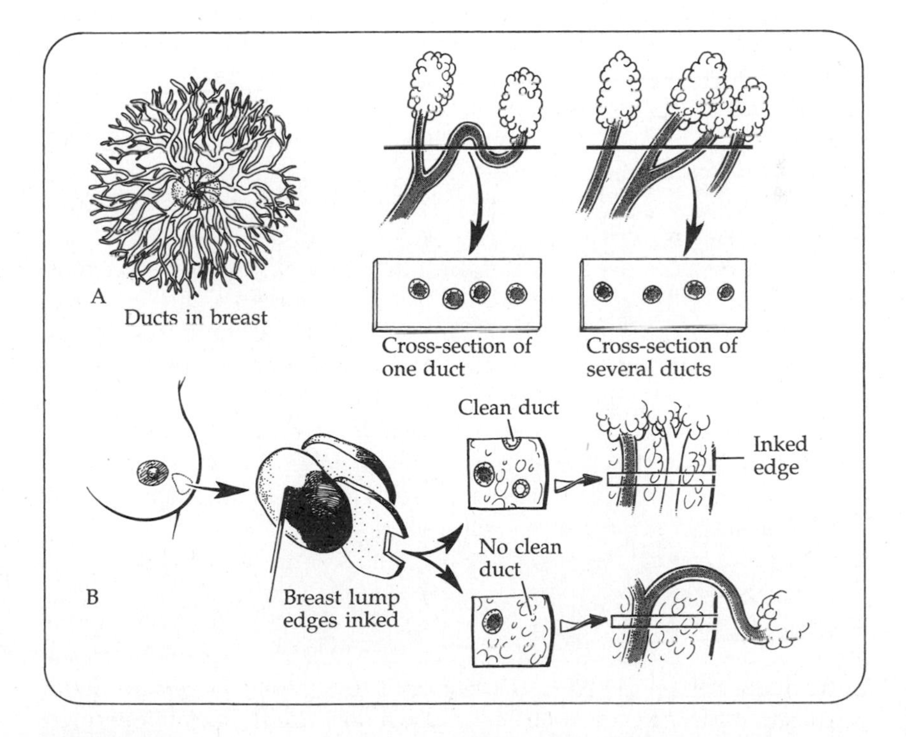

FIGURE 12-5

Most high-grade lesions tend to be continuous and well marked by mammographically visible calcifications. Low- to intermediate-grade lesions, however, can be more sneaky with discontinuous intraductal spread, often having gaps of up to 1 centimeter between areas of involvement.

What we currently do is a wide excision based on our best guess of the extent of disease. We arrive at this guess by looking at the preoperative mammogram and magnification views, and then studying the tissue we remove from the breast. The pathologist examines the tissue and coats the outer surface with India ink. The tissue is then fixed and made into slides (see Chapter 16), which are examined. If there is DCIS near ink it is said to be a "dirty margin." If there is only normal breast tissue next to ink it is a "clean margin." But the pathologists can't look at every margin—it would be more than 2,000 slides. They are only sampling the margins, so it's possible that even if all the margins they look at are negative there will be a DCIS-filled duct crossing into the breast that they have missed. This is a different situation than when we remove a single lump; in which case, knowing precisely where the lesion is, we know that we have gotten out the right surrounding tissue. So when there's a "recurrence" of DCIS, it's probably not a recurrence at all; it's DCIS that we left behind in the first place, in spite of what we thought were clean margins. This doesn't happen frequently, but often enough (about 10–20 percent of the time) to make it significant. That's why mastectomy, though imperfect, tends to give a lower recurrence rate—it's the widest excision possible.

Unfortunately, a "wide excision" has been defined as simply one in which DCIS can't be seen in the ink around the lesion. But because DCIS can go in and out of the plane of a section (see Fig. 12-5), a truly clean margin should show normal breast tissue between the ink and the DCIS. This is why most doctors now do measurements for margins: we say it has to be more than a centimeter. In reality, this isn't true. It could be a millimeter, if we got all the DCIS within that millimeter out. But since we have no way of knowing when that is so, we give ourselves a big rim around the lesion to be certain.

It is also important to look at a postbiopsy mammogram. DCIS usually shows up on the mammogram as calcifications. Even if calcifications have been removed, there are often some left, and this picture can add information about residual disease.

Options

The goal of treating DCIS is prevention. If the precancer is completely removed, it can neither come back nor become invasive. Sadly, though, we can't be sure that we can completely remove it, and most of our efforts go into minimizing the risk of local recurrence. The options for surgical therapy are simple mastectomy or wide excision (we can't call it a lumpectomy when there is no lump). Amazingly, these two approaches have never been directly compared. The recurrence shown in mastectomy studies is about 1–2 percent, probably representing the fact that we can't remove all of the breast tissue. Breast conservation has a 5–10 percent risk of local recurrence. That might be scary, except for the fact that the chance of dying of breast cancer is about the same, 1–2 percent, in both procedures.[31] Most women undergo breast conservation for DCIS. This is because most lesions are small and detected by mammogram. Invasive cancers are also treated conservatively, and there is no survival advantage to mastectomy. The current controversy is not whether mastectomy is necessary for DCIS, but rather whether radiation is necessary. Three randomized controlled studies have compared wide excision alone to wide excision and radiation for DCIS.[32,33,34] Most of the women in these studies had small lesions that were removed with clean margins. At five years of follow-up, excision alone had about a 16 percent risk of recurrence while excision with radiation therapy had 8 percent. In all studies approximately 50 percent of the local recurrences were invasive and 50 percent had more DCIS. The studies in Europe, Great Britain, Australia, and New Zealand showed a decrease of both by half, while the American NSABP showed a greater reduction of the invasive cancer recurrences. This says two things: first, there are fewer recurrences in women who get radiation and, second, and more important, there were fewer *invasive* recurrences. Having DCIS recur is unpleasant, but it won't kill you. Having an invasive cancer show up puts your life at risk.

Can we predict which women with DCIS can do without radiation? After all, 75 percent of the DCIS never recurred. The predictors of recurrence after breast-conserving surgery have been extensively studied. One attempt to make this distinction is to look at the architecture of the DCIS. Researchers have discovered three general patterns (Fig. 12-6). One is called *micropapillary:* the cells fill the duct with a fingerlike mass sticking out into the duct's center. A second is called *cribriform:* it also fills in the duct but then there are punched-out holes like Swiss cheese. These are low-grade patterns sometimes referred to as non-comedo. The third is called *comedo* for its resemblance to a comedo, or whitehead pimple. This is the high-grade pattern. The cells are stuffing the duct, and some of them are dead (necrotic). There is also a lot of apoptosis (cell death), and there are very aberrant cells. If the tissue around the duct is squeezed, white, cheesy material comes out, exactly as if you were squeezing a pimple. The key features that appear to be predictive of recurrence are whether the cells are high-grade and

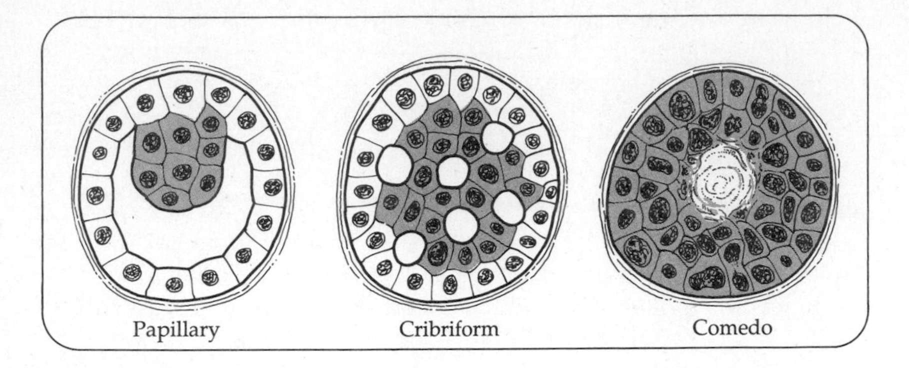

FIGURE 12-6

necrotic. In addition, young women have a greater rate of local recurrence than older ones.

Dr. Mel Silverstein, previously in Van Nuys, California, but now at Norris Cancer Center at the University of Southern California, has been arguing for some time against treating all women with DCIS the same way. He says that if a woman has a tiny, 5-millimeter spot of DCIS that can be cut out with a centimeter of margin all around it, she may not need radiation. At the other extreme, if she has aggressive, widespread DCIS and the surgeon can't get a wide margin, she may need a mastectomy. He and his group have developed a prognostic index (USC/VNPI) in an attempt to distinguish which women needed radiation therapy. They looked at the patient's age, whether the lesion was high-grade or low-grade, the presence or absence of necrosis, the tumor's size, and the size of the margin (how much normal tissue there was between the DCIS and the edge of the tissue that had been removed). They found what we had already suspected: the predictor that trumped the rest was the size of the margins—which translates to "Did we get it all out?" Even with high-grade DCIS, if they get it out with a nice, clean margin, it doesn't come back in the breast.

They were able to distinguish three groups of patients: DCIS patients with USC/VNPI scores of 4, 5, or 6 had the same local recurrence rate whether or not they received radiation therapy. Women with intermediate scores (7, 8, 9) received a statistically significant 12–15 percent survival benefit when radiation was added, and the women with scores of 10, 11, or 12 had the greatest benefit from radiation therapy but still had a 50 percent recurrence rate at five years. It should be noted that this index was based on 706 patients who were not randomized and had not received tamoxifen. Nonetheless some clinicians and patients find it useful in arriving at an informed decision.

So we may be able to select out patients who need radiation. In order for the surgeon to get out a centimeter all around of margin, the lesion has to be small. With a bigger lesion, that large a margin would be a virtual mastectomy.

A 1999 study tested whether adding tamoxifen to lumpectomy and radiation had additional value.[35] Researchers randomized 1,804 women who had been treated for DCIS to receive either tamoxifen or a placebo for five years. All had been treated by excision followed by radiation therapy. Forty women in the placebo group and 23 in the tamoxifen group developed subsequent invasive cancers in the treated breast. In other words, tamoxifen reduced the chance of developing invasive cancer from 4.2 percent to 2.1 percent. There were 47 noninvasive recurrences (more DCIS) in the placebo group and 40 in the tamoxifen group. Tamoxifen lowered the rate of noninvasive recurrences (new ones or DCIS left over from earlier treatment) from 5.1 to 3.9 percent.

Thirty-six cancers (noninvasive and invasive combined) developed in the placebo group and 18 in the tamoxifen group (3.45 to 2.0 percent). Most important, there were 10 recurrences—seven in the placebo group and three in the tamoxifen group—in the nodes, chest wall, or elsewhere in the body (metastases). Although the recurrence rate was less than half as great in the tamoxifen group, the numbers are too small to be statistically significant. There were six deaths from breast cancer (a very rare event for DCIS) in the placebo group, two from cancers in the same breast as the original DCIS. In comparison, there were four deaths in the tamoxifen group, including three that were attributed to cancers in the treated breast.

Overall, the risk of any breast-related event (recurrent invasive disease, noninvasive disease, second cancers in the opposite breast, and metastasis) went from 13.4 to 8.2 percent at five years. Side effects included two cases of phlebitis in the placebo group and nine in the tamoxifen group with one nonfatal pulmonary embolus in the placebo group and two in the tamoxifen group. There was about a 10 percent higher incidence of hot flashes, fluid retention, and vaginal discharge in the tamoxifen group than in the placebo group. There were about 3.5 times as many cases of uterine cancer in the tamoxifen group as in the placebo group, although there were no uterine cancer deaths.

A second study done in the United Kingdom, Australia, and New Zealand looked at wide excision alone, as well as wide excision and radiation therapy both with and without tamoxifen. The study found that the women who received both radiation and tamoxifen had the lowest local recurrence rates. However, the benefits of the tamoxifen were small and statistically insignificant.[36]

One factor in the limited benefits seen with adjuvant tamoxifen may be that it was given to women regardless of the estrogen sensitivity of their lesions. A retrospective analysis of the NSABP study suggests that the women whose lesions were positive for estrogen receptors had a significant reduction in the risk of recurrence (60 percent), while those with estrogen receptor negative tumors had no significant benefit.[37] This suggests that any woman with DCIS should ask to have it tested for estrogen receptors, particularly if she is contemplating taking tamoxifen.

This is obviously a complex issue. The advantages are small, but then so are the risks. Importantly, this study was in women treated with lumpectomy and radiation. In women who underwent mastectomy the benefits are unknown, but are probably limited to a decrease of cancer in the other breast. This risk is about 0.5–1 percent per year, just as with invasive cancers.[38] In a woman who chooses bilateral mastectomy there would be little to no benefit. Each woman will evaluate these risks and benefits differently.

Treatment Options for DCIS

What does all this mean for you? How should you proceed? First, if your routine mammogram has shown a cluster of microcalcifications you'll need to have a core biopsy or a wire localization biopsy (see Chapter 8). This will determine whether you have DCIS. Next, you should have another mammogram to see if the biopsy has gotten rid of all the microcalcifications. However thorough your surgeon has been, a few may remain. If the diagnosis is DCIS, make sure your pathology report includes information regarding the grade, presence of necrosis, margin, and estrogen receptor. Then you've got the four choices described above: wide excision alone, wide excision and radiation, a combination of those with tamoxifen, or mastectomy. Currently doctors differ broadly about the best ways to treat DCIS. Until more studies come out with definitive answers, the controversies will rage. A reasonable approach to treatment options is discussed in the following paragraphs.

You can have that breast removed, which is the ultimate wide excision. Most of the time this will be more than adequate, but there have been reports of DCIS recurring in the remaining breast tissue.[39,40] It happens in about 5 percent of cases. Generally we do a mastectomy only if the DCIS is so extensive that it's the only choice or if the patient strongly wants it.

The next option is a wide excision. This means taking out the area with a centimeter-wide rim of normal tissue around it. Sometimes this has been done on the first operation and other times it is necessary to go back and remove more tissue (a reexcision).

If your margins are less than a centimeter, you can have a wide excision combined with radiation. You can add five years of tamoxifen to any of the choices above if the DCIS is estrogen receptor positive (the biggest benefit of doing this may be not in treating the DCIS but in preventing an invasive cancer or one in the other breast).

There is no reason to remove lymph nodes for small areas of DCIS because precancer can't spread at this stage. But if the lesions are big (greater than 5 centimeters), some experts think they may hide microinvasion and recommend removing the lymph nodes as well. (Sentinel node biopsy is a good option here.) On the other hand, as I explain in Chapter 21, many surgeons will forgo lymph node dissection in this group as well, since even with microinvasion the chance of having positive nodes is so low.[41]

Since DCIS is not capable of spreading, there is no reason to use chemotherapy. The fact that DCIS doubles your risk of getting cancer in the other breast is another factor to consider. But remember that this "double" isn't as alarming as it sounds: it's about the same risk a woman without breast cancer has because of having had a late first pregnancy. (If your general risk at 50 is 1 in 500, it becomes 1 in 250.) Some doctors suggest that you really need double mastectomies. But it's an individual decision. Some women who have mastectomies feel that if they have to lose one breast they may as well lose both and get it over with. Others feel that losing one breast makes the remaining one even more precious and they really want to save it. For the latter group close follow-up alone is the standard, but tamoxifen may be an option.

For the reasons discussed in Chapter 9, I try to encourage every woman to participate in a study, unless she has a definite preference or unless there are reasons to pick a particular treatment. As new studies and information come in, we will refine our understanding of DCIS and have a better basis for determining treatment. Outside of a study, every patient should have the final say in what treatment she gets: some women don't want a mastectomy no matter how big the lesions are, while at the other extreme some patients don't want to gamble even on the smallest lesion. Remember, there is no one single treatment for precancer; there are a number of possible treatments. You don't have to rush into a treatment because your doctor or your friend or anyone else says you should. It's your breast and your life. Take the time to decide what's best for you.

13

The Intraductal Approach: Getting to the Source

The intraductal approach is the area I believe has the most promise. The potential to eradicate breast cancer entirely with the intraductal approach is closer than ever.

We need something like a Pap smear for breast cancer—something that can find abnormal cells, cancerous or not, when they can be treated and the progression reversed before they have developed the ability to spread outside the breast (Fig. 13-1). As I said in the previous chapter, all breast cancer starts in the milk ducts. Since milk comes out of these ducts, I've always felt we need to find a way to go into them to sample the duct lining and see what's happening to the cells inside it. In the mid-1980s I started a research project at the Faulkner Hospital in Boston on the intraductal approach to the breast.

The idea of studying the ducts and their fluid was first mentioned in 1946 when a Uruguayan doctor, Raul Leborgne, described a way to pass a small catheter into a breast duct and squirt saline in, take the catheter out, and collect the fluid as it drips out.[1] He termed his procedure a "ductal rinse." Then in 1958 in the United States George Papanicolaou, the inventor of the cervical Pap smear, described applying suction to the nipple to obtain small drops of fluid from the milk ducts (Fig. 13-2). He termed it a "breast Pap smear."[2] (As I explained in Chapter 7, it's not unusual to be able to obtain fluid from a woman's breast.)

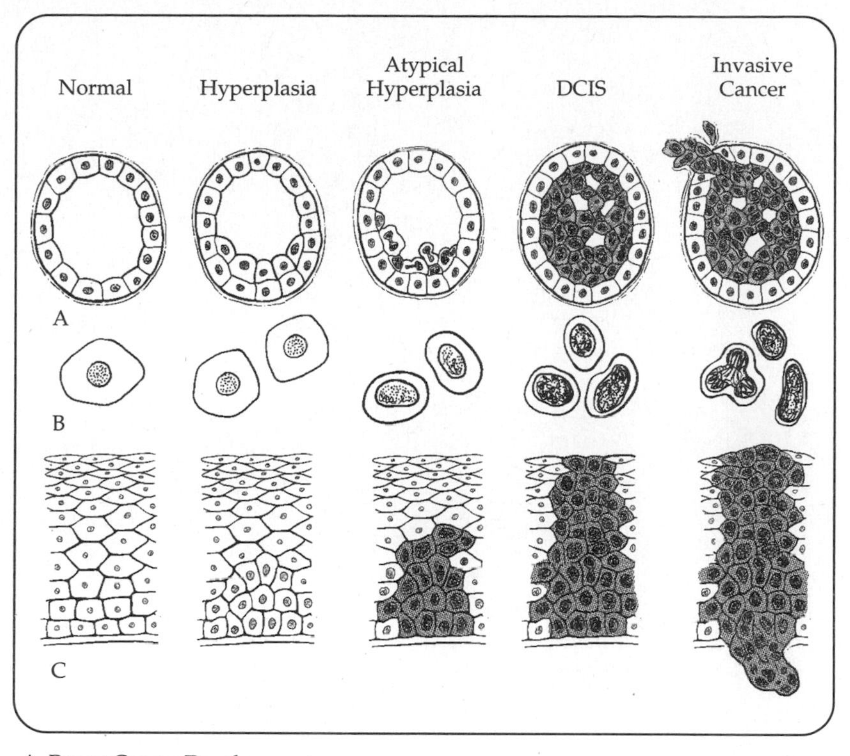

A. Breast Cancer Development
B. Cells from PAP Smear or Ductal Lavage
C. Cervical Cancer Development

FIGURE 13-1

In spite of the fact that Papanicolaou was able to diagnose a case of DCIS in nipple aspirate fluid (NAF), the technique languished for years. This was probably because no one knew in 1958 how the information could be used to help women. But curiosity remained, and in the 1970s, several researchers reevaluated Papanicolaou's approach. Three major series of studies took place, each advancing our understanding in a slightly different way: one by Gertrude Buehring, another by Otto Sartorius, and the third by Eileen King and Nicholas Petrakis.[3,4,5] In all of them researchers were able to obtain breast fluid from about 80 percent of premenopausal women and 50 percent of postmenopausal women by using a suction cup on the nipple.

King and Petrakis took the long view. Between 1973 and 1980 they analyzed the fluid they obtained by aspirating the ducts on a series of women. With a median of 21 years of follow-up, 285 of 3,633 women have developed breast cancer. The researchers compared the outcome

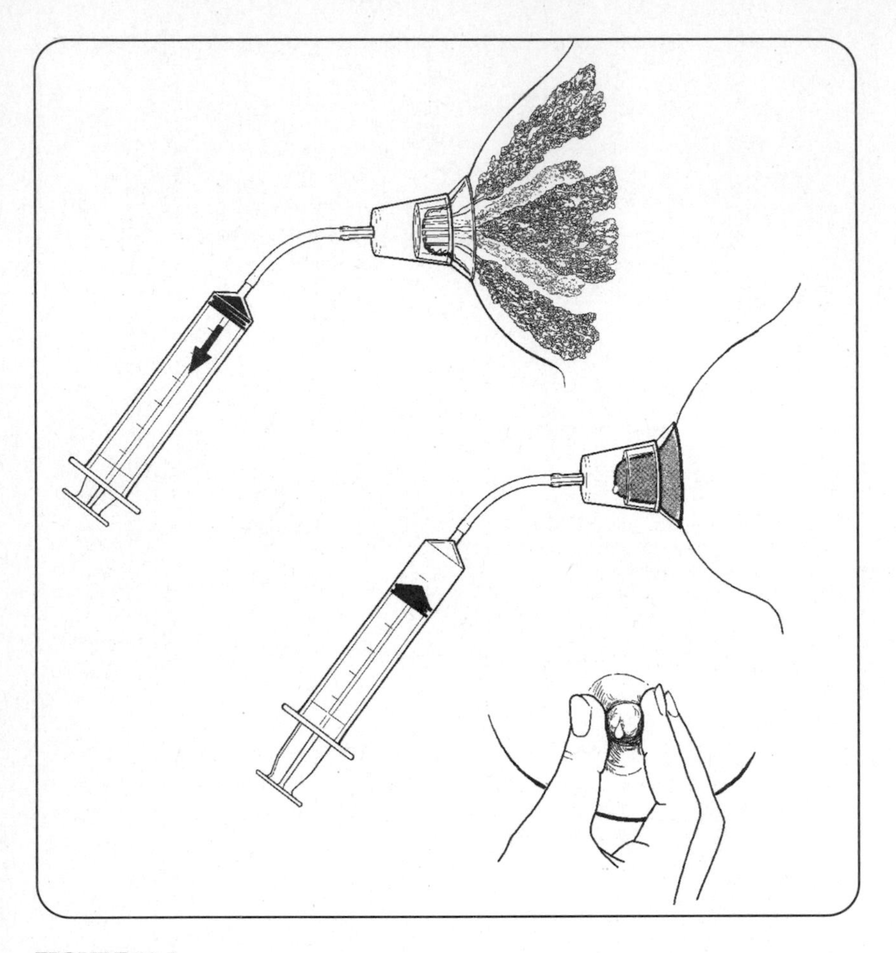

FIGURE 13-2

with their initial evaluation of the fluid they'd taken 21 years earlier. Not surprisingly, they discovered that the women who had had no fluid also had the lowest incidence of breast cancer (4.7 percent). Those with fluid but with normal cells had a slightly higher incidence (8.2 percent) than those without fluid. Those with hyperplasia showed a bit higher (10.8 percent) incidence, and those with atypical cells the highest (13.8 percent). Account was taken of differences in the women's ages and the years they entered the study. The women with atypical cells had nearly three times the amount of breast cancer of the women with no fluid at all.

They also concluded from this study that women with atypical cells and a first-degree relative with breast cancer were nearly twice as likely to develop the disease as were women who had atypical cells but no first-degree relatives with breast cancer. This suggests that if you have both atypical cells and a family history of breast cancer, you have a fairly high risk of getting the disease. Gertrude Buehring recently completed a 25-year follow-up of her series of NAF volunteers and confirmed a higher risk of cancer in those who had both NAF and cells.[6] We are currently doing 20-year follow-up on the Sartorius cohort. So we should soon know how most of the 6,000 or so women who underwent the procedure more than 20 years ago have fared.

Surprisingly, the early experiments with detection of atypical cells didn't catch on with either the public or the medical community. There were two major reasons for this. For one thing, as in the 1950s, we still did not know what to do with the information. If a woman had hyperplasia or even atypical hyperplasia, it was no guarantee that she would get breast cancer; in most cases, neither of those conditions grows into a cancer. What use, then, was the knowledge? Was the woman with hyperplasia going to have a mastectomy simply because she might one day have breast cancer? Or was she to spend years waiting nervously for the other shoe to drop?

Around the time these studies were going on, mammography became more popular. It detected actual cancer and obvious precancer (DCIS), not the processes leading to cancer—and the doctors knew what to do with that information. So the medical community greeted mammography with much more enthusiasm than it did the findings about ductal fluid.

But a few persistent researchers didn't give up. In Santa Barbara, Otto Sartorius didn't stop with NAF. In his surgical practice he routinely attempted nipple aspiration on 2,000 women. Some produced either no fluid or too little fluid for him to analyze. Others were found to have atypical cells. He decided to further probe this latter group of 400 women. He threaded a tiny catheter into a duct opening at the nipple, squirted some contrast material through it into a duct, and took an X ray (ductogram). After this he instilled saline into the duct in an attempt to wash it out. He then removed the catheter and applied suction to the duct to retrieve the saline. He couldn't suction the fluid out through the catheter because the suction caused the flimsy duct to collapse (like someone sucking on a wet straw). He found that washing out the cells with saline usually provided enough cells to make a diagnosis.

Despite this improvement in cell yield, the procedure still was not adopted by the medical community. Doctors thought it was too hard to do and still didn't know what to do with the results.

But timing is everything. By the late 1990s, breast cancer rates had continued to grow and the disease had become known as an "epidemic." Researchers were desperately trying to find a means of detecting the earliest signs of breast cancer risk. They began to review the studies on breast duct fluid, hoping to find in it a sign in the breast duct fluid of the early changes of cancer, something that could serve as a *marker* of what was going on biologically in the duct—a protein secreted by precancerous cells, for example. Ed Sauter, a surgeon from Fox Chase Hospital in Philadelphia, improved the suction technique to obtain nipple aspirate fluid so that he was able to retrieve fluid from close to 100 percent of women.[7] He then looked for PSA (the same marker that is used for prostate cancer) and other markers. As yet the perfect one that can predict who is at risk for breast cancer has not been identified.

In a different approach to the problem of identifying the woman with high-risk changes in the breast, Carol Fabian in Kansas explored the use of fine-needle aspirates (see Chapter 8)—sticking small needles into both breasts on both sides of the nipple and then suctioning out some cells.[8] Although this technique has demonstrated atypical changes in the tissue of high-risk women when compared to those of normal risk, it also has its limitations. The common thinking, as I noted in Chapter 12, is that breast cancer starts in the lining of the milk ducts and only one ductal system goes bad. If this is the case, it is important to identify a ductal system with abnormal cells and check it after an intervention to see if the changes disappeared. If atypical cells are identified by random needle sticks, it is more difficult to ascertain which duct they are in and get back to the very same spot in six months.

I was convinced that the answer to this problem is in accessing the ducts directly, not suctioning the whole nipple or randomly sampling the breast. My research team at Faulkner Hospital first tried using a ductoscope in the ducts to find abnormalities. This was not very successful because the ducts divide into many branches, like a bushy tree (see Fig. 1-4). We tried the nipple aspirate fluid collection with a suction device but were frustrated by the fact that the fluid became pooled before analysis, making it impossible for us to know which duct it came from. I also tried Otto Sartorius's technique with a catheter but was frustrated by the small amount of fluid I recovered. I decided to take a double lumen catheter (catheter with two inner tubes) and thread it through the opening in the nipple into a duct, then squirt saltwater into one lumen and suction it out of the other. After extensive experimentation (on volunteers under anesthesia who were having mastectomies and on freshly removed breasts), I was able to demonstrate that a double lumen catheter could retrieve cells from a duct. This success led me to found a company with an engineering friend, Julian Nikolchev, to commercialize the catheter for washing out the duct, as well as the procedure of ductal lavage. (The company was acquired in 2002 by Cytyc Corporation, which continues to make the catheter, while I am now conducting research through my own foundation.)

With help from a Defense Department grant, my research continued. I was often the guinea pig. We were initially stymied by the absence of a clear map of the ductal orifices. After studying breastfeeding women with the help of La Leche League, we determined that there were between five and nine openings in the nipple and that the pattern was fairly stable (See Fig. 1-6). We also reevaluated the ductograms done by Otto Sartorius and found that the ducts were distributed in the breasts in two concentric circles, with an inner group of three or four and a second, more peripheral, group of three or four (see Fig. 13-2). These anatomical studies helped us find the duct openings, and we confirmed them by injecting blue dye into the nipples of breasts that had been removed by mastectomy and observing the holes the dye emerged from.[9] I even tried it on myself a few times, much to my then 11-year-old daughter's chagrin. I didn't find it particularly unpleasant—but Katie did. The dye turns the nipple blue for several days, and Katie walked into my room one day while I was getting dressed. She glared at me. "Mom!" she said angrily. "Do you know how *embarrassing* it is to have a mother with blue nipples?" I tried to explain to her that there was no need for her to be embarrassed; I had no intention of displaying my nipples, whatever their color, to any of her friends or their parents. It didn't matter. Mom was not to have blue nipples. Luckily we are no longer using the blue dye—so no 11-year-old will ever again be embarrassed by the color of her mother's nipples.

Aside from my daughter's injured dignity, I felt no pain in the process, and this was typical. Some of the first volunteers were moderately uncomfortable, depending on their sensitivity to pain and the ease with which their fluid came out. One woman, whose fluid came quite easily, describes the procedure as "less painful and invasive than a Pap smear," and compared it to going to the dentist. "It's more frightening to think about than to do," she laughs. "I'm pretty squeamish, so I didn't watch them do it, and that helped." In the earlier studies we used injections of lidocaine, and this patient found the anesthetic needle more uncomfortable than the process itself. When the anesthetic wore off, "I felt it—not quite pain, but tenderness: I was very aware that I had a nipple," she says. But she had no bruising or discomfort later.

Another volunteer found the process even less problematic. With both NAF and lavage, she found the sensations strange, rather than painful. "I nursed two kids when I was younger," she said, "and it seemed weird at first, having this pressure at my breast/nipple that wasn't connected to either sexual pleasure or suckling an infant. So you have to get used to the notion that they're messing around with your breast." She didn't like the anesthetic needles but described them as "pinpricks." The discomfort, she said, was "so minor, it didn't matter."

We postulated that the ducts we wanted to study were the ones that yielded fluid on suction. These were the ones we thought most likely to have pathology, according to the earlier studies of Petrakis and Sartorius. The company's first clinical trial designed to demonstrate the utility of this approach involved studying women at high risk for breast cancer. After having the women massage their breasts (Fig. 13-3), we applied suction to their nipples. Once a duct or ducts were identified, a tiny ductal catheter was threaded into a milk duct for a distance of about 0.5 inch (1 cm) (Fig. 13-4). The duct was washed with saltwater and then cells were retrieved from deep in each ductal tree. The fluid was sent to be examined by a cytologist (pathologist who studies cells) and we determined whether there were normal, atypical, or cancerous cells present. These cells were compared to those in the fluid obtained by suction alone. In all, 507 women were studied who

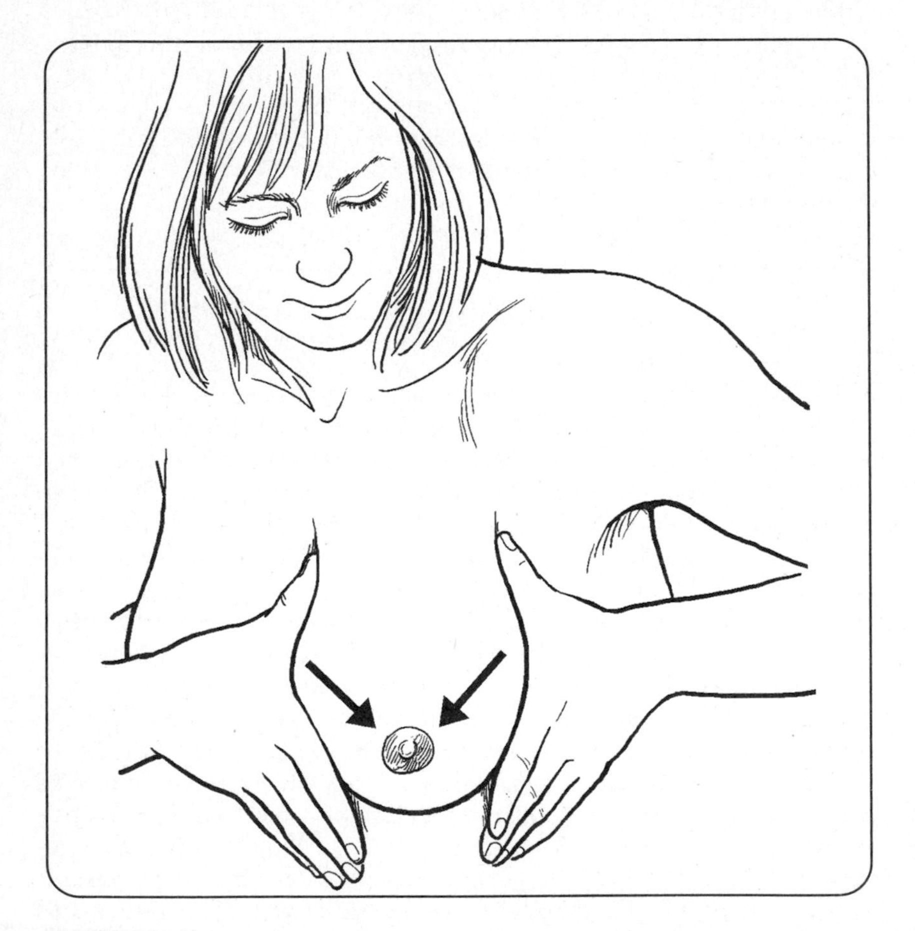

FIGURE 13-3

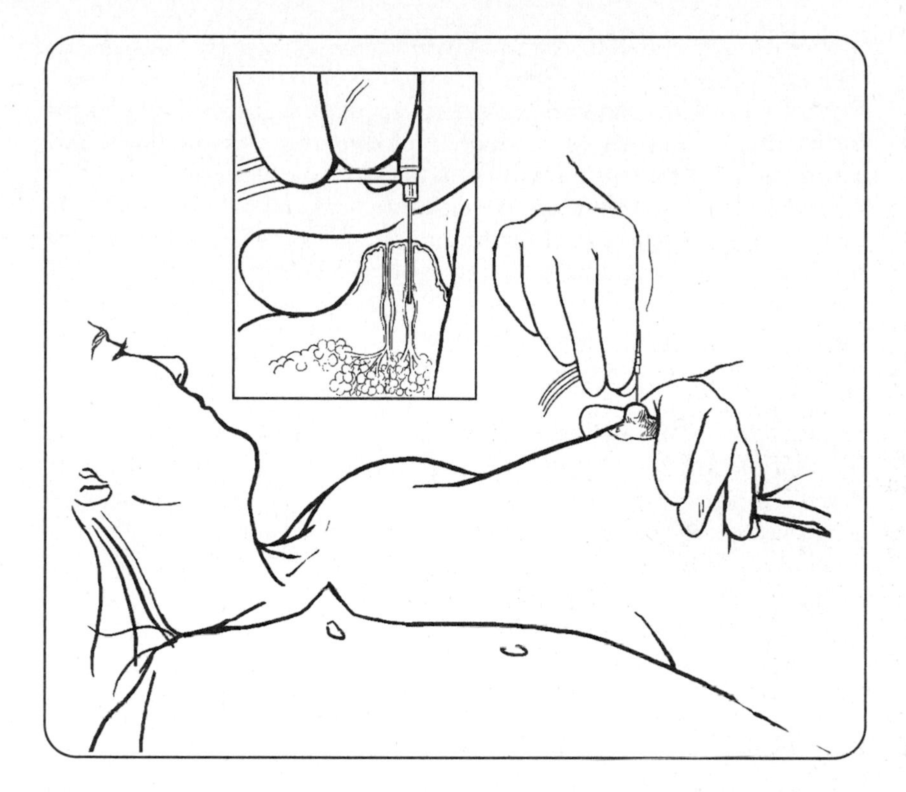

FIGURE 13-4

either had breast cancer in one breast or had a Gail index over 1.7 percent (see Chapter 11). We found that lavage collected a median of 13,500 epithelial cells, compared to only 120 for NAF. It also detected abnormal cells 3.2 times more often than nipple aspiration. There were no serious complications from the procedure.[10]

The procedure was approved for high-risk women. But the question remained: what do you *do* with the information? By the year 2000 we had several options for managing high-risk women. For starters they could be followed more closely with exams and mammograms. Tamoxifen is another option. In the large NSABP tamoxifen prevention study, women with atypical hyperplasia who were treated with tamoxifen had an 86 percent reduction in their chances of developing breast cancer compared with similar women treated with placebo. This makes sense, since nearly all atypical cells are thought to be sensitive to estrogen. A more drastic approach, but one that women with a genetic risk and atypical cells may consider, is preventive mastectomy, which reduces the risk of breast cancer by 90 percent. If malignant cells are found in a woman with a normal mammogram and physical examination, a ductogram or MRI can be done (see Chapter 7) to delineate the area in question for surgery.

In 1999 the Santa Barbara Breast Cancer Institute, now known as the Dr. Susan Love Research Foundation, sponsored the first international conference on nipple aspirate fluid in honor of its founder, Otto Sartorius, who died in 1995 after a lifetime of dedicated work on breast cancer. There were researchers from breast centers in the United States, the Czech Republic, England, and Japan. Since that time we have sponsored three more conferences and the field is growing rapidly. At the fourth conference in March 2005 we had over 100 participants and heard for the first time about intraductal therapy from several investigators.

Ductal lavage is available at some of the top breast centers around the country and is offered to those most likely to benefit from it: women at high risk for breast cancer and women with breast cancer. It has its limits, however. One is that it looks at cells to determine if they are abnormal. In a surgical biopsy you can see not only the cells but what they are doing—invading. (Like catching a criminal committing a crime). In cytology you have only the cells in isolation. Though helpful, this can be misleading. It is like looking at a lineup at the police station and guessing who the criminal is by how he's dressed. Sometimes it's the seedy-looking guy, but it may turn out to be the guy in the three-piece suit. And if you are looking for precancer cells, it's even trickier—like going into the high schools and guessing which students are going to grow up to be criminals by what they wear. At most, you've got a clue. But again, it could be the goth who ends up the law-abiding citizen, and the Barbie doll type who ends up a bank robber. Studies by Dr. Bonnie King looked at not just the cells but the DNA in the cells and found the latter to be more accurate.[11] Other researchers are looking for substances in the fluid that can identify who has cancer or is at risk: patterns of proteins, for example, or hormone levels. I am confident that we will find a good marker of risk in the fluid, which will make it a useful test on a wider level.

Another aspect of this approach is ductoscopy. This involves threading a very small scope through the nipple and down a milk duct. Although many surgeons have identified known cancers through this technique, it is not clear whether it will be a good diagnostic test.[12] Since the ductal system has many branches, it is easy to get lost with the scope.

Being able to get to where breast cancer starts means that we now have the opportunity to figure out what causes it. We have a window on the breast. But first we need to understand how the nonbreast-feeding duct works. When you are breast-feeding, the duct is capable of turning blood into milk. This is magical. But what happens when you are not breast-feeding? What concentrates there and what is absorbed? One of my colleagues postulated that the milk duct is a stagnant pond where toxins can collect, bathing the cells that eventually become cancer. We really don't know. We need studies on normal women as well as women who are at high risk of cancer to start to figure this out. Through my foundation we have started this in Los Angeles with the Normal Breast Study. We are recruiting 100 women who are not at high risk and are willing to undergo ductal lavage. I numb their nipple and lavage approximately six ducts. Then we analyze the fluid for protein levels, hormone levels, and cells. Preliminary results show that each duct is different; some have protein and no cells while others have hormones. We also found that ducts that do not produce nipple aspirate fluid still may be important. We are now trying to develop an ultrasound technique in which we squirt saline with air bubbles that will allow us to tell which duct we are lavaging and correlate it with the findings in the fluid.

Once we understand the functioning of the breast ducts and the local environment that leads to cancer, we will have the potential to alter it and prevent breast cancer once and for all. We could identify women at risk and then either give a drug that is preferentially concentrated in the milk duct and would reverse the situation toward normal, or we could change the environment within the duct, for example, lowering the estrogen levels. All this will be an elegant way to prevent breast cancer but it will take awhile to figure out.

There is a more direct approach that could prevent breast cancer now, even though we don't understand how the breast works or what exactly causes cancer. I call it the fast approach. There is a parallel in heart disease. We don't have to understand what causes heart disease to do a bypass graft and save a person's life. The more subtle approach is to understand and prevent it by lowering cholesterol and blood pressure, but if you have the disease, a bypass works pretty well.

What is the fast approach for preventing breast cancer? Squirting something into the duct which will destroy the cells that can eventually become cancerous. This has been tried by Dr. Sara Sukumar in mice. She has been able to put a low dose of a type of chemotherapy down the milk ducts and prevent breast cancer from developing. At the time of this writing, Dr. Ellen Mahoney and I have just tried this for the first time in a woman in Arcata, California. The woman has had breast cancer in one breast and is scheduled to have a preventative mastectomy in the other. She let us put the same type of chemotherapy used in the mice into her milk ducts and then, when she has her mastectomy in two months, we will see what her ducts look like. It did not seem to cause her any discomfort and we were able to do it under local anesthesia. It is the first time this has been done, and it opens the door for local prevention. A new era is dawning. If this approach continues to have few side effects and is able to prevent breast cancer the way it does in rodents, it will be available to all high-risk women and will provide an alternative to surgical and chemical prevention. We are on our way!

Back in 1958 Dr. Papanicolaou wrote, on the basis if his findings, "examination of the breast in the presence of secretions in patients without symptoms" may help prevent breast cancers from occurring.[13] Those words may well prove to be prophetic.

14

Screening

Screening is the process of looking at healthy people with no symptoms to pick up early signs of disease. The Pap smear for cervical cancer has allowed us to diagnose cancers in women before they have any symptoms. In breast cancer we need something similar. We need a test that's easy to do, widely acceptable to patients (i.e., cheap and painless), sensitive enough to pick up the disease (avoid false negatives), and specific enough not to give false positives. Ductal lavage and nipple aspirate fluid collection may someday fit the bill (see Chapter 13), but it is too soon to tell. Meanwhile, most breast cancer screening is done through one of three tests that vary in effectiveness—breast self-exam (BSE), breast exam by a doctor, and mammography. All these tests attempt to find cancers that are still curable.

EVALUATING SCREENING TESTS

There have been several studies examining the value of screening for breast cancer. Accepting that not all cancers will be found early, what evidence is there that our current tools are making a difference? Before we get into the studies, it's useful to look at a few common biases that complicate the issue of early detection (Fig. 14-1).

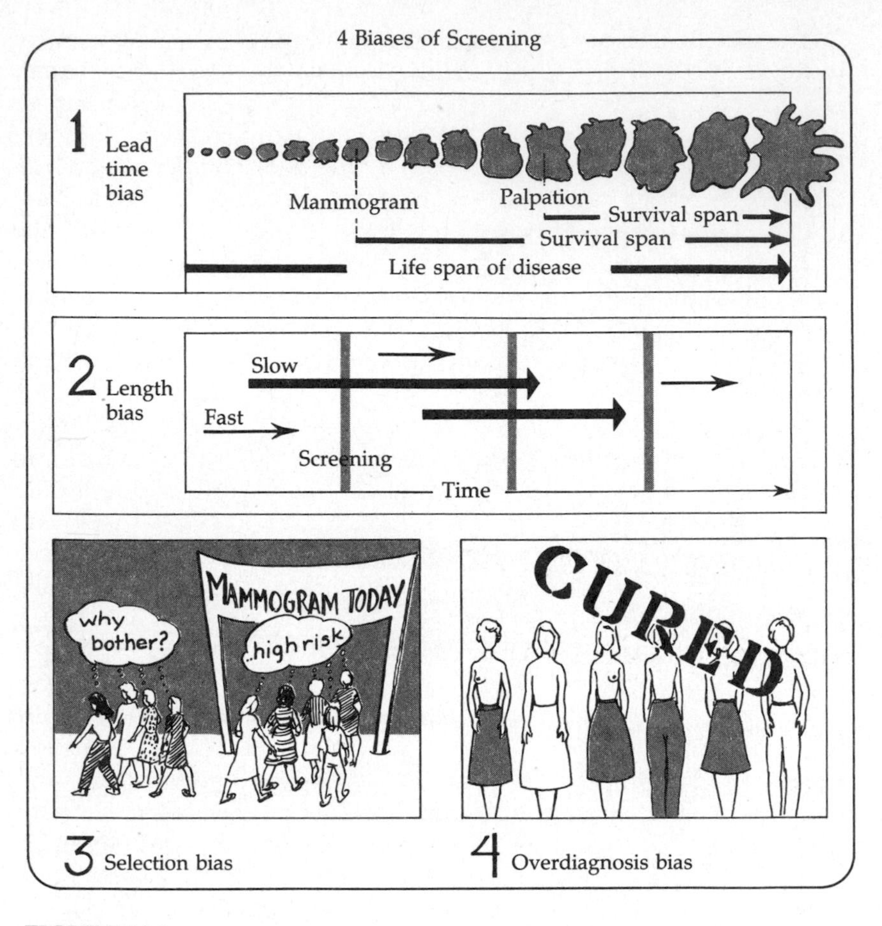

FIGURE 14-1

The first is lead time bias—the assumption that catching a disease early will necessarily affect its rate of progress. This is sometimes true and sometimes not. Let's assume you have a disease that usually kills eight years after it starts. If we diagnose the disease in the fifth year, you'll live three years after the diagnosis. If we diagnose it in the third year, you'll live five years—and we gleefully proclaim that our early diagnosis has given you a longer survival span. Actually, it hasn't—it's just given you a longer time to know you've got the disease, which may or may not be a benefit. So just looking at years of survival after diagnosis isn't enough—we need to know how many people actually die of the disease with and without early detection. Most breast cancers have been around six to eight years by the time they appear on a mammogram, and most women with breast cancer survive many years, so this bias can be very misleading.

The second is length bias. For instance, take a test that is done every two years on a large number of people. Fast-growing tumors aren't around as long, so we have less time to detect them. Slow-growing tumors are around longer, so we have more time to find them. If, for example, one tumor takes six years to become two centimeters and you do a test every two years, you're likely to find it before the six years are up. Another, very aggressive, tumor grows to two centimeters in nine months. You won't find it in your first test, and before you do your second, it's become a palpable lump and has been found. So screening tests are more likely to catch the slow-growing ones, which have a better prognosis. It's like a nighttime security guard patrolling the bank every hour. The guard will catch a slow robber who takes three hours to get the job done, but the fast robber, who can do the job in 20 minutes, will be in and out before the guard shows up. The chances are that the fast robber is also the most efficient one; the guard will only get the slower, less competent criminal.

Then there's the selection bias. If you make mammograms available to all women over 50 and you don't offer any extra incentives to take the test, who's likely to take you up on your offer? For the most part, it'll be the people who perceive themselves as being at high risk—those who have already had breast cancer or whose mother had breast cancer. Women who worry less about getting the disease are less likely to bother getting the test. So usually those who go for screening have a higher risk than those who don't.

Last is the overdiagnosis bias. A mammogram detects suspicious areas that may or may not indicate cancer. Precancer (see Chapter 12) falls into this category: if it were never diagnosed, in many cases nothing would happen and you'd never know you had it. But if it's overtreated (preventive mastectomies are performed wherever it's found), the cure statistics can be inflated. If, as it currently appears, only 30 percent of precancers ever become cancers and mastectomies are performed on all women found to have precancer, huge numbers of women will appear to have been cured, whereas the majority—70 percent—would never have gotten cancer in the first place.

What's needed for a truly accurate study is a randomized controlled study with mortality as its endpoint to take care of the lead time bias. If you take a group of women and pick randomly who'll get the test and who won't, that takes care of self-selection and overtreatment. If you have the same numbers of fast- and slow-growing tumors in the overall group, this counters the length bias and ensures that both the study group and the control group have the same risks of, and the same kinds of, cancer. Studies like this are few and far between. We must examine the data supporting each modality of screening against this standard, however, if we are truly to understand its worth.

Finally, we need to contend with the concept of early detection. As we'll see in Chapter 15, this notion is somewhat misleading. But is it a total falsehood? Not really. There are some cancers that we *can* detect early. What's misleading is the idea that every cancer has the potential to be found early by current techniques. We are unfortunately limited by both our techniques and our understanding of breast cancer. Screening is still our current best tool for changing the breast cancer mortality rate. We need to take full advantage of it while working hard to find something better.

BREAST SELF-EXAM

Until recently, breast self-exam—much touted as the obvious first step in breast cancer screening—had not been scientifically tested to see if it could change the mortality rate of breast cancer. The first randomized controlled study of breast self-exam (BSE) was done in Shanghai and reported in 1997.[1] In the study 267,040 women from 520 factories were randomly divided between a self-exam instruction group and a control group and followed for over five years. The women in the instruction group were given intensive training in breast self-examination. All women were followed for the development of breast diseases and for death from breast cancer. Approximately equal numbers of breast cancers were detected in the two groups (331 in the instruction group and 322 in the control group). The breast cancers detected in the instruction group were not diagnosed at an appreciably earlier stage or smaller size than those in the control group. The death rates from breast cancer in the two groups were exactly equal. Interestingly there was even a downside to BSE. The women in the instruction group detected more benign lesions (1,457 versus 623) than did those in the control group. This means that BSE not only failed to benefit the women in the instruction group by finding cancers earlier, but led them to be subjected to more biopsies than were those in the control group. The researchers will continue to follow all the women in the study to see if there is a late benefit to BSE that can be demonstrated. I must say that I think it's unlikely, since the size and stage of the detected tumors were the same in each group.[2]

The results of the Shanghai study were surprising and led many to discredit BSE. However, numerous women have told me that they found their own tumor doing BSE and thus believed it was important. But further discussion revealed that the exam wasn't formal BSE, but the kind of inadvertent discoveries I discussed in Chapter 2—the woman noticed it while showering or her lover realized something strange was there. This is different from the formalized searches doctors call breast self-exam. In the Chinese study, members of the control group found their own tumors the way most women do. The study simply confirmed that formal, rigorous BSE is no better than the normal poking around we all do.

BREAST PHYSICAL EXAM

Breast physical exam—examination by a doctor or other medical professional—has never been studied by itself in terms of its usefulness in detecting breast cancer. There is, however, at least one good randomized controlled study in which both physical exam and mammography were combined. This study is the basis of much of our understanding of the advantages of screening. In New York in 1962 the Health Insurance Plan (HIP), a health maintenance organization, chose 62,000 of its female members between the ages of 40 and 64 and divided them into two matched groups of 31,000 each.[3] They then offered the women in one group breast cancer screening, including mammography and physical examinations, with follow-up exams and mammograms once a year for three years. The women in the control group received their usual care. (This was before the era of routine mammography, so it's unlikely that many women in the control group ever had mammograms.) The 31,000 women in the screened group were invited to get mammograms; two-thirds of them accepted and had at least one. To avoid selection bias—since the women most likely to attend were those at higher risk—all the women who were invited were included in the statistics, not just those who actually came, which would underestimate the benefit of mammography. One-third of the cancers detected were detected on mammogram only, while two-fifths were detected by physical exam only and one-fifth by both. After seven years of follow-up there was a one-third reduction in mortality in the members of the screened group. After 14 years of follow-up this difference was maintained, and there is now also a significant difference in the mortality of the women under 50 as well.[4] In fact, at 18 years follow-up the decrease in deaths from breast cancer was equal in the older and younger group.[5] This was the first study to show the advantage of screening for breast cancer, and it was done with the rather crude mammography being employed in the early 1960s. It's important to remember, however, that the HIP study included a physician's exam in the screening, and it's interesting to note that physical examination seemed to be more effective in the younger women (40–50), while mammography was more effective in the older group.

A study done in Canada looked at whether, in older women, mammograms added anything to a well-performed medical physical exam.[6] After a seven-year follow-up they found that in women between 50 and 59 adding mammography didn't decrease mortality any more than physical exam alone.

One problem is that most doctors haven't been trained to do physical breast exam. The breast has always been thought to be the property of the general surgeon. So hardly any gynecologists and primary care doctors have formal training in the breast. Yet most women with breast problems go to their gynecologists or primary care doctors. This is the source of many problems because gynecologists and primary care doctors, untrained in breast problems and breast cancer, often don't know what to do. Surgeons always have had the advantage of educated fingers. They examine the breast and then do a biopsy. That way they learn what different breast problems feel like. Primary care doctors do not have this advantage. We need to be sure that every woman has access to a good clinical breast exam as part of her yearly checkup.

MAMMOGRAPHY

The third screening technique is mammography. In Chapter 7 I discussed mammography as a diagnostic tool for women who have breast complaints. Here I discuss it in relation to all healthy women as a tool for finding early disease. We've already considered some of the limitations of screening studies. The only studies we can really count on for answers are randomized controlled studies, where women are randomly assigned to have mammography or not.

There have been eight randomized controlled trials of mammography over the past 30 years, which is an impressive number. The findings are very striking. All eight studies consistently show a reduction in mortality in women between 50 and 69 of about 30 percent—nearly a third. (This means that a third fewer breast cancer deaths occurred in women who were screened.) This is the largest reduction in mortality we have seen in breast cancer. It overshadows by far the reduction in mortality we've seen in treatments with chemotherapy and surgery. In women between 50 and 70 there is no question that mammography screening can be lifesaving. We don't yet know how it affects women over 70 because there haven't been enough studies to tell us, but there is no reason to believe that the result wouldn't be the same. These benefits far outweigh the risks in having mammography (see below). However, mammography is not perfect, and a mammogram that shows nothing unusual is no guarantee that the woman doesn't have cancer.

What is so magical about the age of 50? It isn't actually 50 that matters, but rather menopause. Before menopause breast tissue tends to be denser because your breasts have to be ready to make milk at a moment's notice. After menopause breasts go into retirement and breast tissue is replaced by fat. Cancer shows up against fat tissue but not against dense breast tissue. Further, breast cancer is more common the older you are. These two factors combined make mammography more accurate in postmenopausal women. There is no argument that every woman over 50 should have yearly mammography.

The controversy involves women under 50. In the eight randomized controlled studies (which looked at women between 40 and 74) the data are very clear: for women between 40 and 49 the trials show no effect on mortality after seven years of follow-up.[7] Four of the eight studies followed women for 10 to 12 years, but none found a statistically significant difference. Summary data from five of the eight trials show a trend toward reduced breast cancer mortality (about 16 percent) only after a follow-up period of 10 or more years. In these studies many of the women began mammography in their late 40s and continued to have mammograms after age 50. Consequently, we can't be sure if the women who benefited from mammography in these studies would have had the same benefit if they had started having mammograms at 50. When they combined all of the randomized controlled trials, it was estimated that regularly screening 10,000 women between 40 and 49 would result in extending the lives of between 0 and 10 women. About 2,500 women would have to be screened regularly in order to extend one life.[8] (This also needs to be compared to the risk of unnecessary biopsies and the cumulative radiation risk discussed below.)

One pro–early mammography camp argues that cancers occurring between ages 40 and 50 seem to be the faster-growing ones. They feel the reason many studies are not showing the value of mammography in this age-group is that the mammograms are not being done frequently enough. Thus, they say, we should close up the intervals between mammograms in those years—especially since 40 to 50 are the years when women still have a lot of dense breast tissue, which can mask a cancer. So having a mammogram every year between 40 and 50, and every two years after 50 may make sense. This theory gained some credence from a study in San Francisco that showed yearly mammography was more able to find cancers in younger women regardless of breast density.[9]

The other argument in favor of mammography between 40 and 50 is that none of the randomized controlled studies, except for the Canadian National Screening Study, was designed specifically for younger women. The Canadian study showed no significant effect in women over 50 and actually found an initial increase in mortality in younger women. However, because breast cancer is less frequent in this 40–50 age group, many more women would have to be added to the study to show the same difference in mortality. The Canadian study also suggested that at least one-third of women under 50 have fatty breasts, which are conducive to mammography, and would therefore benefit. These proponents contend that until there is a study that proves mammography is not helpful in this age-group, we should continue to offer it.[10]

The downside of mammography screening in young women has been underestimated as well. Over one-fourth of invasive breast cancers are not detected by mammography in 40–49-year-olds, compared to one-tenth in women over 50. Women with these cancers may be harmed if their diagnosis or treatment is delayed because of a normal or false negative mammogram in the face of a palpable lump. On the other hand, many mammographic abnormalities may not be cancer but will prompt additional testing and anxiety. As many as 3 out of 10 (30 percent) women who begin annual screening at age 40 will have an abnormal mammogram during the next decade. For every eight biopsies performed on this younger age group, one invasive and one in situ cancer are found.

Finally, there is the risk of radiation. It is low but becomes more significant the earlier the initial mammogram is done and the more mammograms you have. Radiation from yearly mammograms between the ages of 40 to 49 has been estimated as possibly causing one additional breast cancer death per 10,000 women. Women with inherited or acquired defects in DNA repair (see Chapter 10) may be even more susceptible to the risk of radiation. Based on statistical models from epidemiological studies of high-dose exposures, this risk is low. The actual risk at lower doses associated with mammography could be higher or lower. It wouldn't matter if the benefit were higher, but limited benefits (compared to risk) need to be considered.

In 1997 the age issue came to a head when the National Cancer Institute (NCI) sponsored a consensus conference. It went to great lengths to convene an unbiased panel of physicians, scientists, and the public to decide whether the recommended guidelines should be expanded to include women in their 40s. After extensive research, presentations, and debate a consensus emerged that there is not enough evidence to recommend universal screening and that each woman needs to decide for herself—with the help of her doctor—whether to be screened.

Although this seemed perfectly logical to me, it stirred up a hornet's nest of protest. The proponents of mammography screening reacted as if this recommendation was an affront to women. One mammographer actually termed it a death sentence. Paying no attention to the science or the carefully reasoned analysis of the panel, politicians began demanding that mammography screening be recommended to all women over 40. Congress passed a bill and Senator Arlen Spector threatened to hold up legislation if the NCI did not change its recommendation. Politics prevailed and the guidelines now suggest that every woman over 40 be screened. I think this is another instance of having nothing better to offer. If we had a screening technique that worked in younger women, we would not be recommending a limited tool such as mammography. I hope that breast duct lavage will be that tool.

Note that these arguments refer to the value of recommending frequent mammography as a public policy: the benefit to the individual woman may be different.

If you have a strong family history of breast cancer, your chance of getting cancer is higher. Statistically speaking, there is more cancer, and therefore more chance of finding cancer on mammography. For you, therefore, mammography screening may be worthwhile.

One of my patients was a woman in her mid-40s whose cancer was detected by mammogram. She had a mastectomy and seemed fine, but she was very concerned by the studies. "I keep hearing that mammography in women under 50 doesn't affect mortality," she said to me. "Does that mean I'm going to die?"

It didn't mean that at all. In her case the cancer was discovered very early and probably cured. She may have been one of the lucky ones for whom mammography was useful, or she may have been cured even if she had not had a mammogram and the mastectomy had been done after finding a lump. Not all women who develop breast cancer between 40 and 50 die from it; even women in their 20s and 30s survive breast cancer, whether it is detected as a lump or on mammogram.

There can be goals other than reduced mortality. With early mammography screening you may find a cancer that's smaller, so you'll be able to have breast conservation and avoid severe cosmetic damage.

One of the problems with our approach to screening is that we are wedded to the hypothesis that early detection matters. Even the newer techniques being proposed, such as digital mammography, thermography, transcan, MRI, and nuclear medicine, are based on the early-detection notion. Because of this we have lost sight of the biology of the disease. If the early-detection hypothesis were correct, then screening would work better. The fact that it doesn't should send us back to the drawing board to understand how breast cancer develops and how we can better intervene to prevent it. (See Chapter 15.)

SCREENING RECOMMENDATIONS

If you want to do everything possible to protect yourself from dying of breast cancer, as well as avoid disfiguring surgery, what should you do?[11] If you're very young you should begin getting acquainted with your breasts. Have your doctor examine your breasts during your regular checkups; after 40, make sure to have this done at least once a year. Consider getting a mammogram every year between 40 and 50. After 50, make sure you have a mammogram every one or two years. (See Chapter 7 for discussion of the procedure.)

Many doctors stress the importance of a "baseline" mammogram. Actually, your first mammogram could be called your baseline. What's more important is that you have serial mammograms: several a year or two apart so that comparisons can be made. This is what makes mammography the most accurate.

I suggest having a mammogram in your early 40s to find out what your breast tissue looks like. Some women discover with their first mammogram that they have very dense breasts, in which case it makes sense to hold off and not do regular mammograms till 50. For women in their 40s with very fatty breasts, it might make sense to have screening mammograms.

Once you're in your 50s (or whenever your breast density makes it feasible), you should have regular mammograms every year or two, so we can compare each mammogram against the previous one. Often that's how we catch a cancer: this year's mammogram has something that wasn't there last year and the year before. There are people who believe they can get one mammogram and that's it. Much as I oppose overdoing mammography, underdoing it is just as bad.

It's important to point out that this discussion has focused on screening mammograms for women who have no symptoms but want to get checked out. If you have a lump, you should have a mammogram regardless of your age. Mammography, whatever its limitations, is still the best tool we have for detecting breast cancer or determining the nature of a lump. We need to make full use of it while we try to find something even better.

PART FIVE

Diagnosis of Breast Cancer and Decisions

15

Introduction to Breast Cancer

For many women the thought of having breast cancer is so appalling that their first reaction is, "I don't want to deal with this—just remove the breast, get the cancer out of me, and let me go on with my life." It's a reasonable feeling; a cancer diagnosis can turn your world upside down.

But if this is your reaction, don't act on it right away. Spend a day or two reflecting on the new reality you're facing. Your panic may subside and you may decide on a less drastic treatment than your original horror dictated. Whatever you decide, you'll have to live with your decision for the rest of your life—and that life won't be shortened by giving yourself a little time to think it over. Obviously, if you've got cancer you want it taken care of as soon as possible. But the week or so you give yourself won't kill you, and it will help you make the clearest decision possible.

In the past, it was common to make the decision—or rather, allow the doctor to make it for you—before the cancer was even diagnosed. You'd sign a consent form before your biopsy, agreeing to an immediate mastectomy if cancer was found. Fortunately that's much less common now, though it still sometimes happens. It's a terrible idea. No woman should be put to sleep without knowing whether she'll still have her breast when she wakes up. If your doctor wants you to sign such a form, don't do it. What you think you'll want when you're not sure if you have cancer may or may not mirror what you really want when you have a definite diagnosis.

Of course, in the old days, there was pretty much only one decision you could make. Mastectomy was all we had. Nowadays, thankfully, we have numerous options; any given procedure, or combination of procedures, may or may not be right for you, depending on the location of the cancer in your breast, its size, and, very importantly, your own thoughts and feelings. This chapter contains an overview of breast cancer treatments, and in subsequent chapters I'll explain how current treatments fit in the big picture and what information you will need to decide between them. Finally we'll consider each different treatment and what it entails.

Since the first edition of this book came out in 1990, we have seen the approach to treating breast cancer shift from surgery center stage and radiation and chemotherapy playing supporting roles, to chemotherapy and hormone therapy as the leads while surgery and radiation have moved into ancillary positions. This shift in treatment has accompanied a shift in thinking. We used to think that breast cancer started in the breast, grew to a certain size, and then moved out to the lymph nodes, which carried it to the rest of the body. All cancers, we believed, resulted from a series of similar mutations that drove their aggressiveness. This meant that we needed to find the cancer "early" and "small" before it had a chance to become aggressive and spread. The treatment of breast cancer was thus viewed as an emergency, requiring immediate and extensive surgery.

This view of breast cancer also led to the concept of early detection: if we just look hard enough early enough we can find the cancers when they are still localized and therefore curable—a simplistic notion that I discussed in the previous chapter. This understanding dominated the 1960s and 1970s and is still extant in popular culture. The problem is that it doesn't always work. Even when we find cancers "early," some women die. And in some cases, cancers found later are not fatal.

Further research has shown that most invasive breast cancers are present for six to eight years before we can feel them or see them on a mammogram. Angiogenesis, the growth of new blood vessels to feed the tumor, is thought to occur around year 2. This means that microscopic spread has probably occurred in most tumors by the time they are diagnosed. In many women, the immune system takes care of these cells. As I explain in Chapter 16, we use a variety of tests to help us guess which women have cancer cells elsewhere in their body. They are given systemic therapy (chemotherapy or hormone therapy) in an attempt to eliminate the cells. Local treatments, such as surgery and radiation, are used to take care of the cancer in the breast. Varying combinations of these have been effective for many women. This view, first proposed by Dr. Bernard Fisher, led to the era of chemotherapy and the notion that just about every woman with breast cancer needs systemic treatment.

But there are problems with this idea as well. For one thing, the increased identification of precancers on mammography has not led to an equal decrease in advanced disease. One-third of women with breast cancer still die of it. If finding and treating these precancerous lesions does not prevent more advanced disease, then the old linear model of gradual progression has to be reevaluated. We need to go back to the drawing board to come up with a new theory of breast cancer that takes all of these facts into consideration.

Such reevaluation has already begun, with important results. For one thing, we are starting to realize that our current method of categorizing tumors according to their appearance under the microscope (see Chapter 16) is inadequate. The most interesting tool in this regard has

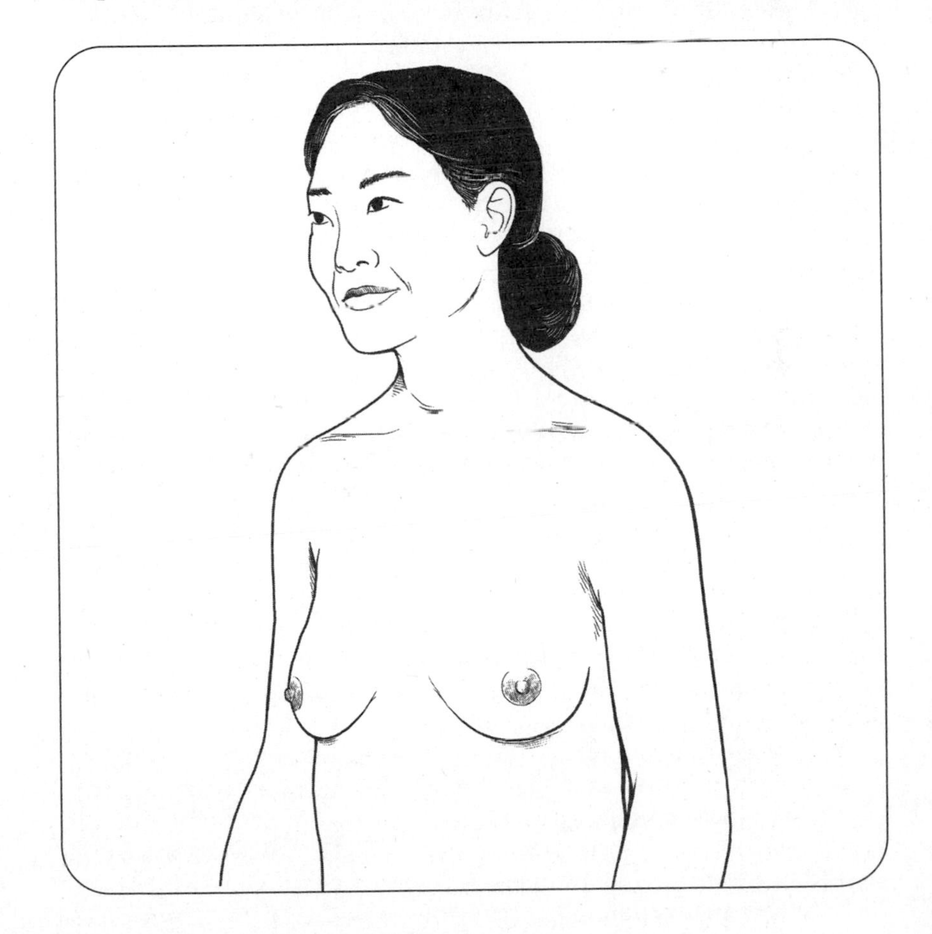

been the DNA microarray analysis. New technology has led to a DNA chip that allows a researcher to look at hundreds of genes in hundreds of tumors at the same time. When this tool is applied to the tumors of patients who participated in previous research, the patterns of gene mutation can be correlated with the known outcome. Initial analysis of a Dutch collection of data has suggested that within the usual two categories of breast cancer (ductal and lobular) there are actually six different types, based on the patterns of tumor DNA mutations.[1] Let's say a gang of boys is caught stealing a car. They are all considered thieves, but if you spend more time with each one you may be able to differentiate personality types within the gang. One may be incorrigible while another might be very susceptible to peer pressure, suggesting that a different environment might help that boy reform. Inside the gang there might even be a couple of kids who tried to prevent the robbery. If you knew all that, you might not treat them all the same way. Looking at patterns of DNA in breast tumors has demonstrated one that has been termed the basal type (ER negative PR negative and Her-2/neu negative), which correlates with aggressive tumors regardless of the size of the tumor. At the other end is what the researchers call the "normal type," which has not been well defined yet. The women with these patterns do well with virtually any treatment. Between these extremes, there are groups who have variable prognoses. This approach of looking for patterns of mutations gives us new insight into both how the tumor can be expected to behave and what may be the best approach to treatment.

In fact, we have already started to use this new type of information. We currently use predictors such as Her-2/neu and estrogen receptors as well as Oncotype recurrence scores to determine whether women need more therapy. (See Chapter 16.) Soon we will also be able to tailor drugs more specifically and, equally important, determine which women need no drugs. Our current guesswork will be replaced by more scientific decisions.

This predestination approach to breast cancer doesn't always paint a rosy picture—just a more accurate one. Does it mean that you're doomed if you have a more aggressive cancer? No. These categories are developed based on mutations in the cancer cells themselves. That alone does not dictate your survival. We are beginning to realize that the environment surrounding the cells can be as important as the cells themselves and potentially easier to alter.

What does all this mean for you, now that you've just learned that you have breast cancer? You will get either local or systemic treatments, or a combination of both, and possibly targeted and complementary therapies as well. The decision making around these options will be discussed at length in the next three chapters. The goal is to choose the combination as precisely as possible for your tumor. It is important to point out, however, that that goal is often still elusive. We have a lot of information from studies but none on you specifically. In the end you and your medical team will have to do the best you can. As you embark on this journey of breast cancer, collecting information and opinions and trying to make some sense of it all, it helps to understand the language that the doctors are using. In this chapter we will review how statistics are collected and how studies are conducted and reported. It can be a bit dense at times, so feel free to jump ahead and then come back on a need-to-know basis.

STATISTICS

As I just mentioned, it is impossible to tell what is going to happen with any one woman. Even if two women had the same genetic mutations, the factors affecting the microenvironment in which those cells live would vary. This explains why a doctor can say that someone has advanced metastatic disease but can still "beat the odds." All our prognostications are of necessity based on large statistical groups of patients. Table 15-1 shows five-year survival rates with only a mastectomy as treatment. This does not mean everyone died at year six or, as some wishfully think, that all who make it to five years are cured. It just means that the researchers checked to see who was alive at year five. These prognostications have some use—as long as you realize they don't absolutely predict the course of your particular disease.

A five-year survival without recurrence is significant, if not definitive. In previous editions of this book I downplayed its importance. However, a recent analysis of several studies has shown that I was probably missing an important point of biology. According to Don Berry, Ph.D., a statistician from Texas, the factors we use to determine prognosis (nodes, tumor size, etc.) have an effect only initially.[2] This suggests that if you have positive nodes and larger tumors and your cancer hasn't recurred within five years, your risk of recurrence is probably the same as everyone else's—no greater but no worse. Although this doesn't give you the assurance of long-term survival that you'd like to have, it does give you reason for cautious optimism.

There are several software programs that add more factors to the survival data shown above. You can go to my webpage (www.drsusan loveresearchfoundation.org) and look under Decision Tools to try one out. Or you can ask your physician to go to Adjuvantonline.com and print out a chart for you. This kind of evaluation of the cancer is what we're currently using to make decisions regarding treatment because it encompasses as much as we are able to know to date about the natural history of the disease and the biology of the tumor.

Sadly, none of this gives us absolute knowledge. All we do is look at

Table 15-1. Five-Year Breast Cancer Survival Rates According to the Size of the Tumor and Axillary Node Involvement

	Patients Surviving 5 Years		
Tumor Size (cm)	*Negative Nodes (%)*	*1–3 Positive Nodes (%)*	*4 or More Positive Nodes (%)*
< 0.5	269 (99.2)	53 (95.3)	17 (59.0)
0.5–0.9	791 (99.3)	140 (94.0)	65 (54.2)
1.0–1.9	4,668 (95.8)	1,574 (86.6)	742 (67.2)
2.0–2.9	4,010 (92.3)	1,897 (83.4)	1,375 (63.4)
3.0–3.9	2,072 (86.2)	1,185 (79.0)	1,072 (56.9)
4.0–4.9	845 (84.6)	540 (69.8)	727 (52.6)
≥ 5.0	809 (82.2)	630 (73.0)	1,259 (45.4)

Source: Carter C., Allen C., Henson D. Relation of tumor size, lymph node status, and survival in 24,740 breast cancer cases. *Cancer* 63 (1989): 181. With permission.

large groups of patients and say, "The majority of women with these signs have this prognosis, and are likely to have this response to this treatment." But you, the individual patient, may or may not fall into the majority category. This has several implications. If 80 percent of patients in your cancer category survive, you have reason for optimism—but not, unfortunately, total rejoicing. You'll probably be in the 80 percent, but you might be in the 20 percent who don't survive. You need to be optimistic but careful. Do everything possible to keep your advantage—careful follow-up and perhaps some of the adjunct, nonmedical techniques discussed in Chapter 25 to complement your treatment.

By the same token, if 80 percent of women in your category die, that doesn't mean you will. While it would make sense for you to think seriously about the possibility of your upcoming death and how you'd best want to prepare for it, it also makes sense to think in terms of being part of the 20 percent who survive. Again, you may find it worthwhile to look into nonmedical attitudinal and nutritional therapies to complement your treatment.

TREATMENT STUDIES: CLINICAL TRIALS AND RESEARCH PROTOCOLS

When you know what your general prognosis is, the next step is to figure out how to improve it. This is where the treatment studies come in. It is important to understand how studies are done and the terminology used in describing these results if you are going to make sense of the next chapters.

As I mentioned in Chapter 9, there are many types of studies looking at factors relating to risk and prevention. The most important studies in the treatment setting are clinical trials. These types of studies (also known as *interventional studies* or *research protocols*) are prospective trials that study a new treatment by having one group of subjects get the treatment while another group, known as the *control group*, doesn't get the experimental treatment. This is where we actually test the hypothesis that a treatment has an effect. The people are followed closely for a given period of time, after which researchers compare the two groups. For example, let's say a new drug (or an older drug used for a new purpose, such as tamoxifen) was now being considered for prevention rather than just treatment. In the study the experimental group would be given the treatment and the control group would be given a *placebo* (an inert pill), and no one would know which group was which. If 20 percent of the women who received the drug developed breast cancer, and 40 percent of those who got the placebo did, we'd know that the treatment did some good. Not all clinical studies use placebos. If there is a standard therapy, the new treatment will be compared to it. In the studies of the new aromatase inhibitors, for example, the inhibitors were compared to tamoxifen, the standard therapy. (See Chapter 18.)

These studies are usually *randomized*. This means that each subject's treatment is picked at random, usually by a computer, so there is no possibility that subjects will be chosen based on situations they're already in. If, for example, all of the women with atypical hyperplasia are put on one treatment regimen to prevent breast cancer and all the women without it are put on another, the second treatment will end up looking an awful lot better than it really was.

It's important that neither the researchers nor the subjects know who's getting the new treatment and who's getting the placebo (or the standard treatment). That way the subjects won't be tempted to alter their behavior based on the treatment they're getting or to unconsciously misreport symptoms, and the researchers won't be tempted to treat one group differently or interpret the results differently. Because neither researcher nor subject knows who's getting the treatment until after the study is completed, these studies are called *double-blind*.

The controlled study that is prospective, randomized, and double-blind has the fewest potential flaws, and so it's the most reliable. It's still not perfect because people who decide to participate in a study like that may not be like most of us—usually people prefer to know what treatment they're getting and don't want to risk being given nothing or a placebo. But it's the closest we can get to good data.

A good example of a randomized controlled study that changed our approach to breast cancer is the Bonadonna study, which looked at the use of chemotherapy in addition to surgery.[3] This study enrolled premenopausal women who had undergone mastectomy and randomized them to receive a certain kind of chemotherapy or nothing. Since chemotherapy was not being used outside of studies at the time of diagnosis, it was perfectly ethical to have an arm of the study in which the women did not receive chemotherapy. (As in all such studies, all volunteered to participate and had been given the pros and cons of the treatment.) Another example is the Veronesi study, comparing radical mastectomy to quadrantectomy (see Chapter 21) for early breast cancer.[4] Surprisingly, this form of extensive lumpectomy had better medical results than mastectomy. (These two studies are also examples of occasions when it isn't possible to include a double-blind approach.)

An example of the problems that can arise when a study is not randomized is the clinical acceptance of high-dose chemotherapy with stem cell rescue after initial studies in the early 1990s. These studies compared women who had undergone this very toxic therapy to what we call historical controls—women with similar cancers that had been treated in the past. The findings suggested that the high-dose chemotherapy was better and appeared to confirm the largely accepted hypothesis that more was better and that killing all the cancer cells was key.[5] When the randomized controlled studies comparing high-dose chemotherapy to standard chemotherapy were later completed, they showed no benefit from the high-dose regimen.[6] How could this happen? We don't know for certain, but probably the women in the original study were screened extremely well to make sure that they had no microscopic spread of their disease before they were enrolled, while the historical controls were not.[7] Also, treatments in general had improved over time; so the new therapy looked better than it actually was. It took the later, randomized study to bring out the truth. Thus the main job of randomized controlled trials is to correct or confirm the results of nonrandomized studies.

What, then, is the good of nonrandomized studies? They are a valuable first step for medical scientists. Randomized studies are difficult and expensive. So we do one only if we have good reason to believe it will contribute to our understanding of the disease. An early study might rule out the use of a randomized study. If, for example, those first studies on high-dose chemotherapy with stem cell rescue had shown no improvement, we could have ruled out the treatments without undertaking larger studies. We are lucky because approximately 200 randomized controlled studies have been done on breast cancer treatments, and our current approaches exist thanks to women who were willing to be randomized. This is a significant benefit to women who are diagnosed today. Ongoing and future studies will continue to improve treatment for women with breast cancer.

End Points of Clinical Trials

So that you can evaluate information from available studies and understand the figures your doctor may quote you, we need to spend a moment looking at what the numbers mean. Research studies about cancer therapy can be confusing. The first thing to look at is a given study's *end point*. End points represent the outcome that is being compared in the two treatments. For example, one study may be looking at whether a cancer came back in the breast, which is very important, but you yourself may be more concerned with whether it prevents the spread of cancer to the rest of the body.

The most important endpoint to most women is overall survival (OS). The time frame is the beginning of the subject's entry into the study to her death from any cause. This may seem odd—if someone who has had breast cancer dies of heart disease, why is that relevant to the study? It may not be—but it is possible that the treatment which cured her breast cancer caused the disease that eventually killed her. An example of this is the postmastectomy radiation therapy that was used in the 1970s. Although the women had fewer recurrences, those treated on the left had more heart disease twenty years later. (See Chapter 17.) This endpoint also takes into consideration the treatment for any recurrence. But the question then arises, How long do you have to follow a woman to measure overall survival? (This is where arbitrary numbers like five years come in.)

Since we want to evaluate the studies as soon as possible, we have other endpoints as well as OS. Disease-free survival (DFS) measures the time from randomization to the first evidence of recurrence or death. This figure reflects the number of women at a particular time who have no recurrence of breast cancer in the breast, chest wall (after mastectomy), or elsewhere in the body. It presumes that the more women who are disease free, the better. Local recurrences (see Chapter 27) aren't as serious as disease that spreads to the rest of the body.

As a result, this is sometimes further modified in a third endpoint, distant disease–free survival (distant DFS), which indicates the time until the first recurrence outside of the breast. Here we are looking at how many women are alive without metastases at a particular point in time.

All of these endpoints have their limitations. DFS is a good measure of primary efficacy of the treatment, but it doesn't consider what happens to the woman after she has a recurrence. Although it usually translates into OS eventually, a treatment could put off recurrence but cause such serious side effects that the woman would die sooner than someone who recurred sooner and lived for a long time with her recurrence. Two treatments might not show a difference in overall survival, yet one might prolong the time the woman is symptom free—something valuable to the woman with cancer. Although lengthening the time to recurrence isn't a cure, it is important. For example, let's say you were diagnosed with a breast cancer that, with the old treatment, would have killed you in one year. A new treatment increases your time to recurrence, or disease-free survival time, by three years and so you die four years after your diagnosis. Your survival at five years would be zero either way, but you have had three extra years of quality time. Improving DFS or OS does not guarantee that the woman will not die of breast cancer eventually; it just makes it less likely to happen within the time frame of the study. Still, a longer life may be worth the side effects of the treatment even if it is not ultimately lifesaving.

When studies are reported in the medical literature, they are often viewed as *survival curves*. This is the percentage of women alive in each arm (treatment) of the study at set time periods (see Fig. 15-1). This graphically shows you the difference between the two curves in general and the absolute difference between them at any one point in time. The overall difference might be that in one arm of the study a large number of women die in the first few years but then anyone who gets past that has a good chance of survival, whereas on the other arm the benefits decrease much more gradually (see above). The absolute difference would be the difference in survival at any one point in time. In our example, the absolute difference in survival at three years may be 40 percent, while at ten years it may be 20 percent because the patterns of the curves are different.

Another way data are presented is in terms of a *hazard ratio*. You see the risk of a recurrence at a particular moment in time for a woman who is still surviving, depending on which of the two treatments she took. You then see the risk for a surviving woman taking the other treatment. These two are compared in the form of a ratio. Using our example above, the hazard ratio at three years would be 40/80 or .5; in other words, only 50 percent of women with treatment B are alive versus those with treatment A. At 10 years, this would also be 20/40, or .5, or 50 percent. Although this is useful for scientists (and drug marketers), it is less so for the woman with cancer. It tells you only that one treatment is relatively better than the other, not whether either is especially good. What is better for you is to look at the absolute difference in the treatments at a point in time. That time needs to be long enough for at least half of the women in the study to have reached it. On our survival curves, the absolute difference at 3 years is 40 women while at

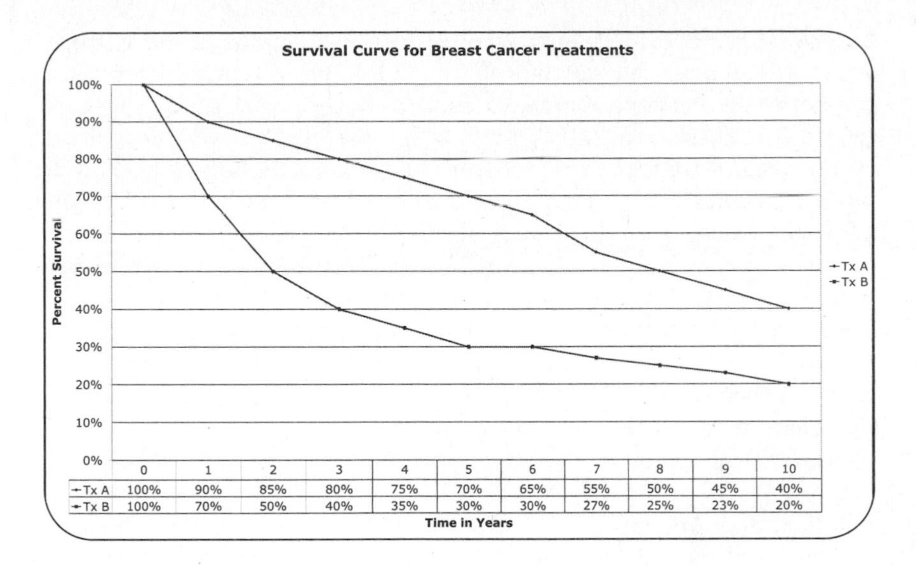

	0	1	2	3	4	5	6	7	8	9	10
Tx A	100%	90%	85%	80%	75%	70%	65%	55%	50%	45%	40%
Tx B	100%	70%	50%	40%	35%	30%	30%	27%	25%	23%	20%

FIGURE 15-1

10 years with the same hazard ratio, it is 20 women. All they say is that A is twice as good as B, but by ten years neither one is that good.

Unfortunately not all studies are reported that way. Some studies refer to the "percentage reduction in mortality." This refers to the percentage of patients who died compared to the number of deaths that were expected. For example, if a study showed that eight patients died in the control group and only six in the study group, there were two fewer deaths than would normally be expected. This is then reported out as a 25 percent reduction in mortality, or two divided by eight. A similar study with more patients might show that 40 patients died in the control group compared to 30 in the study group. The reduction of 10 deaths over a possible 40 is still 25 percent. In the second study, 10 patients' lives were saved, while in the first it was only two. You should always try to get the absolute benefit rather than the relative one if you are comparing treatments. If your oncologist or surgeon does not know the absolute figures, he or she can get them on the Internet at (www.Adjuvantonline.com) and print them out for you.

Even here there are limitations. In the study we are analyzing, women who were dead of cancer by ten years on treatment A still may have had their lives prolonged by the treatment. A way to get at this is to compare median DFS and OS. That is the time that half of the patients in the study had had recurrences or had died. In a study of one particular chemotherapy, the median time to recurrence was 3 years in the control group and 11 years in the chemotherapy group. The difference in median survival was 8 years and 15 years respectively. Clearly there were some women who benefited from a longer time before their cancer recurred who were not measured by looking at the data at 15 years.

Another important study tool is the *meta-analysis*. Sometimes a study is too small to show an effect. For example, let's say that 20 women are studied, 10 on the new treatment and 10 on the old. It appears that there is no difference. But if the study had included 100 in each category, 5 more women would have been seen to survive on the new treatment. By combining many studies looking at the same question, a meta-analysis can come up with more precise figures. The Early Breast Clinical Trialists Collaborative Group combines studies looking at chemotherapy and hormone therapy for a large analysis about every five years and has come up with statistics that none of the small studies found individually. The data from the 2000 analysis reported in 2005 are included in Chapters 17 and 18.[8]

Understanding the value of various treatments will help you understand what your doctor is suggesting, and why. It will also help you decide the treatment *you* want—and they may or may not be the same thing. If, for example, the treatment has comparatively little chance of keeping you alive for a substantial length of time, you might decide that painful chemotherapy will ruin the time you have left to live and that you'd rather risk a shorter, more comfortable lifespan. The writer Audre Lorde, who died in 1992, explained her reasons for making this choice in her book *A Burst of Light*: "I want as much good time as possible, and their treatments aren't going to make a hell of a lot of difference in terms of extended time. But they'll make a hell of a lot of difference in terms of my general condition and how I live my life."[9]

On the other hand, a year or two might feel like "a hell of a lot of difference" to you. You might decide that the possibility of living a little longer is worth the limited suffering chemotherapy entails. There are no right or wrong decisions here; there is only your need, and your right, to have the most accurate information possible, and to decide based on who you are, what choices make the most sense for you.

BECOMING PART OF A STUDY

Learning what studies mean is vital for every woman who is considering using a study as part of a basis for any decision she makes. But you can also take a further step and become part of a study—helping others and very possibly helping yourself. The work that I discussed in Chapter 13 could never have been done without volunteers, both with and without breast disease, who served as subjects in my studies.

As a woman and a physician, I've always been frustrated by the lack of information about women's health. In the past virtually all research was done on men. Even rat research was done on male rats. In the course of reading this book you've probably noticed how often I have said, "We don't know whether . . ." or "More research is needed before we know . . ." You're probably tired of reading it. I know I'm tired of saying it. But the answers aren't there. The data contained in this book is thanks to the women who agreed to participate in studies.

As women, we can't complain that there are not enough data on diseases relevant to us and then remain aloof from studies when they exist. Our demands for research are slowly getting met, and there is important ongoing work that offers women the opportunity to participate. There are several studies on adjuvant treatment for breast cancer—such as testing the use of partial breast radiation (see Chapter 17) at the time of diagnosis and looking at different combinations of hormone therapies. I think women should seek out these studies—especially women who have been underrepresented in research in the past: lesbians, older women, African Americans and other minorities. I realize this may be hard for some people, since I'm asking women who may have already suffered from the insensitivity of the health establishment to involve themselves deeply with that establishment. But the only way to learn about women's health is to have women in studies, and the way to be in studies is to sign up for them.

When you participate in a clinical study, you join a protocol—a program designed to answer specific questions about the effectiveness of a particular approach. The questions can be about methods of diagnosis, types of treatment, dosage of drugs, timing of administration of drugs, or type of drugs used. Let's say you're involved in a protocol for breast cancer treatment to compare two new hormone therapies. You'll be one of a large group of patients who fit the criteria, and randomized to take one drug or the other. Both groups will be followed just as rigorously. What makes it a protocol is the fact that it is asking a question: will the women receiving drug A do better than the women on drug B? By participating in such studies you and the other subjects will get reasonable treatment and at the same time help us figure out the answer.

If you're considering taking part in a study, you have a right to know everything about it. Ask the researchers what exactly they're giving you; find out the possible side effects; find out what they know and don't know. You have to sign an informed consent form, which is often very long. (The form for the study of high-dosage chemotherapy was 27 pages.) Read it thoroughly; it's worth the effort. Write out your questions. Sit down with the doctor, go over questions about anything that's unclear. Also ask to speak to another woman with breast cancer who has gone through the same program ahead of you, if the study has been ongoing.

There are safeguards in most trials. In addition, there is a human subjects protection committee (often called institutional review board or IRB) in every hospital that reviews each protocol to make sure it is safe and well designed. These bodies oversee all clinical trials and make sure that the informed consent is readable and the potential benefits of the study outweigh its risks for the subjects being studied. Of course, you'll always be given the choice. It's both unethical and illegal for a doctor to put you on a protocol treatment or clinical trial without your full and informed consent, and you have every right to refuse. If you're in an experiment and become convinced that it's harming you, you can leave it. You and your doctor both have the right to take you off the study at any time.

There are very good reasons for participating in a protocol. Aside from its usefulness to women in the future, studies assure the patient that she will get the most up-to-date care. For these reasons many women are eager to be part of studies. Susan McKenney, a nurse practitioner and oncology nurse who works extensively with breast cancer patients, talked with many patients at the Dana Farber Institute and found that once they understood they were not just guinea pigs and the treatments could be helpful both to them and other women, they were often anxious to participate. "Breast cancer treatment has changed over the last 20 years because women have participated in protocols," she says.

Patients I've spoken with back this up. One woman who was diagnosed in 1990 with a stage 3 cancer became involved in a phase II study using far higher doses of chemotherapy than the standard—the dose was adjusted upward as far as the patient's tolerance allowed. Along with the treatments in the hospital, which occurred every three weeks, she gave herself nightly injections of a material that stimulated the growth of bone marrow destroyed by the chemotherapy.

She had a difficult time with the treatment, throwing up so often that she slept on the bathroom floor for weeks. "They called me the nausea queen," she recalls ruefully. But her experiment paid off. Although in this study the patients went straight into chemotherapy without having surgery or radiation beforehand, they had been warned that they would probably require both when the chemotherapy course was over. But her tumor shrank so dramatically that she did not need either. "I feel that the only reason I'm alive is because I did that trial," she says. One of the other women in the trial, with whom she became close friends, survived in spite of the fact that she had aggressive inflammatory cancer.

Some studies are actually begun by patients themselves. You can get a group in the community together and initiate a study on your own terms. For example, if you want to research lesbians and breast cancer, you can go to the local medical school or a researcher and say, "This is a study we want to see done. We'll supply the participants—do you have anyone who can work with us?" A number of recent studies have begun that way. For example, a group of women in Long Island were disturbed at the high level of breast cancer in their community. They lobbied the National Cancer Institute and got a study that investigated a possible relationship between environmental pollutants in Long Island and breast cancer. Women on Cape Cod set up a similar study for Massachusetts.

So far, we haven't done enough to encourage women to participate in studies. Only about 3 percent of breast cancer patients in the United States participate in protocols, much lower than in Europe. But we can't wholly blame the patients for this. Many hospitals or doctors don't offer protocols. If you're being treated at a research hospital or major cancer center, you'll usually be offered protocols if you qualify, and large numbers of patients there do participate. Women who choose such hospitals for treatment tend to be those who seek out the most advanced, sophisticated treatments. They feel safer in an environment where the major purpose is to study and fight cancer. But the ability to offer protocols isn't limited to these hospitals. There is now a mechanism allowing community hospitals to offer participation in protocols through a program called CCOP (Cancer Center Outreach Program) that links community hospitals with large medical centers and allows you to participate in the same studies in your local area. Participation ensures that your doctor is keeping up-to-date and that you're getting the best medicine has to offer.

If you're a patient, please seriously think about joining a study. If you ask about trials and your doctor doesn't know of any and doesn't want to bother finding out, you can call 1-800 4 CANCER at the National Cancer Institute or check its website at www.cancer.gov. You can obtain a list of every clinical trial you're eligible for. You'll also find out the trial locations so you'll know whether or not a given study is being conducted near you. Then you can go with that information to your doctor and work with it from there.

The financial aspects of studies vary greatly depending on the nature of the study. For a study that offers no benefit and some inconvenience to the subject, payment may be offered as an incentive—those are the studies college kids often get into to earn a few hundred dollars. (I participated in a study of DES as a contraceptive to help pay my tuition when I was in medical school.) Studies that might benefit the subject or cause the subject no inconvenience involve no financial exchange at all. Occasionally a study of a treatment that can benefit the patient will offer a reduced fee for the treatment, like an asthma and visualization study my coauthor participated in. Finally, as is the case with the chemotherapy studies comparing drugs already approved by the FDA, the patient (or the insurance company) pays the full price for the procedure. When new drugs are being tested, the drug company generally pays for the treatment. Many hospitals will not allow studies involving an experimental drug or device in which the patient must pay. Political action has led some states to mandate insurance coverage and Medicare for standard cancer care as part of a clinical trial.

Unfortunately, even when they're offered protocols, only a small percentage of women accept the offer. Here too there are a number of reasons. Some women are afraid of being randomized. They want to get the best treatment and they find it hard to believe that the medical profession doesn't know what that is. Or they have strong feelings about getting a particular treatment and they don't want to experiment with anything else.

Often women don't want to be in studies because they can't decide which group they'll be in. "I'll be in a study comparing chemotherapy and an aromatase inhibitor," a woman will tell me, "if I can choose which one I'll get." That can't be done in a study, since the treatments need to be chosen randomly for the study to be valid.

Some women don't participate in clinical trials because they think we already have the answers. For example, they assume that the standard treatments will save their lives, and they don't want to rock the boat with something new. But it's precisely because the standard treatments *don't* always work that we do experiments. The courageous women who participated in the phase 1 and phase 2 trials of Adriamycin and Taxol benefited not only themselves but the many women who followed them.

Some women fail to understand the whole idea of a study. They want to choose their own treatment rather than participate in a protocol. After the treatment is finished, they want that treatment and its effects on them to be studied. But of course, that isn't the way it works. For a study of a treatment to give us clear information, it must be done under controlled circumstances, defined by the researchers and strictly followed. After-the-fact statistics have their use, but we can never get the same level of information with this kind of observational study that we can with randomized control studies.

Ironically, some women swing to the other extreme. Once in a while a highly publicized experimental procedure comes along that people think is the miracle we've been searching for. Then the attitude toward being in a study turns around. Instead of fearing being part of an experiment, people demand what they think will be their share of the miracle.

After learning what protocols are available you may decide that none of them offers the treatment you want. But you owe it to yourself and other women to find out what protocols you are eligible for and what they involve, before you decide. My patient who took part in the high-dose chemotherapy experiment says that if she had a friend newly diagnosed with breast cancer she would strongly urge her to look into protocols. "I'd tell her not to jump into anything," she says, "but to explore everything. Find out what's there; weigh it in your mind. 'Latest' isn't always best, and it may be that what you find isn't right for you. But there's a very good chance that you'll find that what's best for you is in a clinical trial."

Whether or not you decide to become part of a clinical trial in terms of your treatment, there's another way you can contribute to breast cancer research and do yourself a favor as well. If you have any surgical procedure—whether a biopsy, a wide excision, a mastectomy, or even breast reduction—make sure tissue removed from your breast is deposited in a tissue bank (see Chapter 8). This is becoming more and more possible because one of the things we're pushing for politically is regional and national tissue banks. You can have this done in any hospital. Both benign and cancerous tissue are useful in medical studies.

We have no guaranteed cures—if we did there'd be no need for trials. But trials ensure that we are doing all we can to help women in the future. Already we see some of the trial results. Not too long ago a woman with breast cancer had no choice but to lose her breast. But a number of women participated in the first breast conservation studies and were randomized to get either mastectomy or lumpectomy and radiation. They were very courageous women, going against the standard thinking to see if there was an alternative. Thanks to them, thousands of women today have saved their breasts. As you make the complex, difficult decisions about your own treatment, keep those women in mind—the brave experimenters and all of us who have benefited from their courage.

16

What Kind of Cancer Is It?

Once you have been told you have cancer, you will want to find out everything you can about *your* cancer. This will be the basis of all your subsequent treatment decision making, so it's worth researching. First, get the pathology report from either your fine-needle aspirate (FNA) or core biopsy, and ask your doctor for a copy of it for your records. If the doctor refuses to give it to you, call the pathology department in the hospital where you had the procedure and ask for a copy. Once you have it, sit down with the next section of this book: it will help you translate your report from "medicalese" into English. There will be a second pathology report after your definitive surgery (lumpectomy or mastectomy and sentinel node or node dissection). It will be a variation on this same theme. It too will be worth obtaining and reading.

HOW TO INTERPRET A PATHOLOGY REPORT

The pathologist is a doctor who specializes in looking at tissue under the microscope. Your surgeon should select a pathologist who has had a lot of experience in diagnosing breast cancer. The language of a pathologist's report can be puzzling and intimidating, and for this reason you should always discuss the pathology report with your surgeon. If you still have questions, you can ask the pathologist directly.

The first part of the report will describe what the pathologist received from the surgeon. It includes measurements and comments on the appearance of the tissue. We call this a gross description, not because the tissue is unappealing but to reflect how the tissue looks to the trained naked eye. The gross description should be distinguished from the microscopic description, which is how the tissue looks magnified 40–400 times under the microscope.

The pathologist looking at the tissue removed can usually tell whether or not breast cancer is present and, if it is present, what kind of breast cancer you have. I say "usually" because sometimes the FNA or core gets only a small piece of the lesion. In this situation the pathologist can report only on what is there. It is important to remember this when reading a pathology report. The pathologist might say that the tumor is "widespread," creating an image of a cancer all over your breast. In reality, it just means it is widespread *in the small piece of tissue* that's under the microscope. On the other hand the pathologist might say that the tumor is small or focal; this reflects only what is in the small tissue piece removed, which is usually, but not always, representative of what is in the breast.

Further, there are limitations in terms of the kind of cancer the pathologist sees in that one piece of tissue. Most breast cancers are heterogeneous—several different types of breast cancer can coexist. The cells are not all alike. It is possible for the biopsy to look like one type of cancer and the lumpectomy or mastectomy to show that other types are also present in the same tumor. When you read your pathology report, remember that a report based on a biopsy may not tell the whole story. Still, it can usually tell if you have cancer—and that is where we will start.

All breast cancer starts in the lining of the milk ducts. Some cancers originate from the duct cells themselves and others from the lobules that populate the ends of the ducts like leaves at the ends of tree branches. Thus your cancer will probably be described as either ductal carcinoma or lobular carcinoma (Fig. 16-1), indicating whether the cells look like they came from the duct or the lobule. Next, the report will say whether or not the cancer is invasive. Invasive cancers are also known as infiltrating cancers—a somewhat sinister-sounding description, which simply means the cancer has grown outside the duct or lobule where it started and into the surrounding tissue. In this case the report will read either "invasive ductal (or lobular) carcinoma" or "infiltrating ductal (lobular) carcinoma." Some cancers contain elements of both ducts and lobules and are considered mixed cancers.

Since lobules and ducts are kinds of glands and the medical term

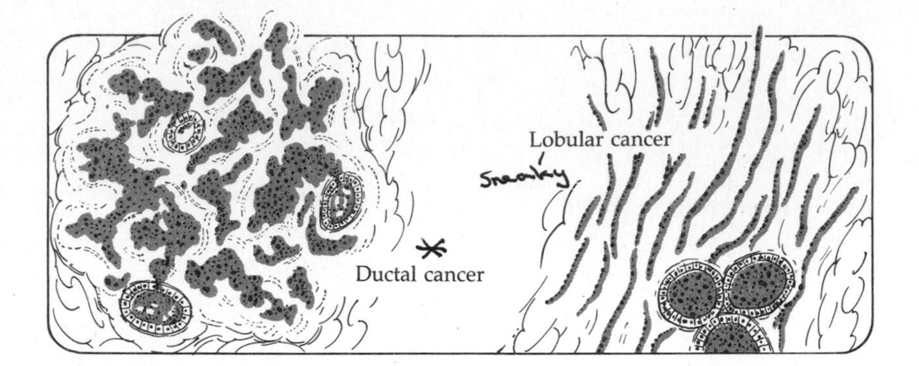

FIGURE 16-1

meaning "related to a gland" is *adeno,* sometimes these cancers are called "adenocarcinomas." Some people are confused by this term, thinking it's a different kind of cancer. It's just a broader category—like calling someone from Los Angeles a Californian.

An infiltrating ductal cancer forms a hard, firm lump because scar tissue (fibrosis) around the cells causes a lot of reaction. This scar reaction is called desmoplasia. Infiltrating lobular cancer, on the other hand, is sneaky. It sends individual cells in little fingerlike projections (cells extending in a line, single file) out into the tissues without inciting a lot of desmoplastic reaction around them, and so you may feel it as a little thickening rather than a hard lump (Fig. 16-2). For this reason it's harder for surgeons to tell if they've got the lobular cancer all out: the little projections can't be felt as easily as a hard lump. Because lobular cancers elicit less scarring, they tend to grow to larger sizes (average 5 cm) than ductal carcinoma (average 2 cm) before they are detected. The prognosis is based on size, not type of cancer. Aside from that, however, one form is no worse than the other; neither has a better or worse prognosis in and of itself. Lobular cancers are almost always sensitive to hormones and seem to be more common in women who have taken hormone replacement therapy. In addition, there's a slightly higher tendency for lobular cancer to occur in the other breast at a later time. Although an infiltrating ductal cancer has about a 15 percent chance of occurring in the other breast over your lifetime, a lobular cancer has about a 20 percent chance—an increase in risk but not an overwhelming one.[1]

If the cancer is not invasive, it is called *intraductal carcinoma* or *ductal carcinoma in situ* or *lobular carcinoma in situ* or even *noninvasive carcinoma* (Fig. 16-3). These are all names for what I call precancer, explained in Chapter 12. Sometimes both cancer and precancer are present in one lump, and the report might read "infiltrating ductal

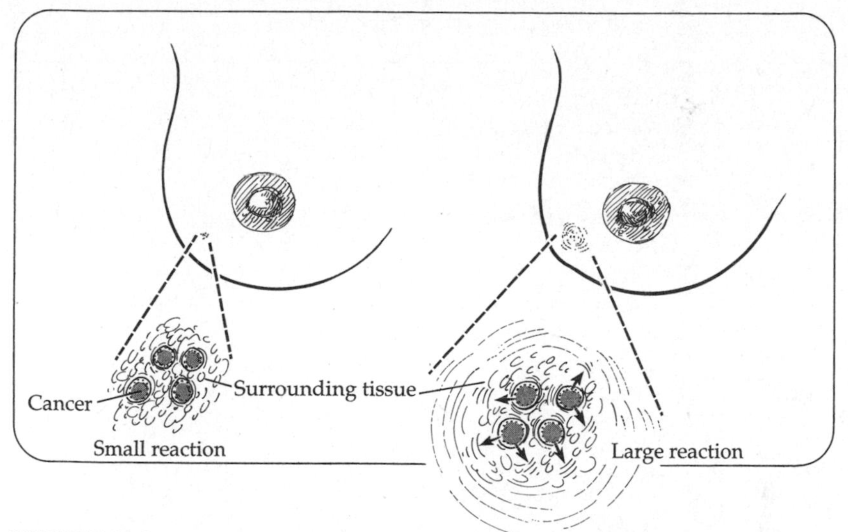

FIGURE 16-2

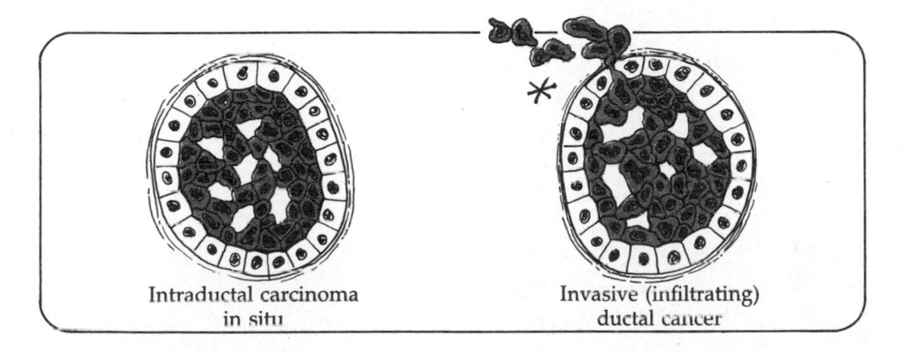

FIGURE 16-3

carcinoma with an intraductal component." This finding will be discussed further in Chapter 17.

Other names for cancers may also appear on the pathologist's report. For the most part they're variations on invasive ductal cancer, named by the pathologist according to the visual appearance of the cells under the microscope. *Tubular* cancer, in which the cancer cells look like little tubes, is very unusual—1–2 percent of breast cancers—and usually less aggressive. *Medullary carcinoma* resembles the color of brain tissue (the medulla), though it has nothing to do with the brain. *Mucinous* (or *colloid*) *carcinoma* is a kind of infiltrating ductal cancer that makes mucus that looks like glue ("colloid" is the Greek word for

Table 16-1. Types of Breast Cancer and Frequency[a]

Type	Frequency
Infiltrating ductal	70.0%
Invasive lobular	10.0%
Medullary	6.0%
Mucinous or colloid	3.0%
Tubular	1.2%
Adenocystic	0.4%
Papillary	1.0%
Carcinosarcoma	0.1%
Paget's disease	3.0%
Inflammatory	1.0%
In situ breast cancer	5.0%
ductal	2.5%
lobular	2.5%

[a]There can be combinations of any of these types.

Source: Henderson C., Harris J.R., Kinne D.W., Helman S. Cancer of the breast. In DeVita V.T., Jr., Helman S., Rosenbert, S.A., eds., *Cancer: Principles and Practice of Oncology*, vol. 1, 3rd ed. Philadelphia: J. B. Lippincott, 1989; 1204–1206.

glue). *Papillary carcinoma* has cells that stick out in little fronds (finger-like projections). (See Table 16-1.) These special cancers tend to have a better prognosis than do typical invasive ductal or lobular cancers, but they are treated according to the same principles. Other types of cancer, such as inflammatory or cystosarcoma phylloides, are a different matter and are discussed in Chapter 19.

After deciding what kind of cancer you have, the pathologist studies the appearance of the cells further to predict how aggressively the particular type of cancer will behave. This isn't 100 percent accurate, however; it's a little like looking at a lineup to pick out the criminal. If one suspect is seedy and scruffy-looking and another is wearing a three-piece suit, you'll guess that the first one is the bad guy. But you could be wrong. Sometimes appearances can be deceiving, both in a police lineup and under the microscope.

Similarly, the pathologist who sees wild-looking (poorly differentiated) cells will predict that such cells are usually more aggressive, while the cells that look more normal (well differentiated) are usually less aggressive (Fig. 16-4). The cells in between are called "moderately differentiated." But poorly differentiated cells aren't a sign of doom—the fact that they look wild doesn't guarantee they'll act that way or can't be treated. Most breast cancers are either moderately or poorly differentiated, but many women who have these cells do fine.

Another thing the pathologist looks for is how many cells are dividing and how actively: this is known as mitotic rate or activity. The most

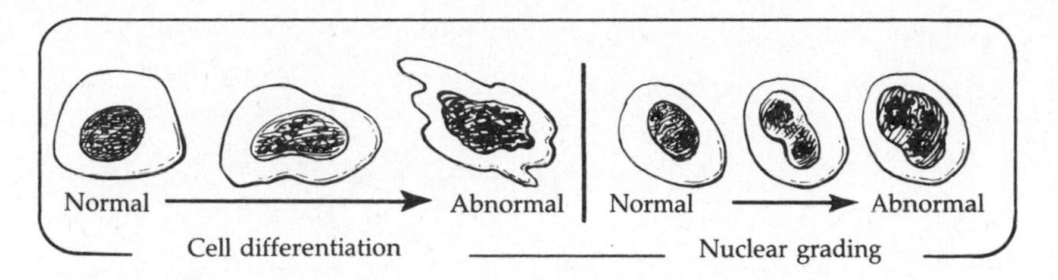

FIGURE 16-4

aggressive cancers tend to have a lot of cells dividing at the same time because they're growing rapidly. Less aggressive cancers tend to have fewer dividing cells. Another feature indirectly related to tumor growth and differentiation is the *nuclear grade*. The nucleus of the cell is the part that contains the DNA, so the grade gives you an idea of how abnormal the DNA is. Pathologists usually grade on a scale of 1 to 3 or 1 to 4, with the higher number being the worst (see Fig. 16-4).

The pathologist will also look for cancer cells inside a blood vessel or lymphatic vessel. If there are any, it's called vascular invasion, lymphatic invasion, or lymphovascular invasion, and suggests that the cancer is potentially more dangerous. In addition, the pathologist sometimes counts the number of blood vessels associated with the tumor. This is because tumors secrete substances that cause blood vessels to grow, a process called angiogenesis. A lot of blood vessels may indicate that the tumor is growing rapidly and thus especially aggressive. I noticed that if I was operating on a lump I thought was benign and there was a lot more bleeding than I would have expected, it was often the tip-off that the lump was cancerous. Another ominous sign can be "necrosis," or dead cancer cells. This usually means the cancer is growing so rapidly that it has outgrown its blood supply (Fig. 16-5). The pathologist checks all of these factors to get as much information as possible about the cancer. None of them is 100 percent perfect at predicting behavior.

Sometimes all of these observations are combined as a score. One commonly used scoring system is the Nottingham histologic score, otherwise known as the modified Bloom Richardson score. It is based on three features: degree of tubule formation (well-formed tubules are good and poorly formed tubules not as good), nuclear grade (regularity in the size, shape, and staining character of the nuclei, with small being better than large), and mitotic activity (few mitosis are good and many mitosis not as good). Each of these gets a score of 1, 2, or 3, with the higher number reflecting poor tubules, large nuclei, and high mitotic rate. The scores are then added up: 3–5 is grade one, 6–7 is grade two, 8–9 is grade three. Grade three is the highest and supposedly the

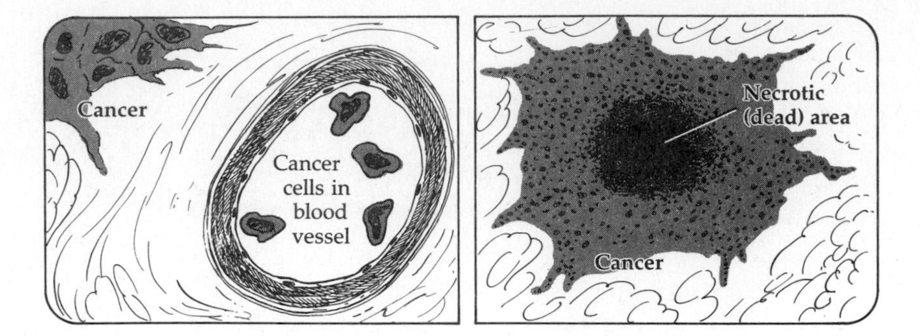

FIGURE 16-5

most aggressive. Unfortunately all of these features are very subjective. A comparison of different pathologists' Nottingham or Bloom Richardson scores on the same cancer showed they agreed only 75 percent of the time. If you see a Nottingham or Bloom Richardson score on your report, you will know what it is and you will also know that it is just a way to quantify how the tumor looked.

In addition, the pathologist should be able to tell you if there's cancer at the margins of the tissue that was removed. This is done by a fairly imprecise technique. Ink is put all around the outside of the sample before it is cut up and fixed, and slides are made. If the slides show cancer cells next to the ink, this means there's cancer on the outer border and presumably some left in the patient. If there are cancer cells only in the middle, away from the ink, there is a "clean margin" (Fig. 16-6). So the report might say, "The margins are uninvolved with tumor," or "The margins are involved with tumor," or "The margins are indeterminate." If the lump has been taken out in more than one piece, we usually can't tell if the margins are clean or not. Also, we can only do representative sections of the margin; to get them all, we'd have to make thousands of slides. So when we say the margins are clean, we're only making an educated guess—we can't be 100 percent sure. (See Chapter 12 for a discussion of margins and DCIS.) Margins are often misunderstood as a black-and-white type of test rather than simply a predictor of the amount of cancer that may remain in the patient's breast. Thus a lumpectomy that shows just one spot of cancer at a margin suggests that there is not a lot of disease behind, while one with a lot of cancer throughout it and one dirty margin probably indicates that there is more disease left in the patient.

How clearly any of these things are seen depends on the pathologist's expertise and effort. Someone who makes only a couple of slides and looks at them hastily is obviously more likely to miss things than someone who makes a lot of slides and looks at them carefully. If you

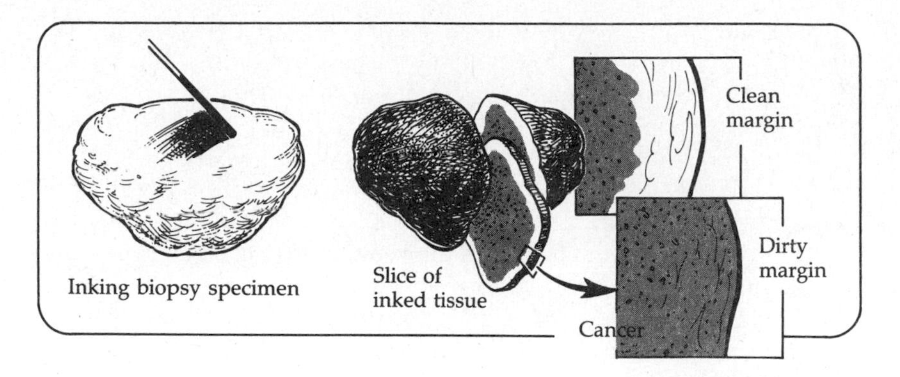

FIGURE 16-6

are at all concerned about the quality of the pathology evaluation, or even if you are not, you may want to have your slides sent to another pathologist in another institution. A breast pathologist with whom I worked at UCLA, Dr. Sanford Barsky, reviewed the slides of all of the women who were seen in the Multidisciplinary Cancer Program. Not infrequently he would change a diagnosis rendered elsewhere. He is now the Senhauser Endowed Chairman of Pathology at Ohio State University in Columbus, Ohio, where he continues his interest in breast pathology.

Some of the things I've described aren't easy to see on the slides. Identification can be somewhat subjective: are these cells bizarre looking enough? Are they invading other structures? It's worth getting a second opinion. Often the pathologists themselves will ask other pathologists on the staff to look at the slides and give their opinions. If you live in a small town with a small hospital, you may want your slides sent to a big university center, where someone sees a lot of breast pathology. You can call the university hospital's pathology department and arrange to have them look at your slides, then call your hospital and have the slides sent. Make sure it is the slides themselves they send, since that's what the second pathologist needs to see—not just the first pathologist's written interpretation. You need to get the best information possible to decide what course of treatment to embark on.

STAGING

The microscopic aspects of the tumor that the pathology report addresses are combined with clinical features of the tumor in a staging system. This classification system, known as the TNM (short for tumor, nodes, and metastasis), categorizes cases so that we can keep statistics and determine long-term survival rates for various treatments. The system is still used, but it is actually a holdover from the past. It doesn't fit very well with our current knowledge of biology because it is based only on the size of the tumor in the breast, the number of lymph nodes involved, and clinically detected spread to other organs. It is like looking at the students who cut classes in high school and predicting that they will grow up to be irresponsible in the workforce. Obviously other determinants of behavior (e.g., parenting, peer pressure, and health) influence future performance in the workforce. Similarly, other determinants of tumor behavior, such as the molecular biology of the tumor or its rate of growth (did it spread to the lymph nodes while small or after it had been around awhile?) are not reflected in the TNM classification system but are important in predicting prognosis and response to therapy. However, since the TNM system is still being used and you will probably be exposed to it, I'm including a detailed explanation here. Just keep its limitations in mind.

The system has been changed various times throughout the years. In an attempt to make it more relevant, a sixth version was introduced in January 2003. The major changes have to do with sentinel nodes and smaller tumors. I will provide a general overview of how it works and a look at the large classifications. In the appendix you'll find a check sheet to help you classify your own tumor.

In this system (Fig. 16-7), the tumor size is first judged clinically, based on the surgeon's exam or an imaging modality such as mammography, ultrasound, CT scan, or MRI scan. If it's between 0 and 2 centimeters, it's T-1; between 2 and 5 centimeters, T-2; above 5 centimeters, T-3 (one centimeter is .39 inch). If it's ulcerating through the skin or stuck to the chest wall, it's T-4. Although the original tumor staging is based on the clinical estimate, it is further refined once it has been removed surgically and examined pathologically so that the full extent of the cancer can be determined. This is called the pathological T stage and is based on the size of the invasive tumor only, without regard to its possible in situ component. If there is more than one tumor in the same breast, the largest of them is used for determining the T size. As we are diagnosing smaller and smaller tumors, subclassifications have been developed. T_{is} refers to the in situ tumors discussed in the precancer chapters as well as Paget's disease (see Chapter 19), while T1mic refers to microinvasion 0.1 centimeter or smaller in greatest dimension; T1a tumor between 0.1 centimeter and 0.5 centimeter; T1b tumor between 0.5 centimeter and 1 centimeter; T1c tumor between 1 centimeter and 2 centimeters.

Then the lymph nodes are examined either by the surgeon or by an imaging test such as CT scan or ultrasound. If there are no palpable nodes, it's N-0; if the surgeon feels nodes but thinks they're negative, it's N-1a; if they're positive it's N-1b. If they're large and matted to-

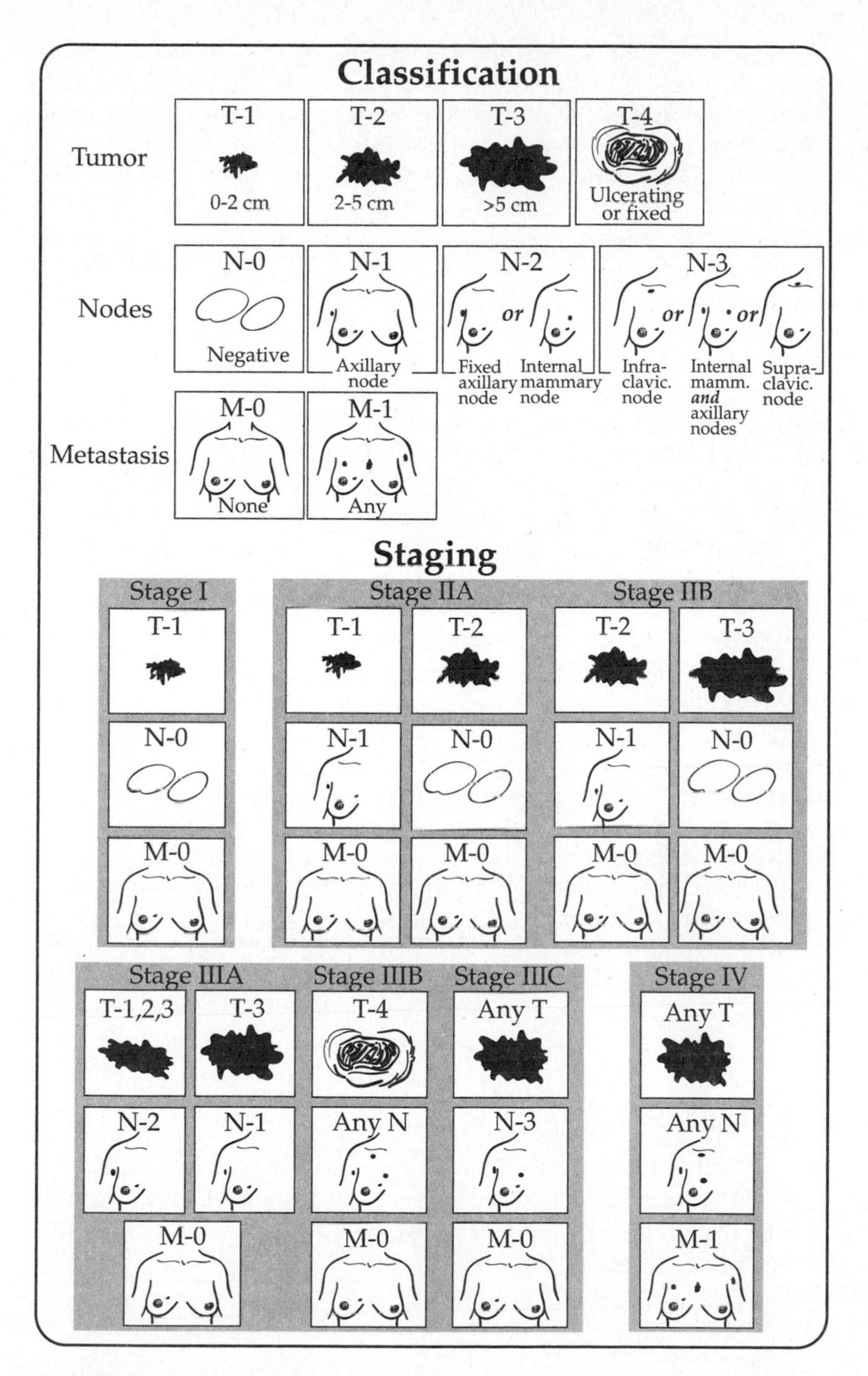
Classification
Tumor
T-1
0-2 cm
T-2
2-5 cm
T-3
>5 cm
T-4
Ulcerating or fixed
Nodes
N-0
Negative
N-1
Axillary node
N-2
Fixed axillary node
or
Internal mammary node
N-3
Infra-clavic. node
or
Internal mamm. and axillary nodes
or
Supra-clavic. node
Metastasis
M-0
None
M-1
Any
Staging
Stage I
T-1
N-0
M-0
Stage IIA
T-1
N-1
M-0
T-2
N-0
M-0
Stage IIB
T-2
N-1
M-0
T-3
N-0
M-0
Stage IIIA
T-1,2,3
N-2
T-3
N-1
M-0
Stage IIIB
T-4
Any N
M-0
Stage IIIC
Any T
N-3
M-0
Stage IV
Any T
Any N
M-1

FIGURE 16-7

gether, it's N-2; if they're near the collarbone, it's N-3. Nodes that have been previously removed are termed $N_{x.}$ Nodes too are reclassified once they are removed. With the increasing use of the sentinel node biopsy, this has been incorporated into the new staging system. For example, if only one or several clumps of cells of breast cancer are found in a lymph node based on IHC staining only (see Chapter 17) or RT-PCR only, they are considered isolated tumor cells and the nodes are still considered negative. This is because we think a few cells may be dislodged during the procedure but that they have no long-term consequence. Only cells that make it to the nodes on their own seem to count. Cancer deposits greater than 0.2 millimeters but less than 2 millimeters are considered micrometastasis and are termed $pN_{1m,}$ while any bigger than 2 millimeters are considered pN_1.The other change in the newer system is subdividing the nodes based on the number that are positive: pN_{1a} 1–3 positive nodes; pN_{1b} 4–9 positive nodes; and pN_{1c} more than 10. These breakdowns are as much to help researchers collect data as they are to improve survival prognostications.

Finally, if an obvious metastasis has been discovered by any of the tests I'll describe shortly, it's M-l: otherwise it's M-0; if we can't tell whether there is metastasis, we designate it M-x.

Then this information is combined into stage numbers. Stage 1 is a T-1 tumor with no lymph nodes. Stage 2 is either a small tumor with positive lymph nodes or a tumor between 2 and 5 centimeters with negative lymph nodes. (Sometimes this is designated as stage 2A.) Tumors between 2 and 5 centimeters with positive lymph nodes or tumors larger than 5 centimeters with negative lymph nodes are also stage 2, but these latter types are designated stage 2B. Stage 3 is a large tumor with positive lymph nodes or a tumor with "grave signs." Stage 4 is a tumor that has obvious metastasis.

The complexity of this system suggests that we still don't completely understand breast cancer. As you will see later in this chapter, the new techniques of DNA analysis are beginning to help us differentiate breast cancers based on the specific mutations in each cancer and on which genes are either over- or underexpressed, and thus to determine more accurately both prognosis and treatment. We are now in a transition between molecular biological and the traditional TNM classification. But in spite of its limitations, the TNM system gives us a conceptual framework for categorizing each case of breast cancer so that different treatments can be compared in the same types of patients.

Has It Spread?

One obvious way to predict a poor prognosis is to find cancer cells in other organs. When the first edition of this book was written, all newly diagnosed women would undergo tests to look for cancer cells in their liver, lungs, or bones. The problem with that approach, however, was that the imaging tests we had, and indeed still have, are useful only for finding chunks of cancer (1–2 cm), not isolated cancer cells. Nonetheless they are still done in women with multiple positive nodes or large tumors. These tests are often called *staging tests*—not to be confused with the stages of breast cancer just described.

A cancer that starts out as a breast cancer remains a breast cancer, wherever it travels, and treatments used for the cancer are breast cancer treatments, not liver cancer or lung cancer treatments (very few cancers travel *to* the breast, by the way). It's a bit like what happens when a Californian moves to Paris. She's living in a new environment, but her language, her personality, her basic approach to life are still those of a Californian. She hasn't become a Parisienne.

To screen for metastatic disease, we can do a chest X ray or a CT scan to find cancer in the lungs. We can do a blood test and/or an ultrasound to see if the cancer has spread to the liver. To learn if the cancer has spread to the bones, we do a more complicated test called a bone scan, one of a group of tests we call *nuclear medicine tests*. A technician injects a low level of radioactive particles into your vein, where they are selectively picked up by the bones. After the injection, you wait a few hours while the particles travel through the bloodstream; then you go back to the examining room where you are put under a large machine that takes a picture of your skeleton (Fig. 16-8). The machine whirs above you, reading the number of radioactive particles in your body. (The husband of one of my patients used to wear a Geiger counter, and right after her bone scan it started clicking whenever she came near it.) In the areas where the bone is actively metabolizing—doing something—the radioactive particles will show up much more strongly than in the more inert areas.

This doesn't necessarily mean that what the bone is doing has anything to do with cancer, however. It can mean there's arthritis (which most of us have in small amounts anyway), a fracture that's in the process of healing, or some kind of infection. All the scan tells us is that something's going on. If the scan is positive, the next step is to x-ray the bone. This will help tell us what it is. We could just x-ray the bone to begin with, but we don't want to expose you to any more radiation than we have to.

Other imaging tests such as MRI or CT scan also may be used, depending on the situation. Some centers use a PET scan of the whole body to see if there are any areas that light up. This relatively new technology (see Chapter 7) is still considered by many to be experimental but holds promise.

Another experimental test looks in the blood or bone marrow for evidence of circulating cancer cells. Although this sounds like the perfect

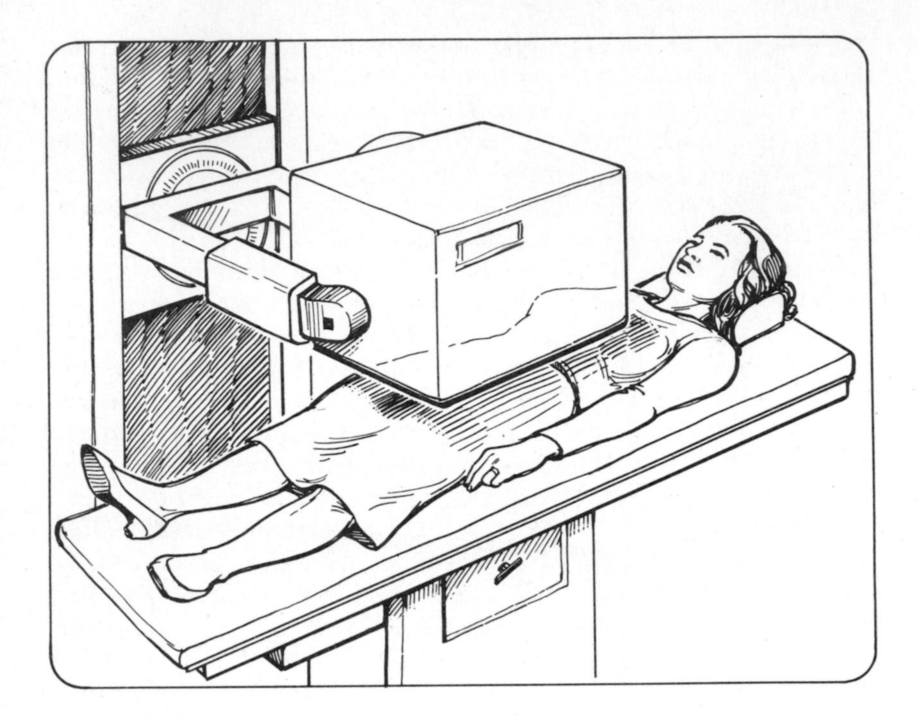

FIGURE 16-8

test to predict the spread of breast cancer, it has a lot of limitations, not the least of which is the fact that we don't have a specific marker on breast cancer cells that we can focus on. This means we are looking for cells that *could* be cancer cells. It's like knowing that the criminal is blond and looking for all the blonds in town. Still, the limited studies that have been done strongly suggest that having cancer cells in the bone marrow is a poor prognostic sign.[2,3] As the method is refined, it will, we hope, permit doctors to detect such cancer cells and later, after the treatment, show that they are gone. Stay tuned to see if this potential is realized.

There are some blood tests for women with breast cancer—CEA, CA 15-3, CA 27.29. All of these are nonspecific markers found in the blood. They can be followed over time and will often go up if metastases develop. It was initially hoped that these tests would detect the presence of a few cancer cells. Unfortunately, we've found that they're neither specific nor sensitive enough for that. But since they tend to go up in people with extensive metastases, they're useful in following women with metastatic disease because they help us adjust treatment.

Remember that all tests have limits. A negative finding doesn't give you a clean bill of health; it simply tells you that there are no large chunks of cancer in those organs. Most people who are newly diagnosed don't have spread of this magnitude. So we no longer do these tests in the usual stage 1 or stage 2 breast cancers. If you have stage 3 or locally advanced breast cancer, or if you have symptoms in any of the organs breast cancer typically spreads to—like low back pain that started right after you found your lump and hasn't gone away—we may do these tests. But we no longer do them routinely.

Since there's no foolproof method for determining the early (microscopic) stages of a cancer's spread, we have to approach it differently. We do have a number of methods of estimating the likelihood of early spread—sort of like trying a case on circumstantial evidence. We do this by looking for other conditions that are often associated with cancer spread. If these conditions exist, we can guess that the cancer has spread; if they don't, we can guess that it hasn't. We go through a series of tests in different sequences to try to determine what the chances are.

The first level is based on how the cancer appears at diagnosis. Certain signs and symptoms statistically indicate a higher chance of microscopic cells being elsewhere. These have been incorporated into stage 3 (T4 lesions) of the TNM system. Cushman Haagensen first described what he called the "grave signs"—findings on physical exam that indicated the likelihood that microscopic cells had spread to other areas of the body (Fig. 16-9).[4] His work was done in the 1940s before chemotherapy was used to treat early-diagnosis cancer. Haagensen's plan was to determine which women would really benefit from a radi-

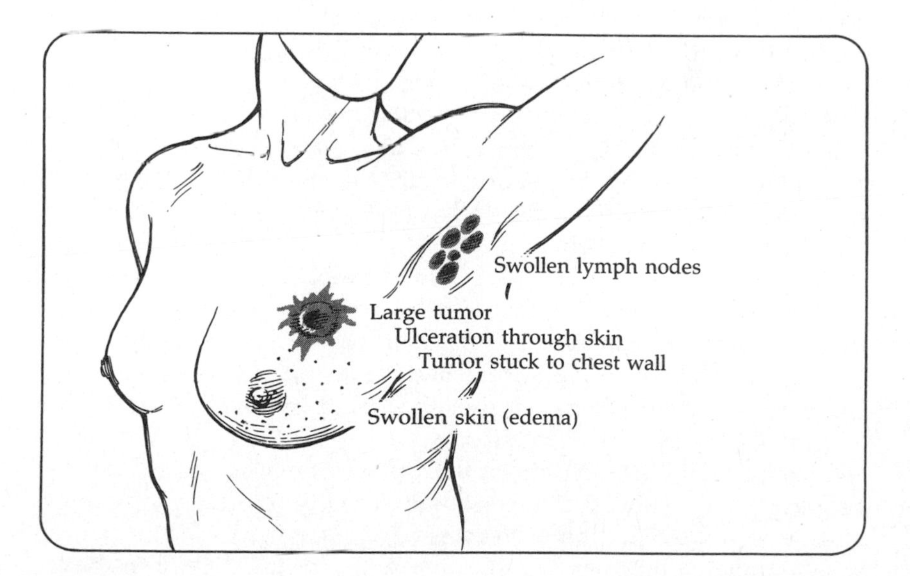

FIGURE 16-9

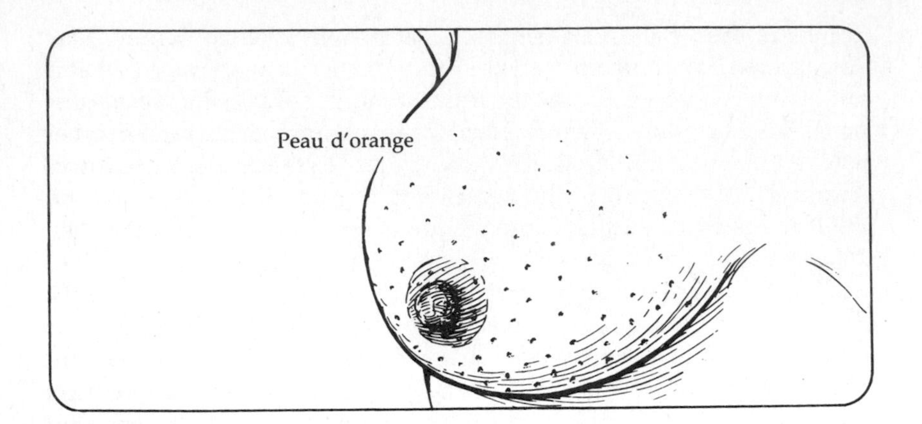

FIGURE 16-10

cal mastectomy. If there was no hope of saving a patient's life, he didn't want to cause needless suffering and destroy the quality of whatever life she had left. His system is still useful in a general way.

One sign that a cancer has probably spread is its size. If it's more than 5 centimeters (about 2 inches), there are probably microscopic cells elsewhere.

Another danger sign is swelling of the skin (edema) where the tumor is. As the skin swells, ligaments that hold the breast tissue to the skin get pulled in, and it looks like you've got little dimples on the area. Because this can look like an orange peel, it's known as *peau d'orange* (Fig. 16-10). If the tumor is ulcerating through the skin, it's ominous. If it's stuck to the muscles underneath so it doesn't move at all, that's also a bad sign. If there are lymph nodes you can feel above your collarbone (superclavicular nodes) or walnut-size lymph nodes in your armpit, that's also dangerous. And if the skin around the lump appears red and infected, it can indicate inflammatory breast cancer (see Chapter 19), which is also likely to spread.

Any one of these signs suggests a high probability that there are microscopic cancer cells elsewhere in the body. If they are present, we plan a systemic treatment (see Chapter 18) as well as a local treatment for the cancer. These tumors are called locally advanced and are often treated with chemotherapy rather than surgery as a first step. (See Chapter 19.)

Most people don't have any of these grave signs, but we still need to figure out the likelihood of microscopic cancer cells existing in other organs. The way we do this is to remove some axillary (armpit) lymph nodes. There are between 30 and 60 lymph nodes under the arm. We try to sample the ones most likely to show cancer cells under the microscope and then examine them. (See Chapter 21 for this surgery.) We look at these lymph nodes because they are a good window for what is going on in the rest of the body. If they reveal cancer cells, we assume there's a high probability that there are microscopic cancer cells in other parts of the body. If they don't show cancer, it means there is a lower probability. Classically pathologists would examine all of the lymph nodes removed in a standard fashion. A more recent technique called *sentinel node biopsy* involves finding the one node the surgeon believes most likely to have cancer cells and to examine it more thoroughly. (Sentinel node biopsy is discussed in detail in Chapters 17 and 21.)

The lymph node evaluation, however, doesn't give us a perfect answer either. Positive lymph nodes don't necessarily mean that there are microscopic cells elsewhere. In fact, they don't in about 30 percent of cases. Conversely even if the lymph nodes are negative, it does not mean that the cancer has not spread elsewhere—20 to 30 percent of breast cancers with negative lymph nodes have spread elsewhere.

To a certain degree, though, the number of positive lymph nodes gives us a sense of the probability of having microscopic breast cancer cells elsewhere in the body. With one or two positive nodes, you're less likely to have them than with 10 or 15, and this is reflected in the new TNM system, which separates N_1 into a, b, and c categories based on the number of positive nodes. However, because with any positive lymph nodes there's a pretty high chance that there are cancer cells elsewhere, we almost always treat women with positive nodes with either hormones or chemotherapy or both (see Chapter 18).

In women with negative nodes, it's trickier. What we want is a way to identify the 20–30 percent who have microscopic cells elsewhere and not overtreat the other 70 percent. At present we don't have a direct way to do this. However, we do it indirectly by examining the primary tumor for the features described at the beginning of this chapter. We look at the size of the tumor; if it's more than 2 centimeters it has a higher chance of spread; if it's less than 1 centimeter it has a very low chance. Then we look for other factors, especially in the gray zone where the tumor is between 1 and 2 centimeters. We look at the biomarkers.

BIOMARKERS

More and more we are trying to identify characteristics of tumor cells—characteristics that cannot be seen directly under the microscope but can be measured with sophisticated molecular tests—that tell us how the tumor will behave. We use a number of biological characteristics of the tumor to help us understand this. We have an enormous list of candidates, but unfortunately we haven't yet figured out which biomarkers may be the best. Every time a new fact about cancer is discovered, somebody will do a test to see whether this new fact can be translated into a good indicator (a biomarker) of the tumor's behavior. These markers are classified into three categories: (1) ones that are used to help determine the prognosis of a particular cancer, (2) ones that are used to predict that a cancer will respond to a certain treatment, and (3) ones that do both. I'll discuss the biomarkers most frequently used.

The most common analysis is for the estrogen and progesterone receptors, to find out whether the tumor is sensitive to these hormones. These receptors are now known to be far less simple than the tried-and-true lock-and-key analogy would imply (Fig. 16-11). What remains true is that tumors lacking estrogen and progesterone receptors are not sensitive to estrogen or progesterone. The implications of the hormone receptor tests are both prognostic and predictive. In general, tumors that are sensitive to hormones—that have receptors—are

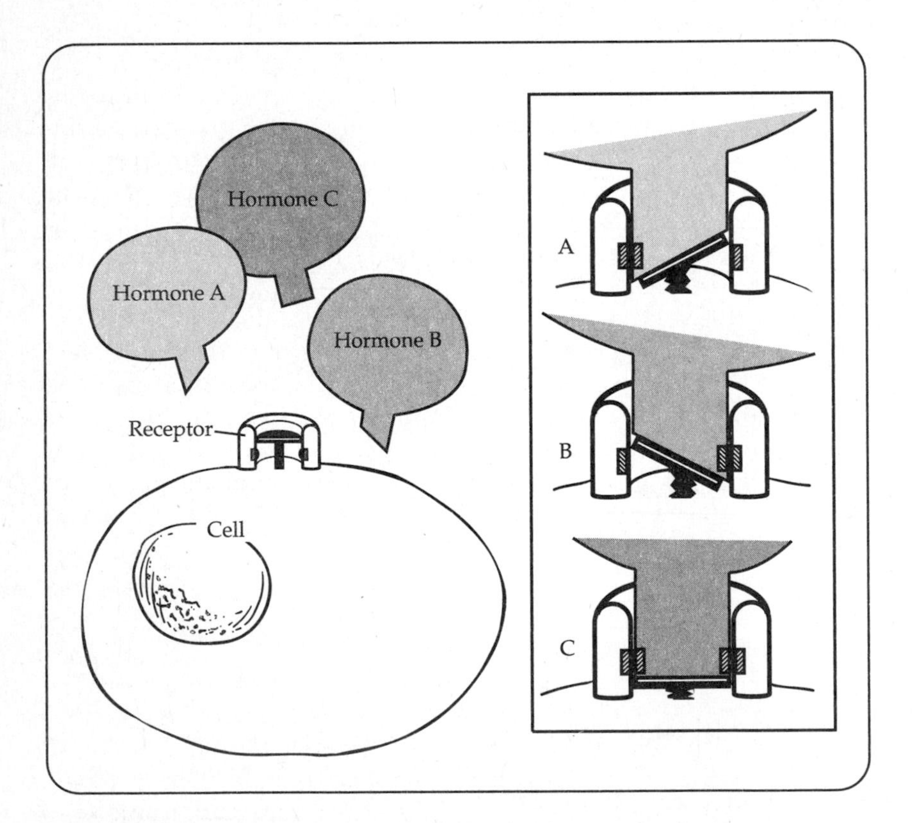

FIGURE 16-11

slightly slower growing and have a slightly better prognosis than tumors that aren't.[5] Generally postmenopausal women are more likely to be estrogen receptor positive and premenopausal women are more likely to be estrogen receptor negative. Second, the test tells whether the tumor can be treated with some kind of hormone blocking therapy. If it's not sensitive to hormones, it rarely responds to hormone blocking treatments (see Chapter 24).

Next, we try to figure out how rapidly the breast cancer cells are dividing or how abnormal they are, based on the idea that the more they divide the more aggressive they must be. We measure these features in a couple of ways. One way is by *flow cytometry,* measuring the amount and type of DNA.[6] If the tumor cells have the normal amount of DNA, they're called *diploid;* if the amount of DNA is abnormal, they're called *aneuploid.* Aneuploid tumors account for about 70 percent of all breast cancer tumors. Diploid tumors behave much less aggressively because they are less abnormal. In addition, these tests can measure the percentage of cells that are in the process of dividing at any one time. This is called the *S phase fraction.* If there are a lot of cells dividing (high S phase fraction), the tumor may behave more aggressively than if there are only a few cells dividing (low S phase fraction). These markers actually give information similar to that of nuclear grade, but they're more reliable because they are objective measurements determined by computer, and they don't depend on a pathologist's subjective interpretation of how bad the cells look under the microscope. Like every test, however, flow cytometry has limitations. For node-positive patients, these tests add little new information. As we'll see in the next chapter, their main use lies in suggesting which node negative tumors need additional treatment and which ones don't.

Another prognostic and predictive biomarker is overexpression (too many copies) of the Her-2/neu (also known as erb-b2) oncogene. Her-2/neu is one of the dominant oncogenes that contribute to cancer by telling cells to grow. Instead of being mutated, however, Her-2/neu is frequently overexpressed and amplified; in other words, there are too many copies of the oncogene so the message to grow is increased.[7] This occurs in about a third of invasive cancers. Having your tumor tested for the Her-2/neu receptor is important because the test can function not only as a prognostic indicator (Her-2/neu positive tumors tend to be more aggressive) but also as an indicator of the best treatment. There are several tests that can be used for Her-2/neu overexpression. One, *immunohistochemistry* (IHC), assesses the overexpression of the Her-2 protein while the other, *fluorescence in situ hybridization* (FISH), assesses whether there are too many copies of the actual gene. It is the difference between measuring the effect or the cause. The initial studies of trastuzumab (Herceptin), an antibody developed to specifically block

Her-2/neu, being used to treat breast cancer (see Chapter 18), used the IHC test.[8] But work in 2000 indicated that FISH may be more precise.[9] Gene amplification appears to be a better predictor of response to trastuzumab than IHC, at least in women who have an IHC result of 2+.

Because FISH is more difficult and more expensive to do, the current practice in the United States is that most samples are first screened with IHC, and those showing overexpression (2+) are retested with FISH. Trastuzumab is currently used in women with metastasis, and it is also useful for women as an adjuvant therapy are ongoing (see Chapter 18). (Almost all DCIS is Her-2/neu positive, but this does not mean it should be treated with chemotherapy. It is still precancer, growing only within the duct.)

A lot of research currently suggests that Her-2/neu can also be used to direct which adjuvant therapy may be best. Preliminary information suggests that Her-2/neu overexpressors are more likely to respond to Adriamycin while Her-2/neu negative women may do just as well with Cytoxan, methotrexate, and 5-FU (see Chapter 18). In addition, women who are both estrogen receptor positive and Her-2/neu overexpressing may be resistant to tamoxifen but sensitive to aromatase inhibitors or ovarian ablation, stopping the hormones produced by the ovary.[10,11,12] (See Chapter 18.)

Urokinase-type plasminogen activator (u-PA) and its inhibitor PAI-1 are biomarkers used more commonly in Europe than in the United States. U-PA is an enzyme that is capable of breaking down the tissue surrounding the ducts (*extracellular matrix* or *stroma*) and is thought to be used by cancer cells to invade. High levels of both u-PA and its inhibitor PAI-1 are indicators of a poorer prognosis. In addition there is a suggestion that it, like Her-2/neu, can predict tamoxifen resistance. A large ongoing study in Germany is using u-PA and PAI-1 to distinguish between high-risk and low-risk women, with only the high-risk women being treated with chemotherapy. When the data from these studies become available, we may see more use of this marker in the United States.

We can now identify many other biomarkers: epidermal growth factor receptor, heat shock protein, nm23, p53.[13] I discuss the basis of some of these in Chapter 27. There are many other emerging biomarkers, and new ones are discovered every day. Most of them are elevated in cancers more likely to recur, but none is sensitive and specific enough to use routinely at the present time.

By putting all of these elements together, we make our best guess. If the tumor looks fairly aggressive and there's a significant chance of having microscopic cancer cells being somewhere in the body, then chemotherapy or hormone therapy may be worth doing. If it looks like there's a low chance, it may not be. We may find out that the important thing isn't whether there are microscopic cancer cells in the body (everyone with cancer may have some), but rather how many and whether they can grow and spread. The ideal set of biomarkers will predict these latter properties.

All of these tests are only tools that, added together, help give us a picture of the cancer, and decide what to do. All any of these tests, and others that are being developed, can do is to give a picture of that particular tumor at one particular time—sort of like a snapshot. They cannot tell anything about how the cancer cell actually acts in a particular woman.

At the end of these tests your tumor will be characterized in a description something like the following: This is a stage 2: 2 centimeter, node-negative, estrogen receptor positive, S phase 10 percent, aneuploid, Her-2/neu amplified tumor.

COMBINED MARKERS

Frustration with the low accuracy of the current prognostic and predictive markers has led to a new approach that combines several into a recurrence score. The first such test to be clinically available, Oncotype DX, is from Genomic Health.[14] Scientists selected 21 genetic markers that held promise for both prognosis and prediction. They then developed a method to analyze these genes in fixed tissue (leftover tissue from a removed tumor that had already been used to make diagnostic slides). They first tested the genes on the tissue from a completed NS-ABP (National Surgical Adjuvant Breast and Bowel Project) study on women with estrogen positive, node negative tumors who were randomized between tamoxifen and placebo. Since this study had been completed, they knew which women had cancer that recurred within the 10-year follow-up. Their test was able to distinguish a high-risk, low-risk, and intermediate-risk group from supposedly good prognostic tumors. The high-risk group had a 30 percent chance of recurrence while the low-risk group had a 6 percent chance. This recurrence score was more predictive than age or tumor size. In fact they found some very small tumors that had a high chance of recurrence and some larger ones that did not. The value of the test was increased with their second report at the San Antonio Breast Cancer Symposium in December of 2004.[15] By applying their test to women who had received chemotherapy in addition to tamoxifen, they showed that the high-risk group benefited significantly from chemotherapy while the low recurrence score women did not. The benefit from tamoxifen was examined using this test in another retrospective study and showed that women with a low recurrence score and high estrogen receptor score had the biggest benefit from tamoxifen while the women with a high recurrence score did not. Oncotype Rx is currently clinically available through Genomic Health, although at the time of this writing it is not covered by many insurance carriers. The data are useful but do not address all the current options. For example, one wonders whether the high-risk estrogen receptor positive women would have done as well with an aromatase inhibitor (see Chapter 18) as chemotherapy. Futhermore, the test does not address risk of recurrence in estrogen receptor negative cancers.

An additional combination test from Europe (MammaPrint), based on the DNA microarray discussed in Chapter 15, was presented at the same meeting in 2004.[16] This test combines 70 genes and predicted which women with negative lymph nodes who had not received chemotherapy developed metastases 14 years later. It is currently being validated in additional studies. Although we still need confirmation that these tests hold up, they are certainly the wave of the not-too-distant future. To judge the prognosis and predict what therapy will work, we are finally moving from the circumstantial descriptive evidence of the past to the molecular, DNA, and gene testing of the future. There is no turning back.

17

Treatment Options: Local Therapy

After you have been diagnosed with breast cancer, you will face several decisions about treatment. As I noted in Chapter 16, there are different kinds of treatment—local treatments to prevent your cancer from coming back in the breast and systemic treatments to destroy microscopic cells we think may have spread into the rest of your body. In this chapter, we'll look at the local treatments, since these usually come first. In the next chapter we'll explore the systemic treatments.

SURGERY AND RADIATION

For years, most surgeons began any treatment course with mastectomy, assuming that this drastic procedure was the most effective way to save lives. But studies in recent years have proven them wrong. Saving lives seems to depend more on the systemic therapies than the local ones. The main goal of therapy to the breast, therefore, is to prevent breast cancer from coming back in the specific area in which the cancer appears. This can be done by taking out as much of the cancer as possible in a lumpectomy and letting radiation destroy any remaining cells. The cancer can also be removed by mastectomy, which in small tumors usually takes out enough tissue to prevent recurrence, so that no radiation is needed. Finally, with very large tumors we use both mastectomy, to remove as much of the tumor as possible, and radiation therapy, to take care of leftover cells. However, you can have a local recurrence, no matter what treatment or combination of treatments we use.

When the tumor isn't so large that it calls for both mastectomy and radiation, the choice of which route to go is very subjective. Large randomized studies with as much as 20 years follow-up have shown that both approaches—mastectomy alone or lumpectomy with radiation—result in the same survival rates. The first study to compare mastectomy and breast conservation surgery was done in Italy in the 1970s. It compared radical mastectomy (a much more extensive operation than the sort of mastectomy we do today) to quadrantectomy (the removal of 25 percent of the breast) followed by radiation, and found there was no difference in the survival between the two methods of treatment.[1] The 20-year follow-up reported in 2002 showed no difference between the two treatments in terms of cancer in the other breast, distant metastases, or new cancers in the same breast.[2] The overall death rates in the two groups were the same, as was the number of deaths from breast cancer. Since then, many other studies have supported this conclusion. The NSABP (National Surgical Adjuvant Breast and Bowel Project) did a study in the United States comparing lumpectomy alone, lumpectomy and radiation, and mastectomy. The 20-year follow-up had similar results: lumpectomy and radiation had the same survival and essentially the same local control rate as mastectomy, considering the fact that the women who had recurrences in their retained breast could have a mastectomy later.[3] (These treatments are described at length in Chapters 21 and 23.)

In June 1990 the National Cancer Institute Consensus Conference concluded: "Breast conservation treatment is an appropriate method of primary therapy for the *majority* of women with Stage I and II breast cancer and is *preferable* because it provides survival equivalent to total mastectomy while preserving the breast" (emphasis mine). (Because of this latter fact, we often refer to this course of treatment as "breast conservation.") What amazes me is that 15 years later we are still doing more mastectomies than breast conservation. Recent studies have shown that only 42.6 percent of women are getting breast conservation.[4]

There is still a tendency to do mastectomy when the tumor appears more aggressive, suggesting that even after 20 years of data to the contrary many people still think of breast conservation as less aggressive therapy—though, as I'll explain later, it isn't. This may be due in part to the American tendency to think that more is always better. If it hurts more or is a bigger operation, people think it must work better. Many of the women I counsel over this decision have that attitude. And too often their surgeons don't try to dissuade them. In Los Angeles growing numbers of women are having bilateral mastectomies for cancers that could be treated as well with breast conservation. The surgeons say it is the patient's choice, but I wonder how often the surgeon is unconsciously influenced by the fact that it is reimbursed better by insurance, it's easier to do, and the burden of responsibility for cosmetic results are shifted to the plastic surgeon. As you are considering your options, be aware that the medical profession has biases that may or may not be in your best interest. It's really wise to get a second opinion.

In some cases, this is as important medically as it is cosmetically. If your cancer is right near the breastbone, the best mastectomy won't allow the surgeon to get a normal rim of tissue around the lump. But radiation will treat the surrounding tissue.

On the other hand, mastectomy is sometimes the best medical choice, for instance, if you have a large cancer in a small breast (although Dr. Gianni Bonadonna's studies with preoperative chemotherapy, discussed in the next chapter, may help here). In short, there are both medical and cosmetic implications to whatever course you choose, and you should be fully informed about both.

After much study, it appears that the most important factor to achieving local control is getting most of the tumor out with surgery. That's the *tumor*—not every speck of cancer. When we started doing breast conservation, many studies were done extensively examining breasts that had been removed, looking for small cancers that might have been missed if the woman had had only a lumpectomy. One study showed 40 percent of breasts had other spots of cancer more than 2 centimeters from the original lesion.[5] This number corresponds closely to the recurrence rate in women who are treated with lumpectomy without radiation therapy[6] and to the identification of unsuspected cancer in women who undergo ultrasound or MRI before their surgery.[7] Radiation has been proven very good at treating these secondary lesions, since the local recurrence rate when radiation is added to lumpectomy is significantly lower than 40 percent. These recurrences are usually at the site of the original lesion, not elsewhere in the breast. Despite what you would think, these tiny spots of cancer elsewhere in the breast do not have to be removed because they can be well treated with radiation therapy. All of this leads me to caution women against having preoperative MRIs or PET scans. These sensitive tests will only show up other spots and lead you on a wild goose chase.

We determine whether we've removed the majority of the tumor by evaluating the margins of the tissue. (See Chapter 16.) If they're free of tumor, breast conservation is fine. This can be affected by the tumor's pathology. Breast cancers have tentacle-like protrusions stretching out into the breast tissue from the original lump. Ductal carcinomas with lots of DCIS (also called *extensive intraductal component*, or EIC), associated with them can reach much farther out. When this occurs, the margins may not be clean on the first try (the surgeon can't see or feel the "tentacles"). A reexcision will sometimes take care of it. But there are some cases in which even a reexcision won't get clean margins, and a mastectomy, the ultimate wide excision, is necessary to get it all out. Infiltrating lobular carcinomas also have a tendency to be sneaky and difficult for the surgeon to find and get around (see Chapter 16). These too need a wider excision and clean margins if they are to be treated with breast conservation, and may still end up requiring a mastectomy.

On the other hand, if the cancer is a distinct lump with short "tentacles," then just removing it is fine. Sometimes the margin is just barely involved in one spot and is otherwise clear. This may still be acceptable for radiation therapy.[8] The key is determining the likelihood of cancer being left behind. In the usual type of cancer, the chance is very low, and radiation therapy can get rid of whatever cells may remain. When lumpectomy with radiation was first employed in Boston, those of us pioneers who were doing it didn't know that margins were important and we just took the tumor out. Reviewing this data in retrospect, we found that in tumors without EIC or lobular carcinoma our recurrence rate was only 4–6 percent over more than 10 years, even though we did not have perfectly clean margins.

Overall there are only five situations that would rule out breast conservation with radiation therapy.[9]

1. The woman has two or more primary tumors in separate quadrants of the breast (although a recent small study questioned this proscription) or diffuse microcalcifications throughout the breast.[10]
2. She has a history of previous therapeutic radiation to the breast region (i.e., Hodgkin's disease) that combined with the proposed treatment would result in an excessively high total radiation dosage.
3. She is pregnant. However, in many cases it may be possible to perform breast conserving surgery in the second and third trimester and treat the patient with radiation after delivery. (See Chapter 23.)
4. There are persistent positive margins after reasonable surgical attempts. A very small sign of cancer in one place on a margin (focally involved margin) may not rule out breast conservation, however.
5. The presence of specific active autoimmune diseases, particularly scleroderma, which can result in severe short-term and long-term complications in the presence of radiation.

In other situations, however, there may be reasons not to choose breast conservation therapy. For example, if the area that needs to be removed is very large compared to the breast itself there will not be enough breast tissue left after a lumpectomy to make it cosmetically worthwhile. (It is commonly accepted that about one-quarter of the breast can be removed and leave a cosmetically acceptable result). If the woman is a carrier of the BRCA 1 and/or 2 gene and has a high risk of other cancers developing in the remaining breast tissue, she may want to consider bilateral mastectomy. LCIS (see Chapter 12), once considered a contraindication for breast conservation, is no longer believed to be one.

Lumpectomy Without Radiation

The NSABP study cited earlier also explored the possibility of getting lumpectomy with no radiation. Researchers discovered that with lumpectomy alone, a woman has a 35 percent greater chance of a local recurrence of her cancer.[11] Twelve additional studies have since been done looking at whether radiation is really necessary. In all of these studies it is clear that the local recurrence rate with radiation is about two-thirds of the recurrence rate without it. None of the studies, however, have shown that the survival rate for breast cancer is different.[12] If only 35–40 percent of women who have wide excision alone will have a recurrence, we're irradiating 60–65 percent of women who don't need it. One group in which this happens is women over 70 with hormone sensitive tumors undergoing lumpectomy and tamoxifen (see Chapter 19).[13,14] At this point we can't figure out which other women might forgo radiation therapy despite several studies attempting to do so, and local radiation is still the best option for invasive cancers treated with lumpectomy.[15,16]

Partial Breast Radiation

One hopeful area of recent study is that of local radiation. Local recurrences after lumpectomy alone are almost all in the area of the primary tumor. So perhaps we can just irradiate the bed of the tumor, sparing the rest of the breast. Further support for this idea comes from the observation that 10 years or so after lumpectomy with radiation therapy, the risk of a new cancer elsewhere in the breast is about the same as the risk in the other breast. So irradiating the whole breast does not seem to decrease the risk of a new cancer developing elsewhere in that breast. Limiting radiation to the tumor bed allows the treatment to be shorter and should limit side effects.

Based on this line of thinking, several techniques have been developed to deliver radiation locally: *interstitial brachytherapy, limited external beam irradiation, intracavitary brachytherapy,* and *intraoperative limited radiation therapy*. These will be described in Chapter 23. So far reports from these techniques have been limited but encouraging. Several randomized controlled trials are under way that will give us the safety data we need before this approach becomes widely adopted. Currently this approach should be limited patients who are older, have no or limited axillary nodal involvement, have clear margins on lumpectomy, and have no pathology showing EIC or infiltrating lobular carcincoma—and with the understanding that the safety is not completely verified.[17] I would suggest that any woman who is interested in this approach try to participate in a clinical trial so that we can get the answers as soon as possible.

Mastectomy

Many people have the misconception that a mastectomy guarantees the cancer will never come back. But as noted earlier, we can never be certain that we have removed *all* the breast tissue, and cancer can come back again in the scar or the chest wall. This is not rare, occurring about 0.6 percent per year, or 5–10 percent over 12 years. I saw one patient with a very small cancer who had bilateral mastectomies because she never wanted to deal with breast cancer again, and a year later she had a recurrence in her scar. No one had ever told her that this might happen, and she felt betrayed by her original medical team.

In my mind mastectomy should be done only when breast conservation is not possible—the particular situations noted above—or when the woman herself has a strong preference for mastectomy, knowing all the statistics.

Reconstruction (see Chapter 22) can be done immediately at the time of mastectomy or later, when and if a woman wants it. Even with this possibility, however, it makes no sense to me to remove a breast and try to reconstruct it when it can be preserved in a cosmetically acceptable way with the same risk of recurrence and same chance of cure.

Sometimes a woman will choose mastectomy over breast conservation because she has been told that if she had breast conservation and the cancer recurred later, she would be unable to have reconstruction at that time. This is silly for several reasons. To begin with, only about 10 percent of women will develop a local recurrence in the breast and require a mastectomy. Further, it is indeed possible to do reconstruction of an irradiated breast, using the woman's own tissue.

Mastectomy with Radiation

With mastectomy, we usually don't do radiation because the tumor has been wholly removed. But studies have shown that in certain situations there is a higher risk of recurrence after mastectomy in the skin or lymph nodes: four or more positive axillary lymph nodes; a tumor over 5 centimeters; close margins (cancer cells at the edge of the mastectomy); and significant amounts of invasion of the lymphatic or blood vessels in the breast tissue. Local recurrence in the skin or lymph nodes after a mastectomy doesn't necessarily increase the patient's chances of dying (although it does signify a more aggressive cancer with a higher risk of systemic recurrence), but getting breast cancer once is upsetting enough, and preventing a recurrence is never a bad idea.

Postmastectomy radiation reduces the chance of local recurrence by 50–75 percent (if the local recurrence rate overall is 5–10 percent, this makes it 3–5 percent). If the chance of recurrence is higher, as in the situations mentioned above, the benefit is also higher. This may be a worthwhile goal in itself, but until lately it was not thought to have an impact on increasing survival. Then three randomized studies of women who had a high risk of local recurrence and positive nodes after mastectomy showed that those treated with a combination of modern radiation therapy techniques to the chest wall, lymph node draining, and systemic therapy had fewer local recurrences than those treated with systemic therapy alone, and their overall survival was significantly better—about 10 percent.[18,19,20] The current hypothesis is that when the systemic therapy has taken care of a microscopic metastasis elsewhere in the body, the microscopic disease left in the breast area becomes more important and has the opportunity to spread. Local radiation therapy is aimed at sterilizing this area.

Why then shouldn't everyone who has a mastectomy also have radiation? Because radiation has its own risks. Studies show that people who had cancer on the left side and got radiation had an increase in heart disease, although this risk has decreased substantially as radiation techniques have improved.[21] (See Chapter 23.) In addition, recent studies have shown a doubling of the risk of lung cancer 10 years after postmastectomy radiation therapy.[22,23] (This risk is related to smoking history as well as the amount of lung that has been treated and, interestingly, does not apply to radiation therapy after breast conservation.) As with all the decisions related to breast cancer treatment, it ends up being a balance of risk versus benefit. When the risk of local recurrence is high enough after a mastectomy, radiation is worthwhile. Most specialists now agree with the idea presented above—that patients with four or more positive nodes or tumors that are larger than 5 centimeters should be treated with radiation.[24,25,26] More controversial is the question of the patient with 1–3 positive nodes. There was a large randomized controlled study in this country that asked whether survival was improved with radiotherapy in women with 1–3 positive nodes.

Unfortunately it closed due to poor patient enrollment (probably due more to physicians' treatment biases). Another study designed to address this question is about to open in Europe. Until we have the answer to this question, any woman with a cancer that requires a mastectomy should discuss with her doctor the advisability of postoperative radiation therapy.

ABLATION TECHNIQUES

As radiation therapy and node testing are becoming less invasive, many researchers have begun to go beyond surgery in their attempt to destroy the tumor, using radiofrequency, cryosurgery (freezing), microwave (yes, microwaves can be used for things other than reheating leftovers) or focused ultrasound.[27,28,29] These approaches are possible because we now can get all the information we need from a core biopsy without having to remove the whole tumor to test it for biomarkers (see Chapter 16). This means that we may be able to destroy the tumor in the breast without removing it. Cryosurgery has the advantage of making a palpable ice ball when treating the tumor. This ice ball can be either removed surgically *(cryo-assisted lumpectomy)* or left in place if the tumor is truly destroyed. Other techniques are also being studied, and your surgeon may mention them to you. If you want to take part in one of these experimental approaches, be sure that it is within an approved study to determine the safety of the technique.

AXILLARY SURGERY

Along with getting rid of the lump, we usually try to discover if there are affected lymph nodes under the arm (axilla). Women do better when these lymph nodes are treated. The improvement in survival is about 5 percent in women whose axilla are routinely treated than in women whose axilla are just observed and left alone unless a lymph node appears cancerous to the touch.[30] What is not clear is that removing the lymph nodes is the only way to treat them. A randomized controlled study comparing radiation of the axilla to surgery in women without palpable nodes showed no difference in survival at 15 years. But there were more recurrences in the axilla of the women who had radiation than in the ones who had surgery. The difference was 3 percent versus 1 percent, so both risks were low.[31]

Aside from preventing recurrence in the armpit, the main purpose for doing axillary surgery is to help decide whether and how much adjuvant systemic therapy to give. Some surgeons have argued that if we are going to give systemic therapy to all women, node negative as well as node positive (a philosophy we'll consider later), there is no reason to dissect the lymph nodes. They feel they can save women the potential complications of this operation (see Chapter 21) by irradiating the axilla instead. The fallacy in this argument, at least at the time of this writing, is that we are not at all sure that every woman *should* be treated with systemic therapy. Until we know who should be treated or we have a better marker of prognosis than lymph nodes, I still think it is an important operation for most women.

Luckily, in recent years, a new variation on lymph node dissection has offered us a better way to find cancer spread. This is known as *sentinel node biopsy.* (See Fig. 17-1.) The concept is pretty straightforward[32,33] and is based on the theory that there are one or more nodes to which a breast cancer is most likely to spread. This was proven by an elegant study done at the John Wayne Cancer Center by Armand Giuliano in Los Angeles. A total of 157 women underwent sentinel node biopsy followed by full axillary dissection. All the nodes

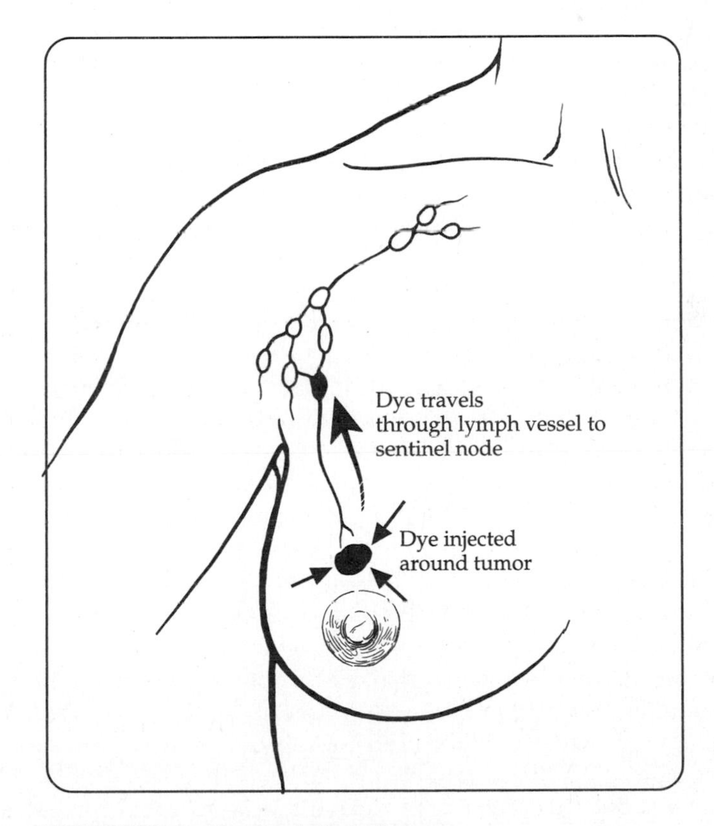

FIGURE 17-1 Sentinel Node Biopsy

removed were studied in the same way—with multiple sections and IHC (imunohistochemistry, a special stain that can identify cancer cells). When the sentinel node was negative, all but one of 1,087 lymph nodes were also negative (the one was questionable).[34] This established the technique as a valid way to identify cancer in the nodes. Indeed, it may even be better than the standard regular dissection. Since there are fewer nodes, they can be studied more carefully. There are now two large randomized controlled studies following women long-range to see if there is a larger number of axillary recurrences later in life among those who had only sentinel biopsy that found no cancer than among those who had a full axillary dissection.[35] These data will tell us whether it is indeed safe to do the lesser procedure and will let us see the potential complications. Because a positive sentinel node often predicts that there will be other positive nodes in the axilla, the current standard of care is for women who have a positive (cancerous) sentinel node to go on to have a full dissection.

Finally there is the question of the special staining. When the sentinel node is examined by the pathologist, the slides are stained in two ways (see Chapter 16)—first with hematoxylin and eosin (H and E) and then with a special immunohistochemistry (IHC) stain for a particular protein (cytokeratin) that's found in breast cells but not in lymph cells. When sentinel nodes are examined both ways, about 6 percent are found to be positive on IHC but not on H and E.[36] Often the IHC shows only a few cells in the node. The controversy is whether these cells are transported to the lymph nodes by surgical manipulation during either the surgery or the biopsy. This concern has been supported by a recent study at Sloan Kettering which found that metastasis discovered in lymph nodes by H and E were related to tumor size and aggressiveness as expected, whereas metastasis found by IHC related more to the type of biopsy than any characteristics of the tumor.[37] As I mentioned in Chapter 16, the new staging system does not consider these cells to be significant and calls them node negative, and the American Society of Pathologists does not recommend doing IHC staining on sentinel nodes. Data on this situation will be collected in the two large studies of sentinel nodes being done and will finally give us an answer.

Experience with sentinel node biopsies has led to guidelines about when the procedure is most appropriate: a tumor that is unicentric, less than 5 centimeters, no previous chemotherapy or radiation therapy, no large resection in the upper outer quadrant (more than 6 cm), and no palpable lymph nodes. Most important is an experienced sentinel node team, beginning with the surgeon. You should always ask questions about the doctor who does the procedure. You want someone who has experience or is working under the supervision of someone with experience, because the procedure is difficult to learn. It has been estimated that a surgeon must do between 20 and 30 procedures to become really good at it. The first few times a surgeon does it, there can be difficulties finding the sentinel lymph node, injecting the dye or the radioactive fluid correctly, and knowing how long to wait before doing the surgery after the injection. So you probably don't want to be someone's second sentinel node biopsy case unless it's someone working under top-notch supervision. Ask how many times the surgeon has done the procedure. In addition, ask what percentage of the time the surgeon has been able to find the sentinel node. It should be at least 85 percent (with experienced surgeons, in fact, it's 90 or 95 percent).

Also ask about the surgeon's false negative rate. When surgeons first learn this procedure, they do it along with a full dissection. They take out what they think is the sentinel node, then do the regular dissection and see whether they identified the sentinel node correctly. A false negative means the sentinel node was negative but there was a positive node someplace else. The false negative rate should be under 5 percent. If a surgeon is unable or unwilling to give you numbers, that's a pretty good sign that you should look for another surgeon. If it turns out to be the surgeon's third or fourth operation, find out who the supervising surgeon is—and get *that* surgeon's numbers. It's also important to make sure that the pathologists are experienced.

In some situations sentinel node biopsy isn't feasible. If you've had extensive breast surgery that may have disrupted the lymphatic pathways—breast reduction or in some cases silicone implants—sentinel node biopsy won't work. If you have nodes that can already be felt, then it isn't necessary; the doctor knows where to go. If you have two lumps in different places in the breast, the sentinel nodes may be in two parts of your armpit and the procedure won't work. It is less successful in older women and in women with extensive DCIS.

In some patients with severe health problems, the risks of general anesthesia may outweigh the advantage of knowing the lymph node status, and in these women it may be reasonable to forgo this operation in favor of axillary radiation. This was in fact my recommendation for my 80-year-old aunt when she was diagnosed with breast cancer this year.

The discussion about axillary dissection is an ongoing one. I think in the future we'll stop doing axillary dissection altogether. Once we've got a better biomarker (see Chapter 16) so we can say, "This is your prognosis," we'll no longer have to subject women to the extra surgery of lymph node removal, with its side effects. At this point, however, I think it's important for every woman to question her surgeon about the necessity of an axillary dissection and make sure she's comfortable with the explanation before proceeding.

TIMING OF SURGERY

There is growing information regarding the timing of surgery in premenopausal women. There have been over 32 retrospective studies looking at this in relation to the menstrual cycle, with most of them suggesting that surgery in the second half of the menstrual cycle is best.[38,39] There is a biologically plausible explanation for this. Scientists have observed that factors influencing the growth of new blood vessels (VEGF) are higher in the first part of the menstrual cycle and lower in the safer second half, possibly preventing cancer cells from escaping. Of course neither studies that observe a phenomena nor a biological explanation are enough to establish cause and effect. Two prospective studies have shown contradictory results.

An interesting study done in Vietnam by my friend Richard Love (no relation) randomized premenopausal women to have an oophorectomy plus a mastectomy or just a mastectomy as their primary treatment for breast cancer. The women who had their oophorectomy in the luteal phase (second half of their cycle) did much better than the ones who had surgery in the follicular phase (first half of the cycle) regardless of their estrogen receptors.[40] I can't help but think that there may be something to this. Three large ongoing studies will answer this question. Meanwhile, this is one piece of information that can be used without risk. If you are a premenopausal woman with breast cancer, it certainly can't hurt to schedule your surgery during your luteal phase—and it may extend your life.

GUIDELINES AND CHOICES

In 1996 the first practice guidelines for breast cancer treatment were published.[41] Since then more have been developed. The most comprehensive are those of the National Comprehensive Cancer Network (NCCN), which can be found free in a patient-friendly version in English and Spanish at www.nccn.org. In general, the guidelines we developed for local therapy nine years ago still stand. Every woman should be considered a candidate for breast conservation unless she strongly prefers mastectomy or has a clear medical reason for it. Any woman whose cancer was picked up with microcalcifications on a mammogram should have a postbiopsy mammogram to demonstrate that all of them have been removed. (As I mentioned earlier, I think preoperative MRIs or PET scans have a role only in special cases of invasive lobular cancers.) If the margins are clean after surgery, she is a candidate for radiation therapy without further breast surgery, although she may still need a sentinel node biopsy. If she has a lumpectomy and the margins are involved in more than one spot or the post-biopsy mammogram shows residual disease, or if she has EIC or infiltrating lobular carcinoma, we suggest a reexcision. A sentinel node biopsy can be done at the same time. This step gathers further information on the cancer. If the new margins are clean she is a candidate for radiation therapy; if not she may need a mastectomy. In addition, if the sentinel node is positive she may need further axillary surgery. The node information will determine the need for systemic therapy. If the tumor is greater than 5 centimeters, she may be a candidate for neoadjuvant therapy, or chemotherapy before surgery, to shrink the tumor before surgery. All women who choose mastectomy should be offered the option of immediate reconstruction.

The first choice you may have to make involves whether you want full axillary dissection, sentinel node dissection, or both. If you want sentinel node dissection and are eligible for it, you may have to search for a doctor with experience doing it. The one thing you *don't* want to do is insist that your surgeon do a sentinel node biopsy. If your surgeon hasn't done the procedure a number of times or doesn't feel comfortable with it, you're better off having the procedure that the surgeon is used to doing.

But it's worth finding out who is available to you if you really want a sentinel node biopsy. In the summer of 1999 I met a 66-year-old woman who was in an HMO, and the doctor she spoke with said that he didn't do the procedure. She was very upset. An active sportswoman, she didn't want to risk injuring her golf arm by having too many nodes removed. I suggested that she ask the doctor if anyone at the HMO did the sentinel node biopsy. She called him, and he willingly gave her a surgeon's name. If your HMO doesn't have anyone, you can explain your need and ask for a recommendation to an outside doctor. Often the HMO will pay the fee for such a specialist; sometimes it will ask for a larger copayment from you.

There are four ongoing clinical trials looking at sentinel node dissection with or without full axillary dissection that you may look into (www.clinicaltrials.gov). There are a couple of good reasons for this. These studies will help us answer some of the questions we have about breast cancer. That's the noble reason. The personal reason is that the doctors working on these trials are well trained and know what they're doing, so you get quality assurance.

If you don't have palpable nodes and have a T1 or T2 tumor (see Chapter 16), I think it's worth having a sentinel node biopsy, even if you're also getting a full axillary dissection. It will allow the doctor to look for which node to study most carefully.

Your next decision concerns *mastectomy* or *lumpectomy with radiation* (the addition of radiation to mastectomy, as I explained earlier in this chapter, is for specific situations that you won't know about until after your primary surgery). What are some of the factors that may influence your choice? There's a tendency to think that mastectomy is more aggressive because it's more mutilating. Actually, the combination of lumpectomy and radiation is more aggressive. Lumpectomy and radiation treat all the breast tissue. The field of radiation may encompass all the tissue that even extensive surgery misses. Some women choose mastectomy because they do not want to make daily trips for radiation therapy; others may want to get it all over with as soon as possible and get back to their lives as though it never happened. However, it *has* happened, and you can never go back to your life exactly the way it was.

There are important drawbacks to mastectomy. It's less cosmetically appealing except with the very best reconstruction and, even with reconstruction (see Chapter 22), leaves you without sensation in the breast or breast area. Lumpectomy and radiation leave you with a real breast that retains its physical sensation.

Some women choose mastectomy because they don't want to take time off from a demanding profession any more than necessary. This makes sense, but now they can also consider one of the partial breast irradiation (PBI) studies, which will allow them to be treated in a few days.

The availability of one kind of treatment or another is also a factor. In some areas radiation is not offered. In others, it is available but is not especially good: a radiation oncologist has to know the technique to get good results. For some women, however, their breasts are an integral part of their sexuality and identity and they are willing (and able) to go to great inconvenience to save them. One of my patients lived in a small town in the Central Valley of California, too far to commute to my breast center in Los Angeles. So she and her husband drove down in their van and lived in the hospital parking lot for six weeks until her treatment was completed. I've had patients whose cancer recurred after lumpectomy and radiation, and even though they finally had a mastectomy, they were grateful for an extra few years with both breasts.

Regardless of the medical facts, however, you need to feel safe with your choice. Some of my patients who had lumpectomy and radiation would wake up every morning sure that the cancer had come back. They probably would have been better off with mastectomies in the first place.

Remember above all that it's your body and no one else's. Don't decide on the basis of what anyone else thinks is best. By all means talk to your friends and your family and your husband or lover, and think about what they say. But make your own decision. Husbands and lovers come and go, but your body is with you all your life. A truly caring mate will support whatever course you think is best for you.

The next issue that may come up in the decision-making time is whether to have a *prophylactic mastectomy* on the other breast at the same time. This is not usually necessary or even contemplated unless the woman is a carrier of the BRCA 1 or BRCA 2 gene, and even then it's certainly not mandatory (see Chapter 9). Women with a new diagnosis of breast cancer and a family history suggestive of a BRCA 1 or 2 mutation could choose to have a lumpectomy and lymph node surgery, then undergo testing and have chemotherapy while waiting for the test result (it can take 3–8 weeks). If the test is positive they can, if they wish, undergo bilateral mastectomy with or without reconstruction following the completion of chemotherapy. If the test is negative they can go on to radiation following chemotherapy. Remember, there is no urgency over prophylactic mastectomy and you may want to get the cancer therapy taken care of first; then, when the timing is convenient, if you still want it, you can have your breasts removed.

The risk to the other breast in nonmutation carriers averages about 0.8 percent per year and an estimated 2–11 percent over a woman's lifetime.[42,43] A recent nonrandomized study compared 1,072 women who had undergone prophylactic mastectomy to 317 who had not. After 5.7 years of follow-up, 2.7 percent of women who had not had the preventative surgery developed a second cancer, compared to 0.5 percent of the women who had it.[44] This suggests a benefit from the surgery; however, prophylactic contralateral mastectomies did not affect the 10.5 percent of women who developed metastatic disease or the 8.1 percent who died. And the current use of hormone therapy in most women with hormone sensitive tumors has the added benefit of reducing the risk of cancer in both breasts by at least 50 percent. It is important to be realistic about the risks and benefits in your own case before jumping to extra surgery in an effort to do "everything possible."

Some plastic surgeons encourage removing both breasts at once because breast reconstruction surgery is easier when they don't have to match an existing breast. While this is worth considering, I don't think it should be the main factor in making the decision, unless you're a Playboy model.

Finally, neither reconstruction nor prophylactic mastectomy must be done immediately. Sometimes all the decisions you have to make are overwhelming and it helps to leave a few for later. A woman I was counseling recently had dirty margins and a positive sentinel node. She needed a mastectomy and axillary dissection on her right breast and was agonizing on whether she should have a prophylactic mastectomy and immediate reconstruction at the same time. Once she realized that she did not have to make that decision right away, she was quite relieved. She decided to go ahead with the mastectomy and axillary dissection and then chemotherapy, while getting genetic testing (she had a family history of breast cancer) to find out what the risk really was to the second breast. After her systemic therapy was over, she would consider prophylactic mastectomy on the other side and research the best type of reconstruction for her.

18

Treatment Options: Systemic Therapy

After you decide about local treatment, you will need to decide about systemic therapy. (The usual order of practice is surgery followed by chemotherapy, then radiation therapy, and finally hormone therapy if indicated.) Systemic means something that creates its effect by circulating throughout your body, unlike local treatments, which are applied just to the area in question. Systemic treatments include chemotherapy (drugs that selectively kill cancer cells and are known as *cytotoxic* drugs), hormone therapies (treatments that are hormones or affect your body's hormones), and targeted therapies (antibodies directed to block specific enzymes or oncogenes). They can also include alternative and complementary therapies (see Chapter 25). Drugs given at the time of diagnosis when there is no known metastatic disease are called *adjuvant treatment.* The same drugs are just called "treatment" when metastatic disease is clearly present. In this chapter we will consider the decision-making aspects of these therapies.

CHEMOTHERAPY

Chemotherapy was originally intended for metastatic cancer only, based on the theory that drugs circulating through the bloodstream could get to all the places a cancer cell was likely to hide. Unfortunately it didn't always work. In time, researchers came to understand that the failure stemmed from two problems: once a cancer became metastatic there were too many cancer cells for the drugs to handle, and some cancer cells became resistant to the drugs. They began to consider giving chemotherapy earlier and earlier when there were fewer cells to treat, and the concept of adjuvant chemotherapy was born. Perhaps the time to give chemotherapy was right after the primary local treatment—either surgery alone or surgery and radiation—when any spread would still be microscopic. And indeed this approach seemed to work. The first studies by Gianni Bonadonna[1] and by the NSABP (National Surgical Breast and Bowel Project) showed that premenopausal women with positive nodes had a significant decrease in breast cancer mortality when given adjuvant chemotherapy.[2] This set the stage for the now common practice of using systemic treatments at the time of initial diagnosis. Today we give adjuvant systemic therapy to all premenopausal women with positive nodes, many with negative nodes, and many postmenopausal women.

What Is the Benefit of Chemotherapy? The Numbers

When you are considering whether to have chemotherapy, it is important to understand what its benefits are. As I explained in Chapter 15, you want to understand not only the benefits of a particular therapy but also the end point being measured.

Chemotherapy reduces the risk of recurrence by about a third.[3] That means that the higher the chance of recurrence, the more beneficial the chemotherapy is likely to be for you. If you have a 60 percent chance of recurrence, a one-third risk reduction means chemo will reduce that chance by 20 percent, but if you have a 9 percent chance of recurrence the one-third reduction is only 3 percent. This is an important concept to understand when trying to weigh risks and benefits. In Chapter 15, I noted that it is always better to look at the absolute benefit of chemotherapy. This can be estimated in Table 18-1.[4] In other words, if your chance of dying by 10 years were 50 percent and you had a treatment that reduced the risk of mortality by 40 percent, your absolute risk at ten years would be 16 percent. And of course you also need to take your age into consideration (see Table 18-2).[5]

Since the mid-1980s the Early Breast Cancer Trialists' Collaborative Group (EBCTCG) has met every five years to perform a systematic review of all randomized clinical trials (published and unpublished) performed in early breast cancer. The 2000 analysis was published in 2004 and included 102 clinical trials that addressed adjuvant chemotherapy questions.[6] Researchers found that multiple drugs were better than just

Table 18-1. Absolute Reduction in Mortality at 10 Years per 100 Women Treated

	Hypothetical Proportional Reduction in Mortality Due to Treatment				
Estimated 10-yr Death Rate with No Therapy	50%	40%	30%	20%	10%
70% (several positive nodes)	25	19	13	8	4
50% (5 cm tumor, neg nodes)	21	16	12	7	4
30% (avg tumor diameter, neg nodes)	14	11	8	5	3
10% (< 1 cm tumor, neg nodes)	5	4	3	2	1

Source: Osborne C.K., "Adjuvant endocrine therapy," Chapter 53 in Harris J.R., Lippman M.E., Morrow M., Osborne C.K., eds. *Diseases of the Breast,* 3rd ed. Philadelphia: J.B. Lippincott, Williams & Wilkins, 2004, p.868.

Table 18-2. Survival Estimates at 10 Years by Age and Risk of Breast Cancer Death, With and Without Adjuvant Therapy

		Alive at 10 yr		
Hypothetical risk of breast cancer*	*Natural mortality without breast cancer, next 10 yr (%)*	*No adjuvant therapy*	*Adjuvant therapy†*	*Absolute benefit*
40 year old				
10% (low risk)	2	88	90	2
28% (intermediate risk)	2	71	77	6
57% (high risk)	2	41	51	10
65 year old				
9% (low risk)	19	73	75	2
26% (intermediate risk)	19	58	63	5
54% (high risk)	19	34	43	9

*Values shown are derived from three different risk estimates and assume exponential death with a constant hazard ratio. The differences between 40 and 65 years of age reflect deaths from other causes.

†Based on a 25% annual reduction in the odds of death, a reasonable estimate of the benefits of chemotherapy in premenopausal patients and tamoxifen in an estrogen receptor-positive postmenopausal patient.

Source: Osborne C.K., Ravdin P.M. Adjuvant systemic therapy of primary breast cancer. In Harris J.R., Lippman M.E., Morrow M., Osborne C.K., eds. *Diseases of the Breast,* 2nd ed. Philadelphia: J. B. Lippincott, Williams & Wilkins, 2000, p. 625.

one and that combinations containing an *anthracycline* (doxorubicin or epirubicin) did better than those that did not. In general, chemotherapy had a greater effect in younger women than older ones. In women younger than 50, polychemotherapy (more than one drug at a time) was associated with a 12 percent reduction in the absolute risk of recurrence at 15 years and a 10 percent decrease in breast cancer mortality compared with no chemotherapy. The 15-year results were more modest in women between 50 and 59 (4.1 percent and 3 percent reduction in breast cancer recurrence and mortality respectively). Obviously there is not a strict cutoff at 50; rather, it's a gradual diminution in benefit. So women between 50 and 55 do better than women between 55 and 60. Premenopausal women may get some of their benefit from chemotherapy by being put into premature menopause, while this effect will not occur among postmenopausal women. In premenopausal women the benefits are about the same regardless of the hormone receptor, but in postmenopausal women chemotherapy decreases the chance of recurrence by 33 percent in estrogen receptor negative women and only 16 percent in estrogen receptor positive women. (Remember that chance of recurrence is not the same as absolute reduction.) Another way to further break down the benefits to women with negative nodes is to look at whether you are at low, medium, or high risk of recurrence. This is determined by all of the biomarkers discussed in Chapter 16. (See Table 18-2.)

The table shows hypothetical breast cancer risks of death for pre- and postmenopausal women. Taking into consideration the other causes of death, we see the 10-year benefit on mortality for adjuvant chemotherapy in the premenopausal women and tamoxifen in the estrogen receptor positive postmenopausal women. Though the table is dated, having been created before we had the current data on the aromatase inhibitors discussed later in this chapter, it is still not far off.

Not all oncologists are current with this way of looking at the figures, and there is a bit of wishful thinking in their approach to chemotherapy. They want it to work and so they start believing it works better than it does. In a 1994 study by S. Rajagopal, oncologists were given certain scenarios and asked whether or not they'd give chemotherapy in each scenario.[7] Then they were asked what percentage of improvement in survival they thought the patient would have. Overall, they estimated a three times greater improvement than was warranted. Thus you need to pin your oncologist down so that you are realistic about the benefits of chemotherapy in your case. If your oncologist is not sure of the absolute benefits, you can suggest she or he go to Adjuvantonline.com or the Mayo Clinic website, where there are tools that can calculate the numbers for you.

Chemotherapy does not guarantee that your cancer will be cured. It just improves the odds a bit. A few years ago a 68-year-old woman with an estrogen receptor negative tumor called me for advice. Her oncologist thought she should be on chemotherapy because her chance of dying in the next five years was 15 percent without it. So she thought she might try it. I asked if the doctor had told her what her chance of dying in the next five years was even if she did take chemo. He hadn't. "I assume it means I have a 100 percent chance of surviving the next five years," she said. I told her that wasn't accurate: her chance of dying from breast cancer, with chemo, was 13 percent. She paused. "Then forget that!" she said finally. "I don't want to go through that for a 2 percent better chance!" However, studies have shown that some women will choose chemotherapy even for a 1 percent improvement in survival. What matters is that each woman has accurate knowledge to work with.

Types of Chemotherapy

If a woman clearly should get chemotherapy, the issue arises of what drugs she should get. The first successful combination was CMF—cyclophosamide (C), methotrexate (M), 5-flourouracil (F). The most recent overview, by the Early Breast Trialists' Collaborative Group, showed a benefit to a combination that included an anthracycline over one that did not.[8] The anthracycline doxorubicin (A) is commonly used in the United States, while epirubicin (E) is used more in Europe. These drugs are often given in combination as FAC or FEC or AC. More recently studies have shown that adding a taxane (T) (paclitaxel or doxcetaxel) after the anthracycline regimen provides additional benefit.

Drug dosage is also an issue. Investigators looked at the dose being received over a period of time. Dose intensity refers to increasing the total dose over a set period of time, while dose density is the administration of a higher dose per unit time. While studies have shown that dose intensity is important, they have indicated that individual agents have a threshold dose that must be achieved. Dose reduction below that threshold appears to be associated with poorer outcome, but dose escalation beyond the threshold increases the danger to the patient while contributing no added benefit. High-dose chemotherapy with stem cell rescue is a good example of this. Commonly and incorrectly called bone marrow transplant, this was an attempt to improve the benefit to women at high risk of recurrence. Women were given such high doses of chemotherapy that their bone marrow was wiped out and they needed stem cells to reconstitute it. Multiple randomized studies showed it to be more toxic but no better than standard regimens.[9,10]

Because high dose was not better, researchers started to look at the schedule the drugs were given on. The standard program has been to give three different drugs with three different mechanisms of action simultaneously. This works but is limited somewhat by the toxicities of one drug, cutting back the maximum dose that can be given of another drug. In the dose dense model, the interval between two courses is shortened, while the dose of each course may be increased, decreased, or made equivalent to a standard dose so that the dose per unit of time is higher. A recent study looked at giving the drugs in sequence rather than at the same time and found that they were equivalent in their medical effect and that the sequential doses were less toxic.[11] In the same study, a dose dense regimen was tried in which the drugs were given every two weeks instead of every three. Preliminary results showed that after three years there was a 4 percent improvement in disease-free survival and a 2 percent improvement in survival compared to the three-week version. This schedule of chemotherapy, however, required that women receive GCSF (granulocyte stimulating factor), a drug that stimulates the bone marrow to recover faster from the chemotherapy. The treatments can be more difficult to take because there is little down time, but they end sooner.

Since there are choices to be made among different chemotherapy drugs, it's especially important for the patient to enter into the decision-making process. Ask why your doctor has chosen a particular treatment regimen and ask to see studies that back it up. Find out exactly what the differences are in efficacy and side effects. For example, as I explain later in this chapter, some drugs are more likely to put you into menopause and thus render you infertile than others (see Chapter 24). Some, like doxorubicin (Adriamycin), can be more toxic to the heart. So you may prefer to stick with the CMF or you may be willing to take a slightly higher risk, hoping that the stronger drug will be better. If you don't feel you are getting straight answers from your oncologist, get a second opinion. If a clinical trial is available, consider participating in it so that we will get some answers (see Chapter 15). You can get accurate numbers for your own case in a number of ways. There are two programs available to oncologists (Adjuvant! at www.adjuvantsite.com or Numeracy at www.mayoclinic.com/calcs from the Mayo Clinic) and one for patients from Nexcura (this can be found on the homepage of my website www.drsusanloveresearchfoundation.org under Decision Tools) that can calculate more precise numbers for you. Ask your oncologist to provide you with the data from the Adjuvant! and Mayo Clinic sites. You are smart enough to take control of this decision.

Timing

Classically, chemotherapy treatments follow local treatments. But another course is now being aggressively studied—*neoadjuvant* (or *pre-*

operative) chemotherapy. This means giving the chemotherapy before surgery, after making the diagnosis with a core or needle biopsy. Because chemotherapy is the most important treatment, dealing with the life-threatening element of the cancer, some of us thought that giving it first might make a difference in survival. Unfortunately none of the studies have shown this to be true. However, we have found two other advantages. First, we can see whether or not the chemo works. If the tumor starts melting away, we know the chemo is working. If it's not working, we can turn to a different chemotherapy. The NSABP study found an 80 percent reduction in the tumor size, and in 36 percent of women the tumor completely disappeared.[12] This allowed doctors to do lumpectomies in 8 percent of women who would otherwise have needed mastectomies (67.8 percent versus 59.8 percent). There's no question now that in tumors over 3 centimeters, most surgeons will do preoperative chemotherapy. In smaller tumors, which would allow a lumpectomy anyway, many surgeons do chemotherapy after the surgery, although there is no reason that neoadjuvant chemotherapy can't be used in this setting as well.

If your tumor doesn't seem to shrink with neoadjuvant chemotherapy, there's no cause for panic. It may still be helping you. As I was writing this chapter, a group of breast specialists at M.D. Anderson Cancer Center who have been doing studies on neoadjuvant chemotherapy for many years made a startling announcement. Looking at the response to chemotherapy according to the type of cancer, they had found that women with lobular cancer (see Chapter 12) were less likely than women with ductal cancer to respond to chemotherapy with tumor shrinkage, though maintaining a better prognosis than women with ductal cancer.[13] Upfront systemic therapy has the potential to teach us many lessons about the behavior of cancer in real life, as opposed to animal models or Petri dishes.

Neoadjuvant therapy is also being used to evaluate the potential of certain drugs for chemoprevention. They are given for a month or so prior to a mastectomy and markers of malignancy are monitored in the tumor. If these markers are reduced, the drug may have the ability to prevent cancers from developing.

Chemosensitivity

A long-standing theory suggests that we could pick chemotherapy the way we pick antibiotics—through sensitivity testing. With antibiotics, the doctors grow the bacteria from your infection in a petri dish that has spots of different antibiotics all over it and then look to see which spots the bacteria grow on and which they die on. Then the doctor can say, "This patient's infection is sensitive to this antibiotic, but not that one, so we'll prescribe this one." This is known as *in vitro drug sensitivity testing* (in vitro means literally "in glass" and refers to any experiment done outside the body).

There have been many laboratory experiments in sensitivity testing for chemotherapy; the problem is that it's never been clear how well it translates to patients. What works in a petri dish doesn't necessarily work in a living body. A 1999 review of 12 prospective studies looked at this in breast cancer.[14] There were 506 patients, 33 percent treated with chemotherapy that had been selected using in vitro techniques. The response rate was a little better—27 percent for the drugs chosen in vitro versus 18 percent chosen by other means. Researchers found no difference in survival rates. Future studies may show a survival rate improvement, but for now we have no certainty of it. It may have a bigger benefit in primary disease than in metastatic disease.

HORMONE THERAPY

Doctors have always been interested in the hormonal manipulation of breast cancers. In fact, the first adjuvant therapies were based on changing the body's hormonal milieu. If a premenopausal woman had a "bad" cancer, her ovaries were removed in an attempt to decrease the total amount of estrogen in her system. The idea was good, and recent studies show a difference in the survival of women who had oophorectomy compared to the control group, which equals that for chemotherapy.[15]

Now we can actually predict who is likely to benefit from adjuvant hormone therapy by using the estrogen and progesterone receptor test mentioned in Chapter 16. In women with hormone-sensitive tumors, we can use a hormone treatment as adjuvant therapy. In women whose tumors are not sensitive to either estrogen or progesterone, hormone therapies are useless and potentially harmful. DNA microarray studies (see Chapter 16) indicate that estrogen receptor negative cancer is a different kind than cancer sensitive to estrogen. This is the first step to individualized therapy.

In addition, we are starting to understand how these hormone therapies work. What they probably do, at least in part, is change the environment around the cell, resulting in control or even death of the cancer cell. (See Chapter 10.) This can happen in a number of different ways. Currently we have two different adjuvant hormone approaches: reducing the production of estrogen or blocking the estrogen receptor on the cell.

Tamoxifen

Tamoxifen has been the mainstay of hormone therapy for breast cancer for many years. It works by blocking the estrogen receptor in the breast and in the metastatic cancer cells, preventing estrogen from getting to them. This is why it has an effect in both pre- and postmenopausal women. Regardless of the source of estrogen circulating in the blood, tamoxifen can block it. One sometimes hears the simplistic notion that tamoxifen throws premenopausal women into menopause. Actually, it's more complicated than that. It stimulates the ovaries to make more estrogen. While blocking estrogen receptors in the breast, it is acting *like* estrogen in other organs, such as the bone and uterus. (See SERMs, Chapter 11.) This trait is responsible for both its side effects, such as uterine cancer and blood clots, and its benefits, such as increased bone density and lower cholesterol.

We initially believed that tamoxifen didn't kill cells the way chemo did—it just blocked them and held them at bay. We thought that if you took tamoxifen for a period of time and then stopped, all those cancer cells that were asleep would start growing again. But follow-up on women who took tamoxifen for five years and then stopped has shown that the benefit persists long after the drug has been stopped. Even taking it for just a year gave benefits that lasted for at least 21 years in one study.[16] The longer a woman takes it, for a period of up to five years, the greater the benefit. Whether it kills some cancer cells, affects the stromal environment they live in, or just puts them to sleep is not clear. What *is* clear is that the effect persists long after a woman stops taking it. Despite this a lot of women don't want to stop taking tamoxifen: it's their lifeline and they feel that losing it will kill them. But that's simply not true.

In fact, taking it longer may harm them. In the past few years, we've discovered that when tamoxifen is used for too many years, the cells can become resistant to it; sometimes it even starts feeding the tumor. The NSABP did a study (B-14) randomizing women who took tamoxifen for five years to either continue taking it or stop.[17] They discovered that after ten years the women still taking tamoxifen did slightly worse.[18] This was quite controversial when it first came out in 2001, and two European studies are addressing this issue. The current recommendation is that women who are prescribed tamoxifen as part of their initial treatment should take it for only five years.

This was a source of consternation for many women until the recent introduction of aromatase inhibitors (see later in this chapter). Now armed with data suggesting the benefit of new drugs following three, four, or even five years of tamoxifen, the question of long-term tamoxifen use is less relevant.

The 2004 overview of treatment for early breast cancer found that in estrogen receptor negative tumors, tamoxifen had no benefit.[19] But in estrogen receptor positive tumors, it had a benefit across the board. The reduction in the yearly rate of recurrence is 40–50 percent, and the reduction in the annual chance of death is 30 percent. This means that while people are on tamoxifen, one of every two recurrences and approximately one of every three deaths are avoided. Looking at absolute reductions, we find an 11 percent decrease in recurrence and a 6.8 percent reduction in death at 10 years for premenopausal women who have taken tamoxifen for five years. For postmenopausal women it is 15 percent decrease in recurrence and 8.2 percent reduction in death at 10 years. As I pointed out earlier in the chapter, the absolute benefit depends in part on the risk. A way to look at that is to consider the difference between women whose nodes are positive and those whose nodes are negative. In node-negative women it is 12 percent reduction in recurrence and 5 percent reduction in death while in node-positive women it is 15 percent reduction in recurrence and 12.3 percent reduction in death after ten years. As usual, the higher the risk the higher the benefit. In case you are wondering why these data are only being reported for tamoxifen, remember they come from a compilation of all the previous studies. We just don't have enough data yet on the aromatase inhibitors to yield these types of statistics.

When I lecture, women will often come to me and say they're taking tamoxifen but having terrible side effects. I suggest they check with their oncologist about why they're taking it and whether one of the other hormone therapies described below may be an alternative for them. The tendency now is for oncologists to put every estrogen receptor–positive premenopausal woman and half of the estrogen receptor–positive postmenopausal women (the rest are starting directly on the aromatase inhibitors) on it because it benefits everyone. But it benefits by different amounts, and if you're in a category in which the benefit is only 1–2 percent and it's making your life miserable, you probably won't want to stay with it. On the other hand, if you're in the 11 percent category, the suffering may be worth that chance. So it's important to ask your oncologist what benefit tamoxifen will offer you, given your specific breast cancer scenario and what benefit something else may have. (Again, you can have your doctor check the websites such as Adjuvant! Or you can check the decision tools on my website www.drsusanloveresearchfoundation.org to get some exact numbers.)

Tamoxifen is the best studied drug for women whose tumors are sensitive to hormones. The question is whether it is the best *working* drug. The past five years have seen several reports on various drugs or combinations of hormone drugs that may improve the odds even further. As we review these, however, it is important to remember how long it has taken doctors to fully understand tamoxifen and not switch to something new just because it *is* new.

Ovarian Ablation

Blocking the estrogen receptor is one way to deprive the breast cancer cell of estrogen; another is to stop the source of the hormones. In premenopausal women this is the ovary. There are three ways to do this: surgery, radiation, or hormonal manipulation—this is known as *ablating* the ovaries. But unless you are a carrier of the BRCA 1 or 2 gene and therefore at higher risk of subsequent ovarian cancer, surgery probably is not the best way of doing this. The surgery is irreversible: if it doesn't work, we can't return your ovaries to you. So you're stuck with all the consequences of having no ovaries (see Chapter 24).

Sometimes doctors can irradiate ovaries instead of removing them, saving the patient the pain of surgery. The problem here is that it's hard to aim precisely at these small organs, and intestines in the area can also get radiated, causing possible problems. Further, like surgery, it's permanent.

Today we can use gonadotropin-releasing hormone agonists (GnRH), originally developed for endometriosis, that block the ovaries and essentially put you into a temporary menopause. This approach seems to work as well as surgery or radiation and has the advantage of being reversible.

The most thoroughly tested drug for doing this in breast cancer is goserelin (also known as Zoladex). In a 1998 study, women were put on goserelin for three to five years to see if it had the same effect as oophorectomy, and it did.[20] In the study, premenopausal node-positive women were randomized to take CMF chemotherapy or goserelin for two years. With 7.3 years of follow-up there has been no difference between the two groups. Most interesting to me was the fact that most of the women on goserelin got their periods back after the therapy was completed and yet did just as well as the women on CMF, who permanently stopped menstruating. In other words, just as with tamoxifen, a short time (2–3 years) of decreased estrogen production was enough to change these women's prognosis. On the other hand, the estrogen positive women who did not become menopausal on CMF did significantly worse than those who stopped menstruating.[21] Obviously part of the benefit of the chemotherapy was that it put these women into menopause. Further studies have shown that adding tamoxifen to the goserelin is even more effective.[22]

Now researchers are asking what would happen if we added ovarian ablation to chemotherapy—would it be improved? Although there are several studies looking at ovarian suppression or ablation after chemotherapy, the results are complicated by the fact that 40–60 percent of women become postmenopausal from the chemotherapy and would not be expected to benefit further from ovarian suppression. One study compared six cycles of CAF alone to CAF with goserelin or CAF plus goserelin and tamoxifen. After nine years there was an improvement in women who received CAF and tamoxifen compared to CAF plus goserelin. However, other groups showed no difference. In a later analysis the investigators suggested that women younger than 40, who were still premenopausal at the end of CAF or had temporarily stopped menstruating but still had a premenopausal estradiol level after CAF, were most likely to benefit from the addition of ovarian suppression to the chemotherapy. The benefit from tamoxifen was most apparent in women who were 40 or older, in those with postmenopausal estradiol levels after CAF, or in those whose periods stopped after CAF.[23] This feeds my bias that ovarian suppression has value in women who are still menstruating after completing chemotherapy and are estrogen receptor positive. Tamoxifen is a good alternative in these women as well. Women who stop their periods can consider the aromatase inhibitors if hormone therapy is indicated.

Aromatase Inhibitors

Removing the ovaries or blocking them with drugs has no effect on women who are already postmenopausal: their main source of estrogen is no longer their ovaries. Instead, the precursors of estrogen, such as testosterone and androstenedione, are produced in the ovaries and adrenal glands and then secreted into the blood stream, where specific organs pick them up and convert them into estrogen through an enzyme called aromatase. This enzyme has been found in the adrenal glands, fat, breast, brain, and muscles, and is responsible for much of the estrogen in postmenopausal women. (Other enzymes such as sulfatase may also be important in this regard.) In addition, recent studies show that postmenopausal women with breast cancer have aromatase in their breast tissue, giving the breast its own supply of estrogen.[24] So, to reduce estrogen levels in the tissues of postmenopausal women we need to block aromatase. A new class of drugs called aromatase inhibitors can do this with minimal side effects.

Three drugs that block aromatase are available clinically. Anastrozole (Arimidex) and letrozole (Femara) work by reversibly blocking this enzyme, while exemestane (Aromasin) binds to the enzyme and inactivates it permanently. These drugs were first tested in women with estrogen positive metastatic disease. All of them had favorable effects (see Chapter 27). The next step was to see whether they were better than tamoxifen in newly diagnosed estrogen positive postmenopausal women. The first trial to be reported was the ATAC study, which compared tamoxifen and anastrozole head-to-head. The study has randomized women, giving one group anastrozole and the other tamoxifen for five years. Another group was given both drugs. After a median follow-up of 68 months, anastrozole was shown to improve disease-free survival by 17 percent, with an absolute improvement of 3.3 percent (575 events vs. 651). Time to recurrence was reduced 26 percent (absolute 3.7 percent) and cancer in the other breast by 42 percent (35 vs. 59). As expected, the effect was only in women with estrogen receptor positive cancer. Overall survival has so far shown no difference between the two drugs, but this is not at all conclusive. The study has not lasted long enough to show such a difference. Still, more and more doctors are favoring anastrozole.[25] It blocks estrogen production and so has fewer effects on the uterine lining than does tamoxifen, but it decreases bone density and increases fractures as well as muscular and joint pain. Other questions about its effects on brain function are still being researched. Interestingly, the women who took both tamoxifen and anastrozole did no better than the women who just took tamoxifen. One theory is that tamoxifen acts more like estrogen when total body levels are low.

The other approach to aromatase inhibitors has been to see whether switching women to them after several years of tamoxifen will give a significant advantage. In the first study reported, postmenopausal women who were completing five years of tamoxifen were randomized to take letrozole or nothing further.[26] Although the study was originally intended to go on for five years, the first analysis of data showed a significant benefit for the women taking the letrozole and the drug company sponsoring the study elected to stop it prematurely. The rate of death due to breast cancer was almost halved. However, the overall survival at two years was 98.9 percent in the group that took letrozole versus 98.6 percent in the group that did not. Because the study was stopped early, the investigators estimated what the benefit might have been if there had been a continuing improvement and if everyone had taken the drug for five years. In that hypothetical setting, the absolute difference between the two groups would have been 2.4 percent for survival and 6 percent for disease-free recurrence. So we know there is only a slight benefit, but we do not know what the risks of taking this drug for five years would be.

A second study looked at exemestane after two to three years of tamoxifen.[27] This showed an absolute benefit in disease-free survival of 4.7 percent at three years. Overall survival was not significantly different between the two groups. (As you will remember from Chapter 15, we can see a difference in disease-free survival but none in overall survival if the women in the control group have a recurrence of disease but have not died yet or if the treatment reduces breast cancer but causes other kinds of deaths, thus evening it out. That said, a decrease in disease-free survival will usually appear as a difference in overall survival if the study goes on long enough.) As in the letrozole study, there was a decrease in new cancers in the other breast as well as in recurrence.

Finally, data were reported at the 2004 San Antonio Breast Cancer Symposium on two studies looking at anastrozole after two years of tamoxifen.[28] The combined data showed that after a mean follow-up of 26 months there was a 3.1 percent absolute difference in all breast cancer events (distant recurrence, local recurrence, or contralateral breast cancer). As in other studies, this showed an increase in fractures (2.1 percent vs. 1.2 percent) in the women on anastrozole compared to tamoxifen. These data suggest that taking an aromatase inhibitor after tamoxifen may help postmenopausal women who are at high risk of recurrence. Now the question is whether tamoxifen for 2–3 years followed by an aromatase inhibitor is better than an aromatase inhibitor alone. In addition, many clinicians are adding *bisphosphonates* (drugs that reduce postmenopausal bone loss) to the aromatase inhibitor, although this approach is still being studied. Clearly tamoxifen is no longer the only option for adjuvant hormone therapy. Many studies designed to answer all our questions regarding the appropriate clinical guidelines for use of all these new drugs will be forthcoming over the next several years. Meanwhile, the American Society of Clinical Oncology suggests in its most recent clinical guidelines that the optimal therapy for a postmenopausal woman with estrogen receptor positive cancer is to take an aromatase inhibitor either right away or after tamoxifen.[29]

As yet we do not have data on the safety of aromatase inhibitors in women rendered postmenopausal with chemotherapy and probably should not use them without further ovarian suppression, since many of these women still have significant estrogen levels. It is also not clear that the results would be the same in women with menopause induced by GnRH agonists like goserelin, although this is actively being studied.

TARGETED THERAPIES

In addition to the efforts to destroy cancer cells or change their hormonal milieu, there is a new form of drug designed to attack a target on the cancer cell in hopes of reducing its malignant potential.

Trastuzumab (Herceptin)

Trastuzumab is the first drug of this category in clinical use. It is the antibody to the Her-2/neu oncogene, which is overexpressed in 30 percent of women with breast cancer. At the time of this writing, it has been tested in women with metastatic disease and shown to have a beneficial effect, both alone and with chemotherapy.[30,31]

As I was in the final drafts of this book two phase 3 studies of trastuzumab (Herceptin) as an adjuvant to chemotherapy in early stage breast cancer announced their interim data.[32] The exciting news was that the combination resulted in a 52 percent decrease in disease recurrence compared to patients treated with chemotherapy alone. Most of the women in the studies had positive nodes and received AC followed by T as well as the targeted therapy. There was a 3–4 percent increase in the incidence of heart failure, however. Nonetheless, this is the first time that a targeted therapy has been shown to affect early breast cancer. It certainly will cause the guidelines to change and suggests that women with positive nodes and Her-2/neu overexpressing breast cancer consider adding trastuzumab to their regimen.

Guidelines and Choices

Should you always choose chemotherapy? If you're premenopausal, with positive lymph nodes and/or a tumor larger than 1 centimeter, I think you should. If you're postmenopausal and hormone receptor negative, maybe. In this case, it will decrease your risk of dying from breast cancer by about 10 percent. That means if your risk of dying is 30 percent, your maximum benefit will be 3 percent. Overall, for postmenopausal women, the improvement rate is 2–3 percent over five years and 4–6 percent over ten years. For most women, many issues enter into this kind of decision. One is quality of life. If you're 80, for example, and have positive nodes, which means the cancer may come back in the next ten years, you may decide it's worth the gamble not to do chemotherapy; or you may decide that any chance of extra time to live is worth it. If you're relatively young and have another life-threatening condition that could be exacerbated by the chemotherapy, such as a heart condition or severe kidney disease, maybe you won't feel the risk is worth it. On the other hand, you may be 50 and just postmenopausal and feel that even a 1 percent chance is worth it to you. Many women who undergo only surgery or surgery and radiation will of course be cured, even with positive nodes, but the benefits of chemotherapy in node-positive women over 10 to 15 years is substantial. Your values and beliefs will play a large part in your decision.

For tumors that are sensitive to hormones, tamoxifen is now used as an adjuvant treatment in premenopausal women with positive nodes or poor prognostic indicators and with negative nodes and continuing menstruation. Estrogen receptor positive women who are still menstruating after chemotherapy may also consider goserelin with or without an aromatase inhibitor. Hormone receptor positive postmenopausal women will probably be offered an aromatase inhibitor, with tamoxifen moving into the second choice position. Decisions about chemotherapy are confusing for women with positive nodes, and even more so for women with negative nodes. We know that between 30 and 40 percent of women with negative lymph nodes will still get metastatic breast cancer and sooner or later die of it (Fig. 18-1). If we give these women chemotherapy for their primary cancer, some of them will have a delay in recurrence and improvement in survival. But 60–70 percent of women with negative lymph nodes won't ever have a recurrence, and if we give them chemotherapy we subject them to an unpleasant process that can occasionally have severe and permanent side effects—including, very rarely, leukemia. The side effects are worth it for women whose alternative is to die sooner of breast cancer: it doesn't much matter that you'd get leukemia at 60 if your breast cancer kills you at 40. But when there's a 60–70 percent chance that your cancer didn't metastasize, should we expose you to the side effects of chemotherapy? Unfortunately we do not yet know how to tell these two groups of women apart. But for women with higher risk node-negative disease, the answer is generally yes. A 40 percent risk of dying of breast cancer is too high, and many women will want to do what they can to decrease it.

Some oncologists suggest women get chemotherapy as "insurance." This doesn't mean it will ensure your survival, but the analogy is good. If you were one of the women who would have been cured by surgery and radiation alone, the chemotherapy would not be a good investment—sort of like buying earthquake insurance when you live in New Jersey. On the other hand, if you have a higher chance of recurrence, the investment may well prove worthwhile—as those of us in Los Angeles have learned with our quakes.

The uncertainty is the reason we put so much time and energy into the new DNA-based tests, which we hope will better enable us to distinguish between those with the more deadly kind of cancer and those with the less destructive kind. The Oncotype Dx test from Genomic Health that I mentioned in Chapter 16 is the first example of this and will help decide which hormone-positive node-negative women really need chemotherapy and which will do fine with hormones. We are currently treating all breast cancer as if it were one of two types—sensitive to hormones or not. But there probably are several different

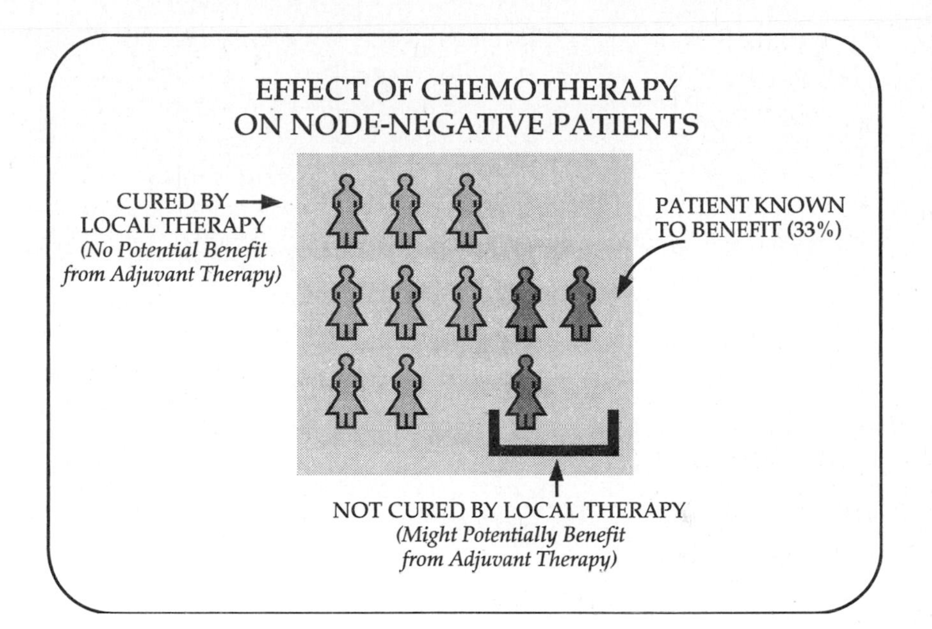

FIGURE 18-1

kinds of breast cancer, and matching the treatment to the type of breast cancer may make a significant difference. My hope is that by the next edition of this book we will be there, but for now we are still struggling with the best choice for the most women. We are left guessing on the basis of probabilities that are not individualized. This usually means that we overtreat, fearing that we may miss someone who could benefit. And you are left with decisions that may feel like a gamble.

All this means that deciding whether or not to have systemic treatment, and if so which treatment, is complicated. You may want to look at the practice guidelines from the NCCN on line at www.NCCN.org to give you a guideline.

Based on risk/benefit estimates, chemotherapy is often considered for otherwise healthy women with node-positive disease of any size or node-negative disease with tumor size greater than 2 centimeters. Women with specific types of breast cancer (see Chapter 19) such as tubular and mucinous carcinoma up to 3 centimeters in size have an excellent prognosis, and adjuvant chemotherapy may not provide additional benefit. The real controversies come in women with stage 1 breast cancer. Up to 20 percent of these women may suffer a recurrence of their cancer, and prognostic factors are used to figure out who they are. In one recent large data set, women with tumors that were stage 1 grade 1 and estrogen or progesterone positive had a five-year survival rate similar to that of age-matched women without breast cancer.[33] Another study included women with tumors less than 1 centimeter or grade 1 tumors less than 2 centimeters and found that these women probably receive little benefit from chemotherapy.[34] Unfortunately we don't know how to add all the factors together, and you still end up making a guess based on the information we have.

So there's no perfect formula, at least so far. I had one patient back in Boston who had a small tumor, negative nodes, and negative biomarkers. But she wanted chemo. Her oncologist and I both argued with her. She was adamant and got chemotherapy. One year later the cancer metastasized and she died. By all statistical predictions she should have survived, even without the chemo, and the chemo should have guaranteed her survival. This isn't meant to depress you: it often works the other way. I had a patient who was diagnosed with 17 positive nodes and had conventional chemotherapy; when I last checked with her 13 years later, she was alive and well and living in Maui. It just illustrates that we have only odds, no certainty; to some extent, it's a crap shoot. You have to just search your heart and make your own choice.

Finally, complementary treatments (the subject of Chapter 25) are actually a form of systemic treatment.

SECOND OPINIONS

Before you decide on which treatment, or treatments, you want, I think it's always wise to consider getting a second opinion, no matter how much you trust your surgeon or oncologist's advice. The preference for a treatment is always somewhat subjective, and you're entitled to consult with more than one expert. Furthermore, special kinds of cancer may require a different approach than your doctor's, and different institutions may be involved in different research with new treatments you may be interested in.

Several breast centers in the country have multidisciplinary programs, in which you can meet with all the specialists involved in your care at the same place. In most of them you can be self-referred—you don't have to be referred by a doctor. I would recommend that any woman with breast cancer research the possibilities of hooking up with one of these centers.

When you call the center, find out what doctors staff it. The opinion is only as good as its weakest link, and sometimes pretty junior faculty are required to participate while senior faculty are seeing private patients. If it seems that the multidisciplinary program doesn't sound optimal for you, try a single expert who knows the field and specializes in breast cancer. A breast surgeon is more likely to be able to talk to you about chemotherapy and radiation therapy than a general surgeon.

If you can't find a multidisciplinary program, don't let that stop you from seeking a second opinion. And don't be afraid of hurting your original doctor's feelings. Most doctors welcome another point of view—and if yours doesn't you should probably be looking for another doctor anyway.

Things are changing constantly in this field. Yesterday's answer may be passé today. I suggest you supplement the information in this book with other sources and especially the Internet. On my website, www.drsusanloveresearchfoundation.org, or on the NIH website, www.cancer.gov, you can find the latest studies and up-to-date information to supplement the overview given here.

19

Special Cases and Populations

So far, I've been discussing "typical" breast cancer—the small lump that forms inside a woman's breast—that is usually discovered by the woman herself or by her doctor, or is detected in a screening mammogram. Sometimes, however, we find a cancer that manifests differently, behaves unusually, or occurs in a special population. This chapter will review these special situations.

LOCALLY ADVANCED BREAST CANCER

Once in a while, a breast cancer isn't discovered until it's fairly big—a stage 3 cancer. It is larger than 5 centimeters (2 inches), with positive lymph nodes. Or it has one of the other features that we think give it a bad prognosis, like swelling (edema) of the skin or a big, matted cluster of lymph nodes. It may be stuck to the chest muscle or ulcerating through the skin. In this situation the diagnosis of cancer is made with one or more core biopsies. These can be used to determine the type of cancer as well as such biomarkers as hormone receptors, Her-2/neu, and nuclear grade (see Chapter 16). Tests such as mammogram, ultrasound, and possibly an MRI are done to rule out obvious spread and document the size of the tumor (see Chapter 7).

The clinical indications, however, suggest that the cancer is likely to have spread elsewhere in your body, at least microscopically. When we find them, we often go straight to systemic therapy to destroy those cells. Surgery and radiation therapy follow chemotherapy. Some women are nervous about leaving the tumor in the breast and want a mastectomy right away. This is a bad idea for two reasons. First, the tumor often shrinks with the chemotherapy, making it possible for doctors to do breast conservation surgery rather than a mastectomy. Second, the tumor's response to the chemotherapy can be a test of whether this tumor responds to chemo. (See Chapter 18.)

Most commonly, chemotherapy is started with AC: doxorubicin (also known as Adriamycin) and cyclophosphamide (also known as Cytoxan). They are given together for three to four cycles or until the maximal response is reached. In one study, in which each woman was treated until she stopped responding, the median number of cycles required to achieve a partial remission was four and to achieve a complete remission, five.[1]

The size of the tumor is measured by clinical exam as well as mammography and ultrasound, so that doctors can determine as accurately as possible whether it is responding. Most studies showed that 10–20 percent of women treated this way will have a complete clinical remission (no obvious tumor remaining), based on exam or imaging. Unfortunately, only about 5–15 percent will also have a complete remission based on examination of biopsied tissue by a pathologist under the microscope once the breast is removed.[2] A recent small randomized trial showed that adding docetaxel (making it ACT; the *T* stands for taxane, the type of drug) after the four cycles of AC increased the pathological complete remission rate, or disappearance of tumor on pathological exam, from 15 to 31 percent.[3] A large NSABP study, B-27, of smaller tumors (2–5 centimeters) also showed an increase in pathological response rates with the combination of four cycles of AC followed by another type of taxane (Taxotere, so *T*).[4] Because of this, the first four cycles of AC are now usually followed by T prior to surgery. If the tumor does not seem to be responding, an alternate chemotherapy such as T can be tried sooner.

Although chemotherapy is most often used for neoadjuvant therapy, occasionally hormone therapy (tamoxifen or an aromatase inhibitor) may be used, especially in older women with hormone receptor positive tumors who may not tolerate the chemotherapy as well. It is also capable of shrinking the tumor and allowing less surgery, as I will explain later in this chapter.

If the tumor has shrunk, we do a lumpectomy; if there is no change, we do a mastectomy. Even when the tumor seems to have disappeared—we can't feel it or see it on a mammogram—there may still be some cancer cells present. So we always want to do a lumpectomy at least on the spot where the tumor had been to see what's actually left. (This procedure is rather imaginatively called a ghostectomy.) If the ghostectomy is clear or shows clean margins, you're a candidate for radiation. Similarly, if we can do a lumpectomy and get clean margins because the lump is small, following that with radiation is sensible. If there is still a large lump or a lot of cancer at the margins, it may be best to do a mastectomy with or without immediate reconstruction. In the case of an ulceration that doesn't leave enough skin to sew together, breast reconstruction provides medical as well as cosmetic benefit: reconstruction takes skin from another part of the body (see Chapter 22). At this time the lymph nodes are also checked. Obviously the significance of negative nodes is not the same after you have received chemotherapy, but it is still a prognostic marker of the likelihood of recurrence. Finally, after either form of surgery, the woman will have radiation therapy to reduce the chances of cancer coming back in the breast or chest wall. And if the tumor tested sensitive to hormones, either tamoxifen or an aromatase inhibitor will be given for five years.

Different hospitals have different preferences in treatment order and combination. For this kind of breast cancer, most centers do chemotherapy first and many then do a mastectomy no matter what.[5] Some of them do breast conservation surgery if the lump becomes small enough and then usually follow with radiation. As we use these combinations of treatments for this kind of breast cancer, we're seeing better response rates. If you have strong feelings about which combination you want, get a second opinion.

In many areas of the country there are protocols studying locally advanced cancers, trying to determine whether different combinations of drugs or different combinations of chemotherapy, radiation, and surgery affect survival rates. I think it's worth your while to consider participating in one if it's available to you (see Chapter 15).

Locally advanced cancers usually fall into one of two categories, though both are generally treated the same way. Sometimes a very aggressive cancer seems to come up overnight as a large and evidently fast-growing tumor (although it's been there undetectable for a while). At other times, the tumor has been present for several years and the woman has tried to pretend it wasn't there, until it's gotten huge or begun ulcerating through the skin, and she finally gets to a doctor. This latter case we call a neglected primary—it's not an especially aggressive cancer, just an especially frightened woman. Patients with a neglected primary cancer often do better than you may expect: if you've had an untreated cancer for five years and it hasn't killed you or obviously spread anywhere, it's clearly a slow-growing cancer.

Few studies, however, have differentiated between aggressive cancers and neglected primaries. Studies of these types of cancer taken together and treated aggressively have shown a median overall survival of 12.2 years and event-free survival of 9.0 years (that means that half of the women in the study have had no recurrences at 9 years and that half are still alive at 12.2 years). Fifteen-year overall survival for women with stage 3A tumors was 50 percent and 23 percent for women with stage 3B. Remember this just means that at 15 years 50 percent were still alive, not that they all died after 15 years. In fact if you are alive at 15 years you are most likely to stay alive. These numbers are from a small study and so should be taken as examples only, but they are the only data we have so far that have followed women for so long.[6] The NSABP is doing a study (no. B-18) that will give us more information.

If you've been putting off seeing your doctor about a lump that's been growing, or if you're suddenly faced with a new large or ulcerating tumor, don't ignore it and assume you're dying—get it diagnosed and start your treatment right away. Your prognosis may not be as good as it would be with a smaller tumor, but it's not hopeless, and the sooner you begin to take care of it, the better your chances are.

INFLAMMATORY BREAST CANCER

Inflammatory breast cancer is a serious kind of advanced breast cancer. Though we see increasing numbers of cases, it is still rare, accounting for only 1–4 percent of all breast cancers. Overall survival is worse in women with this kind of breast cancer than in others. It's called inflammatory because its first symptoms are usually a redness and warmth in the skin of the breast, often without a distinct lump. Frequently the patient and even the doctor mistake it for a simple infection, and she is put on antibiotics. But it doesn't get better. It also doesn't get worse, and that's the tip-off: an infection always gets better or worse within a week or two—it rarely stays the same. If there's no change, the doctor should perform a biopsy of the underlying tissue to see if it's cancer. Two of my patients who have had this cancer had similar stories. One had been breast-feeding and developed what her doctor thought was lactational mastitis (see Chapter 5). It never cleared up and didn't hurt much—there was no fever or other sign of infection. It hadn't gone away or gotten worse in six months. The other patient, not breast-feeding, noticed that one breast had suddenly become larger than the other; there was also redness and swelling. In both cases, the doctors at first thought the women had infections. So if the symptoms continue after treatment, you should ask to have a biopsy done of the breast tissue and of the skin itself. With inflammatory breast cancer, you have cancer cells in the lymph vessels of your skin, which is what makes the skin red; the cancer is blocking the drainage of fluid from the skin.

A study published in 1998 shows that the incidence of inflammatory breast cancer doubled from 1970 and 1992.[7] In white women, it went from 0.3 to 0.7 in 1,000, and in African American women it went from 0.6 to 1.1. (Other races weren't included in the study.) This is reason for concern, but it's still a small number. Women with inflammatory breast cancer tend to be significantly younger than those with other breast cancers, and African Americans with this cancer tend to be younger than whites.

The three-year survival rate from inflammatory breast cancer has improved in recent years. The study published in 1998 shows an increase in survival of 10 percent (42 percent survival vs. 32 percent earlier), while other forms of breast cancer survival only increased 5 percent (from 80 to 85 percent). A recent report followed 61 women with inflammatory breast cancer who had received multimodality (several types of treatment) and found that the 5-year survival rate was 47 percent. Forty percent of the women who received trimodality (chemotherapy, radiation, and surgery) were free of disease at five years.[8] Generally if this type of aggressive cancer does not recur in five years, the woman has a good chance of being cured.

As with all advanced cancers, we start with three or four cycles of AC followed by paclitexel or docetaxel. Then we'll do a local treatment—usually mastectomy followed by radiation. If the tumor is sensitive to hormones, then either tamoxifen or an aromatase inhibitor will be added to the mix. Serious though it can be, inflammatory breast cancer is still an extremely variable disease. It can be especially scary to have inflammatory breast cancer because it is so rare. I would strongly suggest that any woman with this diagnosis check out the two websites dedicated to this disease: www.ibcsupport.org and www.ibcresearch.org for up-to-date information and support. This disease is serious, but great progress is being made and the prognosis is much more positive than when I wrote the first edition of this book.

THE UNKNOWN PRIMARY

"The unknown primary" sounds like the title of a murder mystery; actually, it's the name we give another kind of mystery—a cancer that has spread to a lymph node in the armpit without an obvious primary tumor. In women this type of tumor (also called occult primary) almost always originates in the breast. Previously we would do tests of the whole body to make sure that the nodes really represented breast cancer and not thyroid, colon, melanoma, or some other type. But this is rarely necessary. Not only is it extremely uncommon for any of these other cancers to spread to the axillary lymph nodes, but there are often other tests that can be done on the cancer cells themselves to help determine where they came from.

This is a rare form of breast cancer, accounting for less than 5 percent of cases. Someone shows up with an enlarged lymph node, usually in the armpit. It's biopsied and we find breast cancer cells, but there are no breast lumps. Sometimes we call this axillary presentation of breast cancer and it is staged as T0N1 (see Chapter 16). In the past there were many difficulties in finding the original tumor, but modern imaging has helped significantly. A woman in this situation is first sent for a mammogram and ultrasound. Looking for a cancer that we suspect is there is always different than screening, and many tumors are found on repeat study. If that doesn't show a tumor, then an MRI is done.

As you remember from Chapter 7, MRI is very sensitive but not that accurate. Although this does not make it a good general screening test, it does help in this situation. Recent studies of MRI have shown that it can detect the tumor in the breast in 70–95 percent of women.[9] If the doctors can find the primary cancer, then the patient has the option of getting a lumpectomy and radiation rather than a mastectomy. Several years ago, a woman called me to ask for advice. She was 68 and had been diagnosed with an unknown primary. Her surgeon was insisting that she have a mastectomy, but she really didn't want it. I suggested an MRI and spoke to her surgeon about it. He was reluctant because she had implants and he felt that imaging techniques wouldn't work. I told him that MRI actually worked very well with implants. This was a fairly recent discovery, and he was glad to hear it. She had an MRI, and it did in fact reveal the cancer. It was a 4-centimeter tumor that had draped itself around the implant. This position necessitated the mastectomy after all. But at least the woman knew that the operation was indeed necessary, and not a possibly fruitless hunting expedition.

In situations where no breast lesion can be found, the treatment is more controversial. There's no doubt that a mastectomy would get rid of a cancer if it's there, but we have to ask if it's necessary, given that the primary cancer is so tiny we can't even detect it. It can be devastating to a woman to have a mastectomy and then learn that the primary cancer didn't show up in the tissue after all, and she's had her breast removed for nothing. Three studies have now reported on using radiation for occult primary (T0N1) breast cancers. All showed a decreased local recurrence rate (18 percent in the irradiated group versus 54 percent in the breasts that did not undergo irradiation in the M.D. Anderson group).[10] In all of the studies the survival was the same whether the woman got radiation or not. Obviously it is not the local options that are the most important here but the systemic, and one could argue that doing nothing to the breast is also an option. The local options, therefore, are radiation alone or mastectomy coupled with an axillary dissection and chemotherapy.

Contrary to what you may expect, the survival rate in cancers that show up in the nodes but not in the breast is actually a bit better than it is for cancers that show up as both a breast lump and an enlarged node.[11]

It's unlikely that you have this kind of cancer, but if you do, you should think about what treatment you'll be most comfortable with. If your surgeon comes down with a hard line and tells you there's one sure way to deal with it, be suspicious and insist on a second opinion.

PAGET'S DISEASE OF THE BREAST

Dr. James Paget (1814–1889) has gotten his name on any number of diseases: there's a Paget's disease of the bone and a Paget's disease of the eyelids, as well as a Paget's disease of the breast. The diseases have no relation to one another, except for their discoverer. In the breast, Paget's disease refers to a form of breast cancer that shows up in the nipple as an itchiness and scaling that doesn't get better. As I was researching this section, however, I was amazed to find that the first description of this rare type of breast cancer was by John of Arderne in 1307. John described a nipple ulceration in a male priest, which over several years without treatment (there weren't many treatments available in 1307) went on to become full-fledged breast cancer.[12] Luckily we can now do more than just observe someone with Paget's.

There are two theories about this type of breast cancer. One is that the cancer cells start in the lactiferous sinus (see Chapter 13) and travel up to the nipple openings. This explains why the nipple itself rather than the areola is the first spot of irritation noted in Paget's, as well as the fact that people with Paget's disease often harbor cancers with similar cell types elsewhere in the breast.[13] The other theory is that the cancer cells actually start in the nipple openings. This correlates with the fact that some women with Paget's disease have no sign of cancer elsewhere.[14] Further study will tell us whether either or both theories are correct.

Usually Paget's disease presents as redness, mild scaliness, and flaking of the nipple skin and gradually goes on to crusting, ulceration, and weeping. It can be itchy, hypersensitive, and painful. It's often mistaken for excema of the nipple—a far more common occurrence. Paget's disease is almost never found in both breasts, so if you have itching and scaling on both nipples, you probably have a fairly harmless skin condition. In addition, Paget's usually starts in the nipple and not the areola, so that can be a telling sign. However, if it doesn't get better, you should get it checked out, whether it's on one or both nipples, or even on the areola.

First you'll need to get the skin on the nipple biopsied. This can be done in the doctor's office with local anesthetic; either a nipple scrape or a "punch biopsy" can make the diagnosis. If it's Paget's, the pathologist sees little cancer cells growing up into the skin of the nipple—that's what makes the skin flake and get itchy. Then you will need a mammogram to look for cancer in the breast itself. As with the unknown primary tumors described above, you may want to have an MRI if the mammogram is negative. If these imaging tests detect something, then a biopsy of the lesion is necessary. Paget's can indicate the possibility of a further breast cancer. Carolyn Kaelin, a Boston breast surgeon, combined several studies of Paget's disease and found that out of 965 cases, 47 percent presented with a breast mass and 53 percent had no mass. Of the women with a mass, 93 percent had invasive carcinoma of the breast and 7 percent had noninvasive cancer. Among those with no mass, 34 percent had invasive cancer, 65 percent of the women had DCIS, and 1 percent had only Paget's disease with no cancer in the breast.[15]

The treatment of Paget's disease depends on whether it is associated with DCIS, invasive cancer, or neither. In and of itself Paget's disease is low grade and not aggressive. If there is an invasive or a noninvasive cancer near the nipple, a lumpectomy that includes the nipple and areola can be performed, followed by radiation. Sentinel node biopsy can be added if it is invasive. If the invasive cancer lump is far from the nipple, a mastectomy may be necessary to get both areas out; otherwise wide excision and radiation is a reasonable alternative. If just the nipple is involved, then removing the nipple-areolar complex and adding radiation has an excellent result.[16]

Paget's disease that involves only the nipple has a better prognosis than regular breast cancer.[17] It doesn't tend to be aggressive, and usually the lymph nodes turn out to be negative. Because of its rarity, most doctors do not see many cases of it, and many assume that it requires a mastectomy—they seem to think that if you can't keep your nipple, your breast doesn't matter.[18] Most women, of course, know better.

This has been a campaign of mine, and a few years ago some of us managed to convince the rest of the medical establishment that all that was needed was to remove the nipple and areola, and that many women prefer to keep the rest of the breast if they can.[19,20] True, your breast looks a bit funny after the nipple has been removed, but it is still there. A plastic surgeon can make an artificial nipple (see Chapter 22), though many women don't mind the breast's appearance, as long as they look natural in a bra. Some of my patients with this kind of Paget's disease chose plastic surgery and some didn't bother with it.

CYSTOSARCOMA PHYLLOIDES

This is another rare type of breast tumor, occurring only 0.3–0.9 percent of the time. The most dramatic thing about this kind of cancer is its name. It's usually fairly mild and takes the form of a malignant fibroadenoma (see Chapter 6). It shows up as a large lump in the breast—it's usually lemon-size by the time it's detected. It feels like a regular fibroadenoma—smooth and round—but under the microscope some of the fibrous cells that make up the fibroadenoma are bizarre-looking and cancerous. It's usually not very aggressive.[21] It rarely metastasizes; if it recurs at all, it tends to do so only in the breast. In the past it was usually treated with wide excision, removing the lump and a rim of normal tissue around it.[22] More recently, however, we've learned that it only needs to be scooped out, since the tumor is surrounded by a casing, allowing it to be neatly removed like a pecan from its shell. This is far less mutilating to the breast than wide excision, and studies have shown it to work remarkably well. One study showed a 6.4 percent recurrence rate.[23] In another series of 24 patients there was only a 4 percent recurrence.[24] Cystosarcoma phylloides doesn't require radiation, and we usually won't check the lymph nodes since when it does metastasize it is usually to the lungs and not the nodes.[25] We'll watch you closely to see if it recurs, and if it does, a wide excision usually takes care of it. I had one patient who came to see me because her cystosarcoma phylloides had recurred three times, and her surgeon told her she'd have to have a mastectomy because it kept coming back. I told her I thought we should wait and see if it did come back, and in the six years I followed her, it didn't recur.

The medical literature sometimes talks about a "benign" versus "malignant" cystosarcoma phylloides, based on a subjective interpretation of how cancerous the cells appear. The implication is that malignant cystosarcomas behave more aggressively. About 95 percent are benign. And the 5 percent that metastasize and ultimately kill the patient are hard to predict accurately in advance. Most surgeons suggest a more aggressive approach (mastectomy) if the pathologist feels that it's malignant. These cancers are sufficiently rare that you may want a second breast pathologist's opinion before embarking on a more aggressive therapeutic approach. Recent research has focused on finding a biomarker (see Chapter 16) that will predict this better.

CANCER OF BOTH BREASTS

Once in a great while a woman is diagnosed as having a cancer in each breast at the same time. Typically she finds a lump in one breast, gets a mammogram, and learns there's also a lump in the other breast. A biopsy shows them both to be cancer. A recent review from Milan reported that these tumors are more likely to be small, invasive lobular, low grade, and sensitive to estrogen.[26] Such tumors are thought to reflect a situation in which a woman's particular hormonal environment is conducive to developing cancers.

Is one cancer a spread from the other? Most studies have found noninvasive cancer associated with each of the two tumors, suggesting that it is not. This does not mean that the prognosis is twice as bad. The prognosis is determined by the worse of the two. So they're both treated the same way: we do a lumpectomy or mastectomy and lymph node dissection on one and then the other side. Usually the surgeon first dissects the lymph nodes on the side that appears worse. If the nodes are positive and require chemotherapy, the other nodes won't necessarily have to be dissected if the second cancer has a low likelihood of spreading to the nodes. Unfortunately the surgeon's guess isn't always right. A few years ago I had a patient with three cancers: she had a lump in the top of her right breast, and the mammogram showed two densities in the bottom of the left breast. They'd all been biopsied with needles. She really wanted to keep her breasts, so I did a wide excision of the right breast and sampled the lymph nodes, which were fine. Then I did a wide excision of the two cancers in the left breast, and on the left side she had positive lymph nodes.

You can have radiation treatment on both breasts at the same time, but the radiation therapist has to be very careful that the treatment doesn't overlap and cause a burn in the middle area.

It isn't necessary to do the same treatment on both breasts. You may decide on a mastectomy on one side and wide excision plus radiation on the other, for example.

CANCER IN THE OTHER BREAST

Sometimes a woman who has had cancer in one breast turns up with cancer in her other breast. Usually this isn't a recurrence or a metastasis; it's a brand-new cancer. It's possible for breast cancer to metastasize from one breast to the other, but it's rare. A new primary cancer has a different significance than a metastasis. What it suggests is that your breast tissue, for whatever reason, is prone to develop cancer, so you developed one on one side and then several years later the other side followed along. As with any new cancer, it's biopsied and removed, your lymph nodes are checked, and you're treated. Your prognosis isn't any worse because you developed the second breast cancer; rather, it's as bad as the worst of your two cancers. You can still have breast conservation; you don't have to have a mastectomy if you don't want it. People who have second cancers are more likely to have a hereditary predisposition to breast cancer (see Chapter 10). Some women are so scared of getting cancer in the other breast that they consider having a prophylactic mastectomy to prevent it (see Chapter 11).

BREAST CANCER IN VERY YOUNG WOMEN

Sometimes cancer occurs in an unusual situation. As noted earlier, breast cancer is most common in women over 50, and there are many cases in women in their 40s. It's far more rare in women under 40, but it does occur. We tend to be particularly shocked when it occurs in a young woman. Usually in this situation it's detected as a lump, since we generally don't do screening mammography in young women for the reasons discussed in Chapter 14.

Often a young woman gets misdiagnosed. She detects a lump or a thickening, and she's told it's just lumpy breasts, or "fibrocystic disease," and it's followed for a while until doctors realize it's serious. The vast majority of lumps in women under 35 are benign, and the risk of cancer is very low. Still, it's important for doctors to be vigilant and bear in mind that young women can develop breast cancer.

The youngest patient I ever diagnosed was 23. She was on her honeymoon and discovered a lump. We diagnosed her as having cancer; she had a positive node, and she underwent radiation and chemotherapy. Ten years later she developed a local recurrence that required a mastectomy.

Breast cancer in younger women is more likely to be hereditary.[27] If you've inherited a mutation (and you need only one or two more mutations to get cancer), you're one step closer and likely to get there faster, whereas if you "acquire" breast cancer, you still need to get all of the mutations. That doesn't work all the time. Like older women, the majority of younger women with breast cancer have no family history. But if you have breast cancer in your family you're more likely to get it at a younger age than if you don't.

Many doctors believe that breast cancer in a young woman is more aggressive than in older ones. Two studies shed some light on this theory. Both show that the mortality from breast cancer is higher in women who have been pregnant in the past four years.[28,29] The risk is highest right after a pregnancy and decreases with each year, going back to normal after four years. This makes sense, since pregnancy affects both the milk duct lining cells, making them divide more, and the local environment (see Chapter 13). Since young women are more likely to have been recently pregnant (25 percent of all breast cancers in women younger than 35 are associated with pregnancy), they show more of this effect.[30] This suggests that it may not be the woman's age itself that affects aggressiveness but the changes in her immune system (necessary so that her body won't reject the fetus) and in the hormones that go with pregnancy.

Overall, there is no evidence that breast cancer in a woman under 35 matched for prognostic features (see Chapter 16) is any more aggressive than a cancer in an older woman. Younger women do, however, have a higher incidence of poor prognostic features such as negative estrogen receptors, poor differentiation, and high proliferative (growth) rates. Still, a young woman and an older woman with the same tumors have the same general prognosis.[31]

With younger women, there's some question about whether it's safe to do lumpectomy and radiation. The concern is twofold. One is that we don't know what the long-term (40- to 60-year) risks of radiation are. The other is that there appears to be a higher local recurrence rate reported in young women who get lumpectomy and radiation than in women in their 40s and 50s.[32] However, recent studies show that there's also a higher local recurrence after mastectomy in that group.[33] The treatment for breast cancer in young women is pretty much the same as for older women, with the option of either breast conservation surgery with radiation or mastectomy with or without reconstruction.

Interestingly, chemotherapy works better in younger than in older women. We've decreased the death rate for breast cancer through treatment in this subgroup more than in any other. There are problems with chemotherapy, however. Often it puts a young woman into menopause. The really young woman—in her 20s or early 30s—is less likely to have that happen than the woman in her late 30s or early 40s. The closer you are to your natural menopause the more likely it is to push you over (see Chapter 26). This also varies according to the chemotherapy drugs you take. (See Chapter 18.) The much younger woman will probably get her period back after the treatment course is finished. There is considerable controversy as to whether this is a good thing or not. Some data suggest that a premenopausal woman who is still menstruating postchemotherapy and is sensitive to estrogen may benefit from two to three years of temporary menopause.

A web-based survey of young women with breast cancer revealed, not surprisingly, that fertility after treatment was a major concern. Because of the likelihood of chemotherapy-induced menopause, some women have considered preserving their eggs before the treatment so they can still have children later. There are problems with that, however. With the current state of technology, you can save an embryo but not an egg. So you must choose your sperm donor or partner. While I was writing this edition, an exciting report came out from Dr. Kutluk Oktay at Cornell.[34] He was able to remove some ovarian tissue from a 30-year-old woman with breast cancer before she underwent chemotherapy which, as she had feared, resulted in menopause. Six years later he transplanted her frozen ovarian tissue and ovarian function resumed. He was able to harvest eggs and, with in vitro fertilization, one developed into a four-cell embryo in a petri dish. Whether she will actually be able to get pregnant and carry the embryo and fetus to term is unknown at this writing, but this is a first step toward preserving fertility in young women who need chemotherapy.

The second problem is that a lot of hormones must be administered to make the eggs grow for harvesting. Doctors are often reluctant to give those high doses of hormones to women who have had cancer, especially those with hormone receptor positive tumors. Attempts have been made to retrieve eggs without hormone stimulation, and recently tamoxifen has been used to help harvest eggs from 12 women prior to chemotherapy. Two of the women in the tamoxifen group and two of five women in the no-stimulation group conceived.[35]

This is obviously a moving target. If this is an issue for you, make sure you check out your options *before* undergoing chemotherapy. (The website www.youngsurvival.org is a good source for up-to-date information on this topic.) And remember there are other ways to parent. Losing your fertility does not mean losing all chances to be a parent.

When a young woman has breast cancer, there's an increased risk for her mother, sisters, and daughters, and they should all be monitored closely.

Finding the right support group can be difficult for the younger woman, who can feel out of place among women in their 50s and older. (Check out the www.youngsurvival.org website for support groups for younger women.) Most hospitals have support groups for young women because the issues they face are often quite different from older women's. There are several books on dating after mastectomy, which is a concern to single women of all ages, as are the psychosocial issues we consider in Chapters 20 and 26.

The incidence of breast cancer in the other breast is about 0.8 percent per year, which usually maximizes out to about 10–15 percent. However, women with BRCA 1 or BRCA 2 (about 6 percent of women under 36) mutations can have a much higher chance of developing a second breast cancer in the same or other breast. Since younger women have many more years to get cancer in the opposite breast, their risk is slightly higher than that of older women. Both chemotherapy and hormone therapy reduce this risk.

BREAST CANCER IN ELDERLY WOMEN

Just as very young women can get breast cancer, so can women over 70, and they share some issues. Neither end of the extreme always fits our general modes. There are studies showing that older women aren't treated as aggressively. There's a tendency to restrict the options for treatment: "Well, they're old; they don't really want chemotherapy."[36] I think a special effort has to be made to ascertain what the patient wants, and not permit physicians to act on their own assumptions.

In addition, there's a tendency to do mastectomies on older women without offering them breast conservation treatments, assuming that elderly women don't care as much about their looks. Some doctors tell an older woman that six weeks of radiation therapy will be too much for her, making mastectomy sound less arduous than lumpectomy plus radiation. But radiation isn't really all that hard to go through. As I noted in Chapter 17, for some older women, just as for their younger friends, it's preferable to the emotional trauma of mastectomy.

Not only do many doctors neglect to mention lumpectomy and radiation, they also neglect to offer reconstruction to the older woman on whom they've urged mastectomy, again assuming that she won't care enough about her looks to want it. And again, that assumption is totally off base. I remember one patient in her mid-80s with large, droopy breasts, who had always wanted to have a reduction but thought it was too dangerous. She got a cancer at the upper end of one of her breasts. She wanted breast conservation; she didn't want a mastectomy. But it seemed foolhardy to us to radiate all of this breast that didn't show cancer. So after discussing it with her, we did a lumpectomy and bilateral reductions, and then did radiation. She was delighted; when the radiation was done she went off on a cruise and found a new boyfriend.

So you can't make any assumptions.

A recent study looked at whether radiation was necessary for older women with estrogen receptor positive cancer. Tamoxifen is known to reduce local recurrence, and researchers thought it might be enough. They included women over 70 with tumors up to 2 centimeters and randomized them to lumpectomy plus tamoxifen or lumpectomy plus radiation plus tamoxifen. There was no difference in overall survival or disease-free survival. The only difference was in local recurrence: those who received radiation had a local recurrence rate of 1 percent while those who did not had a local recurrence rate of 4 percent.[37]

Clearly in these women the radiation is probably not worth it, expecially since the current aromatase inhibitors that are being used in place of tamoxifen are even better at local control. More difficult, though less common, is the situation of estrogen receptor negative cancer in women over 70. Here you don't have the local benefits of hormones and radiation is still probably worthwhile.

There's a move, particularly in the United Kingdom, to treat older women with breast cancer—women 70 or over—with tamoxifen alone, without even the lumpectomy. Several studies have examined this, mostly in women who were too frail to undergo surgery. Overall the tumors in 63 percent of the patients treated with tamoxifen alone as a first-line treatment shrink or disappear.[38] About half of the women will experience a response by 13.5 weeks, which lasts a varying amount of time. But in one-third of women the response lasted five years.[39,40] However, two-thirds relapsed within five years and needed additional therapy. Aromatase inhibitors are likely to do a better job with this group; in one randomized study of neoadjuvant letrozole the tumor responded in 55 percent of the cases compared to 36 percent with tamoxifen.[41] This suggests that if you're older and fragile, and you don't want to go through surgery, it's reasonable to start you off on tamoxifen or an aromatase inhibitor alone and hope you can continue to avoid surgery.

Part of the problem in studying women over 70 is that we really can't evaluate long-term survival, since elderly people die from many illnesses. But not all elderly women are frail. I had a 95-year-old breast cancer patient in Boston who was very active. I did a lumpectomy and put her on tamoxifen. Unfortunately she couldn't tolerate the tamoxifen and dropped it. She was fine for about a year and a half; then her cancer recurred locally. I did another lumpectomy, and this time I really tried to get her to stick with the tamoxifen, and she did for a while. The last I heard she was still going strong. So when we look at how to treat "old" women, we need to look at how frail they really are: people vary greatly. Those who live into their 90s tend to be healthy, or they wouldn't live to that age. We can't just assume, as many doctors do, they'll be dead in a year or so and forget it—sometimes they live to over 100.

CANCER DURING PREGNANCY

Once in a very great while a patient develops breast cancer while she's either pregnant or breast-feeding. We used to think that pregnancy-related hormones fired up the cancer and made it worse.

The studies are contradictory. Most show that, stage by stage, it's no worse than any other breast cancer. The problem is that when you're pregnant, your breasts are going through a lot of normal changes, which can mask a more dangerous change. For one thing, breasts are much lumpier and thicker than usual. Similarly, when you're breast-feeding, as I discussed at length in Chapter 1, you tend to have all kinds of benign lumps and blocked ducts, and you may not notice a change that ordinarily would alarm you. Infections are common when you're breast-feeding and can mask inflammatory breast cancer, so the physician may also find diagnosis of inflammatory breast cancer difficult.

As I noted earlier in this chapter, studies have found that women who were diagnosed with breast cancer while pregnant or within four years thereafter did indeed have a higher mortality rate.[42] As more women are having later pregnancies at the age where breast cancer becomes more common, this may become a bigger issue.

Treatment is also a problem. What we can do about your cancer depends on what stage of pregnancy you're in. If you're in the first trimester, you may want to consider therapeutic abortion, depending on your beliefs about abortion and how much this particular pregnancy means to you. Women who abort their fetuses do not have a better prognosis, but it's easier to proceed with treatment. If you continue with the pregnancy, treatment options are somewhat limited. Radiation in the first trimester can injure the fetus. The fetus's organs are being formed at this time, and the data from other cancers suggest a high rate of fetal malformation with chemotherapy in the first trimester. The same applies to general anesthetic, which rules out a mastectomy. We can do a biopsy or a wide excision under local anesthetic. But if further treatment is called for, we usually try to wait until the second trimester.

In the second trimester, since the fetus's organs are already formed and it's safer to use general anesthetic, we can do a mastectomy. We would rather not risk radiation. In recent years, studies have shown that chemotherapy can be used safely in the second and third trimesters. So far, in these studies the babies have appeared healthy, but we won't know if complications will appear later in the child's life. If you're in your third trimester, we can do a lumpectomy, or, if need be, a mastectomy, and possibly chemotherapy, then wait for further treatment like radiation and/or tamoxifen until the child is born. We can begin chemotherapy if it's important to get going right away. If you are close to your due date, your obstetrician can induce labor as soon as the baby can be expected to survive well outside the womb or do a cesarean section, and then start you on chemotherapy and radiation after delivery.

My neighbor in Los Angeles was diagnosed with breast cancer when she was pregnant with her seventh child. Her physicians told her to abort and she had trouble convincing them that she wanted her seventh child just as much as the first. She underwent a mastectomy in the second trimester and did well. Because she had many positive nodes she received chemotherapy during her third trimester. Her delivery went well, and she said for years afterward that this seventh child was the smartest of all, which she attributed to chemotherapy.

In the mid-1990s I saw a woman who had been diagnosed 20 years earlier, when she was seven months pregnant. She had undergone a radical mastectomy and then had radiation with Cobalt while she was pregnant. She said she had to have a dose monitor in her vagina to keep track of the amount of radiation her fetus was receiving. Nonetheless she carried the baby to term and both were fine 20 years later.

BREAST CANCER DURING LACTATION

Breast cancer during lactation isn't quite as complicated, since you can always stop breast-feeding and start your child on formula. Radiation will probably make breast-feeding impossible, and you won't want to breast-feed if you're on chemotherapy, since the baby will swallow the chemicals.

There are some misconceptions about cancer and breast-feeding that need to be addressed. The first is that a child who drinks from a cancerous breast will get the cancer. This theory is based on a study of one species of mouse, which does transmit a cancerous virus to its female offspring through breast-feeding. At this time, it hasn't been found in any other species of mouse, in any other animal, or in humans.

Another notion is that a baby won't drink milk from a cancerous breast. Normally this isn't so. If a breast has a lot of cancer, it probably won't produce as much milk, so the baby will, quite sensibly, favor the milkier breast. There's nothing wrong with this. Many babies prefer one breast to another even with a very healthy mother.

We're not sure yet if lactation affects the cancer. I've had two patients whose breast cancer showed up while they were lactating. Both were treated, both stopped breast-feeding, and both did well without a recurrence for several years. After much debate both women decided to get pregnant again. One had a recurrence during the second pregnancy; the other had a second primary develop while she was lactating. This leads me to wonder whether, if a cancer shows up while a woman is pregnant or lactating, there is a higher risk of a recurrence in another pregnancy. Obviously we can't do a randomized study, and it's too unusual an occurrence to draw any conclusions. Our evidence is purely anecdotal. For now, all I can suggest to someone who has developed breast cancer while pregnant or lactating is to consider seriously not having another pregnancy, in case it affects the chance of a recurrence. An article by breast surgeon Jeanne Petrek in 1997 discussed the question of pregnancy after breast cancer.[43] She looked into a number of published series (articles by doctors reviewing their own cases over a period of time) and found that breast cancer survival didn't change with a subsequent pregnancy. But because there were a number of possible biases (see Chapter 15), the results are inconclusive. It's possible that the doctors selected their patients by telling only the women who were likely to be cured that pregnancy would be safe, and discouraging the others. Or it may be that getting cancer while you're pregnant has a different effect on your body than getting it afterward.[44,45,46] Petrek's point, and I think it's a wise one, is that we don't really know the answer yet. She started a large, multicentered trial at Sloane Kettering in New York. This will look at a number of issues concerning breast cancer and reproduction, and it should give us some of the answers we need.

WOMEN WITH IMPLANTS

There's no evidence that women with implants have a higher vulnerability to breast cancer than other women, and some evidence that it may actually be lower.[47] Sometimes cancer is detected on mammogram, and sometimes the lump is palpable. It's diagnosed in the same way as any breast cancer—with a biopsy. We may be able to do a needle biopsy, depending on where the lump is. We don't want to stick a needle into the sac and release the silicone or saline into the breast.

The treatment options are the same. You can have lumpectomy and radiation.[48] You can radiate with the implant in place. There is a higher incidence of encapsulation (see Chapter 3), but other than that there's no problem. You may think that cutting into the breast would break the silicone cover, but there are a couple of ways around that. For example, we can use the electrocautery instead of the scalpel, and that can't cut into the implant.

If you had injections back in the 1960s when they were legal, the same applies. It's even harder than with implants to detect cancer on mammogram, since it's hard to tell what's silicone and what's something else. So you need to go to a high-quality center where you can be carefully monitored. It's very important to have the mammograms serially, comparing one year to another, because that's what can tip you off: one of these lumps that you were calling silicone is growing. You can have lumpectomy and radiation.

AFRICAN AMERICAN WOMEN

As I explained in Chapter 10, the incidence of breast cancer is different in different ethnic groups. In addition, there is a difference in survival. The most data reported so far are on African American women, in whom breast cancer usually occurs at a younger age and is more deadly. Some of this effect has been attributed to access to care, but more recent studies on molecular markers have established that African Americans are more likely to have an aggressive tumor even when it is small. Significantly more African American women had high grade cancer, larger tumors, positive nodes, and estrogen receptor negative disease.[49,50,51] How these factors correlate to treatment will be important to examine in the future.

BREAST CANCER IN MEN

This book addresses breast cancer in women because it is the most common malignancy in women. Among men it accounts for less than 1 percent of all cancers. Overall there are 1,500 cases a year in men and over 200,000 in women. Many of the men who get it seem to have a family history on their father's or their mother's side.[52] There's also a theory that it's connected to gynecomastia—femalelike breasts (see Chapter 1), either now or during puberty, but so far we have no proof of this. We do have proof that men with Klinefelter's syndrome, a chromosomal problem in which not enough testosterone is produced, are susceptible to breast cancer.[53] Interestingly, risk factors for women such as early exposure to radiation[54] and higher estrogen exposure in utero also seem to be relevant to men.[55]

For a time there was concern that men who got estrogen treatments for prostate cancer were more vulnerable to breast cancer, but this doesn't seem to be the case. Rather, prostate cancer can metastasize to the breast.[56] (Remember that it remains prostate cancer, not breast cancer.)

Breast cancer in men shows itself in all the ways it does in women—usually as a lump—but it tends to be discovered later because men aren't usually very conscious of their breasts. The treatments are the same as well. Men can undergo sentinel node biopsy (see Chapter 17), and either lumpectomy and radiation or mastectomy.[57] There is a tendency to overtreat men with postmastectomy radiation because surgeons see these cancers so rarely. Recent data demonstrate that local recurrences in men are rare even in stage 3 disease and that the same indications should be used as are employed in women (see Chapter 17).[58]

One issue that is often not addressed, however, is the fact that the cosmetic implications are somewhat different for them. On the one hand, they don't tend to regard breasts as crucial to their sexuality the way women do. On the other hand, their naked chests are more likely to be visible. It can be more awkward for a man to have a scar, to lack a nipple, or to have a deformed chest, than it is for a woman. So, like a woman, a man might prefer lumpectomy and radiation to mastectomy. The one extra consideration is hair. After radiation therapy a man loses most of his chest hair on that side. If he is very hairy, a mastectomy with the scar hidden in hair may prove more cosmetic. Depending on where the tumor is, the nipple can often be conserved. If he loses the nipple, a plastic surgeon can give him an artificial one. When I worked at UCLA, a golfer with a small breast cancer came to me. He was distressed that the only option he had been given was a mastectomy. After a lumpectomy and radiation, he was very happy and felt normal on the course.

Treatment in terms of chemotherapy and axillary nodes is exactly the same as for women. Interestingly, tamoxifen works in men with estrogen receptor positive tumors. Recent reports suggest that the aromatase inhibitors work as well.[59,60]

DCIS (ductal carcinoma in situ) is even rarer in men than is breast cancer. In 1999 the Armed Forces Institute of Pathology did a study on male DCIS.[61] Researchers found 280 cases of pure DCIS and 759 of invasive. They studied the pure DCIS cases and found older rather than younger men. It was different from DCIS in women (see Chapter 12) in that it was more frequently the low grade papillary version than either cribriform or the high grade comedo kind. High grade DCIS was especially rare. Occasional cases showed necrosis. The men were treated with wide excision alone without radiation for this low grade DCIS.

Several years ago I got an e-mail from a man who had DCIS. He had a mastectomy and then radiation. Then he was told he had to go on tamoxifen. He wanted to know if tamoxifen could harm him. It's unlikely that it would. There are lots of data on men taking tamoxifen, and it doesn't harm them. They can get hot flashes, but they can't get vaginal dryness or endometrial cancer, or any male version of those. But this man didn't need it. He probably needed a mastectomy without radiation. The only data for tamoxifen with DCIS show a very small benefit, and that occurs only with women who had lumpectomy and radiation, not mastectomy. The doctors were probably inexperienced in male breast cancer and thought it wisest to use every treatment possible.

Usually, however, when a man has a breast lump, it isn't cancer but unilateral gynecomastia, which can happen anytime in a man's life, especially if he's been on some of the drugs used to treat heart conditions or hypertension or smokes marijuana. It's never a cyst or fibroadenoma—men don't get those.

OTHER CANCERS

When I arrived at UCLA in 1992, within the first week or two I got a call to see a patient who had a breast lump. It was soft and smooth, and on the side of her breast. It felt like a cyst, but I tried to aspirate it and that didn't do any good. Then she had a mammogram and an ultrasound, which confirmed that the lump was solid. We took the lump out under local anesthesia, and indeed it was malignant. When I talked to her afterward, I broke one of my cardinal rules—never make absolute promises. I told her that, though it was unfortunate that her tumor was malignant, it was a small tumor and I could guarantee that she wouldn't have to get chemotherapy. Since she was postmenopausal, the most she'd need would be tamoxifen.

Then we looked at it more closely under the microscope, and found that it wasn't a breast cancer at all but lymphoma, a lymph node cancer, showing up in the breast. Lymphoma is treated with chemotherapy. The tale has two morals. One, never break your own wise rules. And two, things aren't always what they seem. It's ironic that my first breast cancer patient at UCLA didn't have breast cancer. (I'm glad to report that she responded well to the treatment and is doing fine.)

Occasionally other kinds of cancer occur in the breast. Since the breast contains several kinds of tissue besides breast tissue, any of the cancers associated with those kinds of tissue can appear in the breast. In addition to lymphoma (since there are lymph nodes), these include a cancerous fat tumor (liposarcoma) and a blood vessel tumor (angiosarcoma). You can also have a melanoma—a skin cancer. Connective tissue in the breast, as elsewhere, can become cancerous. Usually these cancers are treated the same way they'd be treated in any other part of the body—the tissue is excised, and radiation and chemotherapy follow (the chemicals are different from those used to treat breast cancer).

When another form of cancer shows up in the breast, we know it isn't breast cancer from the pathologist's report. As I noted earlier, each kind of cancer has its own distinct characteristics, and we rarely mistake one kind for another. We choose treatment for the particular cancer rather than breast cancer treatment. We didn't, for example, do an axillary section on my lymphoma patient.

Having breast cancer doesn't immunize you from other forms of cancer. You have the same chances as anyone else of getting other cancers. I've had a couple of patients with breast cancer who were also heavy smokers. They were treated for their breast cancer, continued smoking, and ended up with lung cancer. A bout with any kind of cancer can provide a useful time to consider altering your lifestyle in ways that promote overall health.

20

Fears, Feelings, and Ways to Cope

The first thing a woman thinks of when diagnosed with breast cancer is, "Will I die?" This is quickly followed by, "Will I lose my breast?" Obviously breast cancer is a disease with a major psychological impact. Whenever you think you have a lump, get a mammogram, or have a biopsy, you rehearse the psychological work of having breast cancer. Although, as I have pointed out, most women don't die of breast cancer and most do not lose their breasts, these fears remain.

How does the average woman react to this terrifying diagnosis? In my experience, women go through several psychological steps in dealing with breast cancer.

First there is shock. Particularly when you're relatively young and have never had a life-threatening illness, it's difficult to believe you have something as serious as cancer. It's doubly hard to believe because, in most cases, your body hasn't given you any warning. Unlike, say, appendicitis or a heart attack, there's no pain or fever or nausea—no symptom that tells you something's going wrong inside. You or your doctor have found a painless little lump, or your routine mammogram shows something peculiar—and the next thing you know we're telling you you've got breast cancer.

Many women say this is the worst part of their journey. The initial shock can leave you feeling confused and not sure how to proceed.

You're at your worst. But once you get the medical information you need to make decisions, things get better.

Along with shock there's a feeling of anger at your body, which has betrayed you in such an underhanded fashion. In spite of the horror you feel at the thought of losing your breast, often your first reaction is a desire to get rid of it: take the damned thing off and let me get on with my life!

While this is a perfectly understandable emotional response, it's not one you should act on. Getting your breast cut off will not make things go back to normal; your life has been changed, and it will never be the same again. You need time to let this sink in, to face the implications cancer has for you, and to make a rational, informed decision about what treatment will be best for you both physically and emotionally.

Because patients are so vulnerable when they receive their diagnosis, in my surgical practice I didn't like to tell them about all their options at the same time I told them they had cancer. I preferred to tell a woman she had cancer and that there were a number of treatment options that we'd discuss the next day at my office.

But ideally the process starts earlier than that. When a patient came to me with what I thought might be a malignancy, I started talking with her right away about the possibilities, from the most hopeful to the most grim, and asked her to consider what it would be like for her in the worst possible scenario. We used the scary word: cancer. We discussed the general range of treatments we were likely to want to choose from. Then we'd talk about when I would call her with the results of her biopsy, so she could decide where she would be and who would be with her. I was taught in medical school that you should never tell a patient anything over the phone, but I found that it often worked better if I did. If the patient didn't have cancer, why keep her in suspense any longer? And if she did, I preferred that she find out in her own home or in whatever environment she'd chosen to be in beforehand.

Then if it was bad news, she didn't have to worry about being polite because she was in my office and there were all these other people around. She could cry, scream, throw things, deal with the blow in whatever way she needed to. She wouldn't have to lie awake all night hoping I wouldn't tell her something awful the next day but knowing that I would. So I would tell her on the phone and then make an appointment to see her within 24 hours. By that time, the shock would have worn off a bit, and she could absorb information about her options a little better.

Even when it's done this way, it can be very difficult for a patient to take it all in. For this reason I suggest that you bring someone with you when the doctor explains your options—a spouse, a parent, a close friend. Sometimes a friend is best: someone who cares a lot about you but isn't as devastated as you are by the news. The person is there partly to be a comfort and support, but also to be a reference later. So it's good if it's someone detached enough to remember everything that was said at the meeting, or even just someone to take notes while you are busy trying to take in as much as possible. Such a friend is also good for asking questions you may be afraid to ask.

These days, this approach isn't all that unusual. In the past, surgeons were very paternalistic: they told a woman she had cancer and she had to have a mastectomy and when it was over she'd be cured and everything would be fine from then on. It was a lie, of course, but the patient usually believed it because she wanted to—who wouldn't?—and for the time being at least, she was reassured.

WEIGHING THE OPTIONS

Today there's much more emphasis on doctor and patient sharing the decision-making process, and there are more options to choose from. There's also a lot more knowledge available—there are articles about breast cancer and survival rates in both the medical and the popular press and on the Internet; you *know* you have no guarantee that everything will be fine once "daddy doctor" makes you better. All this is good, of course, but it's also very stressful. In the long run, I'm convinced you're better off when you consciously choose your treatment than when it's imposed on you as a matter of course. But in the short run, it's more difficult. The end result is a little more anxiety ahead of time while you are trying to make decisions about your treatment, but less depression afterward.

Of course, different patients have different needs. Some women still want an "omniscient" doctor to tell them what to do. I was involved in a pilot study on how patients decide their treatments and what kinds of decision making had the best psychological results. I expected to find that women coped better when they got a lot of information from their doctors and learned all they could about their disease, its prognosis, and the range of available treatments. But we found this wasn't always the case. Far more important was whether the doctor's style matched the patient's. Some women preferred to deny their cancer as far as possible, and have their doctor take care of it for them. They did better with old-fashioned paternalistic surgeons who told the women what was best for them, giving them minimal information. Others liked to feel in control of their lives and to know all they could about their illness and its ramifications. They did better with surgeons like me, who wanted to discuss everything with them. Still others wanted a great deal of information but deferred to the doctor for decision making. There is no right or wrong style, so don't feel guilty if your needs are not the same as those of your friend or neighbor. Remember, it's about what style works best for you.

I experienced this when I was in practice. There was a well-respected breast surgeon in Boston when I was at the Faulkner Breast Centre in Boston. He was much more in the taciturn, old-fashioned mode, and he and I would lose patients to each other all the time; sometimes we referred patients to each other. It worked out very well, and we were both happy about it, since we were both able to help people while remaining true to our own styles and philosophies.

Sometimes I would get a patient who clearly preferred not to know a lot, and over the years I learned to recognize the signs and to respect them. I'd give such a patient enough information, but not in as much detail as I usually did, and then try to hear what she was choosing and say something like, "It seems to me that you're leaning toward mastectomy, and maybe that's the best decision for you." I still wouldn't tell her what to do, but I'd give a little more guidance than usual.

So if the first stage is shock, the second is investigating your options. (Sometimes, however, it works in reverse, and these stages can vary in order and intensity.) How extensive this investigation is varies enormously among women. Some of my patients simply went over what I told them and discussed it with a friend. Others did research in medical libraries and on the Internet, and then went for second and third and fourth opinions. You can't take forever, but you don't want to hurry yourself either. In my experience, most patients can't handle prolonging this stage for more than three or four weeks.

When you're exploring the options, you should reflect seriously on what losing a breast would mean to you. Its importance varies from woman to woman, but there is no woman for whom it doesn't have some significance. Although many women say, "I don't care about my breast," deep down this is probably not true for most of us. A mastectomy may be the best choice for you, but it will still have a powerful effect on how you feel about yourself. Often the loss of a breast creates feelings of inadequacy—the sense of no longer being "a real woman." In her book, *First, You Cry,* Betty Rollin talks about the first party she went to after her mastectomy.[1] Although she knew she looked pretty with her clothes on, she felt like a "transvestite," only playing at being a woman.

The fear of feeling this way may start long before the mastectomy—indeed, it plays a part in how the woman copes with her breast cancer from the first. Rose Kushner surveyed 3,000 women with breast cancer and concluded that most women "think first of saving their breasts, as a rule, and their lives are but second thoughts."[2]

My experience was different. The first reaction of most of my patients was, "I don't care about my breast—just save my life." Later, when the first shock had worn off and they'd had time to think about it, their priorities remained the same, but they realized they did in fact care very much about their breast. Many women feel robbed of their sexuality when they lose a breast. Betty Rollin found that while her husband still desired her after her mastectomy, her own sexual feelings were gone. "If you feel deformed, it's hard to feel sexy," she writes. "I was dark and dry. I no longer felt lovely. Ergo, I no longer could love." Holly Peters-Golden, on the other hand, points out the importance of distinguishing between the distress caused by mutilating surgery and the distress that comes from having a life-threatening disease.[3] Certainly in my experience with patients, the latter far outweighs the former. The fear of losing a loved one can stress a relationship and affect one or both members sexually.

Sociologist Ann Kaspar studied 29 women between the ages of 29 and 72, 20 of whom had mastectomies, and 9 of whom had lumpectomies.[4] While, as she hastens to explain, she had no illusions that 29 women constituted a definitive study, her findings are interesting. Most of the women with mastectomies had been deeply concerned before surgery that the mastectomy would "violate their femininity." Yet, with only one exception, they reported that after the surgery it was much less traumatic than they'd anticipated, and that they'd realized that being female didn't mean having two breasts. "They got in touch with their identity as women, separate from social demands. Even the ones most determined to get reconstruction didn't feel that the plastic surgery would make them real women—they knew they already were real women," Kaspar says. She did find that anxiety was higher among the single women in her study, especially the single heterosexual women, who worried that "no man will ever want me." Those already in relationships usually found their partners were still loving and sexual, and more concerned with the women's health than their appearance.

Although the experience of these young, single, heterosexual women is consistent with my patients' experience, I've also had many other patients who had different reasons for wanting to keep their breasts. Middle-aged women approaching or just past menopause can have very strong feelings about their breasts. They've experienced the loss of their reproductive capacity with menopause; often their children are leaving home and they are rediscovering their relationship with their spouse. This is no time for a woman to experience yet another loss around her womanhood. Elderly women too often want breast conservation. They're already experiencing many losses and may not want to add the loss of their breasts, which have been a part of them for such a long time. Nothing makes me angrier than hearing of an elderly woman who has been told by her surgeon, "You don't need your breasts anymore; you may as well have a mastectomy." Different choices may make sense at different stages in a woman's life. Your choice should be based not only on the best medical information you can gather but also on what feels right to you. Don't let generalizations about age, sexual orientation, or vanity get in your way.

Many studies have been done comparing conservative surgery and mastectomy with or without immediate reconstruction, looking for differences in psychological adjustment. Interestingly, the important factor often appears to be the match between the woman and her treatment.[5] That is, the way she feels about her body, about surgery, about radiation, about having a say in her treatment, and about a multitude of other factors affects how she reacts to this new and enormous stress.

Most importantly, a woman faced with these decisions cannot make a "wrong" choice. If we give her options it's because these are reasonable options in her situation. In most cases both mastectomy and lumpectomy with radiation work equally well (see Chapter 17). It is not as though if she chooses wrong she'll die, and if she chooses right she'll live.

Along with the fears and stages of recovery, there are also a number of related issues that come up for people with cancer. One of these is the tendency to feel guilty for having cancer—a sense that you've somehow done something wrong. People have a tendency to blame themselves for being ill anyway, and, irrational though she knows it to be, a woman often feels she has betrayed her function as a caregiver by getting breast cancer.

In this connection, the holistic perspectives that I'll discuss in Chapter 25 can have their negative side. The mind-body connection is real, and its validation is important, but it's not the only force at work in any disease.

Most of the studies on the relation between stress and cancer have been done on rats and are equivocal at that—some studies show that stress is a factor in cancer, others that it's a factor in *preventing* cancer. In any case, it's only one factor, not a significant cause. I wish there were some simple, clear cause of cancer so I could say, "Don't do this and you won't get breast cancer." Unfortunately it doesn't work that way. We don't have total control over our own bodies; we don't always, to use the popular New Age phrase, "create our own reality." You didn't give yourself breast cancer, and you won't help your healing by feeling guilty.

FINDING SUPPORT

Having explored the options and their feelings, most women move into a "get on with it" stage. You know all you want to know, you've decided what you want to do, and now it's time to do it. This is the time to make your decision—you understand that you have cancer;

you know the pros and cons of the different treatments; you're not happy about it but you're not still in shock.

How long the treatment lasts depends on what the treatment is. If you're getting a mastectomy without immediate reconstruction, it may just be one or two days. If you have reconstruction, it will be several days in the hospital and a few weeks recuperating at home. If you're having wide excision and radiation, it will go on daily for six weeks, and if you're having chemotherapy in addition to your other treatments it can go on for another four to eight months. However long the treatment process lasts, it's important to have a lot of support around you, and it's important to allow yourself to feel lousy. Cancer is a life-threatening illness, and the treatments are all emotionally and physically stressful; you need to accept that and pamper yourself a bit. You don't have to be Superwoman. Get help from your friends and family—throughout the treatment.

Sometimes, when you're having chemotherapy, the people who were supportive in the beginning start to dribble off. At that point, you may want to get into a breast cancer support group, where there are women who are going through, or have been through, similar experiences. It can be of enormous help to you. (Check with the nearest hospital or branch of the American Cancer Society.) In some parts of the country, away from big cities, it can be hard to find breast cancer groups per se, and you may not be certain about whether a mixed-gender, mixed-cancer group is appropriate for you. It's worth checking, though; sometimes such groups can work well, and often many of the members are women with breast cancer. You can check it out by calling the leader and getting the rundown on who is in the group, asking if your situation allows you to relate to the others in the group. This call would also be a good idea if you have found a breast cancer support group. In that case, you would want to ask the leader about the other women in the groups, specifically where they are in their breast cancer experience. Some women feel most supported and helped in a group where there are women with all stages of breast cancer; others are upset by the stories of women with metastatic disease and would not do well in a mixed-stage group. Also, you can join a support group on the Internet or a bulletin board community.

As stressful as the treatment period can be, it's an improvement over the earlier stages; you're actually doing something to combat your disease. (This feeling is often stronger when you're doing meditation, visualization, diet changes, or one of the other techniques we'll talk about in Chapter 25.) But when the treatment period is done, you're likely to find yourself in a peculiar sort of funk. This is what I see as the fourth stage, what some call the "post-treatment blues." This stage lasts at least as long as the treatment itself. You're experiencing separation anxiety because the experience and preoccupation you've lived with so intensely is over, and where are you now? The routine established during your treatment has helped you feel supported, protected, and active against your cancer. Losing that feeling is hard. It's a little like leaving a job—even one you didn't like. Rationally you're glad it's over, but emotionally you feel lost. The caregivers (nurses, doctors, and technicians) you've come to depend on are no longer a daily part of your life.

The recent news that lifestyle changes including low fat diet, exercise, and weight loss can affect recurrence (see Chapter 26), give women something they can do for themselves after the doctors are finished.

Compounding the situation is a reasonable fear. There's no more radiation going into your body, no more chemotherapy; without them, is the cancer starting up again? It's a scary time. This anxiety may well progress into depression, which is very common and can sneak up on you when you're least expecting it. You find yourself feeling sad and anxious; you can't sleep or you want to sleep too much; you've lost interest and pleasure in people and activities that you used to enjoy. These symptoms are normal. Often they last only a few weeks or months; but if they seem to drag on, you may want to see a counselor or therapist to help you get unstuck and go on with your life. Barbara Kalinowski, a former colleague of mine who ran two support groups at the Faulkner Breast Centre in Boston, finds this one of the most helpful times for a woman to get involved with a support group. She says, "Sometimes it can be too much for a woman before this: she's working at her job, she's taking care of her kids, and she's going for treatment. Adding the extra time commitment of a support group can create even

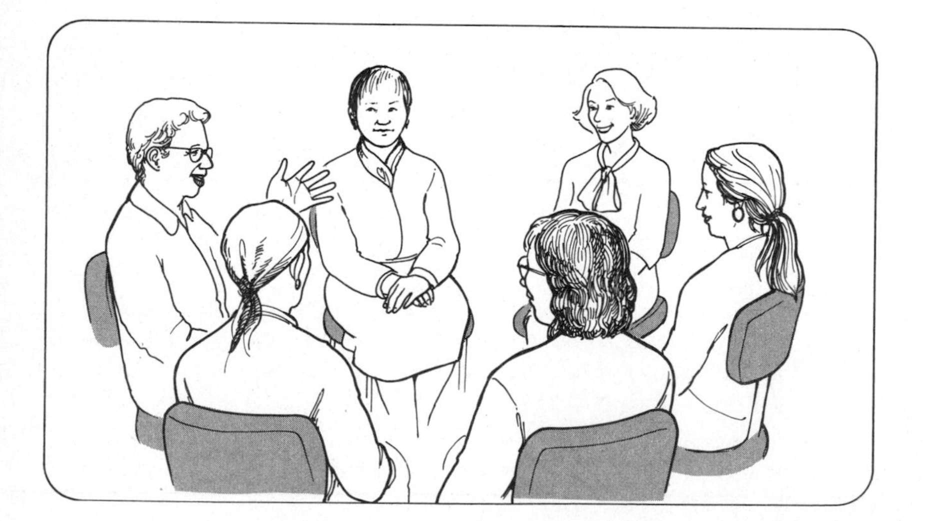

more stress. But when it's done and the depression sets in, you may really need the group."

Such groups can especially help when, as often happens, you feel a little apart from the people you love. You're going through something they can't really understand—only somebody else who's been there can. You'll meet other women who are at various stages of the disease—including some who had it 10 or 15 years ago and are living happy, healthy lives. Often the only people you've known with breast cancer were in an advanced stage—the ones who get better seldom talk about their disease with anyone. Knowing long-term survivors can help you to realize that you're not necessarily doomed. And knowing other women who are at your stage can give you a sense of shared problems, of comradeship with people who understand what's happening to you because it's also happening to them. Indeed, you may want to look into a group before your treatment. Hester Hill Schnipper, an oncology social worker and breast cancer survivor (author of *After Breast Cancer: A Commonsense Guide to Life After Treatment*), has had women join her group before they have surgery, so they can learn about it from those who have already been through it.

Many women find that this period of intense feelings can be a time of emotional growth. They reevaluate their lives; they know their own mortality in a new way. How are they living? Are they doing what they want to do for the rest of their lives? I've seen fascinating changes in some of my patients' lives during this period. One of my patients finally left a bad marriage she'd stuck with for years. Conversely, another decided it was time to make a commitment she'd avoided before—she married the man she'd been living with for a long time. A minister who lost her job because of her cancer left the ministry and got a job selling medical equipment. Another, a breast cancer nurse, left her job to work with a holistic health center. A patient whose husband once had Hodgkin's disease had her first child; faced with life-threatening illnesses, the couple wanted to confirm their faith in life and bring a new life into the world. Several of my patients began psychotherapy, not only to deal with their fears around their cancer but to look into issues they'd been coasting along with for years. They wanted to make the best of the time they had left, whether it was 5 years or 50.

This period of preoccupation and turning inward can last a long time. It's not that you're always completely depressed and out of it; you're just tired, a bit listless. Your body and mind haven't fully healed yet.

For many women the cancer never returns, and they begin gradually to rebuild their lives. But sometimes cancer does return. Because the emotional issues of recurrence are so profound and complex, I've written a separate chapter to address them.

COPING: WHAT TO TELL YOUR CHILDREN

A particularly trying issue people face is the question of what to tell their children. Again, it's an individual decision, and there are no hard-and-fast rules. I do think, in general, it's wiser to be honest with your kids and use the scary word "cancer." If they don't hear it from you now, they're bound to find out some other way—they'll overhear a conversation when you assume they're out of the room, or a friend or neighbor inadvertently says something. And when they hear it that way, in the form of a terrible secret they were never supposed to know, it will be a lot more horrifying for them. By talking about it openly with them, you can demystify it. In addition, if all goes well your children learn about survival after cancer. Kids need to know they can trust you—you don't want to do anything to violate that trust. It's a two-way communication; remember to listen to their fears. If you find it difficult to bring up the subject, there are children's books that can help you begin.

How you tell them, of course, depends on the ages of the children and their emotional vulnerability. With a little child you can say, "I have cancer, which is a dangerous disease, but we were lucky and caught it early, and the doctors are going to help me get better soon." What younger kids need to know is that you're going to be there to take care of them, that you're not suddenly going to be gone. They also need to know that the changes in your life aren't their fault. All kids get angry at their mothers, and they often say or think things like, "I wish you were dead." When suddenly Mom has a serious illness, the child may well see it as a result of those hostile words or thoughts. They must be told very directly that they did not cause the cancer by any thoughts, words, anger, dreams, or wishes. Your children will also be affected in other ways. You may be gone for a few days in the hospital and will need to rest when you come home. You may be getting daily radiation treatments, which consume a lot of your time and leave you tired and lethargic. You may be having chemotherapy treatments that make you violently sick to your stomach. Your children need to know that the alteration in your behavior and your restricted accessibility to them aren't happening because you don't love them or because they've been bad and this is their punishment.

Some surgeons encourage their patients to bring young children to the examining room. I found that it could be very helpful for a daughter in particular to see me examining her mother. If you're being treated with radiation or chemotherapy in a center where your children are permitted to see the treatment areas, it's a good idea to bring them along once or twice. The environments aren't intimidating, and a child who doesn't know what's happening to you in the hospital can conjure up awful images of what "those people" are doing to Mommy.

It is also important to be careful about changes in your older children's roles at home. You don't want to lean too heavily on them to perform the tasks you are unable to do; instead, you want to give kids things they can do that make them feel useful. Wendy Schain, a psychologist and breast cancer survivor, and David Wellisch, a psychologist I worked with at UCLA, did a study on daughters of women who had had breast cancer. They found that the daughters who had the most psychological problems in later life were the ones who had been in puberty when their mothers were diagnosed. This was in part because their own breasts were developing at a time when their mothers' breasts were a source of problems. But interestingly enough, that wasn't the major reason for their problems. Far more damaging was the fact that they were expected to perform many of the mother's traditional household tasks. They were physically capable of this work, but they were not psychologically able to cope with the responsibility and they felt guilty about their resentment.[6]

Hester Hill Schnipper points out that it is important not to make promises that you may not be able to keep. It is a mistake to promise kids, for example, that the cancer won't kill their mother. Instead, if your child asks, "Will you die?" you can reply, "I expect to live for a very long time and die as an old lady. The doctors are taking good care of me, and I am taking good care of myself, and I hope to live for years and years."

Judi Hirshfield-Bartek, a clinical nurse specialist in Boston, usually recommends to couples that the partner take the kids out for some special time together. This gives them a chance to ask questions they may be afraid to ask their mother and know they'll get honest answers. A close relative or friend can also do this.

Frightening as it can be for kids to know their mother has a life-threatening illness, if you're honest and matter-of-fact with them, chances are it won't be too traumatizing. One of my patients decided when she learned about her breast cancer that she would demystify the process for her 7- and 10-year-old daughters by showing them a prosthesis (artificial breast) and explaining what it would be used for. The next day she came into my office for her appointment. When I asked her how her experiment worked, she started to giggle. "Well, they certainly weren't intimidated by it. They listened very carefully to my explanation—and then started playing frisbee with it!"

Breast cancer has particularly complex ramifications for a mother and her daughter. Aside from the normal fears any child has to deal with, a daughter may worry about whether this will happen to her too. It's not a wholly unfounded fear. As I explained in Chapter 10, there is a genetic component to breast cancer. You need to reassure your daughter, explain to her that it isn't inevitable but as she gets older she should learn about her breasts and be very conscious of the need for surveillance.

Often teenage daughters of my patients came to talk with me about their mother's breast cancer and their fears for themselves. It can be very useful to a girl to have her mother's surgeon help her put the dangers she faces into perspective, and it may be worth asking your surgeon to meet with your daughter. This may also be useful years later, if your daughter does develop problems; she's already built a good relationship with a breast specialist, and she's more likely to seek treatment with confidence and a minimum of terror.

Often daughters find themselves feeling angry at their mothers, as though the mother created her own breast cancer and thus made her daughter vulnerable to it. Mothers often feel the same way; their feeling that they caused their own cancer expands into guilt over their daughter's increased risk. Often a patient said to me, "What have I done to my daughter?" These feelings need to be faced and dealt with. Without openness, the cancer can become a scapegoat for all the other unresolved issues between the mother and daughter, putting the relationship at risk.[7]

It's a good idea to let the people at your child's school know about your illness. That way if the child begins acting out or showing other problems, the school knows what's going on.

COPING: FEARS OF YOUR LOVED ONES

Husbands or lovers of women with breast cancer also have feelings that need to be acknowledged. They worry that she might die; they worry about how best to show their concern. Should they initiate sex, or would that be seen as callous and insensitive? Should they refrain, or would that be seen as a loss of attraction to her sexually?

The cancer is affecting your whole family, not just you. While you're in treatment, you focus chiefly on yourself. But as soon as possible you need to deal with how it's affecting those closest to you. Sometimes couples therapy with your spouse or family therapy with your spouse and children can help. They too are feeling frightened, angry, depressed, maybe even rejected, if all your attention is going to your illness, and they may not have as much support for their feelings as you do for yours. It's crucial to communicate with one another at this time, to work through the complex feelings you're all facing.

SEARCHING FOR INFORMATION

Knowing that many women these days want more information, I've set up a website, www.drsusanloveresearchfoundation.org, where I post new information as it emerges. The Internet is a wonderful source of information, but you need to be a savvy surfer. If you are searching the Internet, make sure you follow a few guidelines.

1. Know the site's sponsor and whether it has anything to gain from the information given. For example, a site sponsored by a pharmaceutical company may have good information but may be biased toward its own drugs. Some of the sites pushing alternative therapies are also selling them.
2. Know who is answering questions or giving medical advice. Is it someone you have heard of? What are her or his credentials? Is she or he an expert in breast care? You can get good advice from other women with breast cancer on the bulletin boards but you don't know if their experience is standard or if they have an ax to grind.
3. Check who wrote the information on the site and when it was last updated.
4. Look to see if the information is backed up by references in scientific journals.
5. If information that you get on a site disagrees with what your doctor says, print out the page and bring it to your doctor for discussion.

The same provisos can be applied to books and articles.

WHAT TO LOOK FOR IN A DOCTOR AND MEDICAL TEAM

As women we are socialized not to question authority, especially when we're sick. A good place to begin is to put together a questionnaire that will help you assess your potential doctor or medical team. This doesn't have to be an actual document, but if it helps keep your thoughts, questions, and needs organized and concise, there's nothing wrong with putting pen to paper. What are some of the things you will want to include? The items may vary a bit from person to person, based on insurance coverage (or lack thereof), diagnosis, and so on. The following questions will give you a good start:

Do they listen?

We all know doctors are busy, pulled in many directions, and pressed for time. When you are dealing with people you may otherwise find intimidating, you may be a bit reluctant to make demands. But remember, they are people just like you, and you can bet they'd want someone to pay close attention if they were in your shoes. Never lose sight of this fact—and don't choose a doctor who has.

Do they sit down, look you in the eye, and connect with you?

You should expect your doctors to hear you. As a way of showing they are listening and caring, it is not unusual for doctors to pull up a chair and sit face-to-face while discussing your diagnosis and options for treatment. You need to feel that your doctor sees you as a person.

Do they solicit and answer your questions?

If only one of you is doing the talking, there's a problem. You will want to make certain that your doctor not only answers any questions you may have but also provides you with information that allows you to make decisions or shows you where to look for the answers.

Do they show you your X rays and test reports and explain them if you ask?

Each of us has a comfort level when it comes to facing what lies ahead in terms of surgery, adjuvant therapies, prognosis, and possibilities. You may want to know every detail. If this is the case, you should expect the doctor you select to explain tests and procedures you will be undergoing. However, you should decide in advance how much you really want to know. Some of us need the hard, fast facts; others just want a broad overview; still others want only the information needed to take their first step. One size does not fit all, so feel free to ask about anything that comes to mind.

Do they allow you to tape the visit?

Because you may be nervous or frightened—or simply because you may be asking questions that require lengthy or complicated answers—you may want to tape-record conversations with your doctor. Don't be afraid to ask. This is a great way to make sure you aren't missing anything important. It provides you with the opportunity to review what you discussed, and also allows you to absorb what was said at your own pace, in your own time. If you run into a doctor who doesn't want to be taped, you should seriously consider whether this is someone you feel safe and confident with, or if it's time to move on.

Do they ask you about your use of alternative and complementary therapies?

In this day and age, it is not uncommon for women with breast cancer to seek out therapies that may be considered outside the realm of Western medicine. A growing number of patients feel they need to approach the cancer on more than one level. You may try acupuncture, massage, Chinese herbs, Reiki therapy, vitamins, or many other therapies currently labeled alternative or complementary. Your doctor should want to know about them and may have useful advice about things such as combinations of herbs or vitamins and mainstream drugs that may be helpful or should be avoided. You want to pay close attention to reactions when you discuss any therapies you may be trying or want to try. If your doctor dismisses these therapies without evidence that they are harmful or ineffective, you may want to leave that doctor and find one who acknowledges that alternative treatments can help your physical and emotional well-being. Many women feel that having the option of an alternative therapy provides them with a sense of control when everything else seems to be out of their hands. However, always be skeptical of practitioners who promise a cure, ask for large amounts of money for treatment, or make statements that simply sound too good to be true. (See Chapter 25.)

Do they suggest additional sources of education and support?

Ideally, your doctor will present you with brochures, pamphlets, and the names of books and other resources designed not only to assist you in making decisions about your treatment options, but also to help you regain your equilibrium. You are going to need information that allows you to ask questions when you need to, talk to other women who have faced what you are going through, educate yourself about your specific type of breast cancer, and even have a shoulder to cry on once in a while. You should see a red flag if you are given a diagnosis, told you need surgery, and then sent home to prepare without any of the resources mentioned.

Do they seem to feel threatened when you bring information from the media to discuss?

While not every bit of information you retrieve from the Internet, magazines, newspapers, and so on, may be relevant, it's imperative that your doctor be willing to evaluate what you find, discuss it with you, and assist you in making decisions. Procedures, drugs, and information are changing so rapidly that you may stumble on an article, web page, or even information in a chat room that could have a profound effect on your treatment—and that your doctor may not have heard about. A good doctor won't be threatened by this sort of information but will want to help you interpret it.

Do you feel that they are partners in this journey?

Although no one else can travel the emotional, physical, or psychological path you will be following, it is important that your doctors convey a sincere aura of understanding, support, and partnering. You should feel that any decision you reach is one both of you can agree on, discuss honestly, and then act on in a spirit of hope and possibility.

Do they discuss clinical trials?

A clinical trial (sometimes called a protocol or study) is designed to decide whether a new drug or procedure is an effective treatment for a disease, or has possible benefit to the patient. These trials give doctors and researchers an opportunity to gather information on the benefits, side effects, and potential applications for new drugs, as well as help them determine which doses and combinations of existing drugs are most effective (see Chapter 15).

SECOND OPINIONS

Exploring the options often means getting a second opinion. Some women assume this is just a confirmation of the treatment plan chosen. Often patients came to see me with their surgery scheduled for the next day and became upset if I disagreed with their doctor's plan. But that is the risk you take. As anyone reading this book knows, the treatment of breast cancer is far from straightforward. If you go for another opinion, you may well get one. When the second opinion is different from the first, a patient often assumes that this new opinion must be the right one. Further, having to think about what both doctors have said and make a decision can be extremely stressful. You feel very insecure because your life is on the line and no one seems to know what to do. But the truth is that there are choices. There are different ways to approach the problem and there is no one right answer. It's really your decision: either the first or second opinion can be right. Even getting a third opinion may not prevent the uncertainty. You would like to believe that there is some objective truth: one right way to treat your disease. But this is often not the case. You have to explore all of the possibilities until you find the one you're comfortable with.

Sometimes patients are shy about seeking a second opinion—as though they're somehow insulting their doctor's professionalism. Never feel that way. You're not insulting us; you're simply seeking the most precise information possible in what may literally be a life-and-death situation. Most doctors won't be offended—and if you run into a doctor who does get miffed, don't be intimidated. Your life, and your peace of mind, are more important than your doctor's ego.

PART SIX

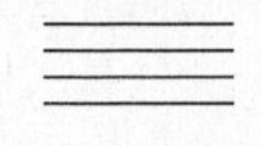

TREATMENT

21

Surgery

Almost every form of breast cancer involves surgery—the initial biopsy and probably a lumpectomy or mastectomy as well as surgery on the lymph nodes. It's always a frightening prospect, but demystifying the process can be helpful. I've already discussed aspects of surgery in Chapters 3 and 8. In this chapter we will go over what you can expect from your surgeon and your operation for breast cancer. I will be fairly explicit because I think the more information you have, the less scared you will be. If you find surgical details unpleasant, you may skip those parts.

When I was in practice, I would talk with the patient a few days ahead of time and explain exactly what I'd do in the operation, and what risks and possible complications were involved. I'd draw her pictures and show her photographs, so she'd know what to expect. (If your doctor doesn't do that, you can check my website and others for photos and descriptions.)

As with any operation, patients are asked before the surgery to sign a consent form. This can be a little scary, especially if you read all the fine print, because it asks you to state that you know you can die from the surgery or suffer permanent brain damage from the anesthetic. This doesn't mean that either is likely to happen, or that by signing the form you're letting the doctors off the hook if something *does* happen.

Rather, it's an acknowledgment that you've been told about the procedure and its risks and that you still want to have the operation. (Obviously you have to balance for yourself the risk involved in the operation against the risks of not having it.)

It's very important to know the risks. Never permit yourself to be rushed through signing the consent form. You should be given the form well before you go in for surgery—it's hard to read small print when you're about to be wheeled in to the operating room. You need to have plenty of time to ask the surgeon questions about risks and complications. If anything confuses you, be sure to ask for clarification.

For the bigger operations (mastectomies and immediate reconstruction with a TRAM [transverse rectus abdominis muscle] flap) I often recommend that the patient donate a couple of pints of her own blood a week or two prior to the procedure. Transfusions are rarely necessary in breast surgery, but it's a nice secure feeling to know that if you do need blood you can get the safest possible—your own. If your surgeon doesn't offer this, you should ask. The Red Cross is more than happy to assist in this procedure.

On the other hand, directed donor blood has not been shown to be safer than blood bank blood, so if you don't give your own, trust the blood bank. I don't think this is needed for mastectomies, but is a good idea for TRAM flaps.

Your surgeon will tell you to stop taking aspirin, aspirin-containing products, or nonsteroidal anti-inflammatory drugs and vitamin E at least one week before surgery. All of these interfere with clotting and cause more bleeding in surgery. If someone has taken a drug of this type we do a "bleeding time" (a test that tells how fast your blood clots) prior to surgery to make sure it's safe to proceed. If not, we postpone the surgery for a week or two until the clotting returns to normal. It is important to tell both your surgeon *and* anesthesiologist about all drugs, vitamins, and herbs you are taking so they can check for interactions.

ANESTHESIA

There are several anesthetics we can use in various procedures: local anesthesia, described in Chapter 8; general anesthesia, described below; and a kind that falls between, called conscious sedation. It puts you into a kind of twilight sleep in which you're somewhat aware of what's happening but you really don't care. (This is also described in Chapter 8.)

Other anesthetics that are midway between local and general—nerve blocks, epidurals, and spinals—don't work well for major breast surgery, although some surgeons use a thoracic epidural (like the block used in childbirth but higher up on your body) to decrease the amount of general anesthesia needed. Local anesthesia doesn't work for extensive breast surgery either: the amount of local anesthesia you'd need to block out the pain would be toxic.

In recent years, general anesthetic has become a complex, sophisticated combination of drugs. The first element in any general anesthetic combination is something to induce sleep quickly—usually propofol. This drug is given intravenously and puts you out immediately. Its effects last about 15 minutes, and it's followed with a combination of other drugs. Sometimes the anesthesiologist uses a combination of narcotics to prevent pain, gas to keep you unconscious, and a muscle paralyzer to keep you from coughing or otherwise moving during the operation. Since the muscle paralyzer prevents breathing, it's necessary to put a tube down your throat and into your windpipe to keep your airway open and hook you up to a breathing machine to ensure that you get enough oxygen into your body during the operation. Sometimes doctors skip the paralysis and put a tube into your throat, letting you breathe yourself. Sometimes rather than use the narcotics, they use gas that can keep you asleep and get rid of pain.

Which of these various agents are used, and in what combination, will be chosen only after consultation with the individual patient. Your medical history will make a big difference here. If you have asthma, for example, a drug that opens up the airways is more suitable so that you don't get an attack under anesthesia. If you have a heart condition, a drug that doesn't aggravate the heart but has a calming effect on it will be chosen.

Since anesthesia and its administration are so complicated, most hospitals will have you talk with the anesthesiologist before the operation. This is usually done during a preoperative screening appointment. Anesthesiologists are highly trained doctors who have gone through at least three years of specialized training after internship. Your anesthesiologist will take your medical history, looking for information that may suggest using, or not using, various anesthetic agents. She or he will ask about chronic diseases you may have, past experiences with anesthetic, and so on and, after thoroughly exploring all this with you, will decide what to use in your operation. If you have previously undergone surgery and had trouble with the anesthesia, try to bring a copy of your anesthesia record from the hospital where the surgery was performed. This interview with the anesthesiologist is very important, since the risk of an operation lies as much in the anesthesia and its administration as in the surgery. When you talk to the anesthesiologist, ask questions and give any information you think may be of importance. Many hospitals also have nurse anesthetists who help administer anesthesia under a doctor's supervision.

Before you're put to sleep, you will be hooked up to a variety of monitoring devices. There's an automatic blood pressure cuff that feels very tight when it's first inflated, but don't worry. As soon as it knows how big your arm is, the amount of pressure used on subsequent inflations is less. There's an EKG monitoring your heart rate. Sometimes a little clip or piece of tape is put on your finger, toe, or earlobe to measure the amount of oxygen in your blood. If the operation is a lengthy one, as with reconstruction, a catheter is put in your bladder to measure the amount of urine output and make sure you're not dehydrated. Thus your bodily functions are all carefully monitored. Large pads are placed over your lower body to maintain your body temperature during the process. If you have had general anesthesia in the past but not in recent years, you will be pleasantly surprised about modern anesthetic techniques. We see less shivering, less nausea, and fewer "hangovers" these days. In fact, most people wake up so gently and promptly from general anesthesia that it contributes to the decision to leave the hospital the same day—a fact that unfairly gets blamed on insurance companies!

Once you're on the operating table, you go to sleep very quickly. Many people who haven't had surgery for 30 or 40 years remember the old days of ether and are nervous about the unpleasant sensations they recall while going under. But sodium pentathol (which is almost never used anymore) and propofol work differently, and most patients report it as a very pleasant experience. You may experience a garlic taste at the back of your mouth just before you go under, and you may yawn. Propofol may burn as it goes into your arm. Pretreatment of the vein with local anesthetics before the propofol is injected helps this considerably, but if you feel it, it is only for a second or two before you go to sleep, and you probably won't remember it. Then you're asleep. People are often reassured to know that they don't talk under anesthesia, even sedation: your deep dark secrets remain safe. With MAC (monitored anesthesia), you may tersely answer a direct question, but you won't chat, and the questions won't be any more personal than "Do you feel this?"

How you wake up from the operation will depend, again, on the drugs that were used. For some drugs an antidote can be given to end the effects. For example, if you've been given a muscle paralyzer, a drug can restore your muscle mobility. But if you've been given gas to put you to sleep, you have to wait slightly longer till it wears off. As soon as they think you're awake enough to breathe on your own, the tube is removed. Occasionally you'll be vaguely aware that this is happening, but usually you're still too out of it to notice. You stay a little fuzzy for a while. When the surgery is over, you're taken to the recovery room, where a nurse remains with you, monitoring your blood pressure and pulse every ten or fifteen minutes until you're fully awake and stable.

Patients often feel cold when they first wake up. Particularly in a big operation, when you aren't covered up, you lost body heat; in addition, the intravenous (IV) fluids going into you are cold. Some of the drugs can create nausea, and you may feel sick when you first wake up. This was succinctly described by a recovery room nurse I once saw on a TV show. She was asked what patients usually say when they first come out of anesthesia, and it was clear the host was expecting something profound or moving. Instead, she replied, "They say, 'I think I'm going to be sick'—and then they are."

You may find that you wake up crying or shivering, but only rarely do patients wake up in great pain. You'll probably fade in and out for a while, and then you'll be fully awake. But expect to be groggy and out of it for a while. It's several hours before most of the drugs are out of your system, and a day or more till they're all gone. If it's day surgery, you'll probably want to go home and go to bed; if you're still in the hospital, you'll sleep it off there.

Even apart from the surgery, anesthesia is a great strain on your body, and it will cause some degree of exhaustion for at least four or five days. People often don't realize this, especially if the surgery is very painful: they attribute all their exhaustion to the pain of the operation. But anything that puts great stress on your body—surgery, a heart attack, an acute asthma attack, or anesthetics that interfere with your body's functions—has a lingering effect. Your body seems to need all its energy to mobilize for the big stress and doesn't have any left over for everyday life for a while. You need to respect that and give yourself time to recuperate from the stress of both the surgery and the anesthetic. I also think it has some effect on brain chemistry that we don't yet understand. Previous experience is not a good guide to how it will affect you the next time, even if the same drugs are used. So don't assume that because you felt fine after your last surgery, you'll feel fine after this one. You may or may not.

There are, of course, risks involved in using general anesthetic, but it's important to keep them in perspective. With the refinements in anesthesia in recent years, the risks are extremely low (about 1 death in 200,000 cases).

Depending on how complicated the operation is, you can now have surgery the same day you're admitted to the hospital, or you can even have day surgery: "outpatient" surgery. In the last few years I was practicing, I tended to do lumpectomy with axillary dissection only on an outpatient basis, so my patient had her two hours of surgery, spent another few hours in the recovery room, and then went home. I frequently did mastectomies as day surgery or just an overnight stay.

Since the rate of infection is twice as high among women who stay in the hospital, I think leaving as soon as possible is a good idea. (I understand the concerns of many patients that managed care companies try to save money by sending people home too soon, but in some cases, leaving the hospital as soon as possible really can be best for the patient.) Many women prefer going home right away, while others feel more comfortable staying in the hospital for a couple of days. A patient who has a mastectomy and immediate reconstruction will be in the hospital for two to five days. If your surgeon wants to send you home earlier than you feel comfortable with, discuss your problems with him or her and see if you can arrange a longer stay.

The main thing that keeps people in the hospital after mastectomy is learning how to manage a drain. If possible, ask your doctor to show you and your family the drain and how to empty it at the preop visit. The main reason to stay in the hospital is advanced age or pain control (except for TRAM [transverse rectus abdominis muscle] flaps, which still require 3–5 days). As soon as you can take oral pain pills, you can go home and not be awakened at 2:00 A.M. for your blood pressure check!

When the surgery is being done under general anesthesia, all the preop procedures are the same, however long your hospital stay. "Twilight sleep" procedures require the same preop preparations, since they need to be monitored, just as general anesthesia does.

PRELIMINARY PROCEDURES

In the operating room, before you are anesthetized, the anesthesiologist will be setting up, and the nurses will put EKG leads and an automatic blood pressure cuff on you. You'll probably wear "pneumatic boots"—plastic boots that pump up and down massaging your calves during the operation to prevent clots from forming during long operations (Fig. 21-1). A grounding plate is put on your skin to ground the electrocautery and protect you from shock. The IV is put in, and then you're given propofol. During this time, your surgeon may or may not be with you. Some surgeons prefer making personal contact before surgery; others maintain a professional distance. Then the surgeon goes out to scrub (wash hands).

After scrubbing, the surgeon goes back in to the operating room. The area of your body that's going to be worked on is painted with a disinfectant, drapes are put around you to prevent infection, and the operation is under way.

All of the procedures I've just described are done regardless of what kind of operation you're having. Now I'll describe what happens in

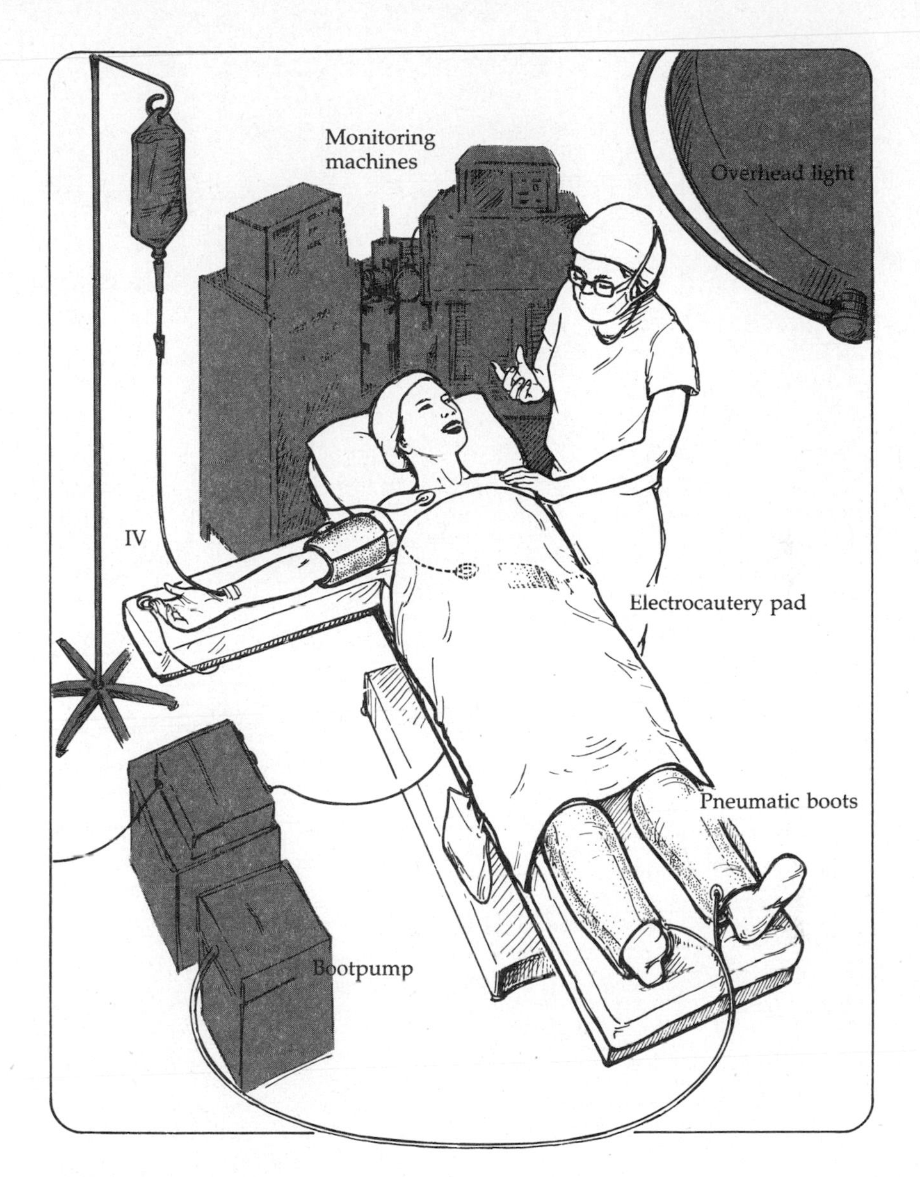

FIGURE 21-1

each different breast cancer operation, starting with the simplest and moving on to the more complex. (Biopsies are described in Chapter 8 and breast reconstruction in Chapter 22.)

Most surgical operations have traditionally been done with a scalpel or scissors. More recently, electrocautery (a type of electric knife) has been used with less blood loss.

PARTIAL MASTECTOMY AND AXILLARY DISSECTION

Partial mastectomy, lumpectomy, wide excision, segmental mastectomy, and quadrantectomy are all names for procedures short of mastectomy and are used virtually synonymously (Fig. 21-2). What each term means precisely depends on the surgeon who's using it. Except for quadrantectomy, none of the terms suggests how much tissue will be removed, and often surgeons use quadrantectomy when they don't necessarily mean they'll remove a fourth of the breast. With a partial mastectomy, the part removed can be 1 percent or 50 percent of the breast tissue. Lumpectomy depends on the size of the lump. Wide excision just says that tissue will be cut away around the lump—not how much will be cut. "Segmental" sounds like the breast comes in little segments, like an orange. But it doesn't, and the segment removed can be any size. Your surgeon will use whatever term appeals most to her or him.

If you're opting for such surgery, you need to make sure your surgeon explains precisely how much tissue will be removed, and what you're going to look like afterward.

As with much of surgery, standard techniques haven't been worked out. One thing that has been determined is that we should choose the direction of the incision based on which area of the breast contains the cancer.[1] In addition, the area of the breast involved should determine the way the tissue is removed and whether it is sewn back together. After years of doing breast surgery, I discovered something that should have been obvious long ago but never occurred to me. Women look at their breasts when they're standing in front of a mirror; surgeons look at the breasts when the patient is lying flat on her back. So the surgeon's impression of the best cosmetic effect may not be the same as the patient's. Plastic surgeons, at the end of an operation on the breast, typically sit the patient up to see how the breast looks with gravity acting on it. But it's not something other surgeons tend to think of. For example, Langer's lines, which are standard surgical teaching, are supposed to be the lines of skin tension that show us where to best make the incision so that the scar will have as little visibility as possible. The pictures of Langer's lines for the breast look like a target—a bull's-eye with concentric circles (Fig. 21-3). But when you think about the breast of a woman standing upright, that doesn't work: the breast is in a U-shape, not a circular shape, because it's pulled down by gravity. So the way we used to make incisions is probably wrong. Most breast surgeons and many general surgeons now understand how the skin changes with position. Ask your surgeon if you are unsure.

When I was at the Faulkner Breast Centre in Boston, we did a study asking patients what they felt were the most significant aspects of cosmetic results. My bias going into the study was that the most impor-

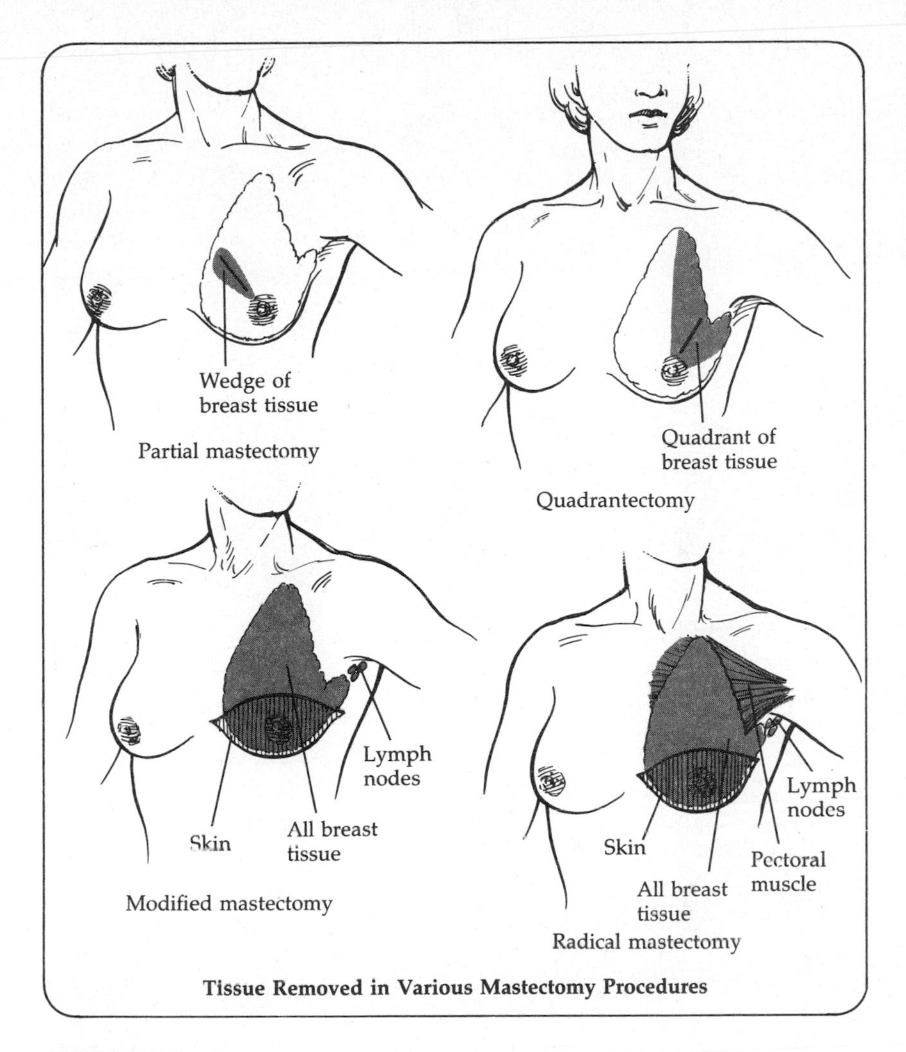

FIGURE 21-2

tant thing for the patient would be that we avoid creating a dent in the breast when we sew her breast tissue back together. It would be a smaller breast, but it would be the right shape. The study showed that I was wrong. What was most important to the patient was size of the breast and the nipple placement. Shape was less important.[2]

When you think about it, it makes sense. If you have one breast a size smaller than the other, it's hard to find a bra that fits at all, or clothing that fits properly. But it's much easier if you've got a breast that's the right size but has a dent in it, because you can push the edges of the dent together inside the bra cup. So I stopped sewing the breast tissue

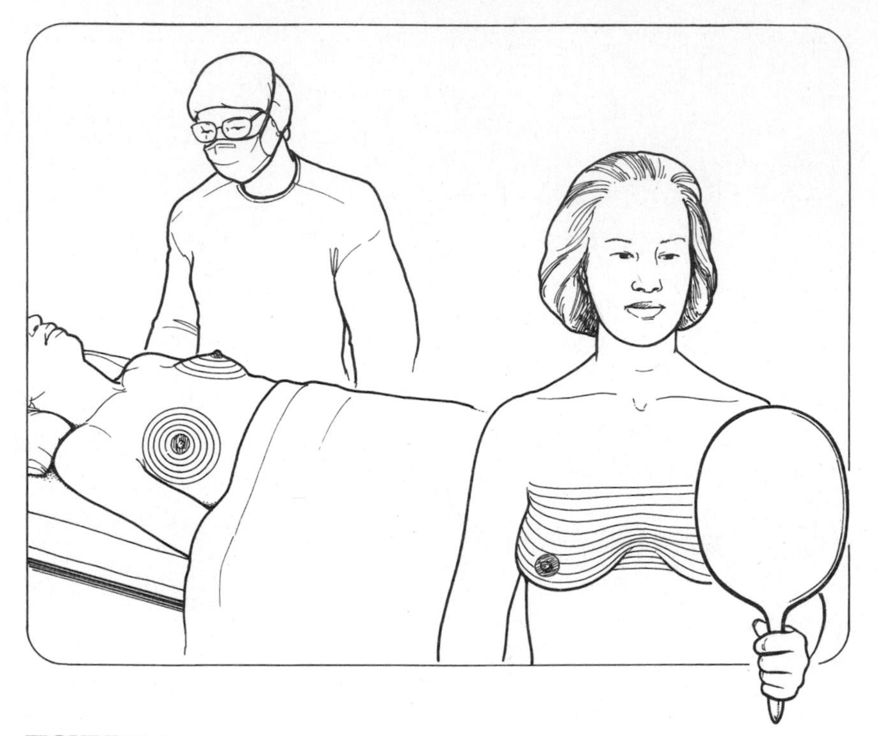

FIGURE 21-3

together and instead sewed just the subcutaneous tissue—the fat and the skin. That would leave the size as close as possible to that of the other breast.

The current trend is to do oncoplastic surgery, a combination of cancer surgery and plastic surgery. This involves using some of the techniques originally developed for reduction mammoplasties (see Chapter 3) to remove the tumor in such a way as to allow the breast to be reconstructed in a cosmetic way.[3] This approach is most important when removing a large area. If your surgeon tells you that he or she cannot remove your tumor cosmetically, you may want to get a second opinion from someone who is trained in oncoplastic surgery. Sometimes this approach looks great but the breasts won't be the same size. In that situation it is possible to reduce the uninvolved breast to match. This solves the mismatch problem mentioned above, without a dent.[4]

Another thing we realized is that if the surgeon does a horizontal incision above or even below the nipple and removes skin, it changes the nipple position, pulling it in the direction of the incision. The same thing happens with a vertical incision: the nipple gets pulled to the side, or towards the middle of the chest. A radial incision, like the spoke of a wheel, leaves the nipple position unchanged. But that too is imperfect.

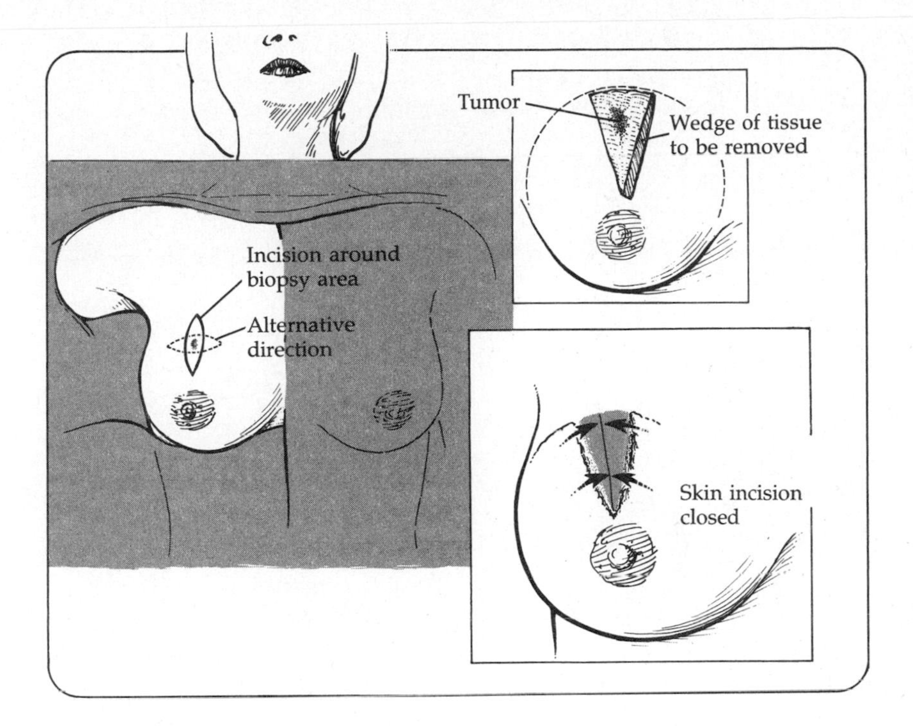

FIGURE 21-4

Radial incisions are likely to be visible in a bathing suit or a low-cut blouse, particularly if it's on the upper part of your breast. So as the patient, you have to decide which is more important: would you rather have your nipples lined up symmetrically, or would you rather have a scar that doesn't show above your bathing suit? The answer to that varies from woman to woman. These are the kinds of questions that we're just starting to look at out in terms of breast conservation. We now have an atlas to demonstrate the best techniques for all surgeons.[5]

The operation itself, however, is pretty standard. It begins with carefully monitored anesthesia, either local with sedation or general anesthetic. If a sentinel node biopsy is going to be done, the surgeon starts with an injection of blue dye. The lumpectomy will be done after the nodes. If a full axillary dissection is being done, then the lumpectomy usually comes first.

Lumpectomy

The surgeon usually starts by taking out the lump with a rim of normal tissue around it. If there is a lot of DCIS the tissue may be removed in a wedge, like a piece of pie (Fig. 21-4). That piece is given intact to the pathologist, oriented with sutures. Then the tissue and skin are sutured together. Some surgeons put drains into the breast to collect fluid afterward. I found this unnecessary and rarely did it.

Sentinel Node Biopsy

A sentinel node biopsy is often done prior to lumpectomy so that the blue dye can be injected and the axillary incision made within five minutes. If a whole dissection is being done (see Chapter for 17 for discussion of options) the surgeon will begin operating on the lymph nodes after the breast surgery is finished (Fig. 21-5). If you are unlikely to have cancer in a node, sentinel node biopsy (see Chapter 8) is likely to be done. It gives you the advantage of being sure there's no cancer in the nodes without the complications of a full dissection. In the rare case when the pathologist then finds a positive node, you can undergo a full dissection at a later date to make sure it was the only one. Sometimes when the sentinel node is removed and is positive, the surgeon proceeds directly to a full axillary dissection. It's important to have the rest of the nodes out in this case because there may be cancer in other nodes and they need to be treated.

The procedure for a sentinel node biopsy is relatively new and the technical details are still being figured out. Some favor using blue dye; others like a radioactive tracer; many prefer to do both. Blue dye can be given at the time of the surgery because it spreads to the nodes quickly. The doctor can inject the blue dye as soon as the patient is asleep. By contrast, the radioactive tracer must be given at least two hours ahead of time, since it takes that long to get from the tumor to the lymph node.

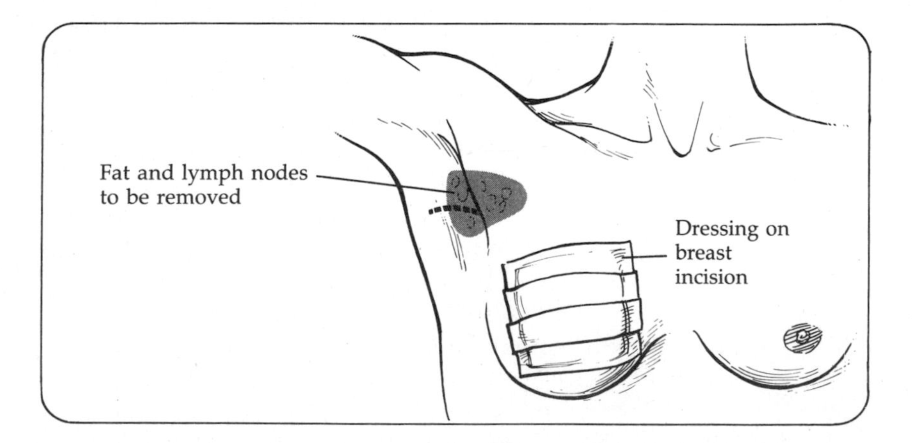

FIGURE 21-5

It's usually injected under local anesthetic, around where the tumor is or was. Most surgeons use both to make sure they don't miss anything. There is a small but real risk of allergic reaction (anaphylaxis) from the blue dye, so be sure to tell your surgeon if you have a severe sulfa allergy, as this may affect the use of the most common type of blue dye.

If you have had an injection of the radioactive tracer, the doctors have no trouble finding the node—the stereo geiger counter tells them where to make the incision. Once the incision has been made, they can then see a blue lymph vessel leading to the lymph node and track it.

Infrequently the sentinel node is not in the patient's armpit but in her chest, beneath the sternum, and here the radioactive tracer has a definite advantage. The absence of radioactivity in the armpit leads the doctor to check for it elsewhere. The usefulness of removing lymph nodes from under the breast bone is controversial, and surgeons need to weigh the pros and cons. It certainly is not clear that it will change a woman's survival rate, but if it shows positive nodes it may affect her decision about whether or not to have chemotherapy or perhaps radiotherapy to the internal mammary nodes. In general, at this stage it should only be done as part of a study.

It's always a good idea to ask your doctor what kind of procedure is being done on you. I know of a woman who had a sentinel biopsy and wasn't even aware of it. She had a lumpectomy and node removal under general anesthetic and assumed that nothing unusual was being done. Doctors removed only four nodes—all of which were tested with the usual method and showed no spread. She left the hospital certain they had gotten out all the cancer. "They told me they were 90 percent sure," she said, "but they'd call me in a few days with the rest of the results." The rest of the results came from the additional scrutiny given the sentinel node, in which they did in fact find more breast cancer. Though she felt devastated, she at least had accurate information on which to base her decisions.

Most doctors tell you what procedures they're planning. Barbara, a flight attendant I met when she volunteered for my nipple fluid studies (see Chapter 13), was happy to have both the sentinel node biopsy and a full axillary dissection. She knew that with sentinel node biopsy as part of the process, doctors would remove fewer lymph nodes. (Not everyone does this. There are still some surgeons who honestly say that they do both because they are not confident about their skills. In that case, ask if they will let another, more experienced, surgeon scrub in for that part of the operation.). Barbara was particularly concerned, since she was afraid that with many nodes removed, she was likely to have lymphedema, which would probably be exacerbated by the constant changes of air pressure involved in her job. So far she has had no swelling since the procedure.

Her doctor injected the radioactive dye before the surgery. "I lay on the table, and the camera doing a lymphoscintigraphy scan came down at me. It looked like a huge diving bell," she said. "When the nuclear medicine was shot in, it was painful." The doctor waited five minutes after the anesthetic and then put the dye into one breast. Because both breasts were affected, the procedure took about an hour. She was lying on a gurney, and every ten minutes the camera took another picture to see if the tracer had moved to a lymph node yet. "This diving bell camera was practically in my face, and I couldn't move at all," she says. "But at least it wasn't as bad as the MRI, where I *really* couldn't move. Here at least I could scratch my nose if I had to in between pictures!"

The surgery lasted several hours, and she stayed overnight in the hospital. "At 9:00 P.M., I had to go to the john, and the nurse helped me. My pee was a bright cobalt blue. I had known about it, but the poor nurse hadn't and she was really shocked." There was also some blue in her breasts, which took about a month to clear out. Rarely the dye can tattoo the breast for a year and still be normal: this happens when it is taken up by the lymphatics in the skin.

They took out a number of nodes—9 in her right underarm and 15 in her left. They had done a test called *immunohistochemical keratin stain* on the sentinel nodes and found micrometastases. (See Chapter 17 for further discussion; if it is only IHC [immunohistochemical] positive and H&E [hematoxycin and eosin staining] is negative, this is not reason for a dissection.)

The operation on her nodes left her with several weeks of discomfort. "I felt like I had a wad of scotch tape under each armpit," she recalls. "For about two weeks, I couldn't stand my arm and chest skin meeting." By the end of a month the discomfort left, and it was never bad enough to make her take the painkillers the doctors had given her.

Full Axillary Dissection

A full axillary dissection is done either because there are palpable nodes or a positive node was found on sentinel node biopsy or the surgeon is not experienced in the sentinel node technique.

The surgeon makes an incision about two inches across the armpit and then removes the wad of fat in the hollow of the armpit, which contains many of the lymph nodes. The lymph nodes, as I said earlier, are glands. Sometimes they're swollen and big, but usually they're small and embedded in fat. This lump of fat is defined by certain anatomical boundaries and usually contains at least 10–15 lymph nodes. We hope, but can't be sure, that we've included in this fat the significant lymph nodes. The tissue is sent to the pathologist, who examines the fat and tries to find as many of the lymph nodes as possible. The pathologist then cuts each node in half, makes slides, and examines each of them for cancer.

This is where we see the advantage of sentinel node biopsy. We find the one or two nodes that are most likely to have cancer, so we don't worry that we may miss a node that's hiding in a corner somewhere. And since the pathologist knows that this is the node to check, it will be checked more thoroughly than the many nodes in a regular node dissection (see Chapter 15). Thus there's less room for error.

Some women have more nodes than others. Occasionally a patient asks me, "How come you got 17 lymph nodes in me and only 7 in my friend?" We are all built differently. This difference was brought to my attention one time after I did a routine axillary dissection. A new pathologist was dissecting out the nodes and amazed me by finding 40 in a specimen that usually would contain 15. She just looked harder than usual.

However, the total number of nodes is less important than the number that are positive. It is important for the surgeon to remove the tissue that probably contains the nodes. Studies have shown that the chance of missing a positive lymph node if we remove the tissue in the lower two levels of the armpit is less than 5 percent.[6]

Some surgeons put a drain in the axillary incision afterward, but I preferred not to—there's not enough fluid to worry about, in my experience.[7] I would put a little long-acting local anesthetic into the wound, so my patient didn't wake up in pain later, and then sew up the incision.

The operation takes from one to three hours. When you go home you'll have a small dressing on your incision. Depending on the practice of the surgeon there may or may not be sutures to remove, but most surgeons like to see their patients ten days to two weeks after the surgery to monitor their progress. An earlier visit can be scheduled to discuss pathology results.

Risks and Complications of Partial Mastectomy

There may be some loss of sensation in your breast after a partial mastectomy, depending on the size of the lump removed. If it's a large lump, there may be a permanent numb spot, but there won't be the total loss of sensation that results from a mastectomy.

Your breast may be different in size and shape than it was before and will probably differ from your other breast. How great the difference depends on how much tissue was removed and how skillfully the surgery was done. If your breasts have become asymmetrical to an extent that disturbs you, you can get partial mastectomy breast pads called shells to wear in your bra. Or you can have reconstructive surgery: a small flap of your own tissue is put in to fill things out (see Chapter 22). Or, depending on how large your breasts were to begin with, you can get the other breast reduced to create a more symmetrical appearance. Usually, however, that isn't necessary. If you have a small lump and medium or large breasts, it's often hard to tell which breast was operated on, except for the scar.

The possible complications resulting from lymph node surgery are more serious. There's a nerve—and sometimes two or three nerves—going through the middle of the fat that is removed. This nerve gives you sensation in the back part of your armpit, though it doesn't affect the way your arm works. If that nerve is cut, you'll have a patch of numbness in the back part of your arm (Fig. 21-6). Most breast surgeons and many general surgeons try to save the nerve. Even if the surgeon does save it, it may get stretched and cause decreased sensation either temporarily or permanently. If the sensation is gone for more than a few months, the loss is probably permanent. This problem is less common after sentinel node biopsy but is certainly not eliminated. (If this happens to you, you may want to give up shaving your armpits, or use an electric shaver rather than a razor, which is more likely to cut the skin and cause bleeding.)

Another complication, one that's not unusual, is fluid under the armpit. Most women have some swelling, but sometimes a woman

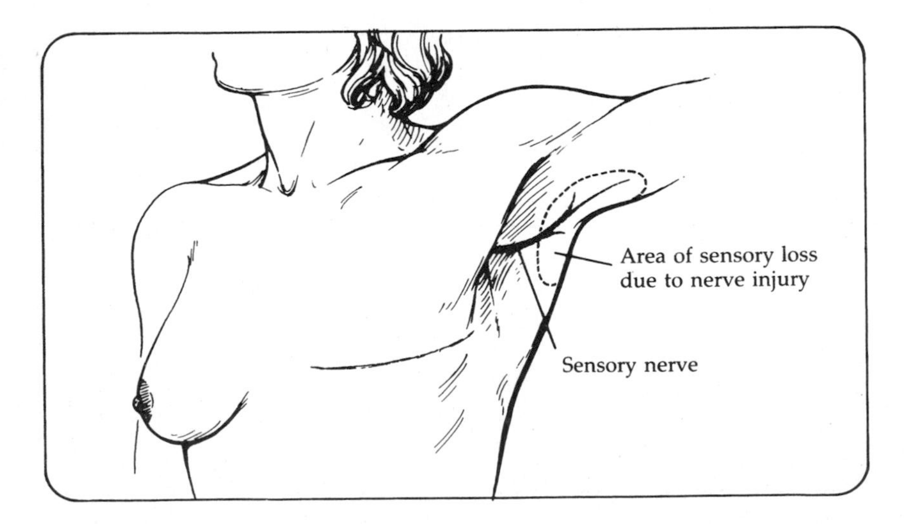

FIGURE 21-6

will get so much that it looks like she has an orange in her armpit. Usually the fluid is aspirated by the doctor in the office.

Very rarely a patient gets a hematoma from surgery and can remain sore and dramatically bruised for several weeks. The surgical dressing tape may cause a rash known as tape burn.

Another early problem can be phlebitis in an arm vein. This usually shows up three or four days after surgery. The woman says, "I felt wonderful after the operation and now I have this tight feeling under my arm that goes down to the elbow and sometimes even to the wrist. And I can see a cord. The pain is worse and I can't move my arm nearly as well as I could before." This has recently been called axillary web syndrome and is very common.[8] I have always felt that it is an inflammation of the basilic vein, but others think it is just a general inflammation from the dissection. It's not serious but it's bothersome. The best treatment is ice and aspirin or an NSAID (nonsteroidal anti-inflammatory drug) such as ibuprofen. It will go away within several days to a week.

The major complication, but fortunately an uncommon one, is swelling of the arm, a condition called *lymphedema,* which we'll consider in Chapter 26.

Another rare complication of lymph node surgery involves the motor nerves (or nerves that go to muscles and control movement) (Fig. 21-7). Two motor nerves can be injured by lymph node surgery. One of them—the long thoracic nerve—goes to the muscle that holds your shoulder blade against your back when you hold your arm straight out. If that nerve is injured, your shoulder blade, instead of remaining

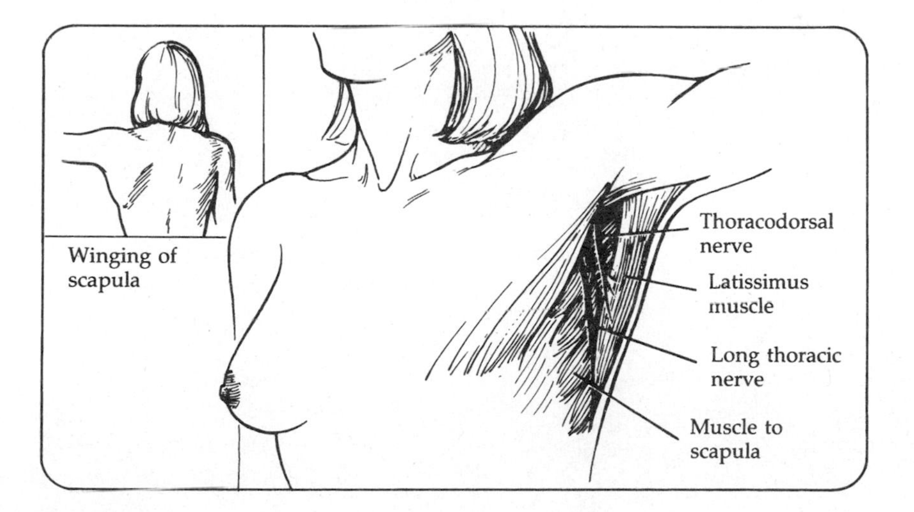

FIGURE 21-7

flat, will stick out like a wing when you hold your arm out. Hence the deformity is called a winged scapula. (There are other causes of winged scapula as well; sometimes it's a congenital condition.) If you're not athletic, it probably won't affect your daily activities, but it affects things like serving in tennis or pitching a baseball.

Permanent winged scapula cases are extremely rare; if the condition is temporary, it should go away in a few weeks or months. Physical therapy can help, especially if an athlete—even a golfer—is affected.

The other nerve is called the thoracodorsal nerve, and it goes to the latissimus muscle. Damage to this nerve is rare and less noticeable than the winged scapula. It is likely to produce a sensation of tiredness in the arm, which won't work quite as well as it did before. This could be a problem for an athlete, since the latissimus dorsi is involved in chin-ups, overhead tennis serves, golf drives, and swimming.

At Home After Partial Mastectomy

Your surgeon may put your arm in a sling to protect the incision from being pulled apart. I never liked to do this; I think the earlier you start moving your arm normally the less chance there is that it will get stiff. Keeping the arm in a sling will cause it to stiffen, even if you haven't had an operation. If your arm is kept immobile for any length of time, you'll need physical therapy to help you start using it again. But if you do use your arm normally right away, you probably won't need the therapy (see Chapter 26). Patients are sore and don't tend to fling their arms about anyway. You shouldn't lift more than about five pounds with that arm for several days, but then you can use it normally.

Once you're home, you'll be exhausted for a while. Respect that tiredness: you've just been through major surgery, anesthesia, and an emotionally difficult experience. The exhaustion often comes and goes suddenly: you'll feel fine and go out shopping; when you get home you'll suddenly feel completely wiped out and need to sleep. It will take a several days for you to feel fully recovered.

You'll have some pain but probably not a lot. Most doctors give their patients pain medication—usually Vicodin or codeine—when they go home, but the majority of women don't finish off the prescription. Occasionally people have a lot of pain, and if that's the case it's a good idea to let the doctor know. It's often a sign of something wrong, like postoperative bleeding or a hematoma.

After a lumpectomy, you should wear a strong support bra day and night for about a week—it hurts when your breast jiggles. Another trick my patients taught me, particularly my patients with larger breasts, is that if you want to lie on your side, you can lie on the side

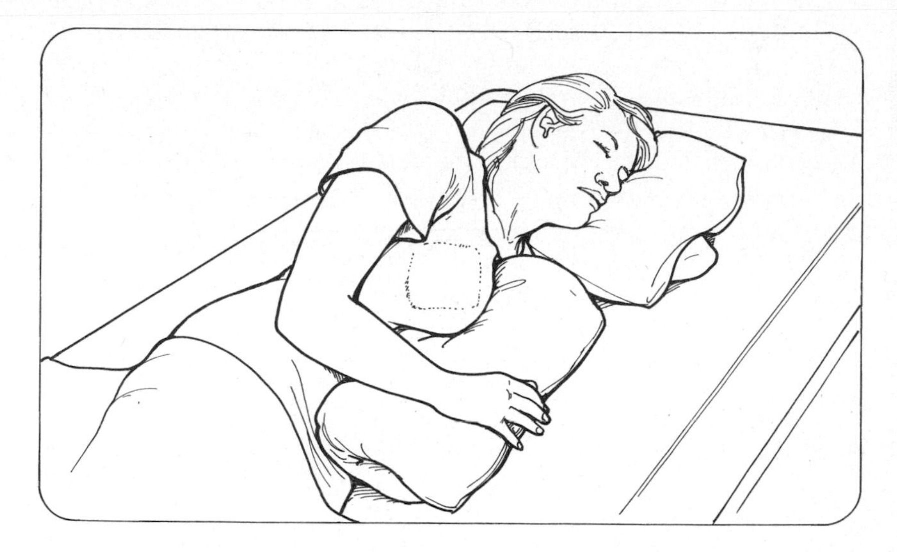

FIGURE 21-8

that wasn't operated on and hold a pillow between your breasts: the pillow cushions the breast that's been operated on (Fig. 21-8).

The pathology results are usually available in a couple of days. The surgeon can then tell the patient what the margins were like and what was actually in her breast tissue and, most important, whether there was any cancer in the lymph nodes. On the basis of the pathology report, you'll discuss the next steps, and whether there is a need for adjuvant therapy.

TOTAL MASTECTOMY

In spite of the availability of partial mastectomy and radiation, which conserve the breast, most women in this country have total mastectomies as their initial therapy for breast cancer.

Total mastectomy should not be confused with radical mastectomy. The latter, once the norm, is now of interest for historical reasons only. The surgical procedure was basically the same as that for the modified radical (described below), but more extensive. In addition to trying to remove all the breast tissue, the surgeon removed the pectoralis major and pectoralis minor muscles (see Fig. 21-9). All of the lymph nodes in the axillary area (up to the collarbone) were removed as well. It was far more deforming than the mastectomy we do now. Today we almost always use neoadjuvant chemotherapy to shrink very large tumors before surgery (see Chapter 19). If the tumor is stuck to the muscle, the

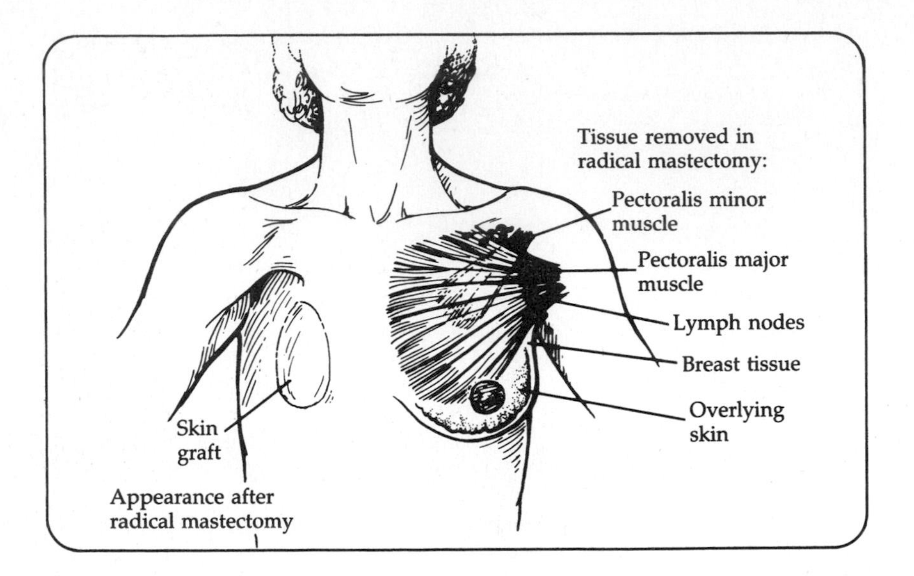

FIGURE 21-9

surgeon must remove the muscle in order to get to the tumor. (In very rare cases the cancer spreads into the muscle.) We used to do radical mastectomies in all of these cases, but now we just take a wedge of muscle under the tumor and leave the rest.

"Total mastectomy," the name usually given to the form of mastectomy used today, is a bit of a misnomer, since we can never be certain the operation is total. Our goal is to remove all the breast tissue, but we can't even be sure we've achieved that. We remove as much of the breast tissue as we can and some of the lymph nodes. It usually takes between two and five hours.

The breast tissue extends from the collarbone down to just below the fold and from the breastbone out to the muscle in the back of the armpit. The surgeon wants to remove as much of it as possible and starts with an elliptical incision that includes the nipple and biopsy scar: exactly where it is depends on where your biopsy scar is (Fig. 21-10).

With the increasing popularity of immediate reconstruction, surgeons have taken to removing as little skin as possible. We used to take out a large amount of skin when we did mastectomies, believing that would help keep the cancer from spreading. It was really a holdover from the old theory of radical mastectomy—take out as much as you can. We also liked the fact that this helped the scar close neatly. If the surgeon leaves a lot of skin and scoops out all the breast tissue, the skin looks wrinkled and baggy. Trimming the skin creates a nice neat line

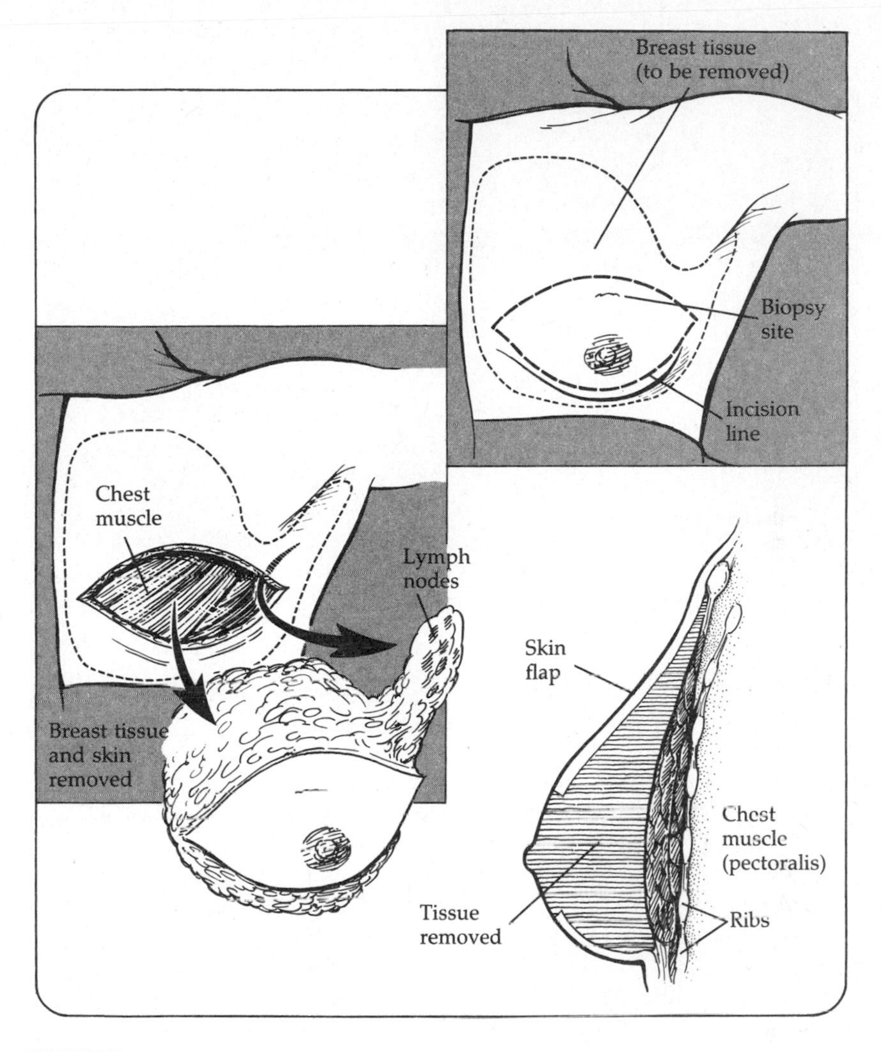

FIGURE 21-10

across the chest. But now, as immediate reconstructions are being done, the need to take off so much skin is being reconsidered. We've moved into the era of skin-sparing mastectomy. Instead of removing a lot of skin around the breast, surgeons remove only the amount that's needed to take the breast off, unless the patient is absolutely sure she never wants reconstruction; then it's nice to be tidy. We've begun to view mastectomy as a very wide excision. Removing every bit of breast tissue isn't possible or necessary: it's getting the tumor out that really matters (Fig. 21-11).

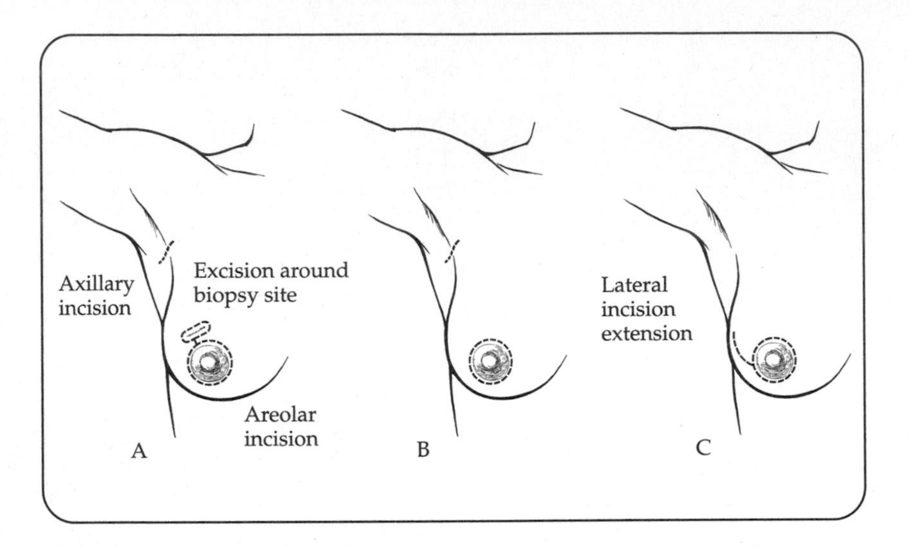

FIGURE 21-11 Skin sparing masectomy Incisions

Next we tunnel underneath the remaining skin all the way up to the collarbone, then down to just below the inframammary fold (see Chapter 2) from the middle of the sternum, and out to the muscle behind your armpit. Once the dissection is done, we peel the breast off, leaving the muscle behind.

When the breast is fully removed, we reach up under the skin to the armpit and do an axillary dissection or sentinel node biopsy as described earlier. We send the breast tissue and the attached fat with nodes to the pathologist, who examines it and begins the process of fixing it to make slides. Meanwhile we sew together the flaps of skin around the incision. You end up completely flat (or, if you're very thin, slightly concave), with a scar going across the middle of that side of your chest. The skin doesn't completely stick down right away; the body doesn't like empty spaces, so the area fills up with fluid. To prevent this, we insert some drains in soft plastic tubes with little holes in them, coming out of the skin below the scar (Fig. 21-12). They help create suction that holds the skin down against the muscle till it heals. Fluid will come out of these drains—it's just tissue fluid, the kind you get in a blister. Initially there'll be a little blood in the fluid, but over time it will become clearer.

If you've decided to have immediate breast reconstruction (see Chapter 22), the plastic surgeon comes in after the mastectomy is finished but before the skin is sewn up and does the reconstruction. Alternatively, the plastic surgeon may be part of the team from the beginning, raising the flap while the surgeon is doing the mastectomy.

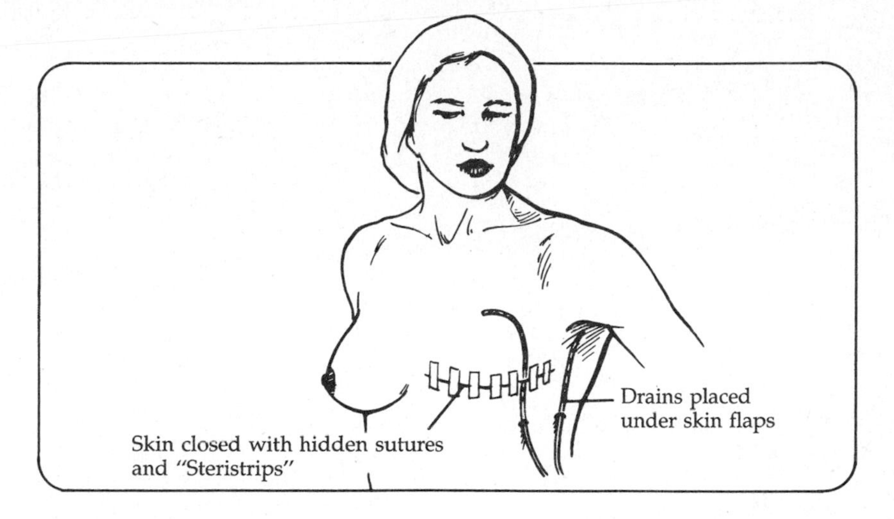

FIGURE 21-12

As with partial mastectomy, the pathology results will be available in a couple of days.

Different surgeons have different styles in postoperative treatment. I usually put a big, bulky wraparound dressing on my patients because it helped them feel protected from the world for a while. My colleague Susan Troyan has switched to a light gauze dressing with a plastic covering so that the woman can shower and move more freely. You'll probably stay in the hospital at least overnight. When there's no longer much fluid coming out of the drains—in about three or four days—we remove them and change the dressing. We used to keep people in the hospital till all the drains came out, but nowadays patients sometimes go home and come back later to get the drains removed.

Some women want to see the wound right away; some prefer to put off looking at it for a week or two. Either way is fine; you need to decide what makes you feel best. But it's important that you look at it at some point. It's amazing how, if you're determined to avoid looking at your body, you can do so when you shower, get dressed, even when you make love. That's okay for a while, but this is the body you're going to be living with, and you need to see it and accept it.

Many of my patients liked me to be with them the first time they saw their scar so that I could offer emotional support and answer any questions they had. If you would like your surgeon with you when you first look at your chest, ask.

Others want to see it alone before showing it to their husband or lover. Again, there's no right or wrong way to face it, as long as you do.

In my experience, most women are relieved when it doesn't look as bad as they feared it would.

Permanent numbness in the area around the mastectomy scar is an unfortunate result of the operation, since the breast's nerve supply has been cut. Some sensitivity remains around the outer borders of the area on which your breast was located. Sometimes the breast area is not entirely numb, however; you can tell if someone is touching you. Unfortunately this usually isn't a pleasant sensitivity. It can be very uncomfortable, like the sensation you feel when your foot is asleep and starts coming back again, with a tingly feeling. This is known as dysesthesia, and it will lessen but will remain with you. Often people who have had mastectomies don't like their scars being touched because it brings about this sensation. Some women will recover sensation over a long time.

Some women also experience phantom breast symptoms—like the amputee who feels itchiness in toes that are no longer there. The mastectomy patient may feel her missing nipple itch or her missing breast ache. This means that the brain hasn't yet realized what's happened to the body. The nerve supply from the breast grows along a certain path in the spinal cord and goes to a certain area of the brain. The brain has been trained over the years that a signal from this path means, for example, that the nipple is itching. When the nipple has been removed, the signal may get generated in a different place farther along the path, but the brain cells think it should be coming from the nipple, and that's the information they give you. This will gradually improve as your brain becomes reprogrammed.

Audre Lorde described these feelings wonderfully well in her book *The Cancer Journal*: "fixed pains and moveable pains, deep pains and surface pains, strong pains and weak pains. There were stabs and throbs and burns, gripes and tickles and itches."[9] In addition, some women feel tightness around the chest as the healing starts. This will ease up over time, and all the weird sensations will start to settle down.

Risks and Complications of Total Mastectomy

Like any operation, mastectomy has its risks. In the process of removing the breast tissue, we sever a number of blood vessels. The only ones left are those that go the whole length of the flap of skin remaining when the tissue underneath is removed. These vessels can barely get to the ends of the flap. Sometimes this doesn't supply enough blood, and the wound doesn't heal right; a little area of skin dies and forms a scab (Fig. 21-13). Once healing is complete, the scab falls off.

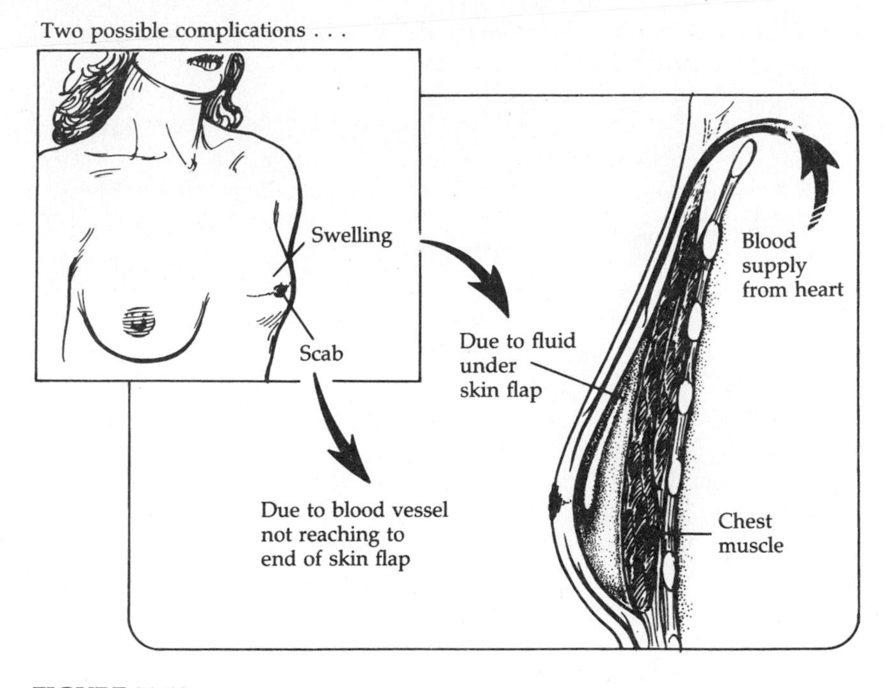

FIGURE 21-13

It's usually not a serious complication. If a big enough area of skin is involved or an infection develops, the surgeon may have to trim the dead tissue so the body can heal the wound.

A second possible complication occurs when fluid continues to collect under the scar after the drains are removed. You'll know this is happening because there's a swelling under the skin below the incision; sometimes you'll hear a slosh when you're walking or you'll feel the fluid on your chest. If it's a small amount of fluid, you can just leave it alone and it will eventually go away by itself. If there's a lot of fluid, you can have it aspirated with a needle: it won't hurt, since the area is numb, and it usually doesn't require local anesthesia. (We try to avoid too many aspirations, since there's always the slight risk of transmitting infection through the needle.) Again, this isn't a serious complication, but it can be annoying.

The risks from the lymph node removal—loss of sensation, phlebitis, lymphedema (see Chapter 26) or swelling and winged scapula—are the same as for partial mastectomy and axillary dissection. Again, it's important to move your arm and keep it from stiffening. Ellen Mahoney, a breast surgeon I admire in Northern California, tells her patients to keep their hand behind their head while reading or watching TV postoperatively to stretch the scar.

Many doctors and nurses send you home with extensive instructions regarding care of your arm after surgery. They are trying to prevent infections, which are more likely to occur when lymph nodes are gone. So they insist that you never garden without gloves because you may get pricked by a thorn, or that you never reach into a hot oven, or cut your cuticles, or have injections in that arm. Be sensible: you want to reduce the risk of infection, but a minor infection isn't going to kill you, and there's no need to live your life in terror of pinpricks. Be reasonably careful, and if an infection does develop, see your doctor as soon as possible and have it treated to prevent lymphedema. Although you should try to avoid significant trauma to the involved arm (blood draws, blood pressure cuffs), this is not as vital as it was in the days of radical mastectomy. By all means avoid carrying heavy objects with your arm hanging down for any length of time, such as a suitcase or briefcase. Try to get your groceries delivered instead of carrying them yourself; if that's not feasible, get one of those little portable grocery carts and wheel them home. Use suitcases with wheels when you travel.

Exercise After Mastectomy

Exercise is important after your treatment, and not only in terms of lymphedema. Again, some doctors can be overrestrictive. After you've

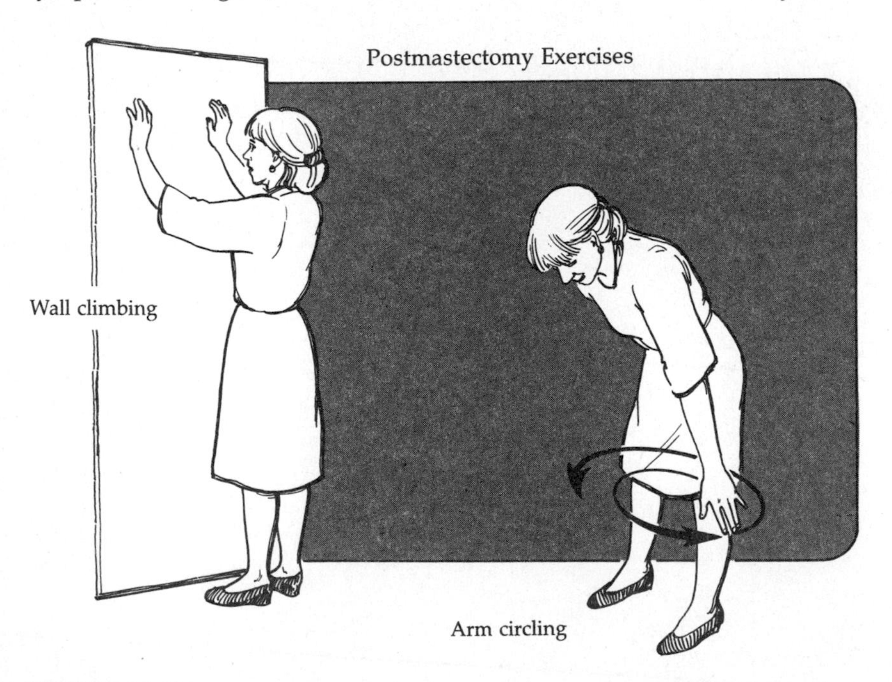

FIGURE 21-14

had a mastectomy or a lymph node sampling, your surgeon may tell you not to move your arm at all. There's a lot of controversy about how protective of the area you should be.

As I mentioned before, if you do keep your arm very still at first, you'll probably find your shoulder extremely stiff when you start moving around.

Certain exercises actually help your shoulder (Fig. 21-13). One is called "climbing the walls." It involves walking your fingers up the wall, stretching a little bit farther each time. You can do it while you're watching TV or talking on the phone. The other one involves leaning over and making bigger and bigger circles with your arm. Swimming is also excellent exercise.

If your arm remains very stiff after two or three weeks, ask your doctor to refer you to a physical therapist. About 10–15 percent of my patients needed physical therapy. It's very important to get your shoulder flexible again, and soon; otherwise you can end up with frozen shoulder, a condition that is difficult to treat successfully. If you already have shoulder problems, see a physical therapist preoperatively for advice.

Any sport or exercise you did before your cancer, you can do now—and you should, if you want to.

22

Reconstruction and Prosthesis

If you're having a mastectomy or have had one, you'll need to decide whether, and how, to recreate the appearance of a breast. Most women take it for granted that they have to appear to the outside world as having both breasts. For years, there was only one way to do that—through a prosthesis, a sort of elaborate falsie designed for women with mastectomies (Fig. 22-1). Nowadays, there is another option, the reconstruction of an artificial breast mound and nipple that, to a greater or lesser extent, appear real.

Before you decide on one of these options, you may want to consider a third possibility—not disguising your mastectomy at all. It's not a choice many women make, but there are a few who do choose it, without regrets. One of my patients thought about her options, then concluded that "a prosthesis sounded too uncomfortable, and reconstruction hasn't been around long enough to see what long-term effects it can have. And then I decided I was comfortable with the way I look." She goes to work, jogs in a loose T-shirt, and feels that "it's other people's problem if they're uncomfortable with it." Once in a while, she feels a need to look more "normal"—especially when she has important meetings with new business associates. Her solution is to stuff shoulder pads from her dresses into her bra. "I never liked

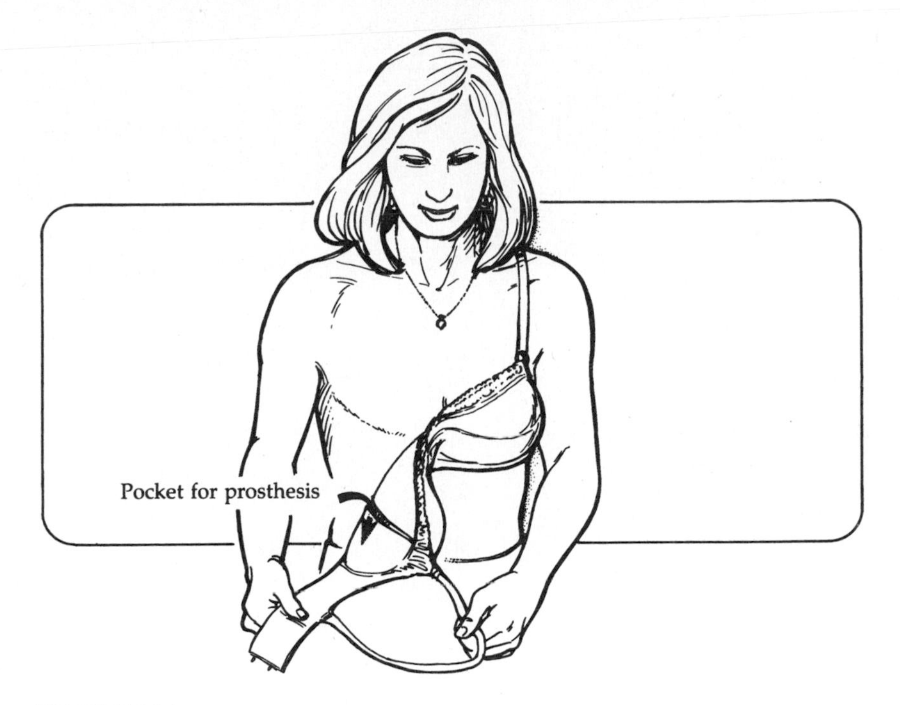

FIGURE 22-1

shoulder pads anyway," she laughs. "Now I get to put them to good use!" For other women, refusing to create the illusion of a breast is part of their feminist beliefs. Artist Matuschka has created photographs of herself in a cutaway gown, showing not her remaining breast but her mastectomy scar. One photograph was on the cover of the August 15, 1993, *New York Times Magazine*. The effect is of harshness and defiance, showing the world what breast cancer does to a woman's body. Writer Deena Metzger, whose book *Tree* addresses her cancer, includes a photograph with a different approach: she softens the effect of the amputation by covering her scar with a beautiful, evocative tattoo of a tree, creating a new beauty where the beauty of her breast once was.[1]

Having the self-confidence to feel comfortable without the appearance of a breast shows wonderful courage, but most of us are products of our culture and need to feel cosmetically acceptable to the outside world. In some cases there are actual penalties for failing to appear "normal." If nonconformity will cost you your job, for example, you're likely to want to have reconstruction or wear a prosthesis (or breast form, as it's also called) at least part of the time.

PROSTHESES

The option of wearing a prosthesis will probably be offered to you right away. In most areas of the country the hospital arranges for someone to visit you to talk about prostheses while you're still there. Your visitor will be from Reach for Recovery or a firm that sells prostheses. You can get a temporary prosthesis first and then shop around for a permanent one. The prosthesis fits into a pocket in a postmastectomy bra. You can shop for them in person or on the web, from catalogs, in medical supply houses, or in fancy lingerie stores. Each supplier has its advantages and disadvantages. You may be put off by the implications of mutilation, the wheelchairs and artificial limbs in medical supply outlets; or you may feel painfully reminded of the breast you no longer have in a lingerie store. Your doctor or the American Cancer Society can help you find the stores, catalogs, or websites to buy your prosthesis, or you can ask friends who've had mastectomies. Y-ME, a volunteer organization of breast cancer survivors, will send you a prosthesis if they have the size required in stock, for a nominal fee.

There are stores that will make a custom prosthesis for you; it's expensive and your insurance company may not pay for it, but you might want a precise match. (It's a good idea to check with your insurance company before buying your prosthesis anyway; different companies have different quirks, and you may want to be sure of what your own expenses will be.) Medicare pays for a prosthesis every year or two years—with a prescription. (Why you need a prescription for a prosthesis, I don't know—I've never met a woman who bought one for the fun of it. But the ways of bureaucracies are mysterious.) There are also specific forms for swimming, though most of the better prostheses are made of silicone and are waterproof.

Prostheses come in a range of prices and quality. If you don't have insurance to pay for one, or if you haven't decided between prosthesis or reconstruction, you'll probably want the least expensive form available, at least temporarily. Catalogs and many stores offer forms for as low as $15 and mastectomy bras for around $10.

Prostheses are made in different sizes and for different operations. If you had a radical mastectomy, you can get a fuller prosthesis. If you had a wide excision that's left you noticeably asymmetrical, you can get a small "filler," or shell that fits comfortably in your bra. In the past, prostheses didn't have nipples, which caused problems for women whose remaining breast had a prominent nipple (Betty Rollin in her book *First, You Cry* has a very funny description of her efforts to make her own "nipple" out of cloth buttons.)[2] Fortunately any prosthesis you buy now has a nipple, and you can get a separate nipple to attach to it if your own nipple is more prominent that the one on the prosthesis.

Some situations may affect what makes a prosthesis right for you. Certain kinds of disabilities, for example, can make a particular form uncomfortable. Judith Rogers, an activist in Breast Health Access for Disabilities, has mild cerebral palsy, and she found that her first prosthesis caused problems. "It was good in terms of matching the size of my remaining breast," she says. "But it was bad for my shoulder: it was too heavy for me. It pulled down, harming my muscles and increasing the effects of lymphedema." When she got a lighter one, she had less pain. You need to take time to consider all the factors involving your body and mind when you choose a prosthesis.

RECONSTRUCTION

Another option is reconstruction—the creation, by a plastic surgeon, of a new and natural-appearing breast. Breast reconstruction has made a big difference both physically and emotionally for many women who have had mastectomies. But it's important to understand its limits before you decide to have it done.

What's constructed is not a real breast. It may look real, but it will never have full sensation, as a breast does. Any surgeon who says, "We're going to take off your breast and give you a new one, and it'll be as good as ever" is either naive or dishonest. The surgeon may tell you that the new breast "feels normal": at best, a half truth. It will feel normal to the hand that's touching it, but it will have little sensation itself. However, feeling is part skin sensation and part mental experience. You may have some slight "feeling" return, but it will never feel completely real to you. As a patient told me, you need time to bond with your new breast.

Is it worth doing, then? For many women, yes. It can make you feel more normal, to yourself and other people, since it looks like a breast. It can make you feel more balanced. And it can make your life a little easier—you can wear a T-shirt or a housedress and not worry about putting on a bra. If the doorbell rings while you're still in your bathrobe, you don't have to deal with whether or not you want the mail carrier to see your asymmetry. Wearing bathing suits and other "revealing" clothes is easier. In *Why Me?* Rose Kushner explains her decision to have reconstruction. She was alone in a hotel room one night, when she was awakened by a fire alarm and the smell of smoke. She jumped out of bed, threw on her clothing, grabbed her glasses, and ran. Downstairs in the lobby with the other guests, she realized that only she had gotten dressed; the others were in their robes. Then she realized why: "This 'well-adjusted' mastectomee wasn't going anywhere publicly with one breast."[3]

A reconstruction can help some women put their cancer experiences behind them. As one of my patients said, "When I was wearing my prosthesis every day, when I looked at my body and it was concave where there had been a breast, I felt that I was a cancer patient, that I was living with that every single day. With the reconstruction I feel that I'm healthy again, that I can go on with my life." Another patient says that after her mastectomy, "I always felt the hollows under my arm. After my reconstruction, I put my arms down, and something was there. That's when the tears came; it was splendid to have that back."

On the other hand, reconstruction isn't right for everybody. One of my patients regretted having it. Displeased with the appearance of her reconstructed breast, she also felt that the reconstruction functioned as a form of denial. "It caused me to postpone the mourning I had to do over losing a breast," she says. "Instead of mourning the loss of a breast, I was thinking in terms of getting a breast. So it wasn't until the process was over, and I saw my new breast, which wasn't like my other breast, that it hit me that I'd lost a breast. If I had the decision to make now, I don't think I'd have reconstruction."

The best reconstructions look like real breasts; but not all operations are equally successful, and some reconstructions look real only through bras or clothing.

Reconstructive surgery is done in a number of ways. There are two basic kinds of reconstruction—those that use artificial substances and those that use your own body tissues. Within these categories there are further variations. In the first category is the implant, which can be either silicone or saline.

Implants and Expanders

Silicone is very controversial, as I explained at length in Chapter 3. Although the FDA banned it in 1992 for use in breast enlargement, women may choose it for breast reconstruction—at least as of this writing. Although there have been 2 million implants used over the past 30 years, there is still very little information about long-term effects. The new government study discussed in Chapter 3 is designed to change that. When the implant is done for breast reconstruction, there is no fear of interfering with mammography, and there is no evidence that implants interfere with the detection of recurrences.[4]

The procedure for both silicone and saline is the same. The disadvantage of the saline is that it may feel more like water than flesh, and when it leaks the reconstruction collapses. The advantage is that it leaks harmless saline into your body and not silicone, with its possible dangers. However, it is encased in a silicone envelope. If the solid silicone is a problem (as of now we have no data), the move to saline will not eliminate it. The same lack of information holds true for other envelope substances now being used in experiments.

The implant is placed behind the pectoralis muscle and the skin is sewn together, which will give you a bulge (Fig. 22-2). The silicone has some weight and bounce to it, which helps it feel real. However, it can't give you a very large breast because it's behind the muscle, pushing everything forward, and everything has to close over the top of it. Also, the implant breast tends to stay firm, while your other breast may not. The implant won't gain and lose weight with you either. It works best in smaller-breasted women or women who have had bilateral mastectomies and are happy with small breasts. It's easier to do than the other operations. With the implant, your hospital stay won't be longer than usual. If you're having it done after your mastectomy, the hospital stay will be about two to three days.

Most plastic surgeons recognize certain categories of women for whom implants may be a better choice than the other forms of reconstruction (discussed later). For an elderly woman who wants something better than a prosthesis, something she can comfortably wear a

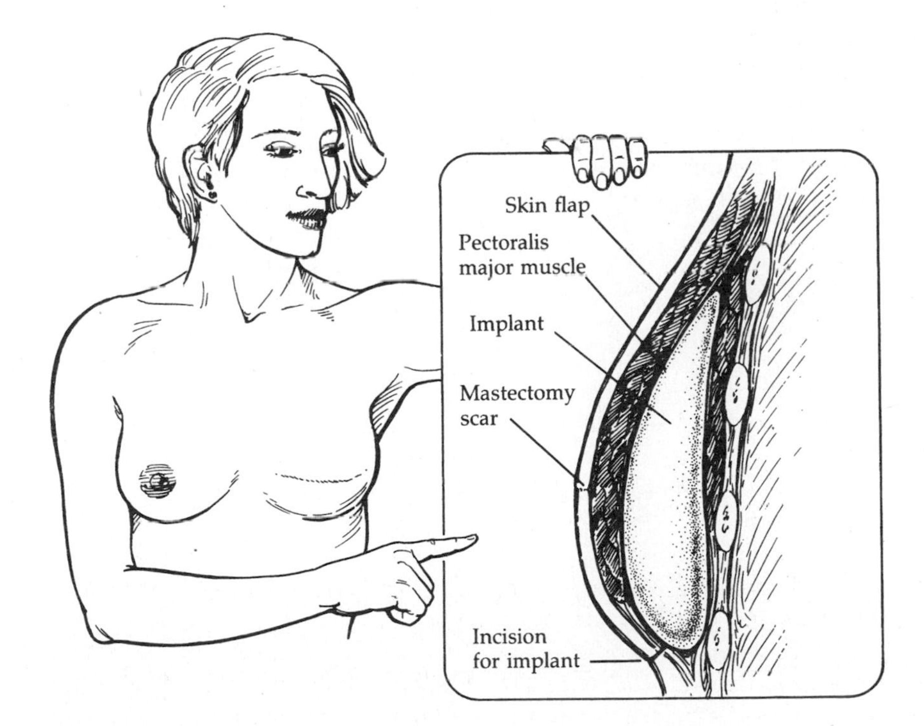

FIGURE 22-2

bra and clothes over, it may make more sense. She is unlikely to be concerned about the problems 15 or 20 years down the line, and it's an easier operation than the others. At the other end of the spectrum is the younger woman with preschool children at home. She may be most concerned with spending all the time she can with her family—and five days longer in the hospital plus the recovery from a flap surgery can make a big difference. Five or ten years later, she may want to come back and have a flap operation—but for now she just wants something to get by with.

A variation on the implant is the expander. An empty sack is placed behind the muscle and everything is sewn closed. There's a little tube and a little valve on the sack, and gradually, over the course of 3–6 months, the doctor injects more and more saline (salt water) into it, which stretches the skin (Fig. 22-3). When it achieves the size you want, the sack is removed and replaced with a permanent saline or silicone sack. The disadvantage is that the process drags out over several months, and stretching the skin and muscle can be uncomfortable. The expander will probably add no additional days to your hospital stay; if done separately, it will keep you in the hospital about two or three days.

Surgery always carries the danger of postoperative infection. An expander or implant can make infection more difficult to treat. Since they are foreign to your body an infection will not heal. One of my patients developed a very bad infection and had to have the expander removed. Moreover, implants or expanders are more likely than other procedures to necessitate your having something done to the other breast to make it match. They're going to give you a nice, perfect, 17-

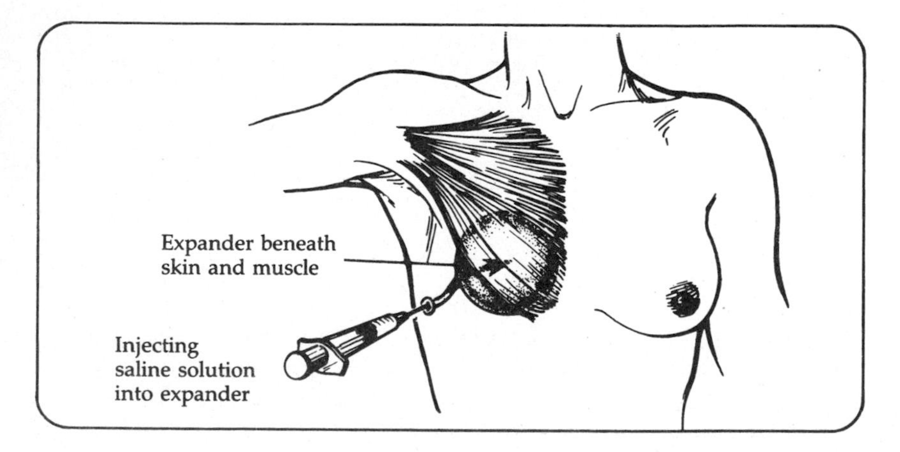

FIGURE 22-3

year-old's breast, but you're probably not a nice, perfect 17-year-old. Since the reconstructed breast doesn't sag much, it may be higher than you want it to be. One of my patients found this particularly displeasing. "The reconstructed breast didn't look like my real breast, and it was much higher," she says. "I had to start wearing a bra, which I don't like at all." So when plastic surgeons tell you implants are the easiest form of reconstruction, requiring the least amount of surgery, it's true as far as it goes. But you need to consider that it may end up involving surgery on the other breast.

It's important to let the plastic surgeon know what size you want to be. I had a flat-chested patient who wanted an implant. She wanted to stay flat-chested; that was what she was used to. But the plastic surgeon was conditioned to think that all women want large breasts. He kept trying to persuade her to let him give her a bigger implant and then enlarge her other breast to match it. Another patient had silicone implants, and the implant on one side encapsulated. But she liked the hard, firm, rocklike texture of that breast, and when she had a mastectomy on the other breast, she wanted the reconstructed breast to match the encapsulated one. The plastic surgeon again had a hard time with that—it wasn't what women are supposed to want. If you know what you want and your plastic surgeon argues with you, argue back or change plastic surgeons. It's your body, not the surgeon's, and it's you who will live with that body.

When the operation works well and the patient's expectations are realistic, implants can make a wonderful difference. As one of my patients says, "I forget it's there—it's a part of me now. It's a little harder than my other breast, but otherwise great. I don't have to worry about what I wear."

There is another important issue with implants: they don't last forever. For the woman who has implants to enlarge her breasts, replacing them can be upsetting enough. For the mastectomy patient, it can be devastating—like losing the breast all over again. Such patients almost always need the flap reconstruction described below. Having problems with the implant suggests the likelihood of having more problems later on. Patients need to weigh the comparative ease of the implant surgery against the inconvenience and emotional consequences of possible later surgeries.

I don't particularly favor either implants or expanders, though of course I would support whatever my patient wanted. But because of the inferior cosmetic effects, the mismatch with the other breast, the possibility of needing them replaced in the future, and the possible health problems with silicone, I don't personally think it's the wisest choice.

Flap Procedures

Several procedures involve using your own tissue, and that's what I tend to favor. In the *myocutaneous flap*, a flap of skin, muscle, and fat is taken from another part of your body and moved. It's better than the silicone implant in the sense that it's your own tissue, and because you've got extra skin, it can make a bigger breast and a more natural droop. You may feel more normal externally since it's real tissue, skin, and fat, though it has little sensation. These flaps can come from the abdomen (transverse rectus abdominis muscle, or TRAM flap), back (latissimus dorsi flap), or buttuck flap (gluteus maximus).

There are two different techniques for the myocutaneous flap. One is the pedicle, or attached flap (Fig. 22-4). Here the tissue is removed except for its feeding artery and vein, which remain attached, almost like a leash. The site from which the tissue was removed is sewn closed. The new little island of skin and muscle is then tunneled under the skin into the mastectomy wound. Since the blood vessels aren't cut, the blood supply remains.

The more recent operation is the "free flap." In this procedure, the tissue is removed and the feeding artery and vein are cut. Then the tissue is moved to a new location and the artery and vein are sewn to an artery or vein in the armpit; the surgeons use a microscope to see what they are doing.

The free flap is not limited to the abdomen. Free flaps can be done by transplanting tissue from other parts of the body to make a breast, such as from the buttock area *(gluteal flap)*, from the hip area (*deep circumflex iliac flap*) from the lateral thigh *(the tensor fascia lata flap)* from the inner thigh (*the gracilis flap*) or from the back *(latissimus free flap)*. This means you can have a flap reconstruction even if your abdomen has been scarred and take advantage of whatever abundance nature granted you (Fig 22-5).

The advantage of the pedicle flap is that it's easier, so more plastic surgeons can do it. A disadvantage is that we can use tissue only from locations that can stretch to the breast—the abdomen or the back. The other disadvantage is that in making the "tunnel" to the breast, we have to disturb all the tissue en route, so we're disturbing a lot of your body surface. This means that you'll have a lot of long-term complications that aren't serious but can be uncomfortable. If we take it from the abdomen, your abdominal muscle will no longer be as strong and you won't be able to do things like sit-ups. One of my patients now has to wear a panty girdle all the time to help support her weakened abdominal muscle. Another has found that since the operation the area around her upper abdomen is so sensitive that she can't wear anything with a waistband. I should add, however, that these problems are rela-

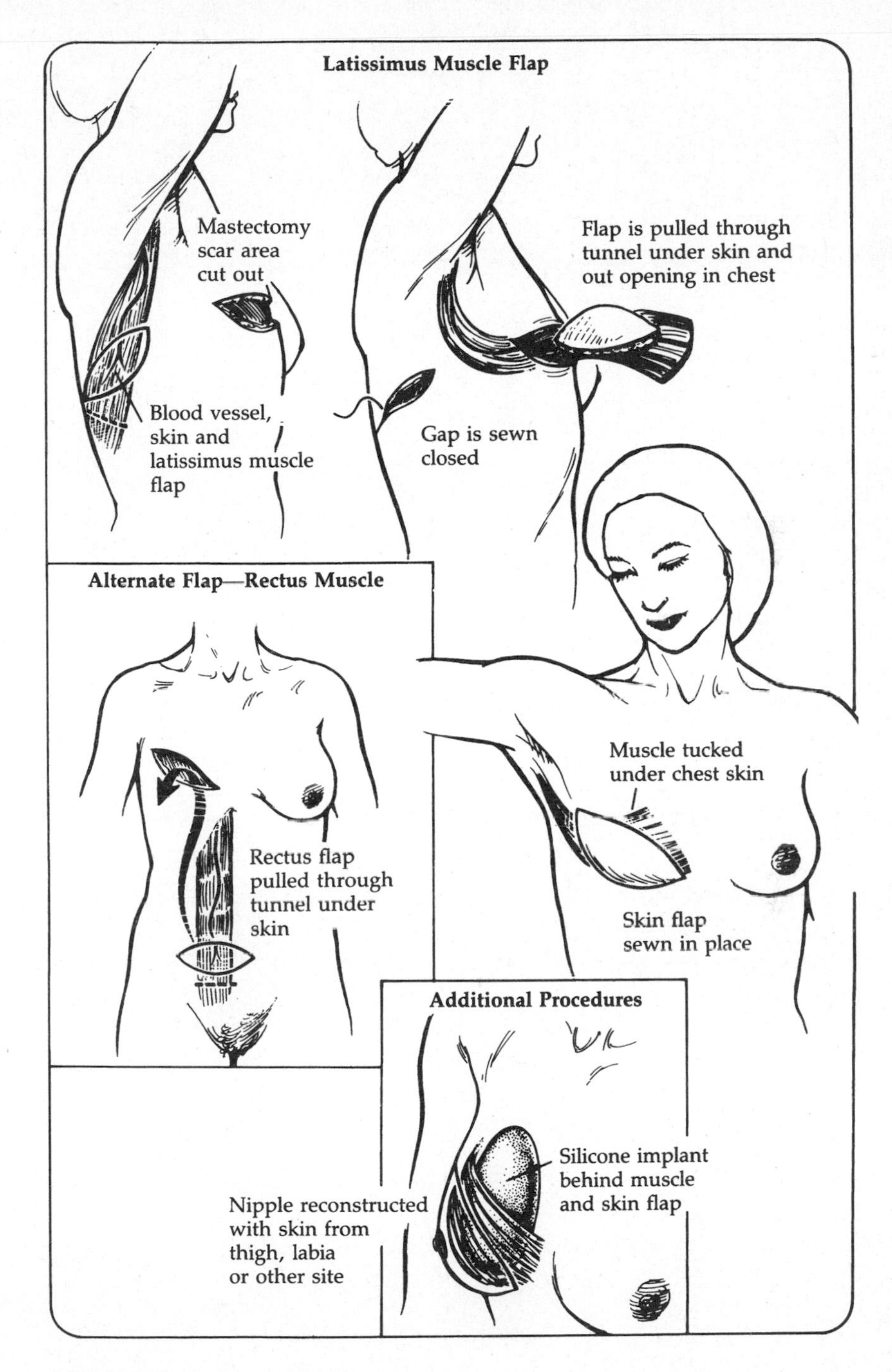
Latissimus Muscle Flap
Mastectomy scar area cut out
Blood vessel, skin and latissimus muscle flap
Flap is pulled through tunnel under skin and out opening in chest
Gap is sewn closed
Alternate Flap—Rectus Muscle
Rectus flap pulled through tunnel under skin
Muscle tucked under chest skin
Skin flap sewn in place
Additional Procedures
Silicone implant behind muscle and skin flap
Nipple reconstructed with skin from thigh, labia or other site

FIGURE 22-4

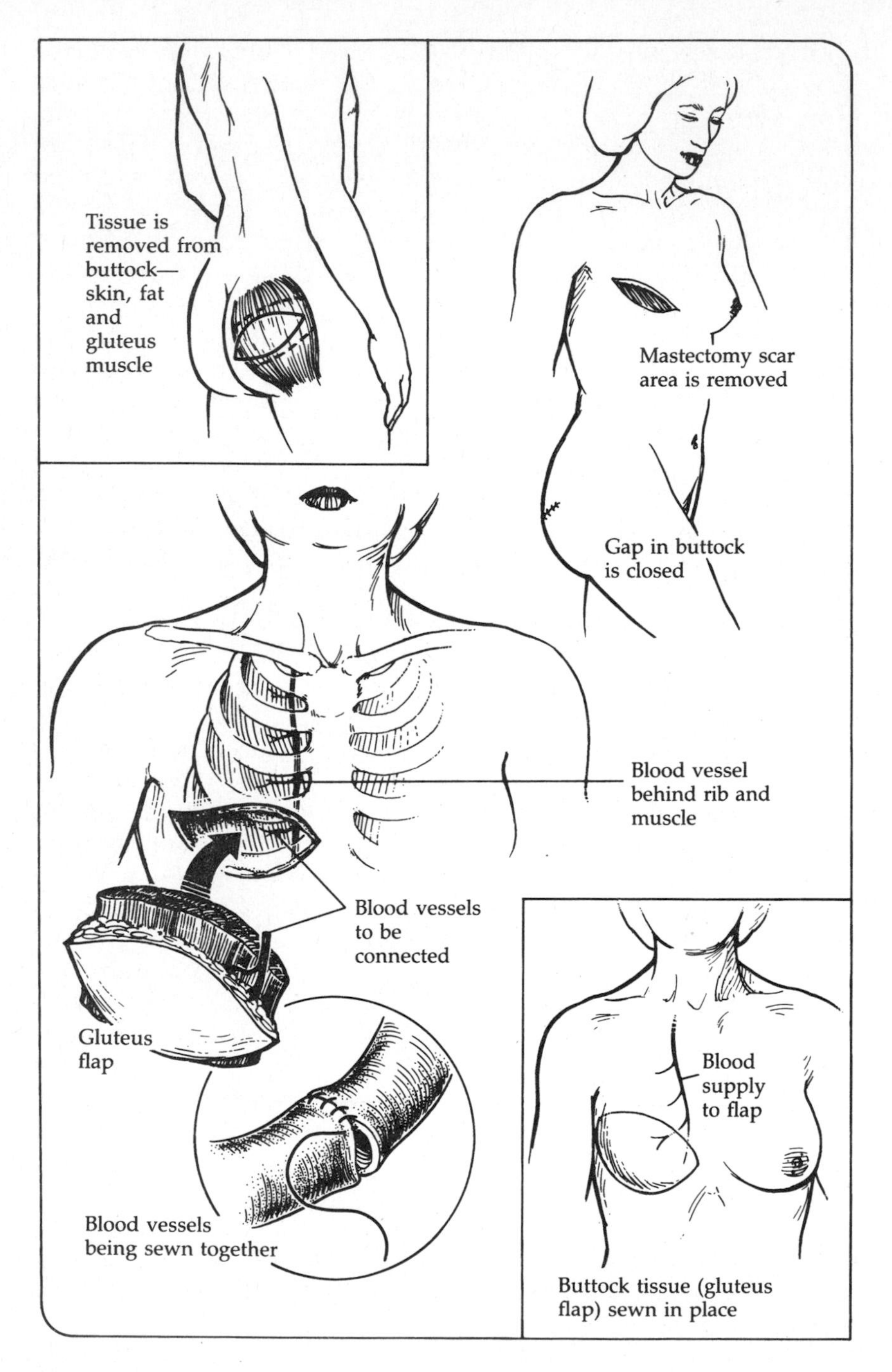
Tissue is removed from buttock—skin, fat and gluteus muscle
Mastectomy scar area is removed
Gap in buttock is closed
Blood vessel behind rib and muscle
Blood vessels to be connected
Gluteus flap
Blood vessels being sewn together
Blood supply to flap
Buttock tissue (gluteus flap) sewn in place

FIGURE 22-5

tively rare, and most patients who have had the procedure have had few problems but much satisfaction. If the tissue is taken from your back, there will be fewer problems, although it may weaken somewhat. This may interfere with shoulder strength for special sports like mountain climbing or competitive swimming. You also may need more physical therapy. Some women have a lot of stiffness and pain after this flap because it throws their whole shoulder girdle off. In either case, you'll have a scar on the area from which the flap has been taken.

With the free flap, the surgeon has to be skilled at sewing blood vessels together under the microscope (Fig. 22-6), and most plastic surgeons aren't. However, in expert hands, there are fewer complications because the tissue in between doesn't have to be disturbed: less tissue is taken out and it's simply removed and sewn closed. It's about five to eight hours of surgery, and you'll probably be in the hospital for four to seven days. If the blood supply is disturbed, part of the flap can die and further surgery will be necessary. The patient I mentioned earlier, who developed an infection from her silicone expanders, was unable to have either the latissimus (back) or rectus (abdominal) procedure because of medical problems in her back and abdomen. The free gluteous flap was the only alternative she had left; though it was difficult surgery that involved a long healing period, she feels it was well worth the pain and inconvenience.

Another variation of the free flap was introduced by Dr. Robert Allen of New Orleans, the so-called perforator flap. Instead of taking some muscle with the free flap, the surgeon dissects out the arteries that perforate through the muscle to the skin and thus spares the muscle completely. It was found that with a sufficient number of perforating arteries to support the skin and fat, there is no need to take any muscle at all. While there may be obvious theoretical advantages of not taking any muscle, it does add some additional tedious dissection through the muscle and possibly a small risk of complications related to this portion of the dissection. Also, because one still has to dissect through the muscle, it is uncertain how much benefit there is in trying to save a small amount of muscle. Thus, in the end, it becomes a practical decision as to whether it's worthwhile to do the extra dissection to save a little muscle. The concept of the perforator flap has been very helpful in focusing our attention on the perforating arteries rather than the amount of muscle. As a result, there's a tendency to take less and less muscle and do a "muscle-sparing" free flap. When there are large perforators that make dissection fairly easy, then it is worthwhile to do a perforator flap.

Another alternative is to do a combination operation, using the latissimus flap and a silicone implant behind it (Fig. 22-4). This can be use-

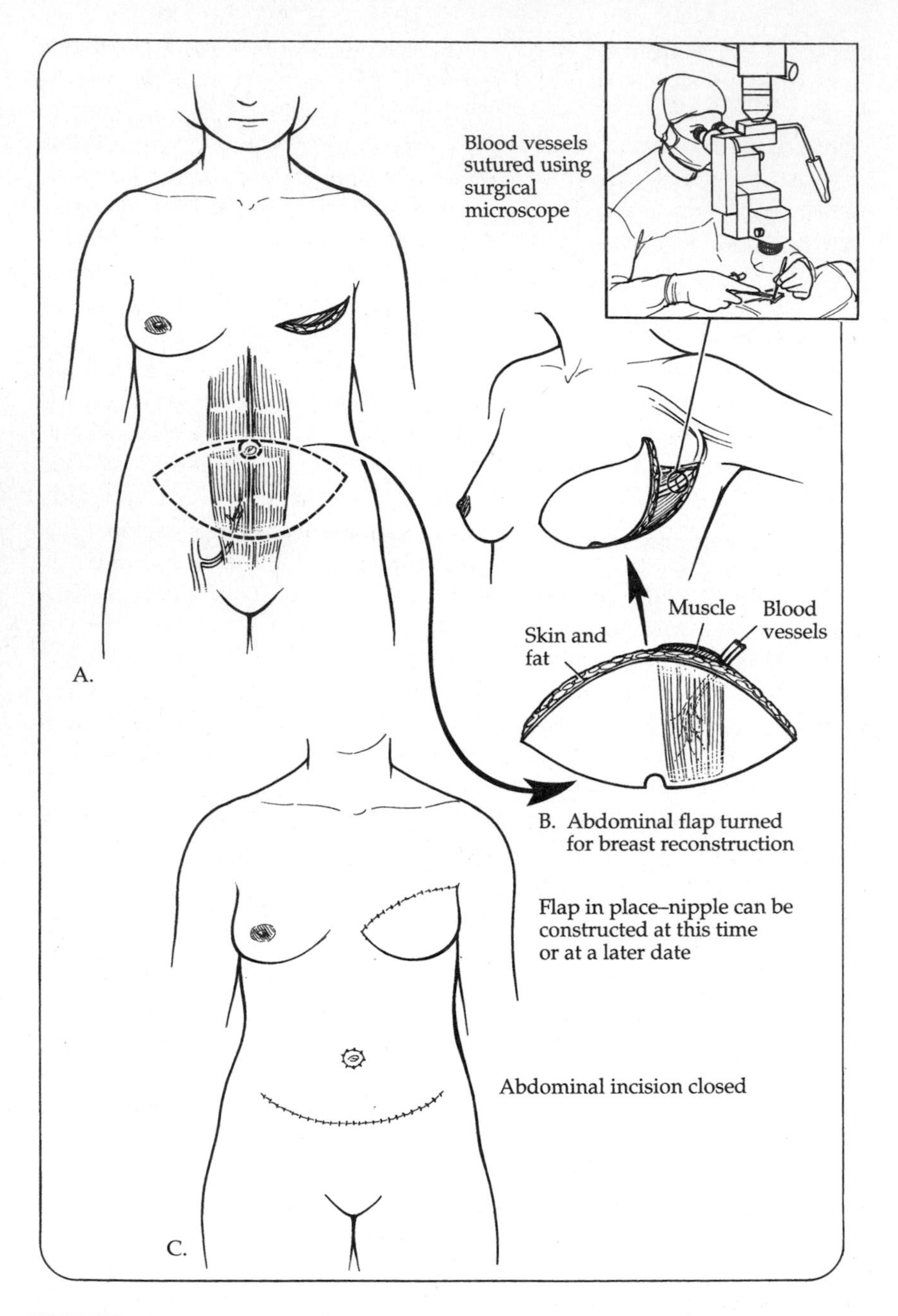
Blood vessels
sutured using
surgical
microscope
Muscle
Blood
vessels
Skin and
fat
A.
B. Abdominal flap turned
for breast reconstruction
Flap in place–nipple can be
constructed at this time
or at a later date
Abdominal incision closed
C.

FIGURE 22-6

ful when there are problems with the abdominal area. The reasons for choosing latissimus flap and silicone implants are twofold: (1) It is technically easier and does not require microsurgery and therefore can be done by more surgeons. (2) Sometimes the abdomen is not suitable because of insufficient volume in a very thin patient or one who has had previous surgery (abdominoplasty or TRAM flap). There is some concern that removing part of the rectus abdominus muscle will weaken the core and lead to back pain. The issue of back problems in the TRAM flap is not significant in most cases. With the current muscle-sparing flap techniques, it's unlikely that the abdominal wall function is altered enough to increase the instance of back problems. With this flap, you'll probably be in the hospital for four or five days; the stitches will be out in two to three weeks, and by five or six weeks, you'll be ready for a fully active lifestyle again.

As I noted earlier, both versions of the flap procedure require highly trained plastic surgeons. There aren't that many of those surgeons around, and it may be virtually impossible for you to find the one you need. There are far more plastic surgeons who can do the simpler procedures of the implant or expander.

To decide what's best for you, you should discuss it with your surgeon and, separately, with a plastic surgeon. They will look at you and your body, see how your body hangs together and how your breasts look before your surgery, and tell you what kind of procedure they think would be best for you. Make sure you ask them which procedures they are familiar with and do regularly. Women have come to me after being told they're not a candidate for a flap, when in reality the plastic surgeon they saw just doesn't know how to do the operation.

The discussion of breast augmentation in Chapter 3 applies here as well. My former colleague Robert Goldwyn, who has done many reconstructions, points out something crucial: you should always be shown pictures of the best and the worst results your plastic surgeon has had. Some doctors will show only the best results—an act comparable to false advertising. It's important for you to know the limits of what the procedure can do for you and the risks you run of having far from ideal results.

Any of these procedures can be done immediately or at a later time. One advantage of doing it immediately is that you don't have another operation later: your regular surgeon performs your mastectomy and then, while you're still under anesthesia, the plastic surgeon comes in and does the reconstruction. Also, when reconstruction is done immediately, the surgeon often performs a skin-sparing mastectomy (see Chapter 21), making it easier for the plastic surgeon to close the incision over the implant or flap. In my experience, though, many women don't have immediate reconstruction because they don't want to go through more surgery. The disadvantages are that it's a longer time in the operating room (usually about six to eight hours), and that it's harder to schedule, since you have to get the surgeon and the plastic surgeon at the same time.

At UCLA, while I did the mastectomy, the plastic surgery team was working on the flap in the abdomen. (If the tissue was taken from the buttocks or back, I operated with the patient lying on her side.) By the time I'd finished the mastectomy they were ready to start moving the flap up. This teamwork approach cut operating time to four or five hours.

When we were done, the patient was taken to the "flap room," a three-bed intensive care unit for the flap—not for the patient, for the flap. The concern was that the blood supply could get blocked, which would cause the flap to turn black and die. So they carefully monitored the flap with temperature probes taped to it. If the flap started getting cold, surgeons were alerted that the blood supply could be compromised.

After mastectomy and immediate reconstruction you come out of anesthesia feeling like a Mack truck just hit you. You've had hours of surgery on both your breast and your abdomen, back, or buttocks. You have continuous pain medication through an IV with a button you can press so that you can control the timing. You're kept in bed rest for one to two days, and you have a catheter so you don't have to go to the bathroom. By about the third or fourth day you start feeling a little better, and you can get out of bed and walk around a bit. You're usually in the hospital about four to six days. There are drains placed in the abdominal scars as well as in the chest. Usually you won't have much pain in your chest, which will feel numb, but your abdomen, or the other area the tissue has been taken from, will hurt a lot.

So the double operation is certainly an ordeal. In addition, you'll probably need a second operation for final touchups. Sometimes after the operation there is a little too much tissue in one place or another, so the surgeon does some fine-tuning. It won't hurt because the area is now numb.

But it's usually worth it and you do eventually recuperate. We've even done this surgery on elderly women with other medical problems, and it's worked for them.

If the free TRAM is the operation you want, you should take the time to research and find out who in your area can do it. If there's no one in your area and you still want a particular form of reconstruction, you can always wait, have the mastectomy first, and then go find the right plastic surgeon when your treatment is done.

MAKING A DECISION

You may not be sure at first whether you want reconstruction. Some premastectomy patients are too upset by the cancer and the prospect of a mastectomy to make yet another major decision at the time. When I come across this kind of ambivalence, I suggest the patient have her mastectomy, take whatever time she needs to deal with it, and then, when she feels ready, come back if she still wants reconstruction.

Although plastic surgeons were initially reluctant to do immediate reconstruction, it is becoming much more popular. I find some surgeons will actually recommend bilateral mastectomies with immediate reconstruction as being the easiest. It probably *is* the easiest for the surgeon, who doesn't have to worry about the cosmetic results of breast conservation. It is also easier for the plastic surgeon, who doesn't have to worry about matching the uninvolved breast. But it may not be easier for you.

Make sure you think it through. The local plastic surgeon may not be the one you want to do your reconstruction, especially if you want a free flap or a muscle-sparing approach. If you delay reconstruction, you may have more of a choice.

There is no time limit for reconstruction. In fact, current techniques have made it a better option than it used to be. If you had a mastectomy in the past and are now thinking about reconstruction, you should feel encouraged. Even with a radical mastectomy, reconstruction is still possible. Or if you originally decided against reconstruction and now want to reconsider, that's also fine. (Some of my patients had their mastectomies in the winter and didn't want reconstruction but changed their minds in the summer, when they wanted to wear bathing suits and sundresses.) Women with bilateral mastectomies can have both sides reconstructed into any reasonable size they like. If you were an A cup and always wanted to be a C, now you can probably do it! Of course, you are limited somewhat by the amount of tissue and skin you have.

Once you have the new breast, you may want a nipple. We don't do it right away because the surgeon needs to be sure it's in the right place. There's a lot of swelling after reconstructive surgery, so we need to wait till that goes down and the nipple is placed on the breast as it will look permanently. It will match the color of your original nipple. Sometimes the skin from your inner thigh is used, since it's darker than breast skin. Sometimes a surgeon can make a nipple from the tissue in the flap and tattoo an areola. Whether or not you want to bother with the nipple depends on why you want the reconstruction. If it's just for convenience, you may decide against it. If you want the new breast to look as real as possible, you'll probably want the nipple. Again, it's your decision—you're the one who'll go through the surgery, and you're the one who'll live with the results. I've had a couple of patients who, before they had the nipple put on, showed their reconstruction to anyone who was curious—then once the nipple was on, they didn't want to show it. Somehow it felt more like a real breast, and displaying it seemed immodest.

Breast reconstruction depends on the patient's goal. Some women are very concerned about symmetry; many others aren't. Do you want to look good in your clothes, or is it important that a new lover won't even know you've had surgery? Do you want to have your remaining breast altered to achieve a more perfect match? These concerns are not foolish, and you should never hesitate to look for what you want out of guilt over "vanity." You've been through an unpleasant and life-changing experience; you're entitled to do what you can to make its aftermath as comfortable as possible. Talk with your plastic surgeon about all the possibilities and decide what's best for you. Dr. William Shaw, a former colleague of mine, warns against looking for one universal operation that's best for every patient. "One of the mistakes surgeons and patients both make is to act as if breast reconstruction is some kind of product you can compare objectively—what's the best airplane? One thing I've learned over the years is that there's no one operation that's best for everyone."

Whatever you decide, check with your insurance company. Some companies will pay for either a prosthesis or reconstruction but not one and then the other, and that may affect your decision.

THE UNACCEPTABLE RECONSTRUCTION

Sometimes reconstruction isn't entirely successful. It may not give you the look you want or it may be a source of pain or medical problems. It can be a source of unpleasant sensations ranging from pins and needles, to burning, to sharp pain. You may just find it hard to adapt to the feel of an implant. An implant may seem solid, even rocklike to the touch. The breast's hardness isn't due to the saline implant but to the scar tissue that has formed around it, encasing it in a tough capsule.

Sometimes plastic surgeons may focus on crafting the "perfect breast," not on replicating the patient's natural breast. Even when an implant matches the breast, the new breast is often heavier because the implant and scar tissue weigh more than breast tissue. The result is often a breast that is too big or feels too big. Also, the new nipple may be higher or lower than the nipple on the other breast.

Because surgeons see women lying on an operating table, they see breasts from a different perspective than do the women, who usually see themselves standing before a mirror. As a result they may misjudge the way a breast will fall when the woman is on her feet (see Chapter 3). If it is a good match for her other breast, which appears flatter when she is lying on her back, it will probably look smaller when she stands up.

You don't have to simply resign yourself to such problems. A plastic surgeon can cut away hard scar tissue and replace implants, exchange an implant for a flap, reduce or enlarge a breast, or lift and reorient nipples. Technology is improving, and so are surgical techniques, as experience with the procedure—and the demand for it—grows. Get a referral to a plastic surgeon from a friend or your breast surgeon, explain your problem, and have the plastic surgeon outline a plan for correcting it. If possible, get a second opinion. Again, ask for pictures of the plastic surgeon's best and worst outcomes.

Occasionally, if the skin has been altered by radiation or is not elastic enough to make additional reconstructive surgery advisable, the best course may be to remove the implant and get a prosthesis instead.

Today, a reasonably good breast reconstruction can be achieved after mastectomy by any of these techniques, using expanders and implants or your own tissue from the abdomen, buttocks, back, or thighs. Achieving symmetry between the nonmastectomy breast and the reconstructed breast, however, sometimes requires reshaping, reducing, or enlarging the normal breast. A large, droopy breast on the normal side can be reduced to match the reconstructed breast. If the breast volume is satisfactory, then the breast can be reshaped by "mastopexy" techniques to lift the nipple and reshape the breast. A normal breast that is too small may be augmented with an implant behind the muscle. This should be done cautiously because the implant-augmented breast tends to be firmer without the natural droop, thus presenting a potential problem for achieving symmetry if the opposite is done with one's own tissue. Also, you should be careful about the potential problems in follow-up of this breast in terms of palpation or mammography. In high-risk patients, this would not be a good idea.

PARTIAL RECONSTRUCTION AFTER LUMPECTOMY

When a patient has a poor cosmetic result from wide excision, a reasonable result can still be achieved by one of two methods. If the breast is large enough in overall volume, the surgeon can often "rearrange" the breast tissue and perform a customized mastopexy to reshape the breast. This usually involves lifting the nipple and moving the breast tissue around to fill in the depressed areas. Usually a similar procedure with a slight reduction is needed in the opposite breast to achieve symmetry. A breast that is distorted or depressed after wide excision can be corrected by replacing some volume in the depressed area. Usually a flap of tissue is taken from under the arm and then transposed into the defect, or part of the latissimus dorsi muscle and the skin and fat over it are moved into the defect. In this way, the reconstructed breast is made up entirely from the patient's own tissue; therefore, it can easily be examined by palpation or mammogram.

The one thing that you shouldn't do—and this is very important—is to get a small silicone or saline implant put in the remaining breast tissue. We can't mammogram through an implant. If you have a recurrence, it's likely to be in the same area obscured with the implant. When women have an implant for augmentation there are techniques we can use to push the implant back and take a mammogram. When an implant is used to fill out the breast after a lumpectomy, it is in the middle of the breast tissue so it is in the way. A flap, however, uses the body's own tissue, which is mostly fat and won't block the mammogram.

THE OTHER BREAST

There is another possible alternative that some women request. If your only aesthetic concern is asymmetry, you can have both breasts removed. While this destroys a healthy breast, it does make it possible to wear loose shirts without a bra. I had only one patient take this route, and she had to fight with her insurance company to get them to pay for the removal of the healthy breast. She told them that since they paid for reconstruction for symmetry they should pay for a contralateral mastectomy for symmetry.

23

Radiation Therapy

The idea of radiation therapy may make you nervous. After all, radiation can cause cancer, and the last thing you want is to find yourself in danger of even more cancer. But, as you saw in Chapter 17, the doses given in radiation therapy rarely cause cancer and often cure it.

As a form of local control (treatment of an original cancer), radiation is more effective in some forms of cancer than others. Luckily it's been very effective with breast cancer.

Radiation for breast cancer is ordinarily used in conjunction with surgery, so you may have had a lumpectomy (or even a mastectomy) before your radiation. It works best when it has comparatively few cells to attack—it's least effective on large chunks of cancer. So we try, if possible, to do the surgery first, getting rid of most of the tumor before cleaning up what's left with radiation.

In the old days, we used cobalt as a source of radiation. Most places now use radiation generated by electricity in machines called linear accelerators. The edges of the beam from this type of machine are "sharper," sparing most of the adjacent tissue. Also, the treatment is planned more precisely, with newer planning machines called simulators. Further, it is aimed in tangents to the breast, so that it goes through the breast tissue of one breast and out into the air, with much less getting into your heart or lung (Fig. 23-1). Even so, there can still be internal scatter, which can affect other spots. Some women who were treated for Hodgkin's disease 10 or 15 years ago now have breast cancer. Unfor-

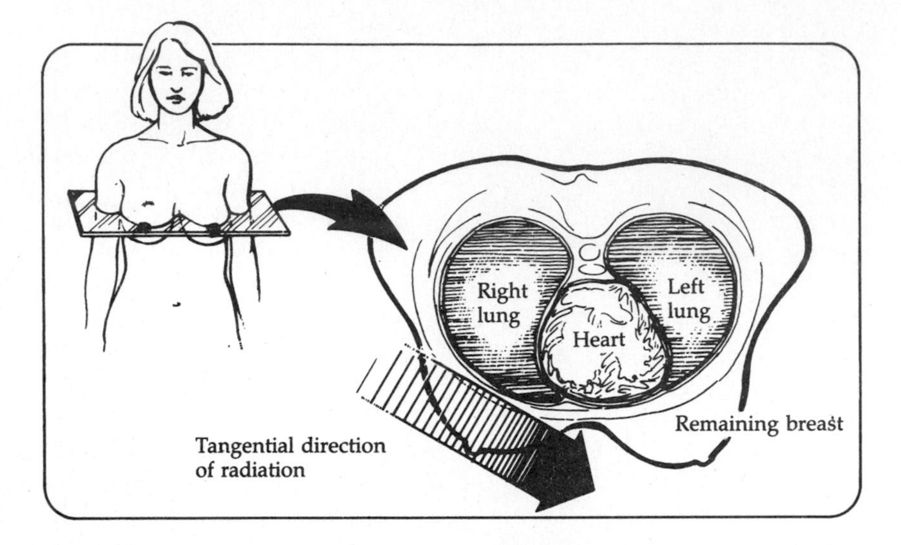

FIGURE 23-1

tunate as that may be, radiation therapy is important. If the Hodgkin's had gone untreated, those women probably would have died long ago.

Like surgery, radiation is a localized treatment. (Chemotherapy, given by injection or in a pill, goes through your bloodstream and affects your entire body.) It's aimed at a specific area and affects only that area. The linear accelerator, as you might guess from its name, accelerates charged particles and shoots them at a target that generates photons. These photons are aimed directly at the body part they're intended for, as a beam. The beam is sharpened in the head of the machine to minimize scatter.

As I explained in Chapter 17, radiation complements lumpectomy as an alternative to mastectomy and may also be used with mastectomy. In the past 20 or 25 years, as adjuvant chemotherapy has improved survival, we're seeing more local recurrences. Chemotherapy, which is so good at stopping cancer that's spread outside the immediate area, doesn't help the immediate area. This has fueled the current trend to do more postmastectomy radiation in certain groups of patients—those most at risk for recurrence after mastectomy, such as the ones with four or more positive nodes, lymphatic vascular invasion, or large tumors. (See Chapter 16.)

INITIAL CONSULTATION

Radiation oncologists (who are always medical doctors) like to see patients soon after the biopsy—ideally while they still have the lump—to get a firsthand sense of the tumor. Sometimes the initial consultation is held in the radiation therapy department and involves a team approach, including a specially trained radiation nurse who inquires into the patient's needs, taking into account her emotional response to her cancer. The consultation involves a physical exam as well as conversation between patient and doctor.

This first visit to a radiation oncologist doesn't mean you'll necessarily have radiation treatment. The oncologist will talk with you and get your medical history, do an examination, review the X rays and slides from your surgery, and talk with your primary doctor, your surgeon, and your oncologist if you have one. They will then come up with a recommendation. Make sure you are offered options. Ask what your risk of local recurrence is with and without radiation therapy. If the choice of radiation seems appropriate to you, you'll be sent for a planning session and whatever X rays are needed after surgery (see Chapters 21–22), if any surgery has been done.

There are issues that affect the decision to use or not use radiation. First, if you have large breasts the available equipment may or may not be able to accommodate them. You may need to find a center that has the correct equipment. Breast size should *not* be a criterion for excluding radiation.

Second, a bit of the lung gets radiated, which can be dangerous if you have chronic lung disease. So with patients who have conditions like chronic obstructive pulmonary disease or emphysema, we often have planning session (see below) just to do the measurements—to see how much lung will be affected and whether or not radiation therapy is safe for them.

In women who have collagen vascular diseases like lupus or scleroderma, the response to radiation can be less predictable, so they may not be good candidates for radiation.

Previous radiation to the chest is usually a contraindication to breast radiation. Your radiation oncologist should carefully review your previous treatment records to assess whether it's safe to give you breast radiation.

In any of these cases, when the potential risks of radiation are greater than the potential gains, a mastectomy should be done rather than lumpectomy and radiation.

THE PLANNING SESSION

Usually you'll wait at least two weeks after surgery before the planning session, to make sure everything's healed and you can get your arm over your head comfortably.

The session takes about an hour. You put on a johnny and lie on a

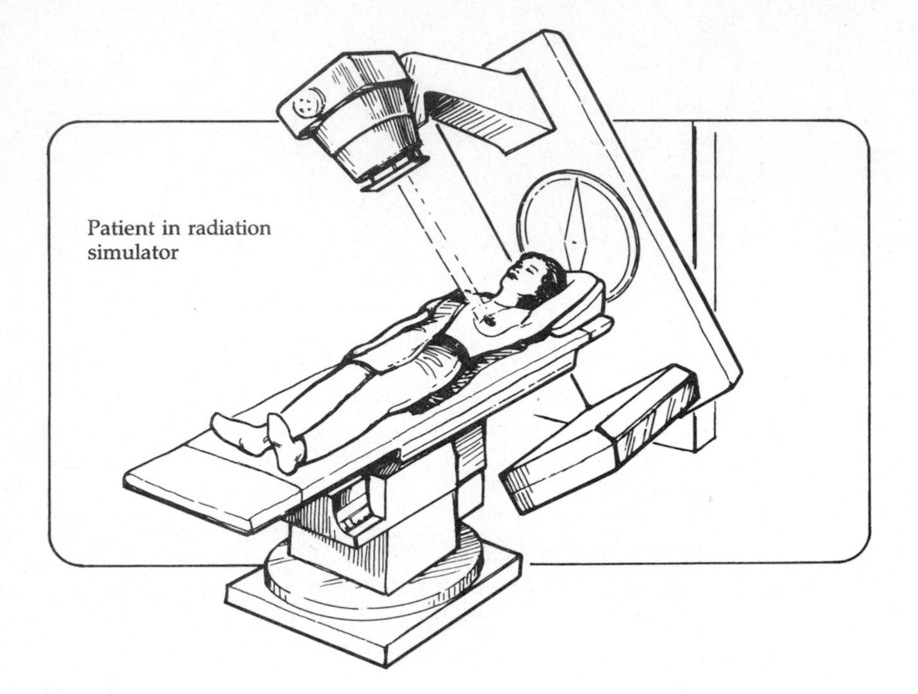

FIGURE 23-2

table with your arm lifted and resting on a form above your head. Over you there's a machine similar to the radiation machine, called a simulator (see Fig. 23-2). It doesn't actually give radiation, but it uses the same energy as a chest X ray machine. You are imaged in the same position you'll keep for treatments. A lot of measurements and technical X rays are taken to map where your ribs are in relation to your breast tissue, where your heart is in relation to your ribs, and so on, figuring out precisely how that area of your body looks (Fig. 23-1). Depending on what area of your body is going to be radiated, you may also be sent for X rays, a CAT scan, or ultrasound to get more information. Then they'll put all the information into a computer that calculates the angles at which the area of your body should be radiated. Some radiation oncology facilities use CT simulators to do the radiation planning so the CT information is readily available. In some cases a mold is made for you to hold your arm in, so that you'll be in the same position every day. Women with very large breasts are sometimes treated lying on their stomachs.

Before the treatments start, the radiation oncologist marks out the area of the body that's going to be treated. In most cases, it is only the breast. Sometimes it's the breast and lymph nodes. You should be

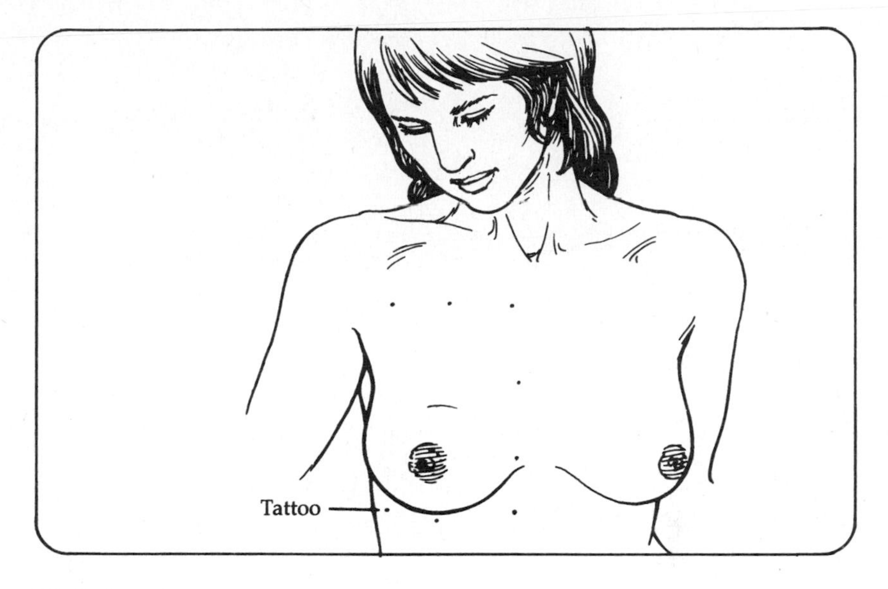

FIGURE 23-3

aware that the breast and the lymph node areas will be treated from different angles, thus covering a fairly large area of your chest. Many doctors use tattoos, which are permanent little blue dots, to outline the area to be radiated (see Fig. 23-3). There are a couple of reasons for that. One is to be sure that during the treatment they use the same "landmarks" and position you exactly the same way. The other is to make sure that in future any radiation oncologist will know you've had radiation in that area, since you can only have it once on any given spot. For example, if you were to get cancer in the other breast and the area was near the previous cancer, the tattoo mark would tell the radiation oncologist where the field that could be radiated ended. I found tattoos useful because often when I was doing a follow-up exam on a patient whose surgery wasn't extensive, I couldn't remember which breast was treated—it could be a year or so after the last exam. So I looked for the tattoo.

Although the dots may be unattractive, they're not going to turn you into Lydia the Tattooed Lady. They're tiny and, depending on your skin coloring, can be invisible. One radiation nurse I know says, "I've had patients call me up and say, 'I've washed my tattoos off—I can't find them!'" Some doctors use Magic Markers, especially if the patient is adamant about not having tattoos; the problem with this is that the markings will wash off, and you don't have this guidance for the doctors working with you in the future. You can limit the number of tattoos to four.

The tattooing can be somewhat uncomfortable, like pinpricks or bee stings at worst. The other discomfort patients sometimes feel from the tattooing procedure is a stiff arm; especially after recent surgery, it can be awkward to lie with your arm above your head for 20 minutes.

THE TREATMENTS

Radiation treatments are scheduled, paced out, once a day for a given number of weeks. There is always a balance between killing as many of the cancer cells as possible and avoiding as much injury to the normal tissue as we can. Recently some centers have been trying higher doses over shorter periods of time: 16 fractions instead of 25–35 fractions (individual doses) with good preliminary results.[1] The treatment schedule varies from place to place. Usually it's given in two parts. First, the breast as a whole is radiated, from the collarbone to the ribs and the breastbone to the side, making sure the entire area is treated, including, if necessary, lymph nodes. This is the major part of the treatment and lasts about five weeks, often using about 4,500–5000 rads—also known as centigrays—of radiation (a chest X ray is a fraction of a rad). If there are any microscopic cancer cells in the breast, this should get rid of them. After this, the "boost" (described later) is given. Recently the value of whole breast radiation therapy has been questioned. Accelerated partial breast radiation (APBI), discussed later in this chapter, is being compared in studies to the standard technique to answer these questions.

How soon after the planning session the treatment begins varies from hospital to hospital, depending on how many radiation patients there are, how much room there is in the radiation department, and how large the staff is. Sometimes the patient waits two weeks to a month and may worry that the delay will allow the cancer to spread. It won't, but waiting can be emotionally hard on the patient.

Radiation may be delayed for other reasons too. Depending on the status of the lymph nodes, you may get chemotherapy right away, and your doctors may not want you to get them both at the same time. As mentioned earlier, with some drugs, such as CMF (see Chapter 18), you can have chemo and radiation together; with others, like doxorubicin (Adriamycin), you usually have the chemo first and then the radiation. Sometimes they're given in a sandwich sequence: chemotherapy, then radiation, then more chemotherapy.

There are important skin care guidelines to follow during your treatment. You should use a mild soap, such as Ivory, Pears, or Neutrogena. During the course of your treatment don't use soaps with fragrance, deodorants, or any kind of metal. All of these can interact with the radiation, and it's important that you avoid them. Don't use deodorant on the side receiving treatment; almost all deodorants contain lots of aluminum. (You can use one of the "natural" ones, such as Tom's, that have no aluminum and come unscented. If you do this, read the label very carefully. Not all "natural" products are the same.) Through the course of the treatment, you can also use a light dusting of cornstarch as a deodorant; it's pretty effective but varies from person to person. But don't use talcum powder.

When you go for your first treatment, you may want to bring someone with you for support. You're facing the unknown, and that's scary. Most patients don't need anyone after the first session.

For the treatment itself, you'll change into a johnny from the waist up. It's wise to wear something two-piece so you only have to remove your upper clothing. You can wear earrings or bracelets during the treatment, but no neck jewelry. After you've changed, you'll be taken into a waiting room; the wait may be longish and varies from place to place and day to day, so you may want to bring a good book or your Walkman. Then you're taken into the treatment room. You're there for about 10 minutes, and most of that time is spent with the technologist setting up the machine and getting you ready. There's a table that looks like a regular examining table, and, above it, the radiation machine (see Fig. 23-4). You lie down on the table, and a plastic or Styrofoam form is placed under your head. This has an armrest above your head,

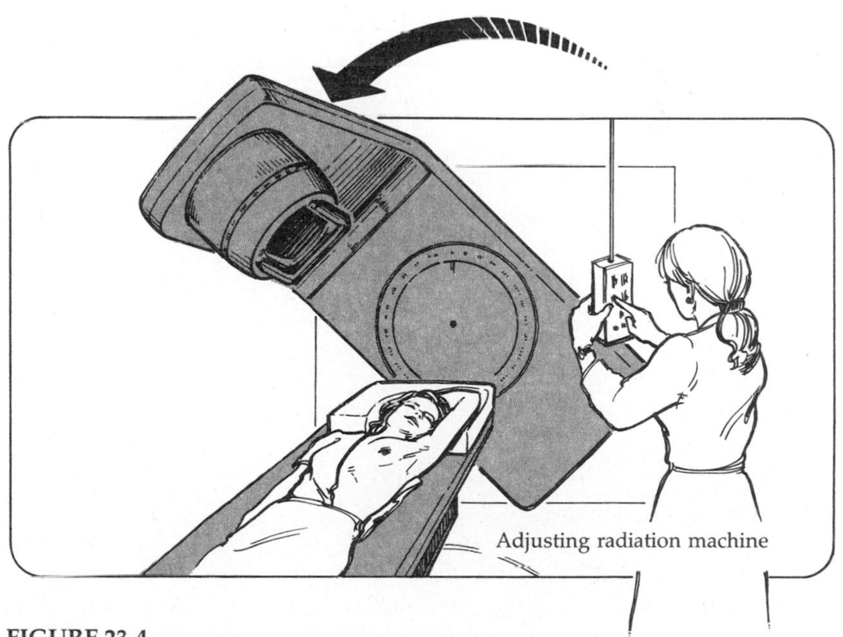

FIGURE 23-4

in which you'll hold your arm during the treatment. After you're set up, the technician will position you, leave, and turn on the machine for a little less than a minute. The radiation isn't given all at once, but is done a number of times from different angles—twice if only the breast is radiated, more if lymph nodes are also being treated. The technician will then come back in, reposition the machine, and go out again. If you're claustrophobic, you may find lying under the machine a little uncomfortable, but it doesn't last long, and the machine never moves toward you.

Radiation therapy units have cameras, so they can see you while you're being treated, and an intercom system so that if you're anxious and need to talk with the technologist, you can. If a friend or family member has come with you, many hospitals allow that person to sit in the room outside the treatment room, watching on the monitor and hearing you through the intercom. If your children are old enough to be curious or are scared at not knowing what's going on, you may permit them to wait outside the treatment room so they can communicate with you. This can demystify the process and alleviate their fears.

The most important thing for you to do during the treatment is to keep still. You can breathe normally but don't move otherwise.

Your blood may be drawn during the course of treatment—once at the beginning of the therapy process or maybe once a few weeks later, to make sure there's no drop in your blood count. This usually isn't a problem with breast cancer, since there's not much bone marrow treated, but we prefer to check, especially in patients who had chemotherapy.

THE BOOST

After a course of radiation to treat your breast, you may be given a boost—extra radiation to the spot where the tumor was. This is usually done by the electron beam. Electrons are a special kind of charged particle that give off energy that doesn't penetrate very deeply, so it's good if the original tumor wasn't very deep. The electron boost is given by a machine; it's aimed at the area where the tumor was. It doesn't require hospitalization. There is some controversy regarding the need for a boost. It was added in the days when we did not demand clean margins from surgery. With the current practice of removing more breast tissue, the boost may not be as important but seems to add a small degree of local control.

What most people find hardest to deal with is the length of treatment—approximately six weeks, five days a week. If your workplace and home are near the hospital, you may be able to come in before or after work. Otherwise, you may have to cut into the middle of the workday or take time off from your job. Some mothers use babysitters; others bring their children to the hospital, along with a friend who stays with them while the mother has her treatment.

PARTIAL BREAST RADIATION

There is increasing interest in limiting radiation after lumpectomy to the area of the tumor bed alone. Several different techniques are being studied, all of which attempt to get the same local control in less time. In general, these new techniques reduce the six weeks to four or five days. This is being done in several different ways: interstitital brachytherapy, balloon-delivered intracavitary brachytherapy, conformal or intensity-modulated partial breast irradiation, and single dose intraoperative radiation therapy. The latter is being done mostly in Europe. Most of the studies done to date have carefully limited the therapy to women with small unicentric tumors excised with big margins. The early results have been promising, with good cosmetic effects and low recurrence rates. Several large randomized controlled trials are now being launched to put this approach to the ultimate test. I will briefly describe what is involved in the various techniques, but I encourage any woman who is interested in exploring this option only to participate in a randomized controlled clinical trial.[2]

Interstitial Brachytherapy

If you are familiar with the earlier editions of this book, you will recognize the description of *interstitial brachytherapy*; it's what we used as a boost before the days of electron beam. When I started my breast surgery practice, we would take out the tumor (without any attention to margins) to prove it was cancer. The woman would then have an axillary dissection to check the lymph nodes, and the radiation oncologist would come into the operating room to implant into the breast the thin plastic tubing that held the radioactive seeds during the surgery. Now the tubes can be placed while you're in the operating room or as an outpatient process (see Fig. 23-5). Thin plastic tubing is hooked like thread into a needle and drawn through a spot on the breast where the biopsy was done. Then the tubing is left in and the needle withdrawn. The number of tubes varies, and sometimes they are inserted in two layers. Small radioactive pellets called iridium seeds, which give off high energy for a very short distance, are put into the tubes, "boosting" the immediate area of the biopsy. This implant is left in for 36–48

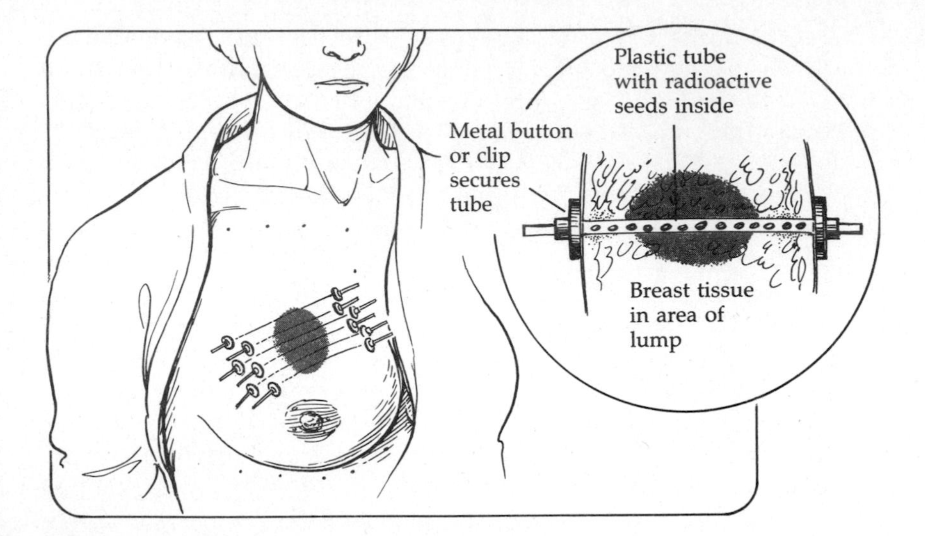

FIGURE 23-5

hours; the time varies depending on how active the seeds are, how big your breast is, and how big the tumor was.

This radiation can be picked up by people around you, although not in large doses. Normally that's no problem, but for some people, such as pregnant women, exposure to even that much radiation could be dangerous. You can't be out in crowds during the time the tubing is in and will be kept in the hospital with a sign on the door that reads "Caution: radioactive." At the end of about 36 hours, both the radioactive sources and the tubes are removed, a process that requires no anesthesia. Unless there's some other reason for you to remain hospitalized, you can go home. Initial results from this approach have been comparable to those achieved with conventional radiation therapy.[3] The second kind of partial breast radiation, *balloon-delivered intracavitary brachytherapy,* is a variation on this theme. At the end of surgery a balloon (Mammosite) is left in the biopsy cavity and later loaded with iridium seeds to deliver the local radiation therapy. There are advantages and disadvantages to this approach since it depends on how well the balloon fits in the biopsy cavity. The third approach uses external beam radiotherapy from a linear accelerator and is called *conformal or intensity-modulated partial breast irradiation* to deliver radiation therapy to the bed of the tumor. This treatment also lasts four or five days. A randomized controlled trial of any of the three of these techniques compared to traditional radiation therapy is now being launched.

Finally there is the single dose intraoperative approach favored in Europe. A lumpectomy is done and then a barrier is placed between the muscle and the breast tissue to protect the chest wall. A mobile linear accelerator made specially for the operating room is used to aim the radiation therapy directly into the bed of the tumor. In a single treatment the breast tissue receives 21 grays of radiation. The first 101 patients treated were followed for approximately eight months, with good results.[4] The study of this procedure is still ongoing.

SIDE EFFECTS

The side effects of radiation depend on the part of the body being treated. Those who receive radiation to the breast and have soft bones may have asymptomatic rib fractures: you don't feel them but they show up on X ray. Depending on how your chest is built, a little of the radiation may get to your lung and give you a cough. Your radiation oncologist will tell you about possible side effects before your treatment starts. Also, it's a good idea to ask to talk to someone who has already been treated.

You'll probably have a mild sunburn effect. The severity varies considerably from patient to patient—one person gets a severe skin rash while another is hardly bothered at all. As you may expect, there is a correlation between skin color and reaction to radiation therapy: the fairer your skin, the worse reaction you're likely to experience.

The other major symptom virtually every radiation therapy patient has is tiredness. I used to attribute this to the length of treatment, but there's more and more evidence that, like anesthesia (see Chapter 21), radiation itself creates tiredness: the body seems to exhaust its resources coping with the radiation and doesn't have much energy for anything else. The fatigue usually gets worse toward the end of the treatment, and its severity depends on what else is going on in your life. You'll probably want to cut back on your activities if at all possible. The fatigue may last several weeks after the treatment has finished, or longer if you have already received chemotherapy; it may even begin after the course of treatment is over.

The extent of the fatigue varies greatly. One of my patients, a lawyer, had no problem working a full day but said she "didn't feel like going out for dinner after work." For others, the fatigue is a bigger problem. One patient compared hers to the effects of infectious hepatitis, which she'd had years before. "The symptoms sound very nondescript," she says. "But I felt really rotten. I was tired all the time—not the tiredness you feel after a hard day's work, which I've always found fairly pleasant. My body just felt wrong—like I was always coming down with the flu. Some days I couldn't function at all—I had to keep a cot at my job." She also experienced peculiar appetite changes. "My body kept craving lemon, spinach, and roast beef—I ate them constantly, and I couldn't make myself eat anything else."

When the breast is being radiated, it may swell and become more sensitive; if you sleep on your stomach, you may feel uncomfortable. As I explained in Chapter 21, one trick is to hold a pillow between your breasts and sleep on the side that hasn't been treated. This sensitivity, like the other side effects, can take months to disappear, and you may find that breast especially sore or sensitive when you're premenstrual.

Few of my patients get depressed during radiation, but many do get depressed afterward—possibly because, time-consuming as the treatments are, there is a sense of activity, of doing something to fight the cancer; once treament ends, there's a sense of letdown. This really isn't surprising. It occurs in other intense situations, like the classical postpartum depression, or the feelings that occur when any time-consuming structure in your life is over—a job you've worked at, the end of a school term. This may be the time to get involved in a support group, if you haven't already done so. You'll have a little more time since you're not going to the treatments, and the company of others who know how you're feeling may help you get through these emotions.

Often the skin feels a little thicker right after radiation, and sometimes it's darker colored. That will gradually resolve itself over time. The nipple may get crusty, but that too will go away as the skin regenerates. This can take up to six months, and in the meantime you'll look like you've been out sunbathing with one breast exposed.

If you have received a lot of radiation to the lymph node areas, it will compound whatever scarring the surgery caused, and the combination can also increase your risk of lymphedema (see Chapter 21). A rare side effect of radiation to the lymph nodes is problems with the nerves that go from the arm to the hand, causing numbness to the fingertips.

Aside from skin reactions and tiredness, there can be later side effects. Some women get costochondritis, a kind of arthritis that causes inflammation of the space between the breasts where the ribs and breastbone connect (Fig. 23-6). The pain can be scary—you wonder if your cancer has spread. It's easy to reassure yourself, though. Push your fingers down right at that junction; if it hurts, it's costochondritis and can be treated with aspirin and antiarthritis medicines. It will go away in a few weeks.

When the treatments are over you'll continue to have tenderness and soreness in your breast that will gradually go away. Some continue to have sharp, shooting pains from time to time—how often varies greatly from woman to woman.

Often patients worry about being radioactive—that they'll harm other people. They ask, "Can I hug my grandchild? Can I pick up my

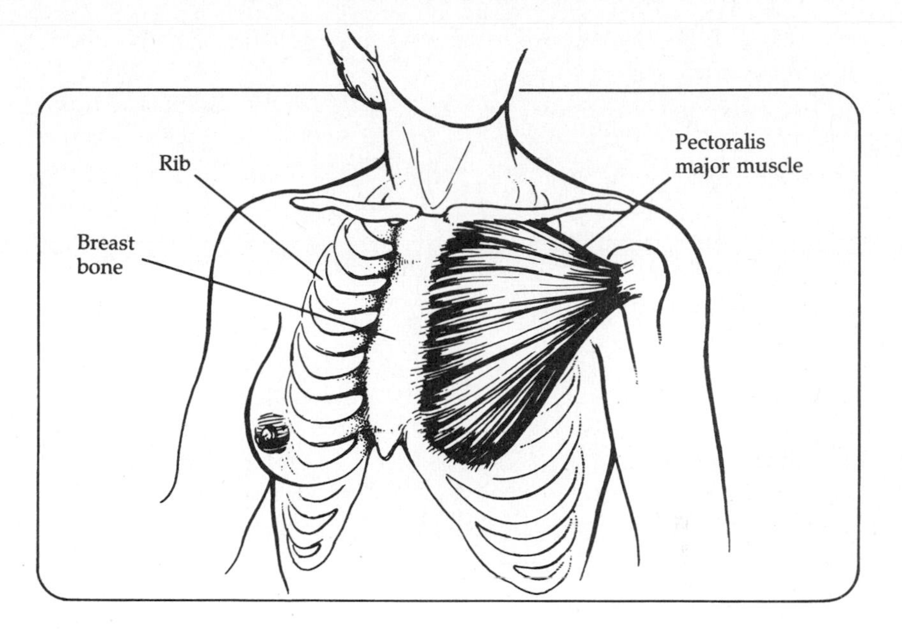

FIGURE 23-6

kids?" Once you leave the treatment room, you can be close to anyone (the implants described earlier are an exception). It's like lying in the sun—once you're out of it, the effects remain, but the sunlight isn't inside you and can't be transmitted to anyone else.

Rarely, radiation can cause second cancers. This is usually a different kind of cancer, a sarcoma, and doesn't occur for at least five years after radiation therapy. Our best guess is that, for every 1,000 five-year survivors of wide excision and radiation, about two will develop a radiation-induced sarcoma over the next 10 years.[5]

Above a certain dosage, radiation given again will damage normal tissue. So if you have breast cancer and it recurs in the same breast, you can't have it radiated again. If you have the tattoos mentioned previously, they will inform future doctors that you've had radiation treatment in that area.

After your treatment is completed, your radiation oncologist will continue to see you, as will your surgeon. In addition to making certain there are no new tumors, the radiation oncologist is watching for complications from the radiation, and the surgeon for surgical complications. These complications are rare, and radiation remains one of our most valuable tools in the treatment of local breast cancer.

24

Systemic Therapy

The hallmark of systemic therapies is their ability to affect the whole body, not just one local area. The systemic treatments used for breast cancer include chemotherapy, hormone therapy, and targeted therapy.

Chemotherapy has had a lot of bad press, and it's a pity, because it's one of the most powerful weapons against cancer that we have. "Chemotherapy" literally means the use of chemicals to treat disease. As we use it, however, it usually refers only to the use of cytotoxic chemicals (those that kill cells).

How does chemotherapy work? Cells go through several steps in the process of cell division, or reproduction. Chemotherapy drugs interfere with this process so that the cells can't divide and consequently die. Different drugs are used in this process at different points, and often more than one kind of drug is used at a time (Fig. 24-1). Unfortunately this effect on cell division acts on all cells that are rapidly dividing—not just cancer cells but also hair cells and, more importantly, bone marrow cells. Bone marrow produces red blood cells, white blood cells, and platelets continuously (Fig. 24-2). Chemotherapy slows this production. When we give the drugs, then, we have to be careful not to stop the production altogether. This is one of the reasons chemotherapy is given in cycles, with a time lapse between treatments to allow the bone marrow to recover.

Another reason the drugs are given in cycles is that not all the cancer cells are dividing at any one time. The first treatment kills one

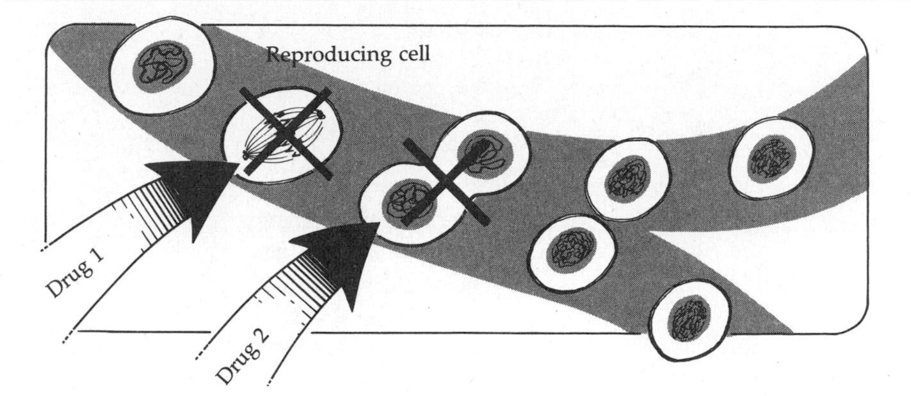

FIGURE 24-1

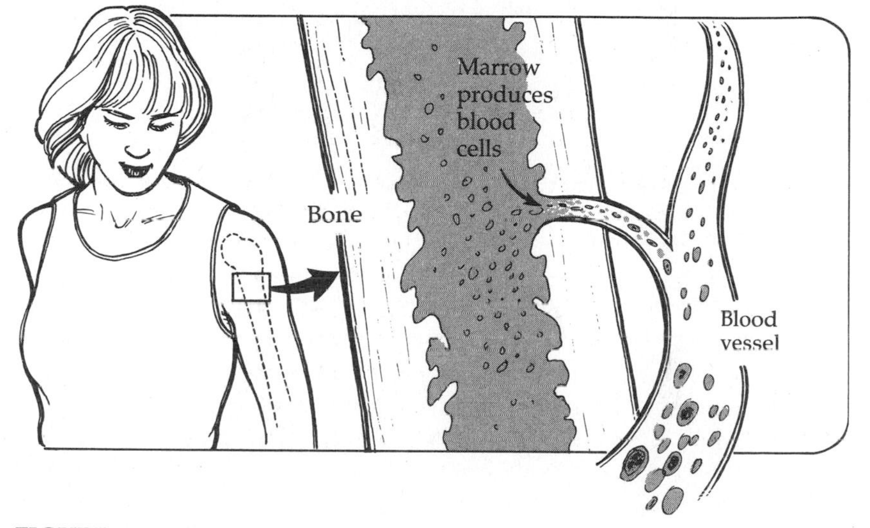

FIGURE 24-2

group of cells; three weeks later a new set of cancer cells is starting to divide, and the drugs knock them out too (Fig. 24-3). The idea is to decrease the total cancer cells to a number small enough for your immune system to take care of, without wiping out the immune system while we're at it. When we first started giving adjuvant chemotherapy after breast surgery, we gave the treatments over a two-year period. Later studies showed that six months was as good as a year, which was as good as two.[1] The extra treatment may have actually harmed the immune system without having any additional effect on the cancer. There probably is a certain key dosage or duration beyond which an addi-

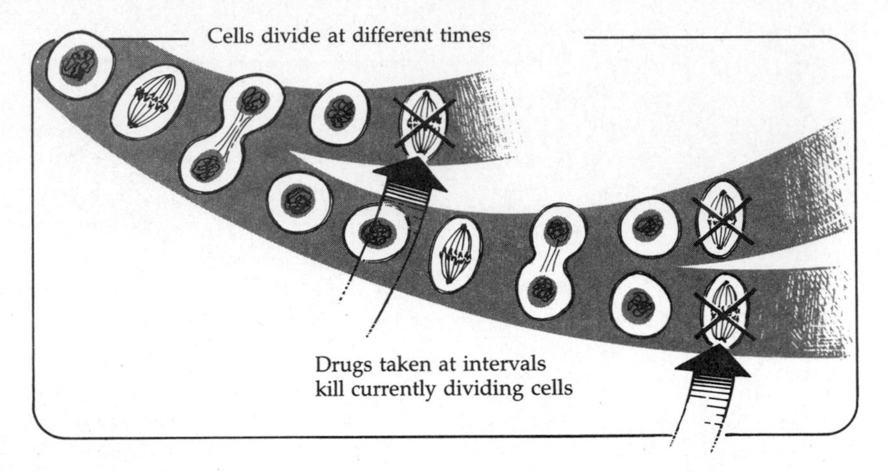

FIGURE 24-3

tional drug is useless, but it hasn't been determined yet. We know now that for some patients, just three months of adjuvant chemotherapy may be best.

Another kind of systemic therapy is the use of hormones or hormonal manipulations to change the body's own hormonal environment in order to affect the growth of hormonally sensitive tumors. This can include surgical procedures such as oophorectomy (removing the ovaries), radiating the ovaries, using drugs that block hormones, or even using hormones themselves. We don't fully understand all the reasons these hormone treatments work, but there is no question that they do work well in certain patients. Since hormone therapy affects only hormonally sensitive tissues, its side effects are more limited than those of chemotherapy. It doesn't kill other growing cells, such as hair and bone marrow. Hormone therapies can kill or control tumor cells by depriving them of the estrogen they require to grow. Without estrogen, some tumor cells will, in effect, commit suicide (apoptosis).

Certain systemic therapies are more targeted, such as trastuzumab (Herceptin), which is being used to treat cancers that overexpress Her-2/neu (see Chapter 18), and bevacizumab (Avastin) (see Chapter 27), which is directed against the growth of new blood vessels (angiogenesis). Several more are in the pipeline, including ones that target epidermal growth factor (EGF).

Systemic therapies are used at two different points in the process of breast cancer. The first is at the time of diagnosis, when it's called adjuvant therapy. The second is at the time of recurrence elsewhere in the body, when the cancer has metastasized. We will consider the latter in Chapter 27.

If you need systemic therapy, you'll meet with a medical oncologist, or cancer specialist, who specializes in systemic treatment. After talking with you at length and reviewing your records, the doctor will decide what systemic program you need and what your options are. These options may vary from place to place. There are general guidelines for breast cancer treatment, drawn up by a group of nationwide breast cancer specialists. At UCLA we developed our own specific guidelines to cover many situations. The field is always changing, however, and it is important that you check with several doctors before you settle on your treatment. You'll want the advantage of the most up-to-date information. Check the Internet for the latest recommendations (www.NCCN.org has patient guidelines for many cancers). You may also want to become involved in a protocol or clinical trial (see Chapter 15).

There are many well-trained medical oncologists throughout the country, and you can usually get very good treatment close to home. You may, however, want to get a second opinion about chemotherapy or hormone therapy at a cancer center before you start. (See Appendix C for a list of comprehensive cancer centers.) Sometimes the cancer center and your local medical oncologist can work together in designing and supplementing your treatment, giving you the best of both worlds.

Your doctor or medical team will also discuss with you the role of systemic treatment in your overall treatment, the expected toxicity, and how the side effects will be managed. Before you make a decision together with the doctor and sign a consent form, all these things must be made very clear to you. (See Chapter 20 for how to pick a good doctor or team.)

The time spent on this depends on the institution and the particular doctor or nurse you're dealing with. Ideally, you'll spend an hour or so, since the information is extremely detailed. Susan McKenney, a nurse practitioner I worked with at the Dana Farber Cancer Institute, gives the patient a written description of everything she needs to know. "I like to translate the information from a didactic, medical form to a written, easily understandable explanation that she can take home and look over at her own convenience; often this is the consent form for a protocol. It's hard to take that much in at one time, and the patient is often overwhelmed—she's dealing with the unknown. I've had a patient sit with me for a hour and the next week when she comes in for her treatment, she can't tell me the names of the drugs she's going to get." Sometimes oncologists spend a lot of time explaining chemotherapy but relatively little on the side effects, risks, and complications of hormone therapy such as tamoxifen. Make sure you understand exactly what drugs you are getting, how you will be getting them and what side effects you can expect, and what can be done to prevent or lessen the side effects.

In addition, says McKenney, it's difficult for a patient to feel that chemotherapy or hormone therapy is really going to help her because she's being told about all the unpleasant things it may do to her in the process. She needs time to assimilate the information about the side effects she'll have to deal with, and written information helps her do this.

You may also want to review the Wellness Community Physician/ Patient Statement in Appendix D and discuss it with your doctor.

In Chapter 18 I talked about the decision-making process and options for adjuvant therapy at length. Now we look at the actual experience of receiving chemotherapy or hormone therapy.

ADJUVANT CHEMOTHERAPY

Once you sign a consent form for chemotherapy, you'll be scheduled to come in for your treatment. It may be in a clinic, your doctor's office, or, rarely, a hospital. A blood sample is usually taken to check your blood count before your treatment, so that the doctor or nurse can determine whether your body is capable of taking chemotherapy—and as a baseline for comparison later. Your initial dose is determined by your body surface area (height and weight). This is a good (but not perfect) guess at what the optimally safe and effective dose of chemotherapy is for you.

The bone marrow's recovery rate helps the doctor adjust the drug dosage. Sometimes when the count is too low, you have to wait for a day or two before treatment to allow your bone marrow more time to recover. When giving adjuvant chemotherapy, your oncologist should be reluctant to administer anything but the standard dosage. Dose reduction (lowering) should only be undertaken for severe, life-threatening toxicities because it is the standard doses that have been shown to be effective.

Think of the bone marrow as a factory churning out red blood cells, white blood cells, and platelets. Chemotherapy injures half the factory's employees, and the factory doesn't work as well till they have recovered. Recently we've discovered drugs that help accelerate the recovery of the patient's bone marrow—keeping all the workers healthy so the factory can get back on track.

The major drug we have for this is GCSF (granulocyte colony stimulating factor), a product you normally have in your blood. It stimulates the bone marrow to make more white blood cells in times of stress or infection, when you need to build up your immune system. Now we've found a way to utilize this in chemotherapy treatment.[2] It's a natural product, which we made from bacteria through genetic engineering. (Although this may sound unnatural, it just a way for bacteria to serve as the production factory.) We found that when we give it to someone, it whips up her bone marrow, so that instead of having a normal white blood cell count of 10,000, she has 40,000 or 50,000. So now when a woman's white blood cell count becomes too low we give her GCSF in an injection and it hastens the bone marrow's recovery. It's like operating on those injured factory workers and getting them back to work. GCSF is thus able to reduce the time it takes your bone marrow to recover after chemotherapy. Because it's important for full doses of adjuvant chemotherapy to be given and to adhere to the the schedule as closely as possible, your oncologist may consider adding GCSF to your chemotherapy if your blood counts are delayed in recovering. Women taking a dose dense schedule of chemotherapy (see Chapter 18) definitely need GCSF because the abbreviated schedule does not give the bone marrow time to recover on its own. Similar types of drugs are sometimes used to boost red blood cells.

If your treatment begins the day the blood count is taken, you'll have to wait for 15–45 minutes for it to begin. In any event, you'll probably have to wait while the drugs are being mixed, though again this will depend on the practice in your institution. Though the wait may be annoying, it can also be an advantage: often this is an opportunity for women to talk to each other and find support in being together. (If you would prefer some time alone, however, you may want to bring a book, magazine, MP3 player, or Walkman with you.)

Standard chemotherapy treatments are given every three weeks, in 21-day cycles or 28-day cycles. If it's a 21-day cycle you may come in for an injection every three weeks. On a 28-day cycle, you come in for treatment on day 1 and day 8, and then go two weeks with no therapy. That's two weeks with therapy and two weeks off. During this time your treatment may be all intravenous or a combination of intravenous medicine and a pill taken orally at home. The treatments can last anywhere from 12 weeks to six months to a year. Dose dense scheduling means you receive the drugs every two weeks for four cycles. This can be sequential: doxorubicin every two weeks for four cycles followed by cyclophosphamide every two weeks for four cycles followed by paclitaxel every two weeks for four cycles; or concomitant: AC every two weeks for four cycles followed by paclitaxel every two weeks for four cycles.

Treatment areas vary from hospital to hospital. Sometimes there's an entire floor for oncology patients and sometimes just a separate area of a larger floor. Chemotherapy can also be given in a private doctor's office. Everyone is aware of patient anxiety levels and tries to make the area as comfortable as possible. Since the process doesn't involve machines, the chemo room doesn't look as intimidating as the radiation

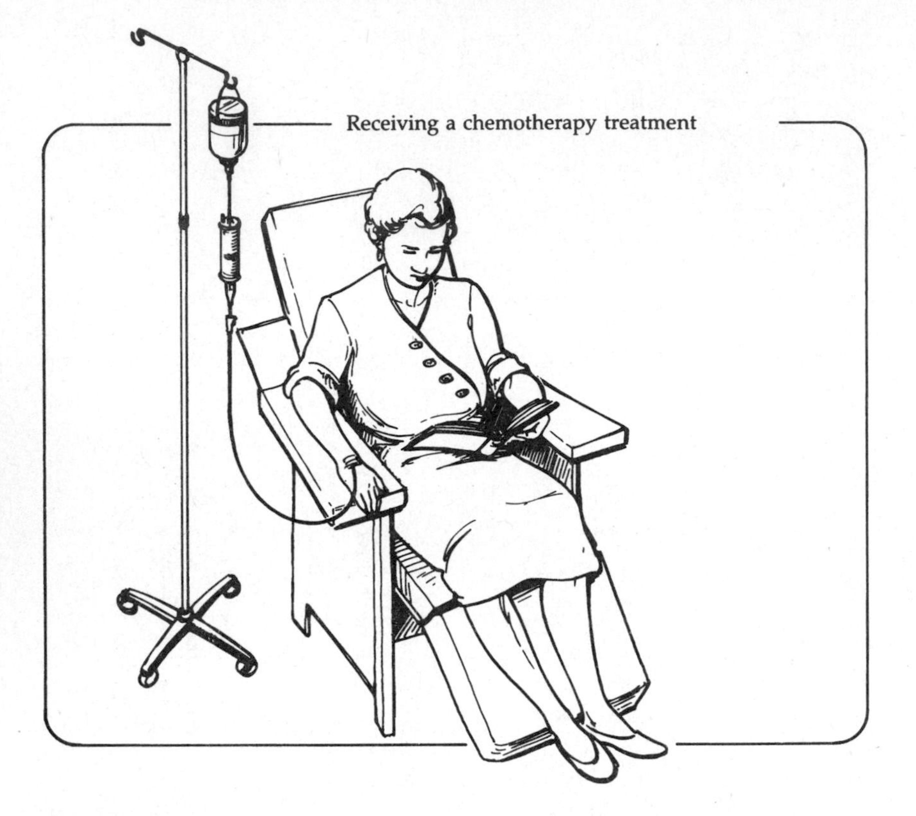

Receiving a chemotherapy treatment

FIGURE 24-4

area. The room is comfortably lit and often has television sets or stereos in it. You may have a room to yourself or may sit among several other patients who are getting their treatments. You'll sit in a comfortable lounge chair for the procedure (Fig. 24-4). Many patients bring books, tape players, or MP3 players with them for the treatment. For a very long treatment, you may want to invest in a handheld TV and watch your favorite talk show or soap opera, or a portable DVD player to catch up on movies. With easily transportable paperwork or a laptop, you can work while the treatment is in progress. If you want to have a friend or family member with you, most hospitals and doctors will permit that. One woman I know would bring her own pillow and blanket from home to help her get through the four hours of her dose dense treatment while friends came along and kept her entertained.

The length of time a treatment takes and the intervals at which treatments are given will vary depending on the type of drugs, the institution giving you the treatment, and the protocol being used. Several different combinations of drugs may be used, each requiring a different time length for administration; in addition, you will likely be given extra fluid as well as medications to control nausea and vomiting. Sometimes a treatment will last 10 minutes, sometimes three or four hours.

The treatments are given by either your medical oncologist or a specially trained nurse. There's nothing particularly painful about the treatment, which feels like any IV procedure. The chemicals come in different colors; in breast cancer, the drugs we use are usually clear, yellow, and red. One woman I counseled told me that she used to have the nurse give the red doxorubicin under the covers because she did not like the color. Never hesitate to ask for something like this: it doesn't inconvenience the staff, and it helps you get through it.

You usually don't feel the medications go into your body, though some patients feel cold if the fluids are run very fast or if they're cold to begin with, or if their bodies are especially sensitive to cold. Cyclophosphamide can cause a weird feeling of pressure in your sinuses, which stops once the infusion is finished. The doctor or nurse will always be there with you, and they're both highly trained specialists in chemotherapy. Sometimes the drugs irritate veins and cause them to clot off and scar *(sclerose)* during the course of the treatment. This can make it very hard to get needles into the veins.

There's a procedure to overcome this—a central access device, a portacath—a catheter-type device placed under the skin into a major blood vessel in the upper chest (Fig. 24-5). Needles can go in and out of that device and spare the patient the discomfort of having peripheral veins (the ones close to the surface, which are normally used for needles) stuck. The catheter must be inserted in the side of the body away from the affected breast, in case you eventually have a mastectomy or radiation therapy. This involves a surgical procedure, usually done under local anesthetic. It can be a bit uncomfortable but it's a trade-off. Patients like the fact that they don't have to get stuck with a new needle each treatment, but on the other hand it can feel a little strange for a while to have a catheter under your skin. The other problem is that the catheter is a foreign body and on rare occasions can cause an infection. It also needs to be flushed occasionally with a blood thinner to prevent a clot. For most women, the decision to use or not use a catheter is reasonable either way, but a catheter is essential for a patient who has trouble with her veins.

There are seven drugs commonly given as adjuvant chemotherapy for breast cancer: cyclophosphamide (Cytoxan) (C), methotrexate (M), 5-fluorouracil (F), doxorubicin (Adriamycin) (A), or epirubicin (E); and paclitaxel (Taxol) or docetaxel (Taxotere) (T). These are usually given in combinations, CMF or AC followed by T or FEC or TAC. In addition there are drugs that are given to maintain your white blood count based on GCSF: filgrastim (Neupogen), and sargramostim (Leukine)

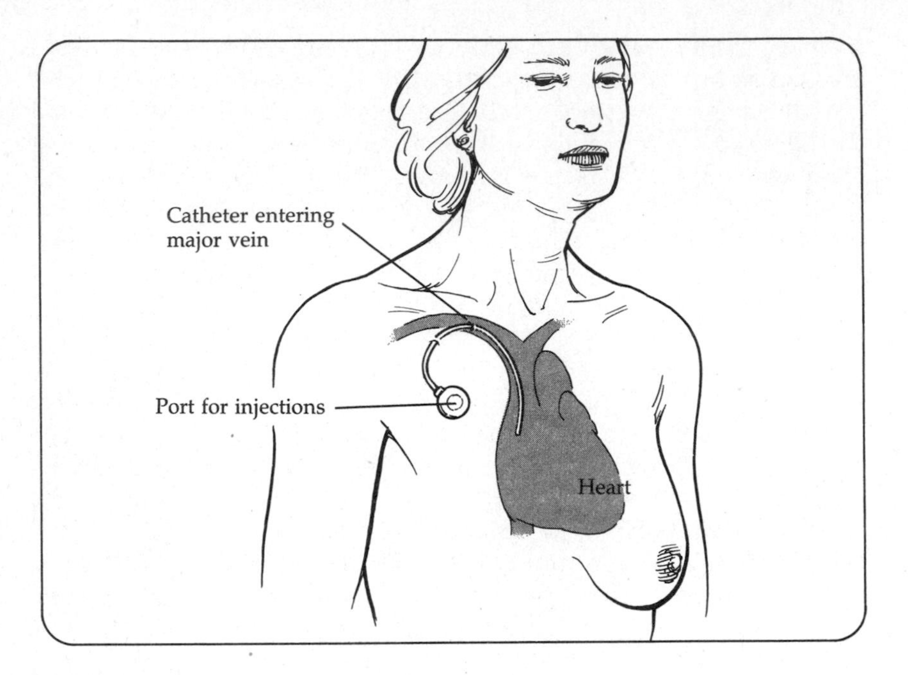

FIGURE 24-5

have to be taken as injections daily over 10–14 days. A new long-acting form called pegfilgrastim (Neulasta), which is only injected once a cycle, may also be used.

Side Effects of Chemotherapy

Side effects vary according to the drugs used. (See Appendix A for a detailed list of some of the drugs most commonly used against breast cancer and their side effects.) The most immediate potential side effect concerns doxorubicin (Adriamycin), which can leak out of the vein and cause a severe skin burn that could require skin grafting. For this reason, it's generally given in a specific way: avoiding weak veins and running in the IV with lots of fluids, so that if it should leak out it won't cause as much harm.

A more common side effect is nausea and vomiting. Overall about 20 percent of women who get CMF, as well as more of the women who receive AC, complain of nausea and vomiting. Recently more attention has been given to this distressing symptom, and as a result we have a much better approach to avoiding it when possible. For one thing, we've learned that not all chemotherapy-induced nausea is the same.

Some drugs are worse than others. Unfortunately the ones commonly used for breast cancer, doxorubicin (Adriamycin) and cyclophosphamide (Cytoxan), are in the high group. Taxanes (Taxol and Taxotere) tend to have less of a tendency to provoke nausea.

The time of nausea differs as well. Cyclophosphamide starts about 6–8 hours after treatment and lasts 8–24 hours, while doxorubicin starts in 1–3 hours and lasts 4–24 hours. Acute vomiting, which usually occurs in the first 24 hours after a chemotherapy treatment, seems to be related to serotonin and responds well to serotonin inhibitors like dolasetron (Anzemet) granisetron (Kytril), ondansetron (Zofran), and plaenosetron (Aloxi). Dexamethasone (a steroid related to, but not the same as, those used illegally by athletes) is also helpful for acute vomiting. Delayed nausea and vomiting are caused by something called substance P and occur 1–5 days after therapy, with a peak effect around 48–72 hours, and respond to a drug called aprepitant (Emend). For treatments with high potential for nausea and vomiting, the National Comprehensive Cancer Network (NCCN) currently recommends starting drugs before chemotherapy with apreptitant, dexamethasone, and one of the serotonin inhibitors.[3] The NCCN website is worth checking (www.NCCN.com). If these approaches are not enough, dopamine antagonists (Metochlopramide, Procholoperazine, domepridone, or Metoprimazine) can be added to the serotonin inhibitors and steroids. Cannabinoid (dronabinol, marijuana) has also been used for both acute and delayed chemotherapy-induced nausea and vomiting, and studies show that it has some effect. (The woman who brought her blanket and pillow to her dose dense treatments swore by it.) It is also available as a pill (Marinol), which is legal but not as effective. Obviously using marijuana has all the downsides—both legal and physical—that you are aware of. If you are going to try it, do so under a doctor's supervision and prescription.

The final type of nausea and vomiting is anticipatory and occurs days to hours prior to chemotherapy. This type can be controlled with benzodiazepines starting one or two days prior to treatment or behavioral techniques. These days most oncologists try to prevent nausea and vomiting in the first place. Make sure you discuss this aspect of your care with your doctor and nurse so that you understand which drugs are being given to prevent nausea and why.

Because the thought of chemotherapy can be frightening, it is a good idea to bring someone with you for your first treatment to see how well it goes and drive you home if necessary. Then if the first treatment goes well and you feel all right afterward, you may not need anyone for the following ones. Usually, if you start off feeling all right and your antinausea drugs are effective, you'll probably get through the rest of the treatments with relative comfort.

In addition to the drugs, some hospitals, like the Beth Israel Deaconess in Boston, incorporate such antistress mechanisms as visualization, imagery, and relaxation techniques into their treatment program. These are often very effective. If your hospital or doctor doesn't offer such techniques, you may want to try some of the ones described in Chapter 25. Many of the techniques are simple and easy for you to teach yourself. In addition, many adult education centers and holistic health institutes in cities and towns all over the country have visualization programs. Acupuncture and Chinese herbs, discussed in Chapter 25, have also brought nausea relief. There are many options, and if what you are receiving from your doctor does not work, you need to ask for something different. There is no excuse for anyone to suffer needlessly.

Sometimes chemotherapy causes you to lose your appetite (anorexia, which is different from anorexia nervosa). In spite of this and the nausea, 21 percent of women will gain weight while on treatment—between 5 and 15 pounds.[4] Food may taste different to you, and some chemicals interact badly with certain foods, though both loss of appetite and chemical interaction are less common with breast cancer drugs than with others. The National Cancer Institute publishes a helpful recipe booklet for people whose eating is affected by their chemotherapy. You may also experience peculiar odors. Barbara Kalinowski, who cofacilitated a support group for women with breast cancer in Boston, describes a woman who talked of constantly walking through her house opening windows so she could get rid of the odor, which she described as similar to the smell of a new car.

Fifty-seven percent of premenopausal women have hot flashes while on adjuvant chemotherapy. The drugs can create a chemically induced menopause, with hormonal changes, hot flashes, mood swings, and no periods.

An article in the *Journal of Clinical Oncology* suggests that the strongest predictors of whether or not you go through menopause with treatment are age and type of chemotherapy.[5,6] The closer you are to natural menopause, the higher your risk. The average age of menopause is 51. A woman of 45 who receives chemotherapy has an 80 percent likelihood of going into menopause as a result, which is much greater than is the case with tamoxifen. A 35-year-old woman has a 20 percent chance of becoming postmenopausal. Many women don't know this ahead of time and have to deal with something unexpected in the midst of their treatment.

With CMF given for six months, the risk of premature menopause is approximately 35 percent in women younger than 40 versus 90 percent in women older than 40. In contrast, less than 15 percent of women younger than 40 who receive four cycles of AC (doxorubicin and cyclophosphamide), and 60 percent of those over 40, will become menopausal.[7,8] Overall, it is the cumulative dose of cyclophosphamide that is strongly related to premature menopause. It is not known what effect the recent addition of taxanes to AC has on the ovaries. Although roughly half of the women younger than 40 may regain some menstrual function, the percentage is much lower in older women. There is some evidence in animals that putting the ovaries into reversible menopause with GNRH agonist during chemotherapy might be more protective, but it has not been tested yet in women.[9,10]

If you do experience early menopause, you will of course be infertile. If your period comes back you can still conceive. Since it's difficult to tell which group you're in, you should use mechanical birth control during treatment if you're heterosexually active. Hormone-based contraception may stimulate the tumor, and the chemotherapy drugs will severely injure a first trimester fetus. (See Chapter 26 for a further discussion of the treatment of menopausal symptoms.)

Chemotherapy treatments used in breast cancer, as in many other cancers, often cause partial or total hair loss. This is somewhat predictable according to the drugs used and duration of treatment. Women who get doxorubicin as part of their treatment always lose their hair, usually soon after the onset of treatment. On the other hand, women who receive CMF only sometimes lose their hair; hair loss occurs about three weeks after treatments have begun, and the hair doesn't fall out all at once. You'll wake up one morning and find a large amount of hair on your pillow or in the shower, or you'll be combing your hair and notice a lot in the comb. This is amost always traumatic, so it's probably wise to buy a wig before your treatment starts. You can ask your oncologist to give you a prescription for a "cranial prosthesis" (wig) and often insurance will cover it. It's best to go to a hairdresser or wig salon at the start of treatment, so the hairdresser knows what your hair usually looks like and how you like to wear it—it makes for a better match. Women receiving CMF often end up not using the wig. (You can always donate it to a local breast resource center.) Patients who don't prepare in advance for the hair loss have a difficult time emotionally if it does occur. Y-ME, a national support organization, sends wigs to women with hair loss for a nominal fee.

Remember, though, it isn't only the hair on your head that falls out. Pubic hair, eyelashes and eyebrows, leg and arm hair—some or all of the hair on your body will fall out, although in most women the eyelashes and eyebrows only thin a bit. Most of the time that isn't a big problem cosmetically—you can thicken your eyebrows with pencil, for example—but it can be startling if you're not prepared for it.

It may take a while after the treatments have ended for your hair to grow back. A little down will probably appear even before your treatments have ended, and within six weeks you should have some hair growing in, though the time depends on how fast your hair normally grows. Often it comes back with a different texture—curly if it's been straight. Eventually the curl relaxes and your hair returns to normal after several haircuts. It may come back in a different color, most commonly gray or black.

Some women experience sexual problems, often related to the vaginal dryness of menopause. And you may suddenly encounter problems with your diaphragm or an IUD due to dryness. In addition there are the physical and psychological effects of the treatment. It's hard to feel sexy when you are tired and bald. This is an important time to communicate with your partner about each other's feelings and needs and to try and find a comforting compromise. (See Chapters 20 and 26 for a discussion of sexual issues and breast cancer.)

Fuzzy thinking and fatigue are common side effects (see Chapter 26) that are just beginning to be acknowledged. Other common side effects include mouth sores, conjunctivitis, runny eyes and nose, diarrhea, and constipation. You may have bleeding from your gums or nose or in your stool or urine, though this is unusual. You may get headaches. Any of these can be mild or severe, or anything in between.

The long-term side effects of chemotherapy include chronic bone marrow suppression and second cancers, especially leukemias. The risk of leukemia is small—0.5 percent in the NSABP series—and probably worth the benefit of the treatment, but you need to be aware that it exists.[11]

Doxorubicin in particular can be toxic to the heart. We believe that it's dose related, and it's rare with four to six cycles, but there may be long-term cardiac effects that we don't yet know about. For example, some people who were treated with doxorubicin several years ago for childhood cancers are experiencing heart failure and need heart transplants.[12] We're only beginning to consider this now because in the past we used doxorubicin only for metastatic cancers, and those patients usually died of the cancer within a few years. Now that we're using it more frequently for women with negative lymph nodes, the patients may well be alive in 20 or 30 years, and we may see more side effects than we did before. It is important not to assume that a drug or treatment that is relatively safe at the time will be safe over the long haul. However, recent long-term studies of doxorubicin in women with breast cancer show that a few have heart problems even 10 years after treatment.[13] Overall, the risk of having a heart problem due to doxorubicin is about 1 in 200 treated women. One of my former patients developed heart disease after being treated with doxorubicin and ended up with a heart transplant. I'm not suggesting that we abandon doxorubicin for adjuvant treatment—my patient, after all, survived long enough to get her heart ailment. Doxorubicin is one of the best drugs we have to treat metastatic breast cancer. If it is indicated, it should certainly be used. But we should not use it indiscriminately in women who are not at particularly high risk for metastases.

Paclitaxel (Taxol) can cause a reversible, dose-dependent, cumulative *neuropathy*. This is a pins-and-needles sensation, often in the hands and feet, which can get worse with each dose but is generally ultimately reversible. Taxol can also cause hand-foot syndrome, an itchy rash on the palms of the hands and the soles of the feet. In about 5–15 percent of women a syndrome of muscle and joint aches and pains can occur, starting about 24–72 hours after the infusion and lasting 2–4 days. It ranges from mild, requiring only occasional nonnarcotic pain relievers, to incapacitating. A woman I counseled through her treatment experienced this and required narcotics to deal with it. The narcotics led to nausea and vomiting. Once you know that you react this way, you can be treated with dexamethasone for several days to prevent the pain. Docetaxel (Taxotere) also causes the neuropathy but is generally milder than paclitaxel. Docetaxel also causes a unique syndrome of swelling and fluid retention; some fluid retention is fairly common but occasionally it can be severe. Fortunately this is reversible but takes a long time.

Though there's no way to know in advance how you'll react to your treatments, your doctor or nurse can tell you how other people treated with the drugs you're on have done in the past.

While it's important to be prepared for the possible side effects, it's equally important not to assume you'll have all, or even any, of them. This assumption can intensify and sometimes even create the symptoms. Sometimes people see the side effects as a sign that their illness is getting worse and consequently contribute to their own negative feelings. Bernie Siegel, the doctor who has worked intensively with mental techniques to reduce pain and help heal diseases, reports in his book *Love, Medicine, and Miracles* on a study done in England in which men were given a placebo and told it was a chemotherapy treatment.[14] Thirty percent of the men lost their hair! Positive thinking and—importantly—exercise, as well as keeping up your normal activities, can significantly reduce the side effects of chemotherapy.

Most chemotherapy treatments are given on an outpatient basis. You will soon know whether you are going to feel sick and, if so, on which day the nausea hits and how bad it is. Most women are able to continue their normal lives and maintain their jobs with minor adjustments while receiving treatment. You won't feel great, but you'll be functional. In 2005, adjuvant breast cancer chemotherapy should be tolerable and you should be able to function well. If it's not, ask your doctor or nurse for strategies to reduce the side effects. Many options are available.

It may, however, be a good time to take up your friends' offers of help. A ride to your treatment can be wonderful, both for the company and the release from worry about traffic and parking. Child care may well give you a breather in a stressful time, as can offers to cook dinner or clean the house. Most friends and family members really do want to help, and this may be the best time to use their support.

Don't expect to feel perfect the minute your last treatment is over. Your body has been under a great stress and needs time to recuperate. It often takes six months or even a year to feel normal again. It will happen, however, so don't despair. (See Chapter 26 for a discussion of rehabilitation after breast cancer.)

ADJUVANT HORMONE THERAPY

Hormone therapies generally have fewer side effects than chemotherapy. The best-known and most widely used is tamoxifen. In terms of administration, hormone therapies are the simplest of the breast cancer treatments. You don't need to go anywhere or have anything done to you—you simply take a pill.

Because we look at hormones in relation to chemotherapy, we tend to minimize their side effects. And indeed they are milder than those of chemotherapy. But they do exist, and for some women they can be significant, including phlebitis (blood clots), pulmonary emboli, visual problems, depression, nausea and vomiting, vaginal discharge, muscular aches and pains, and hot flashes. All of these are rare except for the hot flashes and muscle pains. A lot of women who have these symptoms ask me if they could be caused by their medication. When I say yes, they say, "Thank God—I thought I was going crazy because my doctor said I wouldn't have side effects."

Tamoxifen

The most common side effects are hot flashes, which occur in about 50 percent of women on tamoxifen. Like all hot flashes, they can be severe or mild. They eventually go away, but "eventually" may mean years. New drugs like venlafaxine (Effexor) can reduce the number and intensity of these hot flashes.[15] Alternative choices are discussed in Chapter 25.

About 30 percent of women on tamoxifen experience major gynecological discomforts—anything from vaginal discharge to severe vaginal dryness.

There's some evidence that tamoxifen may, in unusual cases, increase *thrombophlebitis,* a form of phlebitis in the leg in which the vein gets irritated and forms clots.[16] This is rare but very dangerous, as the blood clot can travel to the lung (pulmonary embolus). It can even be fatal. Let your doctor know right away if you develop leg swelling and pain while walking.

The most serious side effect of tamoxifen is uterine cancer. In the NS-ABP prevention study (see Chapter 11), researchers found the risk doubled after five years.[17] It occurs almost entirely in women over 50. This is reassuring because postmenopausal women now have a safer option with the aromatase inhibitors (see below), and premenopausal women can take this drug without worrying about getting uterine cancer.

Premenopausal women have an increased risk of benign gynecological problems, including uterine polyps, fibroids, endometriosis, and ovarian cysts.[18] (See Chapter 19 on the use of tamoxifen to induce ovulation for IVF.) This means that, as with chemotherapy, a heterosexually active woman should use some type of effective mechanical contraceptive while taking the drug. Because tamoxifen can damage a fetus, it's very important not to get pregnant while you're taking it.

If you are premenopausal on tamoxifen, be aware that new gynecological complaints may be related to it.

Some women have an increase in their liver blood enzymes, which goes away once they stop taking tamoxifen. Many women on tamoxifen experience eye problems, including blurry vision and, less commonly, cataracts.

Nonetheless there are several bonuses in spite of these side effects. Tamoxifen raises your high-density lipoproteins and lowers your low-density lipoproteins, which may make you less likely to get heart disease.[19] Tamoxifen often improves osteoporosis in postmenopausal women and sometimes stablizes it, much like raloxifene.[20]

The most important thing about tamoxifen is that it treats the cancer you have, and it reduces your chance of getting cancer in the opposite breast by 50 percent; that is, from 15 to 7.5 percent. So considering all these pros and cons, it is worth taking unless you have had problems with blood clots in the past.

As I explained in Chapter 18, the current data suggest you take tamoxifen for five years and then stop. Much to everyone's surprise, the benefits of decreasing the chance of relapse and of second cancers continue even after you stop taking the drug. Tamoxifen is therefore likely to kill cancer cells or, more probably, put them into a dormant state.

It takes six weeks for tamoxifen to clear from your system after you stop. So if you miss a pill one day, it isn't the end of the world. Just resume taking it the next day.

Other Antiestrogens

Toremifene, a drug that has been approved by the FDA for treatment of metastatic disease, is sometimes used in place of tamoxifen, especially for women who do not tolerate it. Raloxifene is a SERM (see Chapter 11) that has been shown to decrease breast cancer in postmenopausal women with low bone density. Since these women are at low risk of breast cancer, it is not clear if it would have the same effect in women with breast cancer or those who are at high risk. One study of 14 women with metastatic breast cancer showed no effect from raloxifene.[21] A second study showed an 18 percent response rate in metastatic disease.[22] At this time it is definitely *not* an alternative to tamoxifen as adjuvant treatment of breast cancer.

Fulvestrant (Faslodex) is a new steroidal antiestrogen. Unlike tamoxifen and raloxifene, it has no estrogenic effects. In the metastatic setting it appears to be as good as anastrozole and causes fewer joint problems (see below). It is given by intramuscular injection once a month rather than by mouth. It is not clear at this time whether it will be used for adjuvant treatment in the future.

Aromatase Inhibitors

Until recently only tamoxifen was given as an adjuvant hormone treatment. As I mentioned in Chapter 18, aromatase inhibitors are now being used just as frequently. Like tamoxifen they are taken in pill form. Since they block estrogen production and have no estrogenic effects, it is not surprising that some of the side effects are similar and some different. In the study that compared the aromatase inhibitor (AI) anastrozole to tamoxifen head-to-head, the main differences were the endometrial cancer with tamoxifen and the increase in fractures and muscular and joint pain with anastrozole.[23] This is the first adjuvant trial reported, and it is instructive to look at the side effects. Unfortunately the study compares their side effects only to those caused by tamoxifen. Nonetheless the major problems seem to be joint pain, which increased by 32 percent, and fractures, which increased by 50 percent. The fracture problem may not be as bad as we think because tamoxifen tends to reduce fractures; so the difference between the two groups is probably much bigger than if they had compared the aromatase inhibitor to a placebo. When you hear people say that the AIs have fewer side effects than tamoxifen, it is true—but it is also true that we only looked for the side effects that are common with tamoxifen. It will be some time before we know all of women's experiences with these drugs. It is important to note, however, that we have 40 years experience with tamoxifen and know all its pitfalls well, while the longest any woman has taken an aromatase inhibitor is five years. Note how long the tamoxifen section is compared to this one! It is likely that the fracture rate may increase and there are concerns that there may be cognitive difficulties (the brain has aromatase too). Some physicians are giving women taking an aromatase inhibitor a bisphosphonate to attempt to forestall the bone loss, but this combination is still being studied.

When you ask women or oncology nurses what the biggest complaint about the aromatase inhibitors is, they specify bone pain and musculo-skeletal stiffness. Usually these symptoms go away after about three months, but getting through that time period takes patience and endurance. Anti-inflammatories (NSAIDs) seem to help some women, as do warm baths, acupuncture, and massage. Because many women are also coming off hormone replacement therapy, it is sometimes difficult to know which of the side effects are from that and which from the new drugs. A nurse friend of mine says that bioflavinoids help both bone pain and hot flashes in some women. One friend said that sleeplessness was her main problem other than hot flashes. Indeed, in the ATAC study there was a 20 percent incidence of this. More importantly the nurse pointed out that the aromatase inhibitors come in different types and that you can have side effects from one and not another. Don't be afraid to ask to switch.

Goserelin (Zoladex)

This drug is one of the GNRH agonists, which block the pituitary's production of the hormones that stimulate the ovary. The result is that you are put into a reversible menopause. Goserelin is given by a monthly injection under the skin of the abdomen. Since it works by putting you into temporary menopause, it has many of the same side effects. First, your periods will stop. This is not a contraceptive, however, so you should be sure to use another means of contraception as well. Hot flashes, lower sex drive, joint pain, and weight gain are common side effects. Most of the time your period will return when you complete your course of treatment, although in some women close to menopause it will not. Goserelin is sometimes given with an aromatase inhibitor in premenopausal women. Although there are no reports of expected side effects, one would guess that the increased estrogen deprivation this combination results in would cause worse symptoms than either alone. Such obvious side effects as increases in fractures, hot flashes, loss of libido, and vaginal dryness would be expected. In order to deal with the increase in fractures some doctors add a bisphosphonate (see Chapter 11), although we do not yet have data suggesting that this is necessary.

Trastuzumab (Herceptin)

Trastuzumab is now used for both metastatic disease and adjuvant therapy. It is given by injection. The side effects are most common with the first treatment and include fever and/or chills in about 40 percent of women. They are easily managed with Tylenol. Other possible but less likely side effects include nausea, vomiting, diarrhea, headaches, difficult breathing, and rashes. These side effects tend to be worse with the first cycle. Trastuzumab is usually given with chemotherapy; thus all the usual chemotherapy side effects are present. The major concern with trastuzumab is the heart and lung damage that can occur. This is more common when the chemotherapy is given with an anthracycline like doxorubicin that also has potential to damage the heart. Because of these potentially life-threatening side effects, patients are usually evaluated with EKG, echocardiogram, and MUGA (multiple gated acquisition) scan for heart or lung problems before starting treatment and are closely monitored during treatment. Again this is a relatively new drug and we do not have enough long-term experience to know its side effects. The studies demonstrating that it is beneficial in women newly diagnosed with breast cancer who are Her-2/neu positive were stopped prematurely as the final drafts of this book were written. While these women are followed we will surely learn more about the side effects over time. It will also be important to see if the side effects differ with different formulations of chemotherapy. We still have a lot to learn.

Bevacizumab (Avastin)

The other new targeted drug that is currently used only in metastatic disease is bevacizumab (Avastin). Its most common side effects (found in 1,032 patients) were weakness, pain, hypertension, diarrhea, and lowered white blood count. Other side effects include nosebleeds, high blood pressure, and protein in the urine. Again the complications from this drug are compounded by whatever chemotherapy is done in conjunction. These drugs are the first of a new wave of long-awaited targeted therapy. The next few years will show us how much promise they really have.

25

Complementary and Alternative Treatments

Today, most academic cancer centers have Clinics on Integrative or Complementary Medicine, and many cancer patients are combining these techniques with their regular treatments. The Office of Cancer Complementary and Alternative Medicine (OCCAM) distinguishes between complementary medicine—which it defines as any medical system, practice or product not thought of as standard care but used along with standard medicine—and alternative medicine, which is used in place of standard treatments. Most forms of non-traditional approaches can be used in either way.

I think it's very important to be looking at complementary, rather than alternative, treatments if you have breast cancer. For all its limitations, Western medicine is still probably the most important component of any successful effort to cure cancer or to put it into significant remission.

COMPLEMENTARY THERAPIES

Mental Techniques

Many techniques seem to work because of the placebo effect: your mind tells your body that it's getting a certain healing substance, and your body responds as though it were true. As Norman Cousins pointed out in *Anatomy of an Illness*, the effect has worked throughout history—doctors once had some success with such "treatments" as bloodletting and administering powdered "unicorn horns." He calls the placebo "the doctor who resides within," who "translates the will to live into a physical reality."[1]

The application of this concept to cancer treatments was recently examined when Gisele Chvetzoff and Ian Tannock reviewed all the studies in oncology that included a placebo arm.[2] They found that placebos sometimes help with control of symptoms such as pain and appetite but rarely with positive tumor response. In 1989 David Spiegel from Stanford ran a support group for 86 women with newly diagnosed metastatic breast cancer. For a year, the groups met weekly for 90 minute sessions, focusing on enhancing social support and encouraging the expression of disease-related emotion. The study was meant to examine the effects of group therapy on breast cancer patients' quality of life, and indeed it did show benefit in that regard.[3] More surprising, however, were the findings ten years later: the women who had participated in the group survived an average of 18 months longer than the others.[4] This was the first randomized study to show that mind-body interventions could change survival. Since then, nine other clinical trials have been published to test this hypothesis: four show support for the effect and five do not. So it's not conclusive—but it certainly does suggest support for the placebo effect theory.

Prayer

For centuries, people of all religions have believed in the power of prayer—and for some of them it seems to have worked. Estelle Disch, a Boston-area therapist who has worked with many cancer patients, says: "If you're praying for health, on some level you're seeing yourself as healthy, and I believe that makes a difference." Faith in a power that can make you well—whether that's God, or your surgeon, or your own will—can help you to get well. I often pray for my patients, hoping to harness whatever forces I can to help them achieve the result that is best for them.

In the mid-1990s two separate groups of researchers pulled together collections of scientific studies on the effectiveness of prayer, and the results are thought-provoking. Paul N. Duckro, a professor of psychiatry and human behavior at the Saint Louis University School of Medicine, looked at experimental studies conducted over 20 years.[5] One small study involved 18 children with leukemia, divided into two groups. Families from a distant Protestant church were given the names of 10 of the children and asked to pray for them without their knowledge. Fifteen months later seven of the ten were alive, while only two of the eight children in the control group were alive. Larry Dossey, former chief of staff at Medical City Dallas Hospital, reported on similar studies in his book *Healing Words*.[6] In one study, a randomized double-blind trial of 393 heart patients at San Francisco General Hospital, half the patients were prayed for daily and half weren't. None of the patients, their doctors, or their nurses knew who was being prayed for and who wasn't. The patients who received the prayers had fewer complications and needed fewer antibiotics.

Meditation and Visualization

Meditation has been an important part of almost every major religion in history. While there are many forms, the ones most commonly used in conjunction with healing work are variants of that very simple one in which the person sits in a comfortable position, eyes closed, focusing on the inhaling and exhaling of breath, and chanting a mantra, a particular word or phrase. The Eastern *om* is fine, but you can also use different language—"peace," for example, or a brief phrase from a prayer.

Herbert Benson, an M.D. who has extensively studied various forms of nonmedical healing, describes this particular form of meditation as "the Relaxation Response" and it is the basis of his work as director of the Mind/Body Medical Institute in Boston. He and his colleagues run a number of groups for people with various diseases. The technique creates physiological responses that contribute to stress reduction.

Most programs that use meditation combine it with visualization, or imagery. This too is an ancient technique, based on the belief that if you create strong mental pictures of what you want, while affirming to yourself that you can and will get it, you can make virtually anything happen.

The pioneers of visualization in disease treatment were Carl and Stephanie Simonton, an oncologist and a psychologist. Their book *Getting Well Again* recounts their experiences with "exceptional cancer patients"—those who recover in spite of a negative prognosis—and maintains that their visualization techniques have significantly extended patients' lives.[7] However, no controlled studies have either proven or disproven this. Studies *have* proven that visualization and meditation combined can reduce pain and the uncomfortable side effects of cancer treatments, which certainly makes them worth trying.

Visualization typically begins with a meditation-relaxation exercise; then you begin to envision your cancer in terms of some concrete image—like gray blobs inside your breast (or whatever area you're dealing with). Next you picture your white blood cells, or your radiation or chemotherapy treatments, as forces countering the cells. You can do visualization with a group or on your own. I've had patients who've

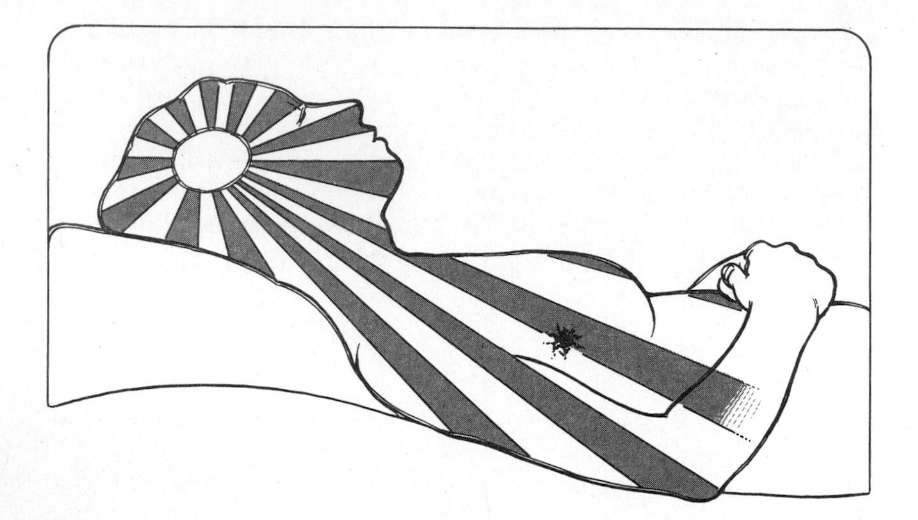

used the techniques in both contexts. The Simontons favored violent images—soldiers attacking the cells, or sharks destroying them, but some prefer different images. A friend with metastatic breast cancer felt much better singing her cells a lullaby to put them to sleep.

Similar to visualization, and often used in conjunction with it, are affirmations—statements affirming one's value and intentions, recited aloud if possible, mentally if not. One of my patients had a list of her favorites, which include, "I am now renewing my body's ability to heal itself" and "I now let the light from above heal me with love." Others prefer to frame their affirmations in terms of choice: "I choose health." They should always be used positively rather than negatively—not "I will not stay sick" but "I am growing healthier each day." Affirmations can be repeated regularly and frequently. You can say them while taking your shower, walking to your car, or unloading your groceries. Susan Troyan, one of my surgical colleagues in Boston, has patients bring in positive sayings, which are read during their surgery. She says that whether or not it helps healing, it gives women a much needed sense of control.

Laughter

Even simple laughter can be a healing tool. When Norman Cousins set about to cure himself of his neurological illness, he "discovered that ten minutes of genuine belly laughter had an anesthetic effect and would give me at least two hours of pain-free sleep."[8] There appears to be some medical basis for this: laughter can stimulate endorphins—chemicals that act like narcotics in the brain.

One of my patients with inflammatory breast cancer said, "I told people I wanted to laugh. Friends send me funny books, cut out cartoons, call me and say funny things." Though she eventually died from her cancer, her multileveled approach to fighting it gave her the strength she needed to live her life fully to the end—including helping launch the breast cancer political movement.

Certainly giving yourself time not to think about your cancer, just escaping into zany humor, can be emotionally healing. Be sure to pick the things that make you laugh heartily, whether it's a P.G. Wodehouse novel or a recent TV sitcom.

Psychic Healing

Psychic healing is another ancient technique, and exists in many forms. Much of charismatic Christian healing involves laying-on-of-hands, a classical psychic healing technique. And the relatively new "therapeutic touch," designed by nurses in the U.S., is similar. Sometimes it isn't even done in person—healers and ordinary people "send healing energy."

Whatever else such healing thoughts can do, they can achieve a twofold benefit. For the patient, it is a reminder of all the love and support that's out there for her. And for those who love her, it can alleviate some of the terrible sense of helplessness they feel in the face of a loved one's suffering. Your friends can't operate on you or administer your chemotherapy, but they can pray or send healing thoughts.

Little research has been done on psychic healing, but studies done in Canada by Dr. Bernard Grad suggest that, even when the subject isn't aware it's being done, it can have an effect on illness.[9] (This echoes the studies on prayer mentioned earlier, suggesting that the placebo effect alone isn't enough to account for the benefits of either prayer or psychic healing.)

Some people attribute healing powers to crystals and other stones. Many believe these can affect different parts of your physical and emotional health, and that using them to meditate, wearing them as jewelry, or simply keeping them around can help you remain healthy or restore health if you're ill.[10] As far as I know, no scientific studies have been done on healing stones, but that doesn't mean they can't work. Some of my patients have great faith in them, and I like to keep a small collection of amethysts in my office. Like the Catholic rosary or the Jewish mezuzuh, they can provide a concrete symbol of your belief in your ability to heal. Amethyst is seen as an all-purpose healer, while sugalite and tiger's eye are considered particularly effective with cancer, and moonstone with women's cancers, but any stone you feel drawn to is useful.

Some patients find their stones so soothing they bring them to their treatments. One of my patients had her favorite crystal taped to her hand during surgery. Another carried her sugalite with her to her chemotherapy treatments, holding it to the parts of her body that the chemicals most negatively affected.

Diet

In Chapter 11, I discussed the fact that studies show diets high in fruit and vegetables can affect breast cancer occurrence and that women who are obese when they're diagnosed with the disease have a poorer prognosis. So there's scientific encouragement for changing to a low-fat diet, and for losing weight once you are diagnosed. A large national study called the Women's Intervention Nutrition Study (WINS) has randomized postmenopausal women to either eat a long-term, very low-fat diet or continue with their usual fare. This study should answer the question regarding dietary change after treatment.

Unfortunately many proponents of dietary therapy go too far, assuming that the observational data suggesting that certain dietary components can decrease risk means they can also cure cancer. They can't.

There are many diets recommended for cancer in general, and some for breast cancer in particular, most of which are low in fat, high in fruits and vegetables. They usually suggest avoiding processed foods, sugar, alcohol, and beef and chicken treated with hormones. If you decide to include a nutrition approach to your healing, you should work very closely with your nutritionist and your physician both to create your particular diet and to coordinate it with your other treatments.

I would suggest avoiding a macrobiotic diet while you're being treated for cancer. Though generally healthful, it can cause problems for a patient undergoing chemotherapy or radiation, or recovering from surgery. It's low in calories and in protein, and when your body is depleted from these processes, that can be dangerous. If you're on a macrobiotic diet while undergoing medical treatments, make certain it's not causing medical problems.

Vitamins, Herbs

The cancer center M.D. Anderson did a survey of their multidisciplinary breast clinic as well as their gynecological malignancy clinic and found that 48 percent of the patients were using CAM (complementary-alternative medicine), most frequently herbal products and multivitamins.[11] The increase in the use of these products, which are essentially unregulated by the FDA, has led to concern about safety and interactions with chemotherapy. A recent review from the National Cancer Institute listed specific herbal remedies that should be *avoided* during chemotherapy.[12] Most relevant to breast cancer patients were garlic, gingko, echinacea, soy, ginseng, St. John's wort, valerian, kava kava, and grape seed. You can still eat garlic, soy beans and grapes but avoid them in supplements while you're on chemotherapy.

Some supplements have been reported to reduce the side effects of chemotherapy. For example Coenzyme Q10 has been used with anthracyclines (like doxorubicin) to protect the heart and liver. A review from the United Kingdom suggested that COQ10 provides some protection against heart or liver toxicity for patients taking anthracyclines, but the results are inconclusive.[13] A preclinical study showed that CoQ10 did not affect the metabolism of doxorubicin.

The best way to stay up to date on this subject is to monitor the website of the National Center for Complementary and Alternative Medicine at the NIH (http://nccam.nih.gov). In addition many of the large cancer centers such as M.D. Anderson, Dana Farber or Sloan Kettering have Alternative and Complementary Clinics that can help you either in person or on the web.

Acupuncture

Some branches of complementary healing involve treatments, such as the ancient Chinese science of acupuncture, which sees healing in terms of "meridians," energy channels that run through the body. Special needles are inserted into the meridians. Acupuncturists have worked with breast cancer patients, usually in conjunction with Western medical treatments.

Marie Cargill, a Boston-area practitioner of Traditional Chinese Medicine (TCM), has used acupuncture with breast cancer patients. "What they've been using in China is a combination of Western treatments—surgery, radiation, chemotherapy—and Traditional Chinese Medicine," she says. Acupuncture, she adds, can strengthen the body when the other treatments cause weakening.

Cargill and many other practitioners of TCM like to combine acupuncture with Chinese healing herbs. Both, she says, can help relieve all the side effects of radiation and chemotherapy. "Cracking toxin herbs" fight the cancer itself and supplement the work of the other treatments, while other herbs help build the immune system. There are particular herbs for breast cancer, which are different from herbs used for other cancers. In addition, some herbs work on the depression and anxiety that often accompany life-threatening illness. If it's hard to find Chinese herbs and herbal practitioners, Cargill says that acupuncture alone can work well, if it's used frequently enough.

Studies are being done on some herbal remedies, with encouraging results. According to Barry Cassileth, several mushroom-derived compounds are approved for cancer therapy in Japan.[14] Another TCM formula of 19 vegetables increased the survival of 12 patients with late stage non–small cell lung cancer. In addition, the nontoxic vegetable brew significantly improved the quality of life.[15] Helene Smith, a researcher from San Francisco who developed metastatic breast cancer, pushed for a study of an individualized Tibetan herbal formula. Although she died of breast cancer, the study is being done.

Homeopathy

Another area of holistic healing is homeopathy, seen as a method of self-healing stimulated by very small doses of those drugs that would produce in a healthy individual symptoms like those of the disease being treated. The drugs are chosen by the patient with the assistance of a homeopathic practitioner, who may or may not also be an M.D. The substances are all legal, and over-the-counter; you can take them on your own, but it's wiser to work with a practitioner who has expertise. Ted Chapman, a homeopathic M.D. in Boston who has worked with breast cancer patients emphasizes that homeopathy doesn't cure cancer. "Doctors work on the end product of the disease, and they come in from the outside. We're working from the inside, on what makes you vulnerable to your disease in the first place." Like many other adjunctive therapies, homeopathy is thought to work on the immune system.

Bioelectromagnetics

Magnets are popular with many people for the treatment of a number of diseases. The theory is that magnetic fields penetrate the body and heal damaged tissues, including cancers. There are no good scientific studies supporting this claim, but none to disprove it either.

ALTERNATIVE TREATMENTS

Some treatments have been proposed to take the place of medical treatments. Most of them have not been studied in any scientifically rigorous way and their risks and complications are largely unknown. I mention them to be complete, but I don't endorse their use.

The best known is laetrile. It hasn't been shown to work in any randomized, controlled studies, but it has a fair amount of nonscientific support. It's illegal in the United States and is currently being used in clinics in Mexico. It contains cyanide, and there have been reports of deaths from cyanide poisoning in patients taking laetrile.[16]

Another treatment, immuno-augmentative therapy, was invented by Lawrence Burton, who practices in the Bahamas since it is illegal in the United States. It is an individualized treatment considered by its advocates to restore natural immune defenses against all forms of cancer.

Metabolic therapies with detoxification are widely offered in Mexico, especially in Tijuana. One variant, the Gerson treatment, claims to counteract liver damage caused by chemotherapy with a low-salt, high-potassium diet, coffee enemas, and a gallon of fruit and vegetable juice daily. The Gonzalez regimen includes a restrictive diet, pancreatic enzymes, and coffee enemas and has had some success with inoperable pancreatic cancer.[17] The National Cancer Institute is now sponsoring a randomized clinical trial of it at the Rosenthal Center for Complementary and Alternative Medicine at Columbia University.

Stanislaw Burzynski has developed antineoplaston therapy, which is available at his clinic in Houston, Texas. Although there have been anecdotal reports on its efficacy, there is no scientific proof. Chemically antineoplastons consist of phenyl acetate, a metabolite of phenylalanine that is being studied for potential anticancer activity by researchers at the National Cancer Institute and elsewhere.[18,19,20]

Shark cartilage was very popular for a time as a cancer treatment, based on its antiangiogenic properties, but a study showed no benefit.[21]

CanCell is a remedy developed by James Sheridan in 1936, composed of common chemicals and is apparently nontoxic. It has not been tested in a clinical trial.[22] Essiac, another popular herbal cancer alternative, is made up of burdock, turkey rhubarb, sorrel, and slippery elm. Data supporting its anticancer effects are lacking; it is illegal in Canada but available in health food stores in the United States. A study in 2004 used Flor-Essence (a variant of Essiac) in a rat model and showed it *promoted* mammary tumor development.[23]

Iscador is a derivative of mistletoe, widely used in Europe. Although there are extensive data in German, the studies are often small or combine iscador with other therapies.[24] It did appear to prolong survival time of some cancer patients and to improve the quality of life. The NCI is currently conducting a trial of mistletoe plus chemotherapy in patients with metastatic disease.

Research

The Center for Complementary and Alternative Medicine is doing studies on shark cartilege, melatonin, ginseng, mistletoe, and oleander for the treatment of breast cancer. The latter appears to have an antiangiogenesis factor. The National Institutes of Health now has a division of alternative medicine set up to help study some of these techniques.

Many time-tested herbal and diet-based therapies are being studied for their abilities to induce or extend remission. For now, the absence of government regulation of supplements means that scores of unproved remedies or inadequate dosages of proved ones are on the shelves of pharmacies and grocery stores. I believe strongly that all treatments—be they bone marrow transplants or laetrile—need to be held to the same standard and should be adequately studied in randomized controlled trials.

Many people go to the Web for information on alternative and complementary healing, as well as on traditional medicine. This can be a good tool, but you need to know how to use it. Check a few things. Is the organization that is giving the information well known? Can you tell who's sponsoring the site, and what their qualifications are? Is it for profit or not for profit? Is the information dated and referenced? Are there data for safety and efficacy, or just anecdotes? Remember that anyone can have a website. On www.drsusanloveresearchfoundation.org we offer links to many of the reliable sites, and will be doing clinical studies of many of these herbs. You can also check your local American Cancer Society Division Office or quackwatch.com. They keep statements on these treatments that describe exactly what is involved, as well as the known risks, side effects, opinion of the medical establishment, and any lawsuits that have been filed. Make sure you are really informed.

Though I am leery of using such treatments without a medical component, I do feel this is a highly personal decision. What risks any of us will take for what reasons depends very much on who we are and what our values are.

In situations in which a particular cancer or stage of cancer has a bad prognosis, refusing traditional treatment isn't really much of a risk. When chemotherapy isn't likely to extend your life for any length of time, the discomforts may not be worth the slight chance of cure, and an alternative treatment may offer both better survival hope and more comfort during the remainder of your life. When Audre Lorde[25] learned her cancer had metastasized to her liver, she decided to forego chemotherapy. She went to homeopathic doctors in Europe for injections of iscador and did visualization and meditation, determinedly living her life to the fullest. She survived for several years—an impressive achievement with liver metastasis. Maybe it was because she chose a treatment that she believed in, and that allowed her to remain as active as possible, doing the work to which she was so passionately committed.

One of my patients, a 46-year-old woman whose cancer metastasized to her bone marrow, also did remarkably well for a time. A devout Catholic, she cherished the advice of a nun who told her to "work as though everything depended on you, and pray as though everything depended on God." She had surgery and tamoxifen therapy, went on a macrobiotic diet, took a mind-body course at Beth Israel and continued a regular meditation and visualization program. Whenever any church had a healing service, she went to it. She carried a rosary made of healing stones. She went to Lourdes. Though she ultimately died from her cancer, her health improved for awhile. In spite of the cancer in her bones, she went mountain climbing and cross-country skiing—and dancing.

PART SEVEN

Living with Breast Cancer

26

After Treatment

You've had breast cancer and you've been treated for it; now it's time to get on with your life. But your life has changed, and you have to adjust to your new situation on a number of levels. One of my patients told me that "it's like your life breaks into a million pieces and when you put the pieces back together they don't quite fit exactly the same."

THE FOLLOW-UP

Survivorship means, for one thing, being followed for the rest of your life. At a minimum, the follow-up involves regular monitoring for a recurrence. It also involves addressing chronic treatment-related results of your treatment (e.g., fatigue, sexual dysfunction, "chemo brain," pain syndromes) and monitoring for potential late effects of treatment such as heart disease, lymphedema, and non–breast cancer malignancies. While this may sound depressing, it shouldn't. It means that we now have enough experience with survivorship to know what to look for and what to do about it.

UCLA and other centers have follow-up programs in which patients are seen every three to six months for the first two years and every year after that. The program includes not just exams and mammograms but also physical therapy, nutritional counseling, psychosocial support, and involvement in research. Usually the surgeon and/or other specialists who did your primary treatment will follow you at regular intervals for a period of time.

In follow-up examinations the doctors are looking at how you are healing, as well as checking for signs of recurrence or problems resulting from the therapy. Surgeons, for example, are looking for lumps in the breast, mastectomy scar, or other breast. They check your neck and the area above the collarbone for lumps that may indicate a lymph node, and feel under both arms.

In addition, they question you carefully about how you're feeling. They ask to see if you've had persistent and unusual pain in your legs or back, a persistent dry cough, or any of the other symptoms described at length in Chapter 27. In general, if you have a new symptom that doesn't go away in a week or two, check it out. Usually that's what most patients do anyway. One study found that a third of recurrences were manifested by the symptoms, a third were detected by physical exam, and a sixth were found by mammogram (for those of you mathematically inclined, the other one-sixth covers everything else).[1]

Patients are often surprised when their doctor doesn't find anything on their follow-up exam; they've been waiting for the cancer to pop up again and tend to be anxious about examinations. Some women start getting nervous days before these visits, and the visits themselves often trigger fears of recurrence. This is normal. However, if worry creeps in weeks before, further evaluation of how you are coping may be useful. You may want to consider seeing a counselor or getting some antianxiety medications.

Studies of a large group of breast cancer survivors by my oncologist colleague Patricia Ganz found that age at follow-up and having received adjuvant chemotherapy (versus other treatments) increased worry about a recurrence.[2] Younger women perceive themselves as having more to lose, and most women consider the use of chemotherapy as a marker of more aggressive disease. Interestingly, the type of surgery did not seem to affect worry: women who underwent a mastectomy worried no more or less than those who had lumpectomy and radiation. Although this seems counterintuitive, since many women say they have a mastectomy so that they won't worry, it probably occurs because women have more choice as to which surgery they will get. Unfortunately the worry does not diminish over time. While some women worry less as they get further from their treatment, others experience constant concern. As one woman said, "Worry just comes with the territory." Unless it is disrupting your daily life and plans, this recurrence anxiety need not be treated.

Not all symptoms mean the cancer has spread. Women who have had cancer are as likely as anyone else to get other diseases as they age. Having had cancer does not make one immune to arthritis or diabetes, for example. Furthermore, aside from ordinary, nonrelated problems, patients may experience conditions as a result of the cancer treatment, such as heart disease, leukemia, and osteoporosis. Then there are the physical changes that your body experiences as a direct result of your therapy. It's important to have frequent checkups because a breast that's been radiated undergoes a lot of changes. There will be a lumpy area under the scar and perhaps some skin firmness and/or puckering. By keeping track on a regular basis, the doctor can assure you that the changes you're experiencing are related to the treatment—and if there's a different, more ominous change, the doctor can distinguish it from the others. As I write this, ASCO (American Society of Clinical Oncology) is revamping its follow-up guidelines to include some of these issues.

For the same reasons your surgeon will probably want you to have mammograms every six months for a year or two, and then once a year. In addition to monitoring the treated breast, the doctor will examine your other breast yearly for the possible development of a new cancer, since women with cancer in one breast have an increased risk of getting it in the other. This is particularly important if you are a carrier of the BRCA 1 or 2 gene (see Chapter 10). MRI may be done as well (see Chapter 7). In non–gene carriers, breast cancer in the other breast is less likely; the risk is about 1 percent per year, or an average of 15 percent over a lifetime.[3] (See Chapter 19 for a discussion of the second primary cancer.) Some types of breast cancer indicate a greater propensity for a second breast cancer to develop. Cancers with a lot of lobular carcinoma in situ (see Chapter 12) have been thought to fit into this category.[4] Even in this situation, however, the increased risk to the second breast is about double, or 2 percent per year, a cumulative lifetime risk of 30 percent. Obviously the younger you are and the longer you live, the greater your chance of developing a second cancer. If this thought is too scary for you, you may want to consider a preventive mastectomy on the other side. But in my experience most women prefer close follow-up to such a drastic step. If you're considering this, it's important to remember that a mastectomy can't guarantee that you won't develop breast cancer again (see Chapter 17).

In addition to your surgeon, you may be followed by your whole team; your radiation oncologist and/or your medical oncologist may also want to check on you regularly. Some patients find this overwhelming and don't want to spend all that time trekking back and forth to doctors. More typically, you'll be followed by one of the members of the team, or even by your local family doctor, if she or he has experience with breast cancer. In a 1996 study, women were randomized to be followed by their primary care doctor or a specialist. Interestingly, specialist care did not lead to earlier diagnosis of a recurrence, improved quality of life, or even lower anxiety levels.[5] Your HMO may affect which kind of follow-up is available. But basically the choice is yours: don't worry about hurting your doctor's feelings. It's your feelings that matter now. Pick the doctor with whom you have the greatest rapport.

Many doctors still do blood tests every three to six months, including not only your blood count (CBC) but also specific tests (for example, a CEA, CA 15-3, or CA 27.29), as well as liver blood tests to catch metastatic disease at the earliest point. Both patients and physicians assume that early diagnosis of metastases improves outcomes. Unfortunately we have lots of data that this is not true. For one thing, these tests don't always succeed. Most are not very sensitive or specific. They go up when there is metastatic disease but they also go up for other conditions. And even when they find metastases, there's no evidence that such detection does you any good.[6] As you will learn in Chapter 27, we still have no guaranteed way of curing metastatic disease—though we can relieve symptoms and perhaps add a few years to your life.[7,8] In terms of quality of life, knowing sooner that you have a metastasis probably doesn't do you much good. These tests can actually interfere with quality of life without affecting its length. Even if they turn out negative, you still may have a metastasis that is too small to show up on the tests. This also holds true for the routine use of bone scans, chest X rays, CAT scans, and liver blood tests. These and other data led to follow-up surveillance guidelines issued by ASCO and NCCN (National Comprehensive Cancer Network) that advised only routine discussion of whatever symptoms you may have plus physical and yearly mammogram.[9,10] If you are taking tamoxifen, you should also have a yearly pelvic exam. The mammogram can make a difference in longevity, since it shows local recurrence in the breast or a cancer in the other breast. So unless you're taking part in a protocol that requires regular testing, you may not want to have the other tests.

With breast cancer, unlike some other cancers, we can't be sure that if it hasn't recurred within a few years, it won't. It's usually a slow-growing cancer, and there are people who have had recurrences 10 or even 20 years after the original diagnosis. In some ways this is similar to a chronic disease. You are never quite sure if or when it will come back.

Time does, however, affect the *likelihood* of recurrence—the longer you go without a recurrence, the less likely you are to have one. So going 10 years without the cancer coming back should give you reason for optimism, if not certainty.

Since problems resulting from treatment can come up years later, it's important to keep records of your treatment and have continued contact with somebody who knows about its delayed effects. Dr. Ganz says, "I've seen women 10 or 15 years after their treatment who have no records of what happened years ago. And we've had to try and reconstruct their history. Survivors need to have knowledge about what they were treated with, so they can remind their family doctor or tell any new doctor about it, and have medical records to show them." In this mobile age, you'd be wise to make sure you get a written summary of your disease characteristics, cancer treatments received, and complications experienced after treatment was completed. In fact, the President's Cancer Panel 2003–2004 report on Cancer Survivorship recommends this be routine. Such information is helpful to different health care providers, so you'll want to copy these documents and file them in a safe place. You can take better care of your records than any hospital or doctor—you have a bigger investment in them. You may even want to keep a copy in a safe deposit box.

At the end of the treatment period you go back to your normal activities; you look fine and you expect to feel fine. Everybody's relieved that things are back to normal again—everybody but you. Physical problems that wouldn't have bothered you before now seem ominous. The slight headache that two years ago you would have dismissed as tension—has the cancer metastasized to your brain? And does the bruise on your arm mean you have leukemia? You're now in the "I can't trust my body" stage. Well, why should you trust your body? It betrayed you once, and you know it can do it again. Every time you go for a checkup, every time you get a blood test, you're terrified. In my experience with patients, this stage usually lasts two or three years, until you've had enough innocent headaches and bruises, enough reassuring checkups and blood tests, to feel somewhat trusting of your body again.

But you probably don't feel fine—not the way you used to, anyway. For most women the end of treatment is accompanied by lingering side effects.[11] However, they are usually thrilled to be through with treatment, and that helps a lot. As a result, women are all the more surprised by the fears that often rear up at this point. Few are well prepared for the end of treatment and the loss of a valued support network. New worries arise: will the cancer come back now that I am no longer being treated (in this regard taking tamoxifen or an aromatase inhibitor may be reassuring)? Who will I call if something comes up? What symptoms should I look for? Who is going to follow me now? You begin to get used to this new set of feelings.

And then, just when you are settling down and starting to forget about it, something pops up in the paper or on the news about a risk factor or new treatment, and it all comes back. You start wondering if it was the alcohol or birth control pills (or whatever happens to be on today's "hit list") that caused your cancer. Or you regret the decision you made, thinking, "With this new information maybe I should have done things differently." Remember, what's past is past. You can't change the way you lived your life in the past based on new information just coming to light today. You have to comfort yourself with the realization that you probably got the best treatment that was available at the time you were diagnosed. If there are improved treatments now, that's wonderful—but you can't waste your energy on what might have been. Read the newspapers and keep informed if you're interested, but don't use it to torture yourself about what might have been. Gradually you will regain your perspective.

Life will never be completely the same as it was before, but eventually you'll stop living in terms of your cancer. The fears and memories will come back occasionally—maybe at your yearly checkups, maybe on the anniversary of your diagnosis, maybe when you find out a friend had a recurrence. But they'll be part of your life, not the center of it.

PHYSICAL ADJUSTMENTS

Since more women are now living for many years after breast cancer treatments, they need as much information as possible about the side effects of treatment. In the following section I attempt to address this need.

Long-Term Side Effects of Surgery and Radiation

Unfortunately your body doesn't always feel the way it did before your cancer began. Radiation can cause delayed problems. A certain side effect can occur between three and six months after you've finished your treatment. The muscle that goes above and behind your breast, the pectoralis major muscle (see Fig. 22-6), will get extremely sore, and it's worse if you grab it between your fingers. That's because the radiation caused inflammation of the muscle, and as it begins to regenerate, it can get sore and stiff, just as it would if you threw it out during strenuous exercise. Most women think it's the cancer spreading—especially since the radiation has been over for months and they're not expecting new side effects from it.

Many women have a stiff or frozen shoulder a month after breast surgery. These arm and shoulder problems result from the lymph node dissection, not the breast surgery. When your armpit hurts, it's natural to try to protect it by keeping your arm immobilized. But when you don't use your arm, your shoulder muscles grow weak and the tendons and ligaments tighten. You may have difficulty reaching and feel pain when you raise your hand above your head. Not using your arm for a long time may lead to frozen shoulder—the joint becomes locked. Frozen shoulder can be more difficult to treat than a stiff shoulder, and it sometimes requires surgery. Bear in mind, however, that arm and shoulder problem are not an inescapable consequence of the procedure. They can be prevented or reversed. Start with gentle exercises, like climbing the wall with your fingers and circling your arms as soon as you feel able (see Chapter 21). The YWCA has a wonderful exercise program, Encore, that focuses on helping women recover. Swimming is also good because it doesn't put weight on the arm. You can resume any exercise routine you enjoyed in the past.

If exercising on your own isn't successful, a physical therapist can assess what you are capable of doing and where you need help and then devise a program to increase your strength and flexibility. The therapist will train you to do exercises properly so that you don't get hurt when you do them. Insurance plans often cover physical therapy after breast surgery, so be sure to ask.

Massage has effects similar to those of exercise. It can help relax tight tendons to get your shoulder back in commission. Acupuncture is another possibility. Although it has been tested for only a few applications in Western medicine, acupuncture hasn't been demonstrated to cause harm. There is some evidence it can help relieve lower back pain, so it may also help shoulder stiffness. However, there are no scientific data about this.

Scarring is an inevitable consequence of breast surgery. Initially, many women are so intent on saving their lives that they don't think about how their body will look after therapy. Of course, the appearance of the scar depends not only on the extent of surgery but on your skin, your body type, the size of your breast, and the type of surgery you had. To avoid being surprised by your body's appearance after surgery, ask your doctor to show you pictures of women who have had a similar operation; you may also go to my website and look at the "show me" collection or read books on the subject. There are several things you can do to make the scar more acceptable to you, from working with the surgeon to prevent surprises to having plastic surgery.

After mastectomy, the incision can take more than a year to heal completely. It may be difficult to know whether a problem that arises is temporary or will be with you long-term. Either way, you should discuss problems that seem significant or unusual with your surgeon. It's also important to remember that you don't need to wait a year to have additional surgery or procedures to correct the problems.

The scar may be raised, seemingly filled with extra skin. This is a keloid scar and results from an overly aggressive effort by the body's immune system to heal the wound. The body keeps filling the scar with collagen long after the wound has closed. The tendency to form keloid scars is probably inherited and can't be prevented. A plastic surgeon may be able to improve the scar's appearance. There is nothing wrong with being concerned about how you look. You've been through a very unpleasant and life-changing experience; you're entitled to do what you can to make its aftermath as comfortable as possible for yourself. Talk to a plastic surgeon about all the possibilities and decide what's best for you.

A mastectomy leaves a fairly large wound. When the surgeon pulls the skin and underlying tissue together to close it, the surface of the chest is drawn taut. In contrast, the surrounding tissue under the arm may seem baggy and excessive and hang over your bra. If fat is a major component of the extra tissue under the arm, it can be removed through liposuction. Excess skin can also be eliminated without increasing scarring.

Even a lumpectomy can change the appearance of the breast you've saved. It may look foreign and disturbing to you; it may have a dent, look shrunken, or appear to be pulled to one side.

If you are still troubled by the appearance of your breast months or years after surgery, you can always have a reconstructive procedure. A plastic surgeon can discuss various techniques to realign nipples, reshape breasts, and make the breasts more symmetrical (see Chapter 22).

Long-term problems may also result from the surgery. While most women experience some pain in the weeks after surgery, especially mastectomy, many will have pain for years. It can even begin years after the operation. Forty-nine percent of patients who have operations for breast cancer say they have some sort of ongoing pain or change in sensation, and 10 percent say it interferes with their daily lives.[12] The biggest complaint is "aching," experienced by 44–47 percent of the women who say they have pain. Many others describe it as a "stabbing" pain. "Shooting," "sharp," "tiring," and "throbbing" are other descriptions. They feel the pain in the mastectomy scar, the arm, even the muscle under the breast. I've known a number of women with this problem and it affects their lives.

Although we don't know precisely what causes the pain, it seems to involve damage to the *intercostal brachial* nerve, which causes numbness in the arm and is usually cut during lymph node surgery. It's also related to the intensity of a woman's postoperative pain. Again, we don't know what that means; possibly these women have a low pain threshold, or perhaps the intercostal brachial nerve was injured.

C.B. Wallace studied pain experienced a year after different kinds of breast surgery.[13] Lumpectomy alone resulted in pain among 31 percent of subjects. Mastectomy plus reconstruction caused pain in 49 percent of the women. Women who had breast reconstruction varied. Those who had implants under the muscle had pain in 15 percent of cases, whereas those who had them above the muscle had pain 21 percent of the time. Mastectomy alone caused pain through the armpit and arm; 82 percent of women had pain under their arms three months after a mastectomy, and in 16 percent, it lasted at least six months. Sometimes the pain was so bad the woman couldn't move her arm and developed frozen shoulder (discussed earlier in this chapter). Women who had breast reduction suffered later pain in 22 percent of cases, and 40 percent of women who had breast augmentation had pain. One study shows that careful surgical techniques reduce the amount of chronic pain.[14] Researchers found fewer pain problems associated with operations performed in centers that do lots of surgery than in those that don't. It makes sense: an inexperienced surgeon is more likely to injure nerves.

This kind of pain has been treated with *myofascial release,* a form of massage.[15] Among my patients acupuncture has helped a great deal. Another pain study suggests that if the pain is caused by damaged nerves, antidepressants can relieve it; this has no relation to the patient's frame of mind but to the specific way such drugs work on nerves.[16] Most large hospitals have pain specialists on staff to consult with patients.

Lymphedema

A major long-term complication is swelling of the arm—lymphedema—which can result from lymph node removal. It can be so slight that you notice it only because your rings begin to feel too tight on your fingers, or so severe that your arm becomes huge, even elephantine (Fig. 26-1). It can be temporary or permanent. It can set in immediately or years after your operation. What causes it? Basically lymphedema—sometimes called milk arm—is a plumbing problem. Normally the lymph fluid is carried through the lymph vessels, passes through the lymph nodes, and is returned to the bloodstream near the heart. The lymph nodes act like a strainer, removing foreign material and bacteria. So if you have surgery in the area and it scars over, some of the holes are blocked and the drainage is affected. The fluid doesn't drain out as well as it needs to, and everything backs up and swells. Protein leaks into the tissue and then scars, causing the condition to become chronic.

This used to be much more common—we'd see it in about 30 percent of cases—because more extensive surgery was done. Dr. Jeanne Petrek reported on 263 women who were alive and symptom free 20 years after their initial treatment for breast cancer. She noted that 13 percent reported severe lymphedema, with 49 percent reporting the

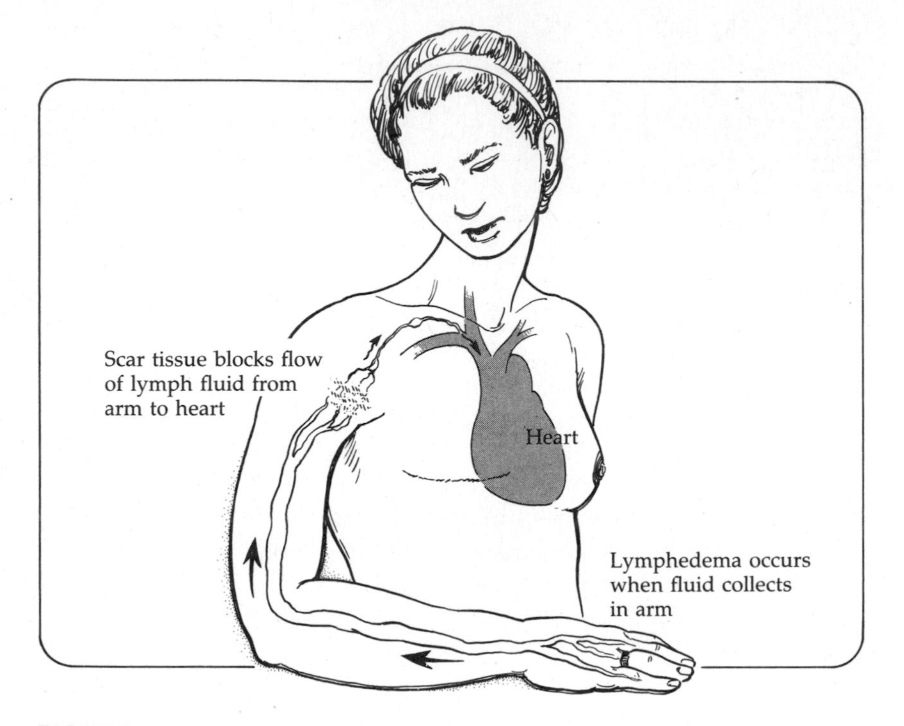

FIGURE 26-1

sensation of lymphedema. Seventy-seven percent of the women with swelling noted it within three years of their surgery, while the remaining developed swelling at a rate of 1 percent a year.[17] Though this is a serious problem for many breast cancer survivors, the current use of sentinel node biopsy promises to decrease women's chances of getting it. Initial studies show that women who underwent sentinel node biopsies had lymphedema 2–6 percent of the time, compared to 17–34 percent for full axillary dissection.[18,19,20]

Most women are cautioned about hand and arm care after surgery so they can prevent lymphedema from happening in the first place. These recommendations are hypothetical and are based on trying to prevent the production of excess lymph and blocked flow. In Petrek's 20-year study mentioned above, the only factors other than treatment that correlated with lymphedema were weight gain after surgery and arm/hand infection or injury. This is yet another reason to try to avoid weight gain. It's a good idea to watch out for infections in the affected arm and have them treated sooner rather than later. You may also want to consider using a compression bandage when doing vigorous arm exercises. In general, however, common sense should guide you. One study comparing women who had had bilateral mastectomies and axillary dissections to those who had surgery on only one side showed no difference in the incidence of lymphedema.[21] Most of them continued to have blood pressures done and blood drawn from one of their arms, suggesting that those procedures are not as dangerous as we might have thought. New studies are being done to determine whether the classical precautions are really necessary.

Lymphedema proceeds through stages. First is the latency stage; the arm is not swollen but the surgery has caused a reduced capacity for transporting lymph fluid. As long as there are no undue stresses on the system all will be well. Stage 1 is reversible, soft swelling. The skin is normal and you can relieve the swelling by elevating your arm. Stage 2 is no longer spontaneously reversible because there are fibrous changes in the tissues that make your arm feel hard. This stage includes frequent infections, which exacerbate the situation. The final stage is "lymphostatic elephantiasis." This is an extreme increase in volume and changes in the texture of your arm, including deep skin folds. Although there is no cure for lymphedema, we can reduce the swelling and maintain the reduction; in other words, bring lymphedema back to a state of latency.

A treatment devised in Germany, called complete decongestive physiotherapy, appears effective in numerous observational studies. It is well known in Europe and, increasingly, in the United States.[22,23] It is usually done by a physical therapist and involves four steps.

1. Skin and nail care, which may include topical and systemic antifungal drugs (making the skin free of infection before treatment)
2. Manual lymph drainage, a special technique of compression
3. Compression therapy using bandaging
4. Decongestive exercises

The treatment is done in two phases. The first is an attempt to mobilize the accumulated protein-rich fluid and start breaking up the chronic scarring. This phase is intense and can last four weeks—ideally, treatment is given twice a day five days a week. The next phase, which immediately follows, includes compression garments and bandaging at night. Although this sounds like a great treatment, it is also expensive and time-consuming. The best results come when the patient is in stage 1. If you are considering it, make sure you find a physical therapist or doctor who has been trained in the technique. The National Lymphedema Network (www.lymphnet.org) can help you locate one in your neighborhood. The National Center for Complementary and Alternative Therapy is sponsoring a study to establish once and for all whether this approach has any validity.[24]

Other therapies include elevating your arm to help reduce the swelling. Physical therapy and exercise can help in early cases. Long support gloves, similar to the stockings used for varicose veins, although unattractive, can reduce the swelling. (Ask for class 2 [30–40 mm Hg] or class 3 [40–50 mg Hg] support.) Although in Australia they initially reported good results with the group of drugs called benzopyrones,[25] such as coumarin, more recent randomized controlled studies have shown them to have no value.[26]

My theory about lymphedema is that we're probably approaching it backward. Patients are advised to go home and elevate the arm if they have a little swelling, to wear an elastic arm stocking for a lot of swelling, and to use the pump for an extreme amount of swelling. But by the time they use the pump, their tissues are so stretched out they've lost all their normal elasticity. It's like putting on a pair of panty hose you wore yesterday. As soon as they get off the pump, more fluid fills up the loose skin. Several operations have been applied to this problem, including liposuction, which is thought to help grow new lymphatics and improve drainage. There are now many lymphedema centers where you can research your options.

I think we should act aggressively when we find a small amount of swelling—physical therapy, manual massage, compression—and try to reverse it. We'd probably be able to reverse the process in more people because their skin would still be elastic.

Lymphedema has been vastly underestimated by the medical profession. Women with lymphedema experience enormous physical and psychological difficulties. Anne Coscarelli, director of the Ted Mann Family Resource Center for Women with Cancer at UCLA, feels that the medical profession underestimates the psychological stress of having lymphedema. It is a constant reminder that the ordeal is not over, and that you can't get back to your old life. On top of this, it generates less support from caregivers and family members because it is not life threatening. Most women with lymphedema benefit greatly from talking to others about the experience, either in a support group or on an Internet bulletin board. In 1995 at UCLA we started what I think was the first lymphedema support group in an attempt to address some of these problems. Lymphedema will end only when axillary dissections are no longer performed.

Cellulitis

Cellulitis is a skin infection occurring in places that have diminished access to the immune system, such as areas of swelling or areas that have been radiated. It can start from any small infection and rapidly spread, often with a red streak up the arm or redness of the arm and/or breast. There is usually a fever as well. Although this type of infection can sometimes be treated with oral antibiotics, usually it requires hospitalization for intravenous drugs. Some women who are prone to recurrent attacks of cellulitis ask the doctor for a standing antibiotic prescription so they can start taking it at the least sign of impending infection. In a series of studies from Memphis, Tennessee, 1 percent of the lumpectomy and radiation patients had cellulitis of the breast.

LONG-TERM SIDE EFFECTS OF CHEMOTHERAPY

In the past, chemotherapy was used only to treat metastasis. Oncologists at that time weren't thinking about long-term effects; they hoped to keep the patient living a few years longer than she would without the treatment. If she lived long enough to deal with long-term effects, she and her doctors were happy. Because we now detect micrometastases and use chemotherapy on people whose cancers haven't significantly spread, this has changed. A woman treated with chemotherapy may now live for many years, and the issues surrounding her long-term well-being are more important. Only now are we beginning to grasp the implications of this development.

"Chemo Brain"

There are many after effects of chemotherapy that we're just beginning to acknowledge, either because they're subtle or because they take longer to materialize. For example, studies show decreased cognitive function (what patients call "chemo brain"). Several studies have been published showing cognitive impairment in women with breast cancer who have undergone adjuvant chemotherapy.[27,28] All of the studies have been criticized for the way they were done; for example, they compared the survivors as a group to healthy controls. Although on the surface this may seem a good thing to do, in fact it is unlikely to pick up subtle differences. Is this the result of the chemotherapy or of the premature menopause brought on by chemotherapy in younger women? How does tamoxifen contribute to the changes? Is it because of depression about having breast cancer in the first place? Or the hot flashes and night sweats that prevent sleep and result from the premature menopause?

In my mind, the best study so far is one recently reported from M.D. Anderson in Texas.[29] Eighteen women who were scheduled to receive FAC chemotherapy underwent comprehensive neuropsychological testing before starting treatment. Interestingly 33 percent of them already showed cognitive problems. This is similar to another report from this center showing 35 percent of women having cognitive dysfunction right before starting chemotherapy.[30] (Of course this could be the anxiety of having breast cancer and facing chemotherapy.) This is important because without this baseline we might have exaggerated the effects of chemotherapy. Even more interesting was the follow-up report on the 18 women. Six months after stopping chemotherapy, 61 percent showed a decrease in function compared to their baseline and reported greater difficulty in maintaining their ability to work. The most common problems were paying attention, learning, and speedily processing. At the 18-month follow-up, approximately 50 percent of the women who had experienced decreases in function showed improvement whereas 50 percent remained stable. Self-reported ability to work also improved. Although this study is small, the way it was done is important in showing the effects of chemotherapy over time. Approximately 46 percent of the women would not have been classified as experiencing a decline in cognitive function based on their postchemotherapy evaluations alone. In other words, compared to their prechemo functioning they had declined, but they were still above the average for healthy women of their age. This study is consistent with published retrospective postchemotherapy reports that identify a subgroup of patients who experienced cognitive decline that improves over time.[31,32]

Research is going on to learn whether specific groups of women are more susceptible than others and whether cognitive retraining can overcome the difficulties.[33]

I doubt that most oncologists warn women who are considering chemotherapy that they may lose a significant part of their brain function. For someone who needs the treatment to survive, it's worth it, but in cases where chemotherapy offers only a minuscule survival improvement, it may not be.

Fatigue

An interesting study looked at fatigue after chemotherapy. (Anyone who's had chemotherapy knows about such fatigue; now we doctors are catching up to the patients!) The women who had chemotherapy suffered 61 percent more fatigue than the women in the control group.[34] I think of it as the "pooped-out syndrome." Your body has been assaulted by surgery, radition, and chemotherapy and is still trying to heal. It needs longer to get back to normal than we previously understood. One patient says it takes as long to get back to normal as it took to get the treatment: if you have six months of chemotherapy, you have six months of fatigue.

There are two ways you can approach this fatigue: drugs and exercise. Much of the fatigue on chemotherapy and after is caused by anemia. This can be treated by transfusions or by erythropoietin (Epogen), which stimulates the bone marrow to produce more red blood cells.[35]

Several studies show that aerobic exercise decreases the fatigue.[36,37,38] This may be hard to force on yourself—the last thing you feel like doing when you're exhausted is exercise! But it's worth pushing yourself. Probably it works by increasing endorphins. And it can help prevent the next side effect: weight gain.

Weight Gain

Although the cause of weight gain with chemotherapy is not clear, one study revealed that 50 percent of patients gained more than 10 pounds.[39] This was independent of type of chemotherapy, age, and menopausal status, although the women who gained weight did have a decrease in activity. Some data suggest that overweight women have a higher mortality than lean ones.[40] This has stimulated interest in nutritional and exercise programs for survivors. (See Chapter 20.)

Bone Loss

Women with breast cancer tend to have high bone density. The problem is that chemotherapy (by putting some women into premature menopause) and some of the current hormone therapies accelerate the normal bone loss that occurs with aging. But others, notably tamoxifen and to a lesser extent toremifene, help maintain bone by preventing its loss. They have about the same effect as raloxifene (Evista), improving bone density by 2–3 percent and preventing vertebral fractures. Goserelin induces temporary menopause for two years, resulting in a 5 percent decrease in bone density, which started improving once the therapy was withdrawn. Women who took tamoxifen while they were on the goserelin showed only a 1.4 percent decrease in bone density.[41] Since use of the aromatase inhibitors results in an increase in fractures compared to tamoxifen, we do not know what the effect of combining goserelin and an aromatase inhibitor will be on the bone. At a minimum women who have had breast cancer should follow the general recommendation from the National Osteoporosis Foundation: first bone density test at 65 or at most at the end of therapy. It is not clear that the decrease in bone density with treatment is permanent. A study of two years of the aromatase inhibitor exemestane showed that after the drug was stopped, the bone density of the lumbar spine improved and that of the hip stabilized, suggesting that the effects of these drugs are not permanent.[42] The bone densities after treatment were greater in the treatment group than the placebo group, a reminder that all women lose some bone. Bone does not change fast and the test itself is not that precise, so the current recommendations are to repeat a bone density test only after a minimum of two years.

Most fractures occur late in life and there is no evidence that treating osteopenia (low bone density short of osteoporosis) reduces your chances of having one. The thinking is that by the time you're 65 we know where your bone density stabilized and have lots of opportunity to treat you if you indeed have osteoporosis. Although women who have been treated for breast cancer may accelerate this process and fracture at an early age, this is certainly not proven. It doesn't make sense to test bone density before, though it may be good to have a bone density test at the conclusion of therapy to see what you ended with.

Based on this thinking and on the absence of data, I am not sure why many oncologists give bisphosphonates to women who are taking adjuvant hormonal therapy or are in premature menopause. These drugs may prevent bone loss, but there is no evidence suggesting that they help prevent fractures in women who do not already have osteoporosis.[43] If you decide to have a bone density test, be careful of falling into the trap of thinking that you should take a bisphosphonate if you have osteopenia; don't confuse bone density with fractures. These drugs are meant to prevent fractures, not treat bone density. The trend is not to give drugs to women to prevent bone loss but to reserve them for those at high risk of fracture (5–10 percent) in the next 5–10 years. All women should be taking calcium and vitamin D and getting enough weight-bearing exercise and weight training. This is the first step to preventing fractures in old age.

MENOPAUSAL SYMPTOMS

A woman can arrive at menopause in one of three ways: naturally, simply by living long enough; surgically, by having her ovaries removed; and chemically, through chemotherapy. This is as true for the woman with breast cancer as it is for everyone else. The difference is that the options for dealing with her symptoms are dictated in part by her history of breast cancer.

Someone treated with a mastectomy but not chemotherapy or tamoxifen may find that she goes into natural menopause right on cue. Or she could be thrown into menopause by a hysterectomy that includes oophorectomy (removal of ovaries) for bleeding or some other problem unrelated to her cancer. In these situations she will have the same symptoms as those who have not had breast cancer (which means they can range from nonexistent to severe). The only difference is that the estrogen question looms larger for her than for someone who is not at any particular risk of breast cancer or recurrence.

She may be thrown into menopause by chemotherapy. Or she may have been taking hormone replacement therapy only to have it abruptly discontinued. The symptoms that arise in these situations will be doubly hard to sort out, since chemotherapy and tamoxifen add their own symptoms or side effects to the mix. Similarly, a woman may be prescribed goserelin (Zoladex), which creates a state of reversible menopause.

With natural menopause the ovaries continue to produce hormones, albeit at a much lower level. Obviously a woman who has gone through surgical menopause—removal of her ovaries—has no ovarian production of hormones afterwards, although her adrenal glands may produce some very small level of estrogen, as well as testosterone and androstenedione, which are converted by fat, muscle, and breast tissue into estrogen by aromatase. However, we don't know what happens with women who have chemical menopause. Does the chemotherapy destroy the ovaries so they never produce anything again? Or does it simply throw the woman into regular menopause, so she gets postmenopausal levels of hormone production? We do know that women around 30 who receive chemotherapy often go into temporary menopause and then get their periods back (see Chapter 24). This may mean that the chemicals don't totally wipe out the ovaries'capacity to produce hormones but simply push the middle-aged woman in the direction she's already heading. Thus women who are apparently thrown into permanent menopause may still have some ovarian hormone production. Or maybe some of them do and some don't. This is an area we need to study more.

There are two aspects of menopause that a woman needs to consider. The first is that symptoms can come with a sudden or an erratic change in hormones. These symptoms, as I explained in Chapter 18, are usually transient, lasting for two to three years on average. They need to be treated specifically, and there is a large menu of options.

The second is the way menopause is often portrayed by the media and the pharmaceutical companies—as the cause of diseases that occur in later life, especially heart disease and osteoporosis. There are several global approaches to these problems, and there are specific remedies for specific symptoms and prevention of specific diseases. Before I launch into an analysis of the pros and cons of the options, I think it is important to point out that doing nothing is an acceptable choice. You don't have to "treat" or "manage" menopause unless it is interfering with your life.

First let's talk about hormones. As I explained at length in Chapter 11, the data are pretty compelling that taking HRT (hormone replacement therapy) increases the risk of breast cancer. This alone should be enough to cross it off the list as an option for the woman who already has the disease. Recent studies have added further data leading to the conclusion that such women should never use HRT. The HABITS trial began in 1997 to recruit volunteers willing to help investigate whether a two-year HRT treatment for menopausal symptoms was safe in women with a previously treated breast cancer.[44] Women with in situ to stage 2 breast cancer were eligible, whether or not they were on tamoxifen (21 percent), if they had menopausal symptoms they felt needed treatment. A total of 434 women were randomized, and 345 had at least one follow-up. After a mean follow-up of 2.1 years, 26 women in the HRT group and 7 in the non-HRT group had a new breast cancer. Of the women with a new cancer in the non-HRT group, two had been taking HRT on their own. (This, by the way, was unfair: if you are part of a study group and decide not to abide by its rules, you should always let them know and leave the study.) Because of this, the researchers stopped the trial and announced that HRT posed an unacceptable risk to women with breast cancer.

A more recent treatment for menopausal symptoms is bioidentical hormones—hormones identical to the ones your own body makes when it is premenopausal. The studies aren't conclusive yet, but there is no reason to believe that bioidentical hormones are safer than synthetic ones. As we saw in Chapter 19, women with high levels of their own hormones—estrogen and testosterone—are at greater breast cancer risk. A recent abstract by a group at Northwestern indirectly implicated the body's own progesterone.[45] Researchers measured salivary levels of progesterone and breast tissue density (a strong risk factor for breast cancer mentioned in Chapter 9) over six months. Only the women on tamoxifen who had an increase in progesterone had an increase in breast density. I should point out that the PEPI study discussed in Chapter 9 also showed an increase in breast density in the women on natural progesterone.[46] Indeed, the mere fact that the women who go through menopause late have a higher risk of breast cancer should suggest that even your own hormones are not all that good for you after a while. So the fact that we don't yet have any data suggesting that bioidentical hormones are dangerous does not mean they are safe. A review of estriol and bioidentical formulations of estrogen (Triest) confirmed that estriol causes endometrial stimulation, just as HRT does, and that it stimulates breast cancers to grow (6 of 24 women).[47] A recent review of bioidentical hormone therapy concluded that hormones specially compounded for a woman may well decrease her symptoms, but there is no evidence that they are safe.[48] It is likely not the type of hormones that you are taking but the fact that you are taking "replacement" hormones that puts you back in premenopausal range. To date there is more hype than science about bioidentical hormones, including over-the-counter natural progesterone creams.[49]

Finally there is tibolone. This is a nonestrogenic drug available outside of the United States. Studies are investigating its use in breast cancer patients, but the Million Women Study, which looked at women in England on various forms of HRT, found that it too increased breast cancer risk as well as endometrial cancer. The jury is still out.[50,51]

TREATMENT FOR SYMPTOMS

If HRT is out, what can you do for menopausal symptoms? Although there are sometimes symptoms during the postmenopausal years, most of the symptoms that cause discomfort come in the transition when your body is experiencing shifts in hormones. So treatments may only last for only a few years rather than a lifetime. Treatments vary with symptoms.

Hot Flashes

A behavioral approach can help. For one thing, you can avoid triggers. These vary greatly among individual women, but you can soon figure out what yours are by keeping a daily "hot flash diary." Spicy foods, caffeine, stressful situations, and hot drinks are among the more common triggers. Once you've identified them you can choose to avoid them. Sleep in a cool room; carry a hand fan (I keep one in my briefcase); dress in cotton and in layers; do paced respiration exercises (practicing deep, slow abdominal breathing); try acupuncture; eat a serving of soy foods (see later in this chapter) and ground flax seeds daily; walk, swim, dance, or ride a bike every day for at least 30 minutes. If none of this helps, try vitamin E (800 mg) or the herb black cohosh (Remifemin, see later in this chapter). If nothing helps symptoms, you can join or create a support group to help you deal with them.

How well do these treatments work? There are data from randomized controlled studies supporting acupuncture and paced respiration. In addition, there are good data from randomized controlled double-blind studies on black cohosh, using both conjugated estrogen (Premarin) and a placebo as the controls. These studies found that the herb reduces hot flashes and helps vaginal dryness. Many U.S. researchers aren't aware of these studies because they were done in Germany.[52,53] There are randomized placebo-based data on dietary soy (*not* isoflavone pills) as well. Fredi Kronenberg and Adriane Fugh-Berman published a great review of all the randomized controlled trials of complementary and alternative therapies for menopausal symptoms and concluded that black cohosh and foods that contain so-called phytoestrogens show promise, but clinical trials did not support the use of other herbs or CAM (see Chapter 25) therapies.[54]

Soy Protein: A Natural SERM? When I lecture on either menopausal hormones or breast cancer, the question I am asked most is about soy. Soy is a food source of isoflavones. Sometimes it is called a phytoestrogen. This is a poor word choice. Although soy acts like estrogen in some organs it blocks estrogen in others—so it's more like a phytoSERM (selective estrogen receptor modulator; see Chapter 11) than a pure estrogen. In addition, it has many effects besides hormonal ones. It blocks tumor cells in a petri dish, whether or not they're sensitive to estrogen. We are only beginning to study the properties of this natural substance. Several randomized controlled studies on hot flashes and soy have shown a reduction in hot flashes not only in countries where soy is a large part of the diet, like China and Japan, but also in the West.[55]

In addition, soy not only decreases bad LDL cholesterol but increases good HDL cholesterol significantly. And unlike conjugated estrogen (Premarin), which increases triglycerides, soy decreases them.[56] It also increases bone density.

Soy seems to act in a couple of different ways on the breast. In the lab genistein (one of the active ingredients in soy) stimulates estrogen receptor positive cancers at low doses and blocks them at high doses. Then there are the nonestrogenic effects of blocking invasion and angiogenesis (growth of new blood vessels), which may be more important in preventing breast cancer. In petri dishes and in animal models, soy definitely inhibits breast cancer growth. And a recent study out of Sanford Barsky's lab at UCLA shows that it has this effect on cancer cells that are both estrogen receptor positive and negative.[57] Clearly soy is more than just a plant estrogen.

Occasionally a woman with breast cancer says to me, "My tumor is estrogen receptor positive: does that mean I can't take soy?" I reassure her that soy is not estrogen—it is an isoflavone and has many effects. I do not think there is a risk in having one serving of soy a day. I am often asked whether a woman who's taking tamoxifen can also take soy, or if the soy counteracts the tamoxifen. A study in mice with chemically induced cancers showed that soy inhibited the tumor incidence, and when researchers added tamoxifen, the combination reduced both incidence of tumors and the number of tumors that developed.[58] So it appears that, at least in this study, soy and tamoxifen work synergistically. In another study in mice, genistein seemed to interfere with the effects of tamoxifen.[59] A study published in March 2004 in the *American Journal of Clinical Nutrition* indicated that soy isoflavones had no biological effect on the indicators of estrogenic activity in postmenopausal women.[60] Another small study by my colleague Mai Brooks at UCLA was also reassuring.[61] She gave soy tablets to women with breast cancer for two weeks prior to their surgery and examined the rate of cell death and of cell division in the tumors on biopsy and again after they were removed—in other words, before and after soy. She also compared the women on soy to historical controls (see Chapter 15)—women who had similar characteristics to those taking soy. She compared their tumors and found no difference between the two. The cancers were not growing any faster in the women on soy. At this point the data are not sufficient to be sure. Barrie Cassileth from Memorial Sloane Kettering Cancer Center feels strongly that women with estrogen receptor positive tumors should not eat soy at all. On the other hand, Mark Messina, Ph.D., who has devoted his career to studies of soy, feels that it is safe to eat soy if you like it but there is still no evidence that it will improve your survival from breast cancer. I tend to side with Dr. Messina. I think it's probably safe for women with breast cancer, but the final answers aren't in yet. You will have to decide for yourself whether to try it. If you do, try eating one serving (40 grams) of soy protein daily. I am confident enough to have a soy drink for breakfast every day, which has vastly decreased my hot flashes, fuzzy thinking, and sleepiness. (Then again, maybe these symptoms would have stopped anyway.)

How should you take the soy? Ideally you should consume it as tofu, soybeans, or soy milk. There are many soy cookbooks around. (It also helps prevent prostate cancer and thus is good for the whole family.) If you do not have time to cook, then try one of the soy protein powders such as Healthy Source or Revival. However, I'd advise against taking soy capsules or capsules of isoflavones or genistein. Although these two are ingredients of soy, we do not know which one is more important. Nor do we know whether they work the same in isolation as they do in food. Also, it is much easier to overdose on soy in capsule form than as tofu. Always remember moderation.

Black Cohosh. Black cohosh (Remifemin) is a promising natural alternative to treat menopausal symptoms, but its mechanism is not understood. The question for breast cancer survivors is whether it is estrogenic. On this front we actually have some data. First, there is no known phytoestrogen in black cohosh. Second, there is no evidence that black cohosh binds to the estrogen receptor. Finally, in a petri dish, breast cancer cells were exposed to black cohosh in the absence of estrogen, in the presence of estrogen, and in the presence of tamoxifen.

They found that the black cohosh given alone inhibited cell growth. When estrogen was added it blunted the growth usually seen and it enhanced the effects of tamoxifen.[62] This effect has been replicated in four other studies on cell lines.[63,64,65,66] Studies in women have confirmed this lack of estrogenic effect.[67,68]

So it sounds safe. But does it work? On this front the data are mixed. A randomized study of women with breast cancer on tamoxifen showed that black cohosh was not statistically more effective than placebo in controlling hot flashes. A pilot study by the group at the Mayo Clinic of 21 women (13 of whom were breast cancer survivors and 6 of whom were on tamoxifen) showed a 50 percent decrease in hot flashes over 4 weeks.[69] Overall it appears safe for the breast cancer survivor and worth a try.

Nonhormone Drugs. A group at the Mayo Clinic has done a good study of menopausal symptom relief in women who have had breast cancer, which can also be used by other women.[70] This group, the North Center Cancer Treatment Group (NCCTG), studied more than 650 women with breast cancer and reported a number of findings. First, researchers found that a placebo alone appeared to cause a 20–25 percent reduction of symptoms in four weeks. This may show a psychological component to hot flashes, or it may reflect the nature of hot flashes: they tend to come and go on their own. My own example is fairly common and serves to illustrate the capricious nature of hot flashes. I had ten and a half weeks of horrible hot flashes and no period. "This is it," I thought. "These things will go on for a few years, my periods will stop, and—if I don't end up in an insane asylum first—so will the hot flashes." All of a sudden, on a Sunday while I was at a medical convention in Atlanta, the hot flashes stopped, and I found myself wondering what had happened. I'm sure if I had been started on a new treatment or had been on a placebo in a study, I would have thought happily, "I'm not in the placebo group, and this blessed treatment works!" Since this wasn't the case, I just whispered a prayer of devout gratitude to my guardian angel. Four weeks later, my period was back, and of course that was why the flashes had stopped.

Clonidine, which has been used for years as an antihypertensive, reduced hot flashes by about 15 percent more than the placebo in the NCCTG study. However, there were a lot of side effects: fatigue, nausea, irritability, headache, and dizziness. The group then looked at Megestrol acetate (Megace), a progestin used in higher doses to treat breast cancer. (This dose difference is found in lots of drugs such as estrogen and treatments like radiation therapy.) They found an 80 percent reduction of hot flashes, and there were no side effects. But this was a short study, and there's no way of knowing whether it will prove safe in the long run. Some researchers are concerned about using progestins, particularly in women with breast cancer, because many breast cancers have progesterone receptors and the low doses used in the study may be more dangerous than the high doses used to treat.

The Mayo Clinic study also found that 800 international units of vitamin E taken daily statistically decreased hot flashes. But the statistics boiled down to an average of one hot flash per woman per day—which may not help much. They also did a pilot study looking at a new antidepressant called danlafaxine (Effexor). They found that low doses, in addition to helping alleviate depression, decreased hot flashes by 50 percent. Since then they have studied other SSRIs (a group of antidepressants) and confirmed that venlafaxine, paroxetine,[71] and fluoxetine all reduced hot flashes by about 50 percent when compared to placebo.[72] This may be especially helpful to women whose symptoms include both hot flashes and depression. The newest candidate is gabapentin, a drug used for epilepsy and migraines that has shown a 54 percent reduction in hot flashes.[73]

There are lots of options for hot flashes. Some work in some women and some in others. If this is a significant problem for you, find a doctor (oncologist or gynecologist) who will stick with you and help you sort through the options to find something that works in your case.

As a flashing woman myself, I think there is one key component to getting through this temporary disruption in life—a sense of humor. If you can laugh at yourself and revel in this change you will, as the saying goes, turn the hot flashes into power surges.

Vaginal Dryness

Vaginal dryness as a result of vaginal atrophy is perhaps the most distressing and least talked about symptom of menopause. It occurs in about 20 percent of women, sometimes transiently and other times permanently. Sexual activity, including masturbation, reduces vaginal atrophy. The problem is that if you're sore from vaginal dryness, you don't want to have sex, and if you don't have sex, your vaginal dryness gets worse—a classic catch-22. There are two approaches. Water-based lubricants like KY jelly and Astroglide don't cure the basic condition, but they can help the immediate problem of painful intercourse. The other approach is to try to increase the vagina's own moisture. Replens, which can be purchased over the counter, causes your vagina to absorb water and become more supple. In one study 61.5 percent of patients preferred Replens, 26.5 preferred a lubricant, and 12 percent had no preference. In fact the use of both a moisturizer and a lubricant may provide the best results.

Both black cohosh and soy have been reported to reduce vaginal dryness. Vitamin E capsules have been used vaginally with some success as well. (You break open the capsule and rub the vitamin E on the lining of your vagina.)

If nothing else works, you may decide to try estrogen to improve the quality of your life. You should use the smallest amount necessary and apply it to where the problem is (interestingly, estrogen by mouth often doesn't relieve vaginal dryness). There's a vaginal ring (Estring) that releases a very small amount of estrogen over a long period of time. In the first 24 hours after you've had it inserted (or inserted it yourself, like a diaphragm), you have a little spurt of estrogen; beyond that it doesn't increase hormone levels because it is low-dose and sustained-release; it is not absorbed. You keep it in for three months and then change it. It's a great solution for women with breast cancer and vaginal dryness. As a last resort you can try vaginal estrogen creams. If you go that route, however, ignore the instructions on the label, which tell you to use an applicator full. Since estrogen as a cream is well absorbed from the vagina, you'll end up with blood levels that rival what you would get with estrogen pills. All you really need is a little dab on your fingertip. If you apply it every day for two weeks, then two or three times a week, it will solve your problems. (But don't use it as a lubricant at the time of sex; it won't help that way and your male partner may grow breasts!)

If you have not had intercourse for a while, you may find that along with dryness your vagina can become tighter as it loses elasticity. A dilator can help with this by stretching things out again. If problems persist despite all of these suggestions, ask your doctor to refer you to a counselor with sex therapy training for further help.

Insomnia, Mood Swings, and Fuzzy Thinking

Although insomnia is often related to night sweats, it is also true that you don't sleep as well when your hormones are awry. Some easy measures can help. Keep your bedroom cool, exercise (but earlier in the day; exercising right before going to bed will keep you awake), avoid caffeine and liquor, take warm baths or showers, increase soy intake, have cereal and milk products at bedtime, and take black cohosh.

To counter mood swings and anxiety, try using the relaxation response (see Chapter 25), exercising (including yoga), eating a plant- rather than meat-based diet, going to a psychotherapist, and finding creative outlets.

For fuzzy thinking, soy seems to help. Other possibilities are exercise, low-fat diet, nonsteroidal anti-inflammatories (Motrin), and vitamin E. The best thing to do for your brain is use it, for example, work, study, crossword puzzles, chess, reading, and card games. A recent study showed that people who stayed socially active had less cognitive decline with age. Remember, menopausal symptoms do not last forever. On average their duration is about two to three years off and on. The best approach to both symptom relief and prevention is to live a healthy lifestyle.

LIFESTYLE CHANGES

As I have said many times, doctors can treat you and sometimes cure you, but *you* are in charge of your healing! The experience of having breast cancer will change you forever. The trick is to use it to improve your life. One of the ways to do that is to look at your lifestyle and see if there are changes that could make it better for you.

One of the few lifestyle factors that appear to be important in dictating survival is weight. Women who are overweight at the time of diagnosis and/or gain weight after diagnosis have a higher risk of recurrence.[74,75] A large study (2,437) looking at low-fat diet compared to a normal diet in postmenopausal breast cancer survivors showed a reduction in recurrence of 24 percent overall with the greatest benefit in the estrogen receptor negative women (42 percent). The absolute reduction in recurrence was about 3 percent in addition to that with standard breast cancer treatments. In this study dietary fat was held to less than 33 grams a day (20 percent of calories), which is doable with a largely plant-based diet.[76] It is hard to know whether the effect is the low fat, the plant-based diet, or the resulting weight loss—but for a survivor it really doesn't matter. Here is something you can do to make a difference that is worth it and that lies in your control. You've heard it all before: eat less and exercise more. An additional observational study lends even more support to this approach, showing that exercises the equivalent of walking 3–5 hours per week at an average pace reduced the risk of recurrence of breast cancer by 6 percent.[77] A review of nutrition and survival after a diagnosis of breast cancer concluded that healthy weight control with an emphasis on exercise to preserve or increase lean muscle mass and a diet that includes nutrient-rich vegetables is recommended.[78]

Not surprisingly, these recommendations are also suggested to decrease chronic diseases of aging. Further, and most relevant here, increased physical activity has been shown to decrease the symptoms of menopause as well as improve the quality of life for breast cancer survivors.[79] It has even been shown to improve brain function![80] There are many ways you can increase your physical activity, many of which can be fun. (Make sure you obtain your doctor's approval first, since some drugs, such as doxorubicin, can have insidious effects on your heart, and this may affect which exercises are safest and best for you.) You can start walking or running regularly; you can even combine exercise and activism by participating in one of the ubiquitous breast cancer fund-raisers. Running a marathon for the first time may be a great way to celebrate being alive. You can join a dragon boat team and train to participate with other survivors rowing a dragon boat. These are very popular in Canada and catching on in the United States. You can start a walking group with close friends, or dance, or roller blade. If there's a sport you've thought of starting, this is a good time to do it. The key is to find something you will do, and happily!

What about diet? The best diet is one that works for you. Currently we have the most data on the Mediterranean diet, which encourages an abundance of food from plants, ideally fresh and locally grown; olive oil as the principal fat; daily consumption of low to moderate amounts of cheese and yogurt, weekly consumption of low to moderate amounts of fish and poultry, limited sweets and red meat and low to moderate consumption of wine. This diet, along with physical activity, will not only help you lose or maintain your weight but has been shown to decrease mortality from other causes. With all the diet fads out there, don't fool yourself. A diet high in any fat or sugar—the usual baddies—is never "best for you," no matter how good it tastes. You don't need to give up all the goodies you enjoy, but you do need to limit their place in whatever food plan you embrace.[81,82]

HEALING THE MIND

Emotional healing techniques are more varied and individual than physical ones, and many have proved helpful to my patients and other women with breast cancer.

Psychotherapy can be a tremendous tool at this time, as it is in any time of great emotional stress. About a quarter to a third of women have post-treatment symptoms that warrant evaluation. Persistent feelings of sadness, loss of self-esteem, lack of interest in things that brought you pleasure before you had cancer are *not* typical and should be followed up.

This may be the time to try a support group (see Chapter 20), especially if you were too overwhelmed to do it during therapy. Or you can join an online chat group. Check out www.acor.org for listings. Sometimes brief one-on-one counseling helps, particularly if you are finding it difficult to move on from the aftermath of your illness.

Many women keep a journal of their experiences to refer to later and to help them cope with their feelings. Some take their healing beyond themselves—reaching out to other women who are going through what they've been through. Writers like Audre Lorde, Linda Ellerbee, and Katherine Russel Rich, and performers like singer Melissa Etheridge and skater Peggy Fleming have spoken out or written about the experience. Indeed, much of the success we've had comes from early pioneers such as Shirley Temple Black, Happy Rockefeller, and Rose Kushner, who publicly fought the stigma attached to breast cancer.

Often the need to "give back" and find a positive side to this experience can be channeled to helping other women with breast cancer. Sometimes this can be done through your work. Two of my patients are psychotherapists who now specialize in breast cancer therapy. Another has begun doing breast cancer workshops at her corporation. If you're a sales clerk, you may want to work in a store selling prostheses, since you now have a special understanding that may help your customers.

If your profession isn't one that can be adapted to some form of working with breast cancer, or if you don't feel drawn toward spending your work life dealing with the disease, you can still help other women—and thus yourself—on a volunteer basis. For example, you may want to get involved with Reach for Recovery or a similar group that works with breast cancer patients. You know how frightened you were when you were first diagnosed. The presence of someone who's survived the disease can be enormously reassuring to a newly diagnosed woman.

You can also become involved in political action, possibly with the National Breast Cancer Coalition (www.stopbreastcancer.org). You can define the level of your participation according to your own energy, time constraints, and degree of commitment: anything from writing an occasional letter to your congressperson to organizing demonstrations and fund-raising events. Jane Reese Colbourne, a former NBC vice president, found that in her own experience political activism was "a very good way to channel anger at the fact that you've had this disease. For me, it was the next step after a support group. Talking about it with other women was important, but I wanted to do something about it."

Finally, make sure you don't feel ashamed of what you've been through. Cancer still carries a stigma in our culture, and breast cancer can have especially difficult associations. You need to demystify it to yourself and to others. You don't have to dwell on it, but it's not a good idea to repress it either. You need to have friends you can talk freely to about your disease and your feelings about it; you need to know you can include it in casual conversation, that you don't have to avoid saying, "Oh, yes, that was around the time I was in the hospital for my mastectomy."

One of the newest areas of survivorship research is called "benefit finding." As usual, it takes doctors and researchers awhile to catch up to what the patients have known all along—that there are many positive things that you can take from this experience. I often hear women say that while they would not wish cancer on anyone, they find themselves living more fully: they "don't sweat the small stuff," they cherish their families, and they truly value each day.

RELATIONSHIPS AND SEX

One of the least discussed subjects about life after breast cancer is sexuality. Your surgeon won't bring it up if you don't; in fact most surgeons will assume that if you're not complaining, everything must be fine. Yet most women find sex hard to talk about—especially when it concerns feelings, perhaps only half recognized, about losing both their sexual attractiveness and their libido when they lose a part of their bodies so strongly associated with sexuality. Doctors need to learn how to open the subject delicately, in a way that doesn't feel intrusive to the woman but communicates that she has a safe place to discuss sexuality concerns. I remember one surgeon who had referred a patient to me on his retirement. He said that after her mastectomy she had surprised everyone with her rapid recovery and exclaimed over how well she had "dealt with it." I took over the case, and in my first conversation with her I found out that, however well adjusted she seemed on the surface, she had not yet looked at her scar—and this was five years after the operation. She had never resumed sex with her husband and even dressed and undressed in the closet so he couldn't see her.

Many women have difficulties with sex and intimacy following a breast cancer diagnosis. Aside from feeling that your body has betrayed you, there is a feeling of invasion from the treatments. All these strangers have been poking and prodding you for weeks; you may almost feel as though you've been violated, and you forget that your body can provide you with pleasure. It takes a while to feel good and in control of your body again. You need to communicate these feelings to your partner so he or she can help you in your healing.

Some women find that after surgery, whether mastectomy or lumpectomy, a sexual relationship becomes even more important in helping them regain their sense of worth and wholeness. There may, however, be changes. One patient of mine who had had bilateral mastectomies felt that all the erotic sensations she had formerly had in her breasts had "moved south," and that her orgasms were doubly good. Other women miss the stimulation from a lost breast so much that they don't want their other breast touched during sex. Dr. Patricia Ganz, who has both worked with and studied the problems of women with breast cancer, talks about the problems women who have had lumpectomy

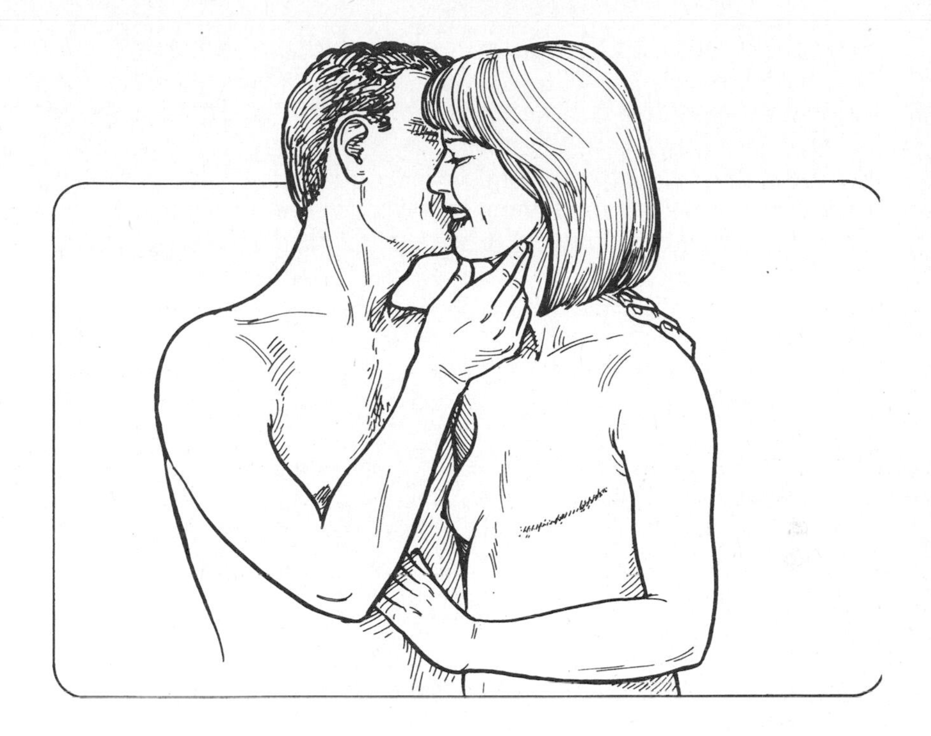

and radiation may experience: "Especially with women who had radiation a number of years ago, they often find the breast isn't as soft and beautiful as it was before the radiation." These changes in the conserved breast can carry over into their sexual relationships.

Some of the changes may be more practical than emotional. Your arm or shoulder may not be as strong on the side of your surgery, and this can make certain positions more difficult during intercourse, such as kneeling above your partner. You may feel uncomfortable lying on the side of the surgery for many months. It is important that you communicate with your partner so that together you can explore new ways of lovemaking that you both enjoy.

Chemical menopause can also affect a woman's sexuality. Menopause, like aging itself, often lessens sexual desire, and when that combines with other breast cancer issues a woman can find that her libido is abruptly and seriously lessened. Studies are now being done to see whether the libido loss of women with chemically induced menopause is more severe than that of women who have experienced menopause normally.

Dr. Ganz adds that it's difficult to separate out the physiological and emotional aspects of libido loss. "Sex is at least partly in the brain," she says, "and the hormones circulating in the body affect the brain and thus sexual arousal. Psychological distress can affect hormones; we've found in our work that women who have a lot of psychological distress have more sexual dysfunction."

There are no aspects of sexual intimacy that cause cancer or increase the chance of recurrence. Nor can cancer be "caught" by sucking on a nipple. Barbara Kalinowski, who once co-led support groups with me at the Faulkner Breast Centre in Boston, finds that "sometimes women who have had lumpectomy and radiation have a fantasy that the breast still has cancer in it, and don't want it fondled because they fear it will shake things up and send the cancer cells through the rest of the body." Even when your intellect knows such fears are groundless, your emotions may not, and that's bound to affect both partners' sexual pleasure.

Sheila Kitzinger in her book *Woman's Experience of Sex* writes that for some women having a brief affair was an important part of their healing process.[83] They said it was all well and good for a husband of 35 years to still love them without a breast, but they needed confirmation of their sexual attractiveness to feel whole again. That might work for you, though it could also put a severe strain on your marriage. At the very least, however, you'll want to be in touch with whatever feelings you're having about sex and decide which ones to act on and which ones to simply fantasize about.

This brings up another issue. If you are single and dating, should you tell or not? Again, this is an individual decision. Some women will tell a prospective lover way in advance, preferring to have it out in the open before the moment of passion. Others will wait until the last instant when there is no turning back to disclose their secret (never a good idea). For the woman who has had a small lumpectomy or has had mastectomy with a natural-looking reconstruction, the need to tell a casual lover about her situation may or may not arise. However, in a long-term relationship, it's important to be honest. For the woman whose surgery leaves visible alteration, dating can be a matter of concern. Yet it doesn't mean you have to resign yourself to a life of celibacy. Barbara Kalinowski found that several women in her support groups were able to form new romantic relationships shortly after surgery. She recalls one woman who had never married and had a mastectomy with reconstruction in her 50s. "I got a call from her a couple of years ago. She was as giggly and happy as a teenager. 'Guess what!' she told me. 'I'm getting married!' They were planning a honeymoon in Paris and she was ecstatic." Another woman from one of Kalinowski's groups was happily married to a man who was wonderful to her during treatment. Two years later he died of a heart attack. Soon after his death she met a widower and they fell in love. "They decided not to wait," Kalinowski says, "because they both knew how chancy life was. She told me, 'We both learned that we don't want to wait for anything anymore.'"

Many women worry that their partner will be turned off by their condition and new body. There are many horror stories of husbands and significant others who opt out of having sex or even walk out entirely. The impact of cancer can be as devastating to the partner as to the patient herself. Partners may feel angry, ashamed, and vulnerable to illness themselves. Their lives and dreams have been changed, but they typically get less support. They feel guilty complaining when they are not the ones undergoing treatment. Some people have problems dealing with serious illness, and others may use it as an excuse to get out of a relationship they thought was not working anyway. Most important is the quality of the relationship and the level of communication. Work by David Wellisch at UCLA indicates that the husband's involvement in the decision-making process, hospital visitation, early viewing of scars, and early resumption of sexual activity were important for couples to function optimally.[84] Open dialogue is critical in this process, for nonmarried and lesbian couples as well as married ones.

Another study found that patients' and partners' levels of adjustment were significantly related; when one partner was experiencing difficulties in adjustment, the other was also likely to be having problems.[85] Difficulties in communication and sex need to be addressed promptly. Patricia Ganz found that most sexual issues were resolved by one year; if not, they were never resolved.[86] Counseling—where you can talk about your feelings in a protective environment—can be important in preventing serious problems. Hoping a situation will get better on its own rarely works and usually causes the problem to become chronic. You should request help for such problems as decreased libido and vaginal dryness; you may even consider seeing a sex therapist.

PREGNANCY

If you are still menstruating, a question that nearly always comes up is whether or not you should risk getting pregnant once you've had breast cancer. There are two areas to consider—the ethical implications and the health-related implications.

In the past doctors (usually male) tended to impose their own value judgments on patients and told them not to get pregnant for least five years after having breast cancer. If you survived five years, they reasoned, there was a good chance you'd won your bout with breast cancer; otherwise, they didn't want you bringing a child you couldn't raise into the world.

This is a moral decision for the patient to make, not the doctor, and there are two equally valid ways of looking at it. Some women do not want to have a child they're not reasonably sure they'll be around to raise. Others feel that even if they do die in a few years they'll still be able to give a child the love and care needed in the early years, and they want to pass on their genes before they die. Considerations of a husband's or partner's ability to nurture a child and support from family and friends will weigh on the decision as well.

Having a child is never a decision anyone can make lightly, and a life-threatening illness complicates it further. Think it through carefully and get the thoughts of people whose opinions you respect—and then make your decision.

The other question is medical. Can getting pregnant decrease your chances of surviving breast cancer? I wish I knew. Although there are no randomized studies, cancer centers that have reported on the outcome of women who have had pregnancies following breast cancer have shown no difference in survival (see Chapter 19).[87,88]

We do know that getting pregnant won't cause the cancer to spread; either it has spread or it hasn't before you become pregnant. But if you had a tumor that left microscopic cells in your body, it's possible that pregnancy, with its attendant hormones, could make them grow faster than they would have if you weren't pregnant. This could reduce the time you have left; for example, if you would have died of breast cancer four years from now, you'll die in three years instead.

So the question is, Do you want to take that risk? If you had a lot of positive nodes, a very aggressive tumor, or some other factor that increases the likelihood of micrometastases, you'll want to take that into consideration. It might be worth the risk to you, or it might not. Again, that's a very individual decision.

If you get pregnant, how will your breasts react? If you've had a mastectomy, obviously nothing will happen on the chest area where your breast was, but your other breast will go through all the usual pregnancy changes I described in Chapter 3. If you've had lumpectomy and radiation, the nonradiated breast will probably go through the normal changes. Radiation damages some of the milk-producing parts of the breast, so the radiated breast, while it will grow somewhat larger, won't keep pace with the other breast, and will produce little or no milk. You can nurse on one side only if you want. The problem with that is increased asymmetry; the milk-producing breast will grow and may stay larger after you finish breast-feeding. If you wish, you can have the larger breast reduced later through plastic surgery (see Chapter 3). One of my patients got pregnant shortly after finishing radiation treatments and successfully breast-fed the baby. But one breast ended up twice as large as the other. Knowing she wanted another child, she decided to wait till after her next pregnancy to get the breast reduced.

It's probably a good idea to wait till a year or so after your treatment to get pregnant. It's a stressful process and you won't want to add morning sickness to the nausea you're likely to get from the chemicals.

On the other hand, I had a patient who inadvertently got pregnant right after finishing chemotherapy. After talking it over with her husband and her caregivers, she decided to have the baby; last I heard, mother and daughter were both doing fine.

We have been talking about having a child after breast cancer when you are still fertile, of course. I discussed this at length in Chapter 19, including new research on transplanting ovarian tissue and using tamoxifen and letrozole for in vitro fertilization (IVF). But the fact that we *can* do it does not mean it is safe to do. As the numbers of young women who are breast cancer survivors increase, we need more studies to answer these questions. (Two good places to research the latest information on this are www.fertilehope.org and www.youngsurvival.org.)

The decision is up to you. If the stress of dealing with cancer and its uncertainties is too great, you may not want to have a child. On the other hand, if you do want to have a child and feel prepared for it, perhaps creating a new life can help you to cope with the knowledge of mortality that a life-threatening illness carries with it—a reminder that death isn't the end.

INSURANCE AND GETTING A JOB

Unfortunately, medical and emotional problems aren't the only ones you'll have to face. People with cancer often experience what amounts to discrimination, and there are some precautions you need to take.

First, you don't want to let your insurance lapse. Your company can't drop your policy because of your illness, so you're safe on that score. But many insurance companies won't take on someone who's had a life-threatening illness, and others will take you on but exclude coverage in the area of your illness. If you change jobs and go from one company's coverage to another, you'll probably be all right (but make certain of this before you accept the new job). If you quit for a while, make sure you keep up your insurance on your own. It's costly, but not nearly as costly as having no coverage if you get a recurrence.

Life insurance and disability insurance are also harder to get if you've had breast cancer. More and more cancer survivors are fighting to get this changed, and it should get better in the future. But for now, be very alert.

One of the hardest questions is whether or not to tell employers and coworkers about your cancer. There are pros and cons either way. Federal law prohibits federal employers, or employers who get federal grants or federal financial assistance, from discriminating against the handicapped or anyone mistakenly thought to be handicapped. The Americans with Disabilities Act (ADA), which was passed in 1992 and amended in 1994, extends this concept to the private sector. Any employer with 15 or more employees is prohibited from discriminating against qualified applicants and employees because of any disability. Cancer and other diseases are considered disabilities under the terms of this legislation. The employer must also make reasonable accommodations to the disability; for example, if you have trouble reaching a high shelf because of pain from your mastectomy your employer must make material accessible on a lower shelf, or even build you a lower shelf if feasible. A recent follow-up study from Canada showed that slightly more survivors than controls were unemployed three years after diagnosis, but among the women still employed no one noted a change in their working conditions because of their cancer diagnosis.[89]

Many women fear employers will find subtle ways to discriminate against them if their cancer is discovered. One of my fellow breast cancer activists tells a great story of how she handled the loss of her job after her mastectomy, before the ADA was passed. Furious, she stormed into her boss's office, reached into her dress, pulled out her prosthesis, and slapped it on his desk. As he gaped at her in horror, she snapped, "Sir, you are confused—I had a mastectomy, not a lobotomy!" Then she calmly walked out, leaving her boss to buzz his secretary and ask her to remove the prosthesis.

The other possibility is that your boss and coworkers will offer you increased support if you are open. More and more attention is being given to cancer survivors in the workplace, and you may find a career counseling center that can give you good advice.

If you are looking for a new job, there is even more difficulty. Some companies are reluctant to hire someone with cancer. This too is illegal under the ADA, but there is always the fear that an employer will find some excuse not to hire you. You may want to be open about your cancer because you don't want to work for someone with that attitude. On the other hand, you may need the job too much to risk being turned down. But if you don't tell and then end up missing a lot of time for medical appointments or sickness, you could run into problems that might have been avoided if you'd been frank in the beginning. It's a tough delimma, and there are no easy answers. (A good place for information is the National Coalition for Cancer Survivors, www.cancer advocacy.org.)

27

When Cancer Comes Back

When breast cancer cells reappear in the area around the breast (local or regional recurrence) or in other areas of the body (distant metastasis), you have a recurrence. For the most part, these are the microscopic cells that presumably got out before your diagnosis and found a niche elsewhere in your body. The cells can get out through the bloodstream or the lymphatic system or other organs, where they can remain dormant for years. Finally something happens to wake them up (Fig 27-1). If we could figure out what puts these cells to sleep and then what wakes them up, we'd be a long way toward eliminating breast cancer.

It may be that radiation or chemotherapy kills some cells and injures others, knocking them out. Then after a long while the ones that survived recover and begin doubling again. Another possibility is that the surviving cells were put to sleep by tamoxifen or chemical menopause and are now awakening. Or perhaps the local environment controlled the cells for a time and then ceased.

Being diagnosed with a recurrence can be devastating. The process of psychosocial adjustment starts all over again; learning to trust your body may take longer when you've been doubly betrayed by it. The feelings you experienced the first time around are intensified because now you not only don't trust your body, but you begin to wonder about your doctors and treatment in general. This is a common feeling.

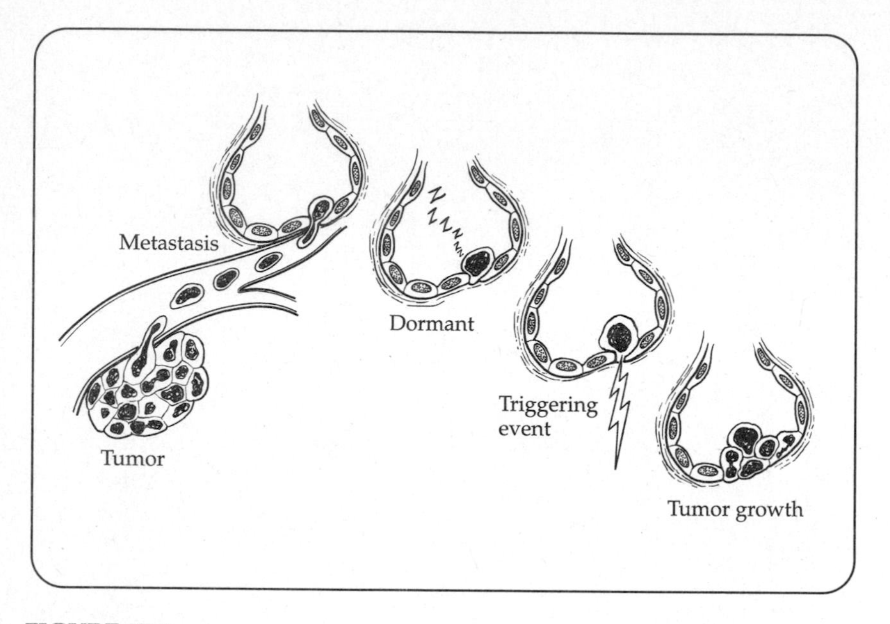

FIGURE 27-1

But remember that a recurrence is not your fault; it's the result of factors that we do not understand and cannot control. You should discuss your feelings with your caregivers. In addition, you'll want to get support and help from friends and family, counselors, therapists, and support groups.

The kinds of support groups that are available vary widely, depending on where you are. Even general cancer groups can be very helpful, but most women find breast cancer groups better. In big cities you may want to search out groups for women with recurrences or with metastases. There are advantages to each type of group. Barbara Kalinowski, a clinical nurse specialist, co-led both a first-diagnosis group and a recurrence group that went on for several years. In the recurrence group, the women all faced similar issues for three years, but the dynamics changed as the women with metastases began to worsen. "The women who are sick are very happy for the women who are getting better, and the women who are getting better are very supportive of the women who are sick," Kalinowski says. One of the women who was well had lunch with one of the others whose metastasis was worsening. Jackie Onassis had just died, and the sick woman said she wanted white and pink flowers at her funeral, the way Jackie had. The next week the other woman sent her a gorgeous bouquet of white and pink flowers, with a note saying, "You don't have to wait until you die for your flowers."

At the same time, Kalinowski says, women with metastatic cancer have more in common with each other as the illness progresses, and she would like to do a separate group for such women. For those who can't find a support group for women with metastatic disease nearby, there are many choices on the website www.drsusanloveresearch foundation.org.

In order to better deal with your recurrence, you need to know more about the nature of breast cancer recurrences. In the rest of this chapter we'll examine the types of recurrences, their symptoms, and their treatments.

LOCAL AND REGIONAL RECURRENCE

What kind of disease recurs is important in terms of prognosis. If the recurrence is precancer (see Chapter 12), it's most likely left over and just needs to be cleaned up with further surgery. On the other hand, if the recurrence is invasive, it may have had a second opportunity to spread. In addition, women with invasive local recurrences generally have more aggressive disease. Exactly how these recurrences appear and are treated is based in part on what the initial therapy was.

Local Recurrence After Breast Conservation

Most local recurrences after breast conservation occur in the area of the original tumor (46–91 percent), on average 3–4 years after the initial therapy.[1] If your initial treatment was a lumpectomy followed by radiation, the first sign of a local recurrence can be a change in how your breast looks or feels. Changes in the physical exam that occur more than 1–2 years after the completion of radiation therapy should always be looked into immediately. Retrospective studies show that the woman herself detects 76–86 percent of local recurrences.[2,3] Less commonly, a mammogram reveals something suspicious. Although MRI has been used to try to distinguish between a local recurrence and scar tissue, only a biopsy can show for certain. Usually a core needle biopsy is sufficient, though sometimes the procedure shows that further surgery is necessary.

Once a local recurrence has been diagnosed, we do tests (see Chapter 16) looking for signs of cancer elsewhere in the body, possibly including bone scan, chest X ray, CT scan, MRI or PET scan, and blood tests, some of the latter looking for tumor markers. If the tests are normal (only 5–10 percent of women with local recurrence have signs of disease elsewhere), then we have to figure out how best to eradicate the tumor from the breast. Usually in these cases we do a mastectomy, since the less drastic surgery and radiation didn't take care of it. Some centers try to preserve the breast with additional limited surgery, but the survival rates are inferior to those of women who undergo mastectomy after a local recurrence. Early studies of breast surgery and reirradiation locally (see Chapter 17) are more encouraging.[4] Overall the prognosis is better in women who are older, have smaller lesions, and have gone a long time between the initial treatment and the recurrence. After mastectomy for a local recurrence, the prognosis is still pretty good, ranging from 50–88 percent.[5] The higher numbers refer to when the disease is limited to the breast while the lower numbers refer to instances of spread. The role of systemic therapy after a local recurrence in the breast is still not clear, but it is often considered in high-risk women. If your tumor is sensitive to estrogen and you were on tamoxifen, it is reasonable to switch to an aromatase inhibitor, or vice versa. The role of chemotherapy, especially if you were previously treated with it, is not clear and is still being studied.

There's something else we call a "local recurrence" that actually isn't a local recurrence at all—it's a new cancer in the breast (often referred to as a new primary). This typically occurs many years after the original cancer and in an entirely different area of the breast. Its pathology is often different—lobular instead of ductal, for example. These second cancers are not common, but they are possible as long as you have your breast. Though they are often counted as recurrences in the statistics for breast conservation, they have a different meaning. They should be treated as completely new cancers, much as with second cancers in the opposite breast. Most often the local treatment will be a mastectomy, since you can receive radiation therapy only once to any area. However, the newer approaches to partial radiation may change this. The addition of chemotherapy and/or tamoxifen will depend on the size and biomarkers of the tumor (see Chapter 16).

Local Recurrence After Mastectomy

You can also get a local recurrence in the scar or chest wall after a mastectomy. Actually the term "chest wall" is inaccurate here because it implies that the cancer is in the muscle or bone. But usually such a recurrence appears in the skin and fat sitting where the breast was before; only rarely does it include the muscle (see Fig. 27–2). In fact 40–60 percent of local recurrences occur where the breast was before, and the risk of this happening is about 10 percent. Ninety percent of these recurrences happen within the first five years after the mastectomy. Approximately 20–30 percent of women with local recurrences after mastectomy have already been diagnosed with metastatic disease and

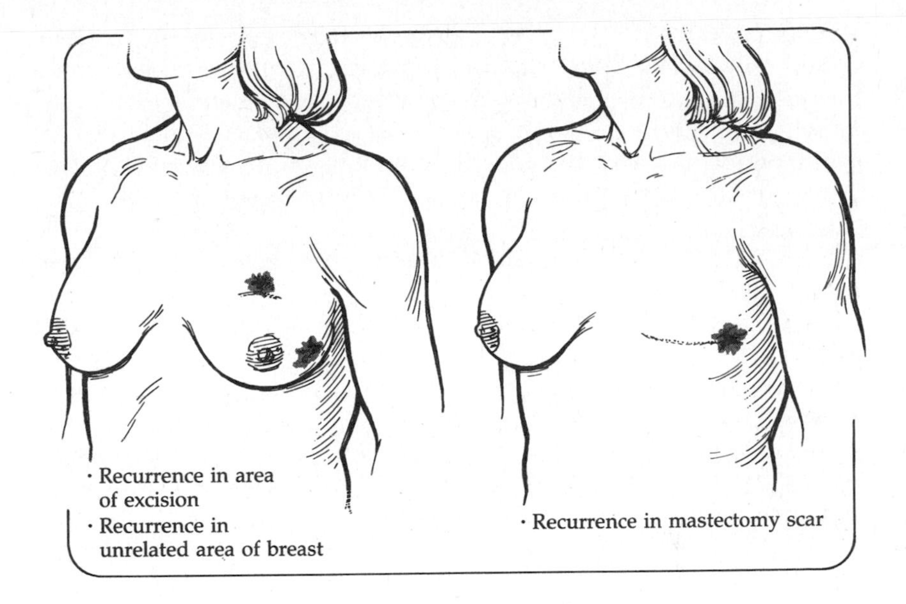

FIGURE 27-2

another 20–30 percent will develop it within the a few months of diagnosis. Therefore, just as with local recurrences after breast conservation, tests should be done to look for distant disease.

Local recurrence after mastectomy usually shows up as one or more nodules on or under the skin in or near the scar.[6] After reconstruction a recurrence can appear at the suture line of the flap or in front of the implant. A local recurrence after mastectomy will usually show up as a pea-size lump in your scar or under your skin. Sometimes it's in the skin itself, and is red and raised. It's usually so subtle the surgeon is likely to think at first that it's just a stitch that got left in after the operation. Then it gets bigger and needs to be biopsied. That can be done under local anesthesia, since the area is numb. Reconstruction rarely if ever hides a recurrence. With implants, the recurrences are in front of the implant. With a flap the recurrences are not in the flap itself (tissue from the abdomen) but along the edge of the old breast skin.[7]

The treatments for a local recurrence are also local. Most commonly the lesion is removed surgically and followed by radiation to the chest wall if the woman has not previously had radiation. Occasionally larger areas are surgically removed, including sections of rib and breastbone. Although this approach has not been shown to increase survival, it can improve the quality of life by preventing further local spread, which can be difficult to manage.

Despite aggressive local treatment, 80–85 percent of women with an isolated local recurrence following mastectomy eventually develop distant metastases. Studies, both randomized and nonrandomized, have suggested, however, that if the recurrence can be removed and radiation given, the addition of systemic therapy such as tamoxifen or chemotherapy can lead to five-year remissions of 36–52 percent.[8,9] The current recommendation is similar to that for a breast recurrence described above. Look for a clinical trial you can participate in to help us answer the questions about chemotherapy. The biggest predictor of overall survival is the length of time between the original therapy and the recurrence, or disease-free interval.[10] The later the recurrence, the better.

Rarely a woman has extensive local recurrence after mastectomy, with many nodules in the skin. They merge and act almost like a coat of armor across the chest and even into the back and the other breast. At this point we call it *en cuirasse,* a French word meaning "in casing." Some women have large tumor masses on the chest wall that weep and bleed. Both of these situations are rare, but they're very distressing because you are watching the cancer grow on the outside. We feel there must be a different genetic mutation for this type of local recurrence than for distant metastasis because these women usually do not have extensive disease in the rest of their body for a long time. Unfortunately we lack a good therapy for it. Surgery cannot cut out enough tissue to clear it, and radiation therapy is limited in extent as well. Some have tried hyperthermia (very high heat) in an attempt to burn off the tumor, but its effect has also been limited. Sometimes chemotherapy will give some relief, but not always. These cases are very upsetting for the doctor and patient, and we are still searching for the right treatment approach.

Regional Recurrence

A regional recurrence is one in the lymph nodes under the arm or above the collarbone. Now that we are taking out fewer lymph nodes from the axilla (see Chapter 21), a cancerous node can be left behind. This is rare, occurring in about 2 percent of breast cancers. Further treatment to this area with either surgery or radiation often takes care of the problem, although systemic therapy may also be used. Regional recurrence in lymph nodes elsewhere, such as the neck or above the collarbone, is more likely to reflect spread of the tumor through the bloodstream. Akin to local recurrence following mastectomy, it usually warrants a more aggressive approach.[11]

As physicians we tend to downplay local and regional recurrences because they are not as life threatening as metastatic disease can be.

Nonetheless, for the patient they can be devastating. When a woman gets a local recurrence, she finds it much harder than she did the first time not to think of herself as doomed. She gave it her best shot and it didn't work—how can she trust any treatment again? This became obvious to me when we first set up our support group for women with metastatic disease at the Faulkner Breast Centre. I wanted to exclude women with local recurrences because I thought their situation wasn't serious enough for this group. My coworkers and patients convinced me that this was not true, and they turned out to be right. The overwhelming feelings are the same. Barbara Kalinowski describes the difficulties women with recurrences have, even around other women with breast cancer. "They find themselves being 'polite' in mixed groups. One woman was talking about having just had her sixth chemotherapy treatment, and the woman next to her said, 'Oh, good, you're almost through!' And she didn't have the heart to tell her this was her second time around." A woman who has gone through the tough round of surgery, radiation, and chemotherapy, thinking she has put it behind her, can feel overwhelmed to find out that she has to go through it all over again. (I discuss ways to cope with this situation later in this chapter.)

DISTANT RECURRENCE (METASTATIC DISEASE)

When a cancer spreads to a different organ, it's known as a distant recurrence, or a metastasis. If a metastasis is detectable at the time of first diagnosis, the patient is described as being in stage 4 (see Chapter 16).

As hard as it is to face a local recurrence, metastatic disease can be even more devastating. It causes the same feelings that go with any recurrence, compounded by the knowledge that the chance of cure is slim. Here you need to face the fact that you are not immortal and create the best quality of life for yourself in the time you have, while maintaining hope. Contrary to common belief, metastatic breast cancer is rarely an immediate death sentence, and with good treatment women with metastisis often live for a number of years, with reasonable quality of life. To quote Andrew Seidman, a medical oncologist from Memorial Sloan-Kettering Cancer Center in New York, you need to remember that "metastatic breast cancer often behaves biologically . . . like a novel with many chapters, fortunately, rather than a short story."[12]

As I mentioned in Chapter 16, when breast cancer shows up in your lungs, liver, or bones, it's still breast cancer—not lung or liver or bone cancer. We can usually tell which it is by looking at it under the microscope.

It's important here to differentiate "metastatic" from "micrometastatic." "Micrometastases" is the term we use when we discuss the likelihood of small cancer cells remaining in the rest of the body at the time of an initial diagnosis and treatment. They are cells that we presume are there but are so small we can't detect them. We believe that such spread, if it exists, can often be cured (see Chapter 24). But when we talk about metastatic disease, we mean growth of cancer cells that often cause symptoms and can be detected on an X ray or scan. At the time I'm writing this book, nothing we know of can guarantee a cure for metastatic breast cancer. However, as new therapies are continuously being developed, we have reason to hope that, as with AIDs, we can one day convert metastatic breast cancer to a chronic disease. Recent studies suggest that in certain situations where the recurrence is limited and the woman can be rendered disease free with multidisciplinary treatments, 3–30 percent of women with metastatic breast cancer can be put into remission for over 20 years.[13] Is that a cure? I suspect it doesn't matter to those women what you call it—what matters is that they are alive and well.

Unfortunately the average survival of women with metastatic breast cancer from the time of the first appearance of the metastasis is between two to three and a half years, according to most studies. But 22 percent of patients live five years, and about 10 percent live more than 10 years. And 2–3 percent are cured.[14] Remember that these numbers are averages, or means. There will always be women who are "above average." There are cases in the medical literature like that of the woman who had metastases throughout her bones, had hormone treatment, and was well 24 years later.[15] I wish we could take credit for such rare and wonderful occurrences, but we have no idea what causes the cure in any of them. It could be that these patients have cancers that remain extraordinarily sensitive to the available therapies, while most metastatic cancers have so many genetic changes that they develop resistance fairly quickly. Alternatively, occasional long survival may occur because the cancer is just very slow growing and has little or nothing to do with the therapy.

On a hopeful note, one population study from British Columbia, Canada, looking at survival after breast cancer recurrence documented a steady increase in two-year survival from 34 percent in 1991 and 1992 to 45 percent in 1999 and 2001. The median survival increased from 435 days to 661 days, or 7.5 months, which suggests that our improved therapy is at least increasing the length of time women live with metastatic disease if not the cure rate.[16] This trend has been confirmed by the group at M.D. Anderson.[17] There are many factors that can help predict who will live a long time, but they're not absolute. One is the length of time between your original diagnosis and your metastasis. If the metastasis shows up six months after your diagnosis, it suggests that you have a much more aggressive cancer than if it's six years after your diagnosis.

Still another is whether or not your tumor was sensitive to hormones. We also look at how many places it's metastasized to—if there's only one, or if you have multiple organs involved. Where it recurs is also a consideration. Metastasis to the bone or the skin is less serious than metastasis to the lung or liver.

All this is just statistics and, as I noted above, what happens to an individual woman may or may not conform to the norm. I've had patients with metastatic disease who have far outlived the most optimistic prognosis. One patient developed lung metastasis while she was getting her adjuvant chemotherapy. That means she had hardly any disease-free interval, and the cancer seemed resistant to chemo. Statistically, she should have been dead within a year or two. She was treated with hormones and the cancer disappeared for two years. It came back at that point and another treatment made it disappear for another two years. When it came back that time, we gave another hormone. Ten years after her initial diagnosis, she died of breast cancer. When she was diagnosed she had an eight-year-old son, and she was able to raise him almost into adulthood. So we can't accurately predict the course of any individual's illness. This is true of initial disease, and metastatic disease is even more unpredictable.

Usually I find that women who have just finished breast cancer treatments don't want to think about the possibility of its spreading. They're busy dealing with the healing process and a metastasis is too painful to think about. But of course it's always somewhere in the back of a woman's mind. Usually about a year after initial treatments the patient will start asking me about symptoms of metastasis. (This is an observation, not a guideline. If you want to know right away or two months later, talk to your doctor. There's nothing particularly brave about toughing it out when you're worried. Every woman's pace is different.)

In medical school, we were taught that we shouldn't tell people who had been treated for cancer what to look for if they were worried about recurrences, because they'd start imagining that they had every symptom we told them about. I've never liked that idea. It doesn't soothe people at all; it just means they'll be afraid of everything, instead of a few specific things. When you've had cancer, you're acutely aware of your body, and any symptom that's new—or that you never noticed before—can take on terrifying significance for you. Anything unexpected in your body has you petrified. Inevitably this will mean a lot of fear over symptoms that turn out to be harmless.

But if you know that the symptoms of breast cancer metastasis are usually bone pain, shortness of breath, lack of appetite and weight loss, and neurological symptoms like pain or weakness or headaches, there are at least limits to your fear. You'll probably be frightened when anything resembling those symptoms comes up, even if it turns out to be nothing but a tension headache or a mild flu. But at least you won't be terrified by a sore spot on your big toe or an unexpected weight gain. Knowing what symptoms to look for reduces fear; it doesn't increase it. Dr. Daniel Hayes, the clinical director of the breast cancer oncology program at the University of Michigan and an old friend of mine, puts it this way: "I tell patients it is common sense: if you stub your toe, and it hurts just like it did before your diagnosis of breast cancer, it is normal. If you have a new symptom that is particularly unusual, severe, and lasts longer than you expect then you should see your caregiver. And be sure he or she remembers you had breast cancer, even 10 or 20 years ago. (I frequently see late metastases that get missed because doctors forget the patient had breast cancer once a long time ago.)"

Most women whose breast cancer has metastasized don't show any symptoms until the disease is quite extensive. It doesn't involve years and years of terrible suffering, the way TV melodrama likes to show it.

Like other cancers, breast cancer can spread anywhere, but it's more likely to show up in the bones, lungs, liver, and occasionally brain. Why this is we don't know. Researchers are studying it and perhaps one day will give us a better understanding of it. The cancer cell may be making some sort of "homing" receptor for a particular organ, or perhaps the environment of certain organs is more conducive to growth for this type of cancer cell.

As I pointed out earlier (see Chapter 26), most recurrences are diagnosed because of symptoms noticed by the woman. Diagnosing metastatic disease early on a scan or blood test does not make the treatment easier or more effective. This means you do not have to kick yourself for not complaining sooner. If you have a symptom that feels abnormal, get it checked out but don't feel it is an emergency.

Symptoms

Symptoms appear differently in different areas of the body. Next we consider some of the most common sites of metastasis.

Bone. In a quarter of the cases, the bones are the first site where metastatic disease is detected. This is true partly because it's more common there than in other places, and partly because it creates definite symptoms. Even if it first appears elsewhere, as the disease progresses it usually reaches the bone at some stage.

Metastasis to the bone is usually diagnosed when the patient experiences pain. Sometimes it's hard to know if the pain is ordinary low back pain or some other condition, like arthritis. Usually the pain you get with breast cancer in the bones is fairly constant and doesn't improve over time. With arthritis, you wake up in the morning and feel stiff but get better as you move around during the day. Also the location is important. Pain in the feet, ankle, and hands is usually caused by arthritis or even by your treatment: tamoxifen and especially the aromatase inhibitors can cause muscle and joint pain. With some muscular problems that cause bone pain, the more you do the worse the pain gets. But the pain from cancer is steady and usually persists during the night, when you're not doing anything. The pain is probably caused by the cancer taking up room in the bone and pressing on it, and it can be worse in different positions. If you're standing up, you may be compressing the bone and causing more pain than if you're lying down. If you have pain that lasts for more than a week or two and doesn't seem to be going away, and isn't like whatever pains have become familiar to you, you should get it checked out.

We usually check bone pain by doing a bone scan. This is a radioactive test I described in Chapter 16. It's not very specific because it can be positive for a lot of different conditions, but it's quite accurate for showing when a cancer may be present.

If the bone scan is suspicious or suggestive, the next step is an X ray. If there's metastasis, this will show one of two things: either lytic lesions (holes where the cancer has eaten away the bones) or blastic lesions (an increase of bone where the growth factor of the cancer has caused the bone to get more dense). CAT scans and MRI, described in Chapter 10, can also be used to confirm a diagnosis of cancer in specific bones.[18] PET scanning is also being done more, although its accuracy is unproven.

A woman I know shared her experience with discovering bone metastasis. She experienced generalized pain around her rib cage and groin and called her internist. He was out of town and so she was seen by a nurse practitioner, who attributed her pain to tendonitis and ordered an anti-inflammatory drug, which relieved the pain. Later when she saw her surgeon, he suggested it could be bone metastases and ordered a PET scan (a bone scan would have been as good). But she was feeling better and did not follow through until four weeks later, when she was hiking and experienced severe pain. She was found to have bone metastases and was started on a hormonal therapy and a bisphosphonate. She has been feeling well since but now wishes that she had followed up on the scan sooner. The result would not have been different, except that she would have had pain relief sooner.

When women have cancer in their bones, we worry about the possi-

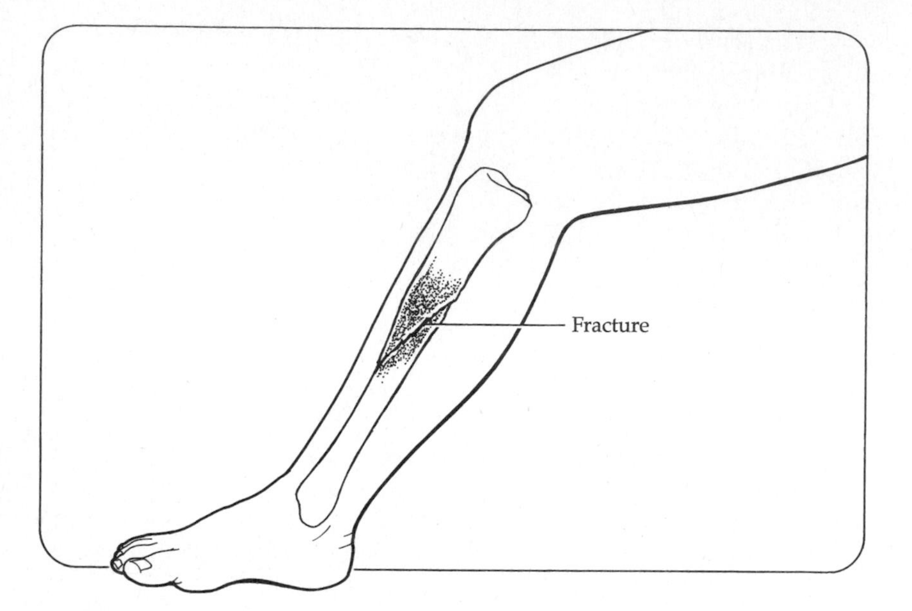

FIGURE 27-3

bility of fractures. If the cancer eats away enough bone, it will no longer be strong enough to hold you up. Then you can get what's called a "pathological fracture," which is caused by something wrong in the bone itself, not by a blow from outside (Fig. 27-3). It's similar to osteoporosis in that it doesn't take much to cause this fracture because the bone is so weakened. A slight pressure that usually wouldn't even cause a bruise triggers the fracture. (It's different from osteoporosis, however, in that it doesn't affect all your bones.)

Luckily the use of intravenous bisphosphonates, pamidronate (Aredia) and zolendronic (Zometa), has dramatically lowered the risk of bone fractures.[19] We try to make sure that the key bones are not at risk. The ones to worry most about are the ones that hold you up—your leg or hip bones. The upper arm can also fracture, but it's less likely because you don't put as much constant pressure on it. You can also get a fracture in your spine. If X rays show that a bone in a critical place has metastatic disease that is a risk for a fracture, we can do surgery ahead of time to pin the hip or stabilize the bone. Again, the idea is to keep you stabilized and functional, with as high a quality of life as possible for as long a time as possible.

Lung. We also see breast cancer metastasis fairly often in the lungs (Fig. 27-4). Usually the symptoms are shortness of breath and a chronic cough. Among patients who die of breast cancer, 60–70 percent have it

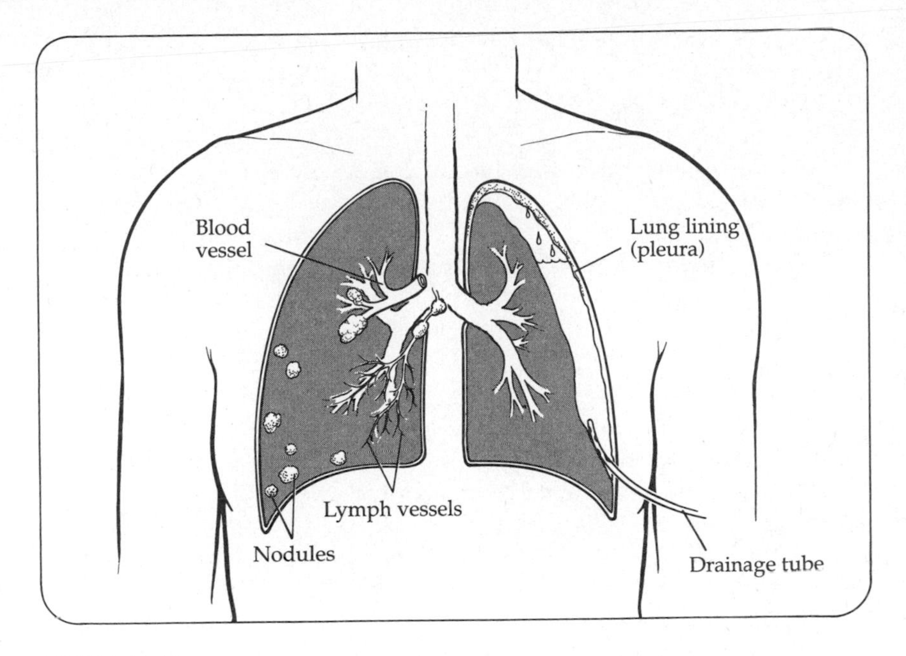

FIGURE 27-4

in their lungs. The lungs are the only site of metastasis in about 21 percent of cases. There are a couple of different ways it can form. One is in nodules—usually several—that show up on a chest X ray. If it shows only one nodule, we can't tell if it's lung cancer or a breast cancer spread. So we do a needle biopsy or a full biopsy to find out. (Lung cancer usually starts in just one spot, but a cancer that has spread to the lung through the bloodstream or lymphatic channels is likely to hit multiple spots in the lung.)

If your breast cancer has spread to your lungs, you may experience shortness of breath on less exertion than normal. It can be fairly subtle. It comes on slowly, since the cancer has to use up a lot of your lungs before you develop shortness of breath.

Another form of metastasis in the lung is called lymphangitic spread. Here the cancer spreads along the lymphatics. Instead of forming nodules it occurs in a fine pattern throughout the lung. It's subtler and harder to detect on a chest X ray. It ultimately causes shortness of breath, since it takes up room and scars the lungs, making them less able to expand and contract and bring oxygen into your bloodstream.

The third way it can show is through fluid in the pleura, the lining of the lung. That usually indicates that the spread is in the pleura rather than in the lung itself. (The lung sits in a sac with a smooth lining around it, so that it can move without sticking to the chest wall.)

The cancer creates fluid around the lung (effusion), and the fluid causes the lung to collapse partially (see Fig. 27-4). Here again, you'll experience shortness of breath. Usually breast cancer in the lungs doesn't cause pain.

If we think your cancer may have metastasized to your lung and the chest X ray doesn't show nodules, fluid, or any of the other signs, we can still do a CAT scan.

For lung metastases the treatment is usually systemic; fluid in the lung can be treated by sticking a needle into the chest and draining the fluid. This works immediately, but only temporarily. Often the fluid comes back right away. In order to prevent the reaccumulation, we fasten the lining of the lung to the lung. When I was in medical school we used to open up the chest, take a piece of gauze, and rub it against the lung to irritate the spot. That got it red and raw and so it stuck together and created a scar, leaving no room for fluid. A less invasive approach is to drain the fluid through a tube and then put in material that will scar up the lining of the sac. The installation of talc powder irritates the pleural surfaces and causes them to scar together so that fluid can't accumulate between them. However, often an effective hormonal therapy or chemotherapy will keep the fluid in the lung from reaccumulating, at least for a while. Eventually many women with recurrent pleural effusions do receive the scarring procedure with talc and chest tube drainage. Occasionally women with recurring fluid will have a catheter left in so that they can be drained as needed.

Liver. The liver is the third most common site for metastases. Again, this can be subtle. The symptoms occur because the cancer takes up a lot of room in the liver, and that takes some time to happen. About two-thirds of women who die of breast cancer have it in their liver, and about a quarter have it initially. The symptoms are common—weight loss, anorexia (loss of appetite), nausea, gastrointestinal symptoms, and pain or discomfort under your right rib cage. You may have some pain in the right upper quadrant of your liver, which occurs when the liver's covering tissue is stretched out.

A diagnosis of liver metastasis is often suspected from blood tests and confirmed by CT, MRI, PET scanning or, on occasion, ultrasound. The major treatment for extensive liver disease is chemotherapy, especially if your liver function blood tests are elevated. Hormone therapy can work well on hormone receptor positive- and slower-growing liver metastases, and the decision to use it usually depends on the extent of damage present to the liver. In certain kinds of cancer, like colon cancer, liver metastasis can be single or just a few, and thus sometimes can be cut out. But with breast cancer there is usually more than one spot involved and surgery becomes impossible. In the uncommon exceptions when there is only one spot, we can surgically remove part of the liver to relieve symptoms or use X ray therapy. There are also new techniques for a small number of liver metastases that involve putting hot (hyperthermia) or cold (cryosurgery) probes into the tumors and burning or freezing them. This can help the obvious spots but must be followed with systemic therapy to control the rest of the micrometastatic liver disease.

Sometimes when patients have a lot of pain we radiate the liver to shrink it. But we do this only for particularly severe symptoms that are not responding to systemic therapy or for the rare case of a woman whose only apparent disease is in the liver. At one time we put chemotherapy directly into the liver through a catheter in the artery leading into the organ, to achieve a more direct treatment of the metastases. But we get just as good a response with less drastic and more comfortable forms of chemotherapy, so we don't do this much anymore. Liver transplants do not work in this situation because the disease is usually more extensive, not just in the liver.

Brain and Spinal Cord. Neurological metastases are less common but very serious. Breast cancer can spread to the brain and the spinal cord. It's still fairly uncommon—about 6 percent. Adjuvant chemotherapy does not get into the brain as effectively as it does into the rest of the body. Because of this, we are seeing brain metastases with somewhat greater frequency as systemic adjuvant therapies have become better at eradicating disease outside the brain. This is particularly true in women with Her-2/neu-overexpressing breast cancers, whose disease outside the brain is well controlled with Herceptin. The most common symptoms are headache, visual changes, and/or persistent nausea. I almost hate to say that, since most people get a lot of headaches during their lives, and I'm afraid any reader with breast cancer who gets a tension headache will be terrified. But if the headache doesn't go away in a reasonable time, check it out. In some patients it's the kind of headache that occurs with a brain tumor. It begins early in the morning before you get out of bed, improves as the day goes on, but then gets worse and worse over time.

Behavior or mental changes are sometimes, though rarely, caused by the tumor. You can have weakness or unsteadiness in walking or seizures. It can resemble a stroke: you suddenly can't talk, part of your body is suddenly very weak, or you can't see out of one eye. Those kinds of symptoms occur when a portion of your brain is blocked, which the cancer growth can cause. The best way to diagnosis it is through CAT scan or MRI. About half of patients have one lesion; the other half have several.

Another kind of brain metastasis you can get is a form of meningitis called *carcinomatosis meningitis.* This affects the lining of the brain rather than the brain itself. It causes weakness in the eye and mouth muscles, headaches, stiff neck, and sometimes confusion, the way any form of meningitis does.

For brain metastases the treatment is usually radiation, which shrinks the metastasis. If there's only one lesion, surgery is indicated, followed by radiation therapy has been shown in a randomized controlled trial to improve survival.[20] Unfortunately this is only useful for single lesions. The "gamma knife" is a new technique for removing a lesion; it permits a higher radiation dose but has not yet been proven to make a difference in overall survival.

You'll also be put on steroids—dexamethasone—right away, to reduce the swelling of the brain. Since the brain sits inside a hard bony shell (the skull) there isn't much room for swelling before important structures are injured. If you're having seizures, you'll also be put on antiseizure medication. Unfortunately chemotherapy and hormone therapies don't work well on brain metastasis, although responses can occur with both.

Metastasis to the spinal cord is also very serious. This is the one area where early detection makes a big difference. The tumor can push on the cord and cause paralysis. Sometimes this happens because the bone metastasis is in the vertebrae and pushes against the spinal cord as it grows out of the bone into the spinal canal (Fig. 27-5). Sometimes

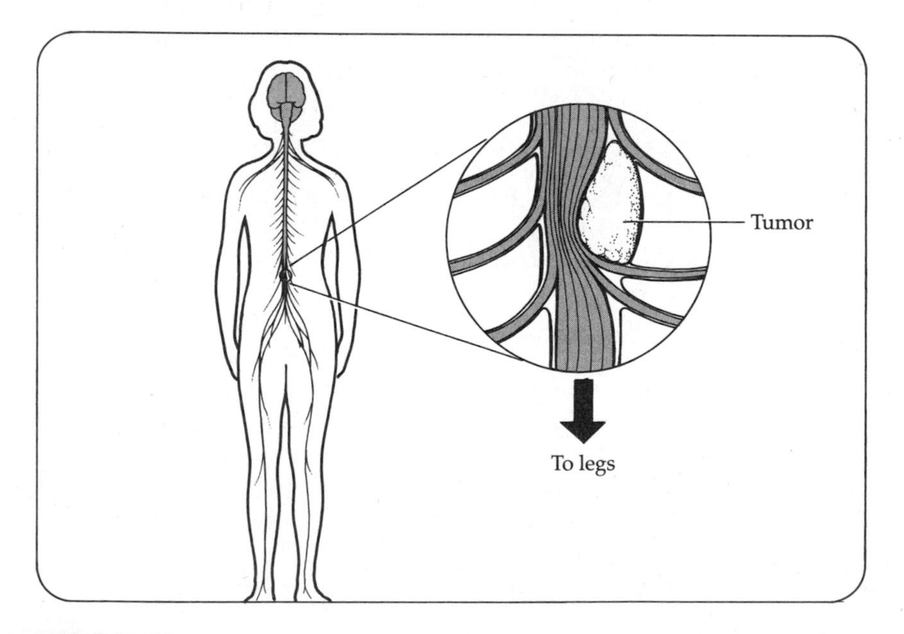

FIGURE 27-5

the tumor grows directly in the spinal cord itself. Before the paralysis, however, there are earlier symptoms—pain, weakness, sensory loss, and bowel or bladder disturbances. Pain is the most common—85 to 90 percent of patients with spinal cord metastasis have pain. It may be the only symptom for months. The problem is that if you have cancer only in the bones and the back, you'll also have pain. So we have to be able to differentiate, or at least be extremely alert, to be certain that the patient with bone metastasis in her back isn't on the verge of spinal cord compression.

Most of the pain is aching and continuous. Its onset is gradual and it gets worse over time; it often becomes severe as it pushes on the spinal cord. And it's very localized: you feel it exactly on the spot where the tumor is. There is another kind of pain that goes downward the way sciatica does, when a disk compresses the nerves and goes down your leg, getting worse if you cough or sneeze. You may also feel pain in your shoulder or back from spinal cord compression. Seventy-five percent of patients with metastasis to the spinal cord have weakness in their muscles from the tumor pushing against the nerves, and about 5 percent have spots of numbness. Anyone with metastatic breast cancer who has unrelenting pain in one spot, and any neurological symptoms, should be concerned. If you have no other signs of metastasis, it probably isn't spinal cord compression, since that's rarely the first sign of metastatic disease, although it can be. We diagnose it with CAT scan or MRI. We used to do a myelogram, in which dye is injected into the spinal column, but we rarely do that anymore. The treatment is generally emergency surgery if there is any evidence of nerve damage, muscle weakness, or a large tumor pressing on the spinal cord. If it's one spot, we may be able to remove the tumor and decompress the spinal cord. Surgery, if performed, is then followed by radiation therapy. Alternatively, the treatment could be emergency radiation alone; it is one of the few instances in which radiation is used as an emergency treatment. The radiation shrinks the tumor and steroids prevent the spinal cord from swelling.

Breast cancer can also metastasize to the eye, though again it's rarely the first place such spread occurs. The initial symptoms are double or blurred vision. It's diagnosed by CAT scan or MRI. It's also treated with radiation, which can often prevent loss of vision.

Another area is bone marrow. The main symptom is anemia, caused by a decrease in the number of red blood cells, and the white blood cells and platelets can also decrease. Though it sounds grim, metastasis to bone marrow often responds very well to treatment, either with hormones or with chemotherapy. This remission can last for several years.

Breast cancer in all its manifestations is an unpredictable disease. These are general descriptions. As I write this, many women come to mind whose cancer didn't follow the rules. Use this information to help understand your own situation and ask questions. Your situation will be unique to you no matter what happens.

Treatment

The treatment approaches to metastatic disease are different from the approaches to primary breast cancer. As I already noted, with metastatic cancer there isn't a reliable method of cure, and our goal is twofold.

First, we want to prolong your survival as much as possible. Hormone therapies, immunotherapies, and even chemotherapy have been demonstrated to induce remissions that last about one year on average but can last as long as 10 years. Some of the newer treatments for metastatic breast cancer are being shown to improve women's overall survival better than some of the older chemotherapy and hormone options. Studies of aromatase inhibitors, which block the production of estrogen in women's bodies, show longer duration of disease control than tamoxifen.[21,22]

Trastuzumab (Herceptin) and the taxanes paclitaxel (Taxol) and docetaxel (Taxotere) have also been shown to substantially improve patients' survival, more than older chemotherapy regimens.[23] As the final draft of this book was being written, the new antibody therapy bevacizumab (Avastin) when given with paclitaxel was shown to improve progression-free survival compared to paclitaxel alone.[24] This is an important first step—one we hope is the beginning of a new era in the treatment of metastatic disease.

However, no one knows how long someone with metastatic breast cancer will live. Therefore our second, main achievable goal is called palliation—keeping you feeling as good as you can for as long as you can. Palliation is achieved by choosing the therapies with the best chance of working and the fewest side effects. What the term "working" means depends on the situation. If the metastases are significantly involving a major organ such as the liver or lungs and compromising its function (major organ dysfunction), then you need something to melt the tumor away as fast as possible. If on the other hand the problems are bothersome but not life threatening, you may use something that takes more time but has fewer side effects. Dr. Hayes tells his patients that "there is bad news and good news. The bad news is you have *metastatic* breast cancer, meaning that it is unlikely that you will be cured with any therapy, no matter how aggressive." He stresses that both the doctor and the patient must understand this or there will be mistrust. Indeed, the reluctance to abandon high dose chemotherapy and stem cell transplant, even with little data to support it, grew out of a lack of acceptance of the fact that we don't have a cure. He continues, "The good news is you have metastatic *breast cancer.*" He explains that there are numerous therapies available to achieve palliation and they are growing yearly. They include local treatments such as surgery, radiation, cryotherapy, and phototherapy. Systemic therapies include at least 10 to 15 drugs (both IV and oral) as well as at least five categories of hormonal therapies and now two biologic therapies. In addition there are new supportive therapies such as bisphosphonates (which treat bone metastasis), erythropoietin (which combats anemia), antinausea drugs (see Chapter 24), white blood cell growth factors (which prevent infection), and better pain medications. "The challenge," he says, "is judicial application in sequence of these treatments to optimize feeling as good as you can for as long as you can."

One of the things most difficult for patients with metastatic cancer is having no clear idea of what to expect—how long they will live and how much pain they are likely to be in. Two things are important to consider. One is dealing with your own emotions, through counseling, a support group, religion—whatever works best for you. (I discussed this at length in Chapters 20 and 26.) The other important thing is to get as much information as your doctor has about the probable progress of your illness and what it entails. Some doctors are very uncomfortable with death; they see their job as fighting even the thought of death until the last minute; therefore they deal with your fear of dying by pretending it won't happen. Sometimes doctors deal with the patient's fear by using every kind of therapy as rapidly and in as great a dose as possible, in an attempt to ward off the inevitable. Often the patient also goes along with this approach. But it's as dangerous as the opposite extreme of shying away from any treatment at all. In the rest of this chapter I'll explain the treatments specific to metastatic disease, and what you can reasonably expect from them.

During and after your treatment for metastatic disease you'll be followed with the staging tests—bone scan, chest X ray, and blood tests—as well as a few other tests such as CAT scans, PET scans, or MRI. These can help determine if you're indeed responding to treatment, although your symptoms are the best test of effectiveness.

HORMONE (ENDOCRINE) TREATMENTS

We've known for a long time that breast cancer in women is often an endocrine disease—the endocrine glands are the ones that make hormones. We can test the cancer when the tumor is first removed and tell if it's sensitive to hormones by doing the estrogen receptor test described in Chapter 16.

In women who have metastatic disease and a tumor that's sensitive to hormones, using endocrine treatments first often makes more sense than chemotherapy. When a patient has responded to one hormone therapy, we know she's likely to respond to a second and possibly a third one, so we use them serially.

The first hormone treatment was used in premenopausal women and consisted of oophorectomy—surgically removing the ovaries. Now we can either do this surgically or use drugs (ablation). In menstruating women who are estrogen receptor positive, the response to oophorectomy is 35 percent. An additional 25 percent will have improved symptoms and a prolonged period of stable disease.

Removing your ovaries puts you into menopause right away, complete with mood swings and hot flashes (see Chapter 27). But it also can relieve your metastatic breast cancer symptoms almost immediately, often by the time you leave the hospital. This approach went out of fashion with the introduction of chemotherapy, but it has resumed an important place in the treatment of metastatic disease with the introduction of several new drugs that can turn off the ovaries' ability to make estrogen and can be just the right treatment for a woman with bone metastasis and an estrogen receptor positive tumor. Whether we remove the ovaries or inactivate them with drugs, the treatment is effective. Reversible menopause can be induced by using GnRH agonists such as goserelin (Zoladex; see Chapter 11), which block FSH and LH and stop your periods.

Another way to block estrogen is to block the receptor that it fits into in the cell in the breast. This is the way antiestrogens such as tamoxifen and toremifene work. They can be used in both premenopausal and postmenopausal women whose tumors are sensitive to estrogen. If you were on tamoxifen in the past and then stopped, it's worth trying again to treat your metastatic disease. On the other hand, if the metastasis became apparent while you were on tamoxifen, you're probably resistant and you should try something else. Note that toremifene (Fareston) and raloxifene (Evista) work the same way that tamoxifen does. Consequently if you are on one of these and your cancer comes back or grows, it is useless to switch to another one.

In women who are postmenopausal (whether by chemotherapy or naturally) estrogen is principally made by the enzyme aromatase, which converts testosterone and androstenedione to estrogen. This enzyme is found in the adrenal glands, fat, muscle, and breast tissue. The first aromatase inhibitor used was aminoglutethimide, but it isn't very potent. In addition, it causes other symptoms by blocking the adrenal glands' production of other hormones. The most recent aromatase inhibitors—anastrozole (Arimidex), letrozole (Femara), and exemestane (Aromasin)—are more potent and specific blockers of aromatase; they are therefore much less toxic than aminoglutethimide and have very good response rates. They are currently the drugs of choice once a tumor becomes resistant to tamoxifen or even if a patient has never received tamoxifen or stopped it years ago. The aromatase inhibitors are well tolerated and have been shown to improve women's overall survival better than the standard hormone therapy, megestrol acetate (Megace) discussed below. The common side effects are hot flashes (30 percent) and weight gain (20 percent), as with tamoxifen; musculoskeletal pain (40 percent), and gastrointestinal complaints (5 percent). But the aromatase inhibitors work only in postmenopausal women. For premenopausal women they are ineffectual and potentially dangerous.

Fulvestrant (Faslodex) is a new estrogen receptor blocker that does not have the estrogenic effects seen with tamoxifen. It benefits 20–30 percent of women after the women have used an aromatase inhibitor and is equivalent to tamoxifen and anastrozole.[25,26,27]

Megestrol acetate (Megace) is a kind of progestin. Its biggest side effect is increased appetite, which leads to weight gain. This occurs in about half of patients, and they gain between 10 and 20 pounds. Twelve percent of women gain more than 30 pounds. (In fact, megestrol acetate is so likely to cause weight gain that researchers tried using it to treat people with AIDS and other wasting diseases.) Megestrol acetate works for about 20–30 percent of women and is now generally used after the aromatase inhibitors, tamoxifen, and fulvestrant.

You might think that if all these hormones work separately they'd work even better together. As I mentioned in Chapter 18, the ATAC study did not show a synergistic effect between tamoxifen and anastrozole in the adjuvant setting. Several studies of combination hormone therapy versus single agents have shown increased likelihood of response but no increase in overall survival except perhaps in premenopausal women, for whom the combination of ovarian ablation and tamoxifen may be beneficial. A current trial is studying anastrozole versus anastrozole plus fulvestrant. But sequential use is a different situation: patients who respond to one therapy are more likely to respond to the next one. Once a woman stops responding to hormones, it is likely that chemotherapy will be effective.

Some women experience a phenomenon called "flare" with hormone treatment of metastatic breast cancer: within the first month of therapy there is an exacerbation of the patient's disease. It actually indicates a good prognosis. Typically it occurs with someone who has bone metastasis and is put on tamoxifen. Suddenly her pain is worse than ever. But then she's back to normal soon after. We think this happens because tamoxifen actually works initially as a weak estrogen in some women, stimulating their cancer, before it starts to function as an antiestrogen. But you need to be aware of this because a flare can be very scary. We also can see a flare in the tumor markers. This is important to know because your doctor, seeing a rise in the markers, might assume that the treatment is not working, instead of recognizing the flare as a sign that it *is* working.

The overall effectiveness of all the hormone treatments is about 40 percent. But it doesn't work out equally for all women. If your tumor is strongly estrogen and progesterone receptor positive, you'll have a 60 percent response rate. That means in over half the cases symptoms are alleviated for a significant period of time. Women with lower levels of estrogen (ER) and progesterone (PR) have a lower response rate, but it is still significant. Only 5 percent of women whose breast cancers are truly ER and PR negative by modern tumor-staining techniques have no chance of benefiting from hormonal therapy. It is reasonable to try a hormone therapy in a patient who has no symptoms and whose disease is slow growing.

Usually the effects of endocrine treatments last for 12–18 months, but many women stay in remission for 2–5 years, and some are free of disease for as long as 10 years. The 24-year survivor mentioned earlier was treated with hormone therapies only. A widely held belief among medical oncologists is that chemotherapy works faster than hormone therapy in reversing symptoms. One reason for this belief may be that chemotherapy often results in faster tumor shrinkage, as seen on X rays. Another reason may be that patients who respond to endocrine therapy are usually those with the more slowly growing disease. There is probably a relationship between the rate at which the disease grows and the rate at which it disappears. When the tumor does show up again, especially if the patient is on tamoxifen, sometimes just stopping the drug can give a secondary response. We think this is because the antiestrogen tamoxifen can, after long periods of treatment, sometimes become estrogenic and eventually stimulate tumor growth; therefore, stopping tamoxifen can halt the growth of the tumor cells again. This "withdrawal" therapy has not been reported for the aromatase inhibitors or fulvestrant, and it is not used anymore because there are so many effective, low-toxicity agents to use after stopping tamoxifen.

For the premenopausal woman, we usually start by trying ovarian ablation, by either surgical or chemical means. If she has a response, we stay with it until the symptoms recur and then go on to one of the other hormone agents not used the first time (tamoxifen or an aromatase inhibitor, depending on whether she is still menstruating). Then, if she has had her ovaries removed, we may try fulvestrant, then megestrol acetate or one of the other hormone treatments. With postmenopausal women we start with an aromatase inhibitor (since ablating the ovaries of a postmenopausal woman doesn't change much); if that works for a time the next step is fulvestrant (an estrogen blocker) or tamoxifen, megestrol acetate, fluoxymesterone, and finally estradiol. If a woman was on tamoxifen adjuvant therapy at the time of her metastasis we would start with anastrozole for postmenopausal women and goserelin (Zoladex) or oophorectomy for premenopausal women. Only when a woman stops responding to hormones do we go on to chemotherapy. As hormonal options are increasing rapidly, we suggest you check the practice guidelines of the NCCN for up-to-date information (www.nccn.org).

The woman with metastatic breast cancer whose tumor is sensitive to hormones is comparatively lucky, since she has more avenues of treatment that are less toxic than does the woman whose tumor is resistant to hormonal influence. As I noted earlier, however, even a woman with hormone receptor negative tumors occasionally responds to hormone therapy. This may be because the older methods of measuring ER and PR were somewhat inaccurate and women whose cancer was called negative were actually low positive. Most oncologists feel that a woman with any degree of ER or PR positivity, however small, should be given treatment with hormone therapy at some time during the course of her metastatic disease. All women with metastasis should question their medical oncologist about the possibility of hormone treatment. It may not occur to them to try a hormone maneuver first unless you bring it up. The best quality of life is associated with less toxic but successful hormone treatments. It is always a discussion worth having, although chemotherapy is probably the better choice if you have moderate to severe symptoms or life-threatening organ dysfunction.

CHEMOTHERAPY

For women whose tumors are not responsive to hormone therapy or those whose estrogen receptor positive tumors are resistant to hormone treatment, the alternative is chemotherapy. This is usually used in women with ER and PR negative tumors, and women who need a rapid response because the metastases are causing organ dysfunction. The percentage of patients who respond at least partially to the commonly used single-drug chemotherapy treatments is 20–59 percent, and about 10–15 percent have a complete response: their tumors vanish on X ray examination for 6–12 months. The average time to respond is around six weeks, although symptoms generally improve within a few weeks. The average duration of the response is 5–13 months, but individual patients' responses can last longer. The maximum duration that we've so far found is over 180 months—which means, in effect, that it's over 10 years and thus could be called a cure.

(Unfortunately this length of survival is very rare.) The average survival of the responders is 15–42 months. It is generally less for women whose cancers are resistant to chemotherapy. So chemotherapy, like hormone therapy, can help you live with symptom improvement for anywhere between one and four years, and there's a small chance it can give you 10 or more years of quality life.

More than 80 cytotoxic drugs—drugs that kill cells—have been tested. Thirteen are used commonly in breast cancer treatment. Interestingly, breast cancer creates the kind of tumor that is responsive to the greatest array of drugs—most other cancers don't respond to as many chemicals. The standard drugs are the same ones I discussed in Chapter 24 in terms of adjuvant treatment: cyclophosphamide (Cytoxan) (C), methotrexate (M), 5-fluorouracil (F), doxorubicin (Adriamycin) (A), epirubicin (E), and paclitaxel or docetaxel (T). These drugs have the highest antitumor activity among all the patients studied, and only limited cross-resistance.

What is used depends on what was used at the time metastatic disease was diagnosed. If you already had CMF, then doxorubicin may be tried. If you had doxorubicin when you were diagnosed, paclitaxel or docetaxel may be the next choice. Fortunately there are other drugs as well. These include capecitabine (Xeloda), mitoxantrone (Novantrone), vinorelbine (Navelbine), gemcitabine (Gemzar), irinotecan (Captosar), cisplatin or carboplatin, and nab paclitaxel (ABranxane), all of which have documented antitumor activity in breast cancer.

Each drug has limitations. With doxorubicin, we can give only a certain dosage, and then it becomes toxic to the heart. Once you reach that point you can't ever use it again. Some of the other drugs you can take indefinitely.

Many of the chemotherapy drugs produce the standard side effects (vomiting, bone marrow suppression, etc), and when the drugs are combined they tend to be worse. For this reason, giving one chemotherapy drug at a time can significantly reduce side effects. On the other hand, there have been recent suggestions that some combinations do better: docetaxel and capecitabine[28] and paclitaxel and gemcitabine.[29] At this point a reasonable approach may be to use a sequential single agent in situations where there is no organ dysfunction and mild to moderate symptoms, saving the combinations for cases with organ dysfunction and severe symptoms.

As I mentioned in Chapter 24, there are now terrific antinausea drugs that have almost eliminated this problem. Most chemotherapy drugs involve some hair loss. Several have a very low potential to cause leukemia down the road. Since you're dealing with metastatic breast cancer, though, that's not a reason to eliminate them. Most will decrease your white cell count. Attempts have been made to test the tumor cells against a variety of drugs in a test tube to predict the right drug or combination of drugs. Although it sounds like a great idea, it hasn't worked in practice as well as we would like.

While cancer cells can build resistance to a particular drug, they don't always do so. Sometimes we treat metastatic cancer with a drug and get a response; then the disease recurs and we use the same drug again, and again it works. It always amazes me how often we find a drug that doesn't work for the majority of patients but turns out to be exactly what one particular person needs. I had one patient with horrible lumps all over her chest. We treated her with just about everything, including experimental drugs, and nothing seemed to work. Then we went back and tried straight 5-fluorouracil, which usually works only modestly in breast cancer—and everything disappeared. So we sometimes can't predict what the right drug is for a particular person, and if you have metastatic disease, you need to keep that in mind. You may feel discouraged if particular drugs don't seem to be working, especially if they're the standard breast cancer drugs. But you never know when we'll hit on the one that will alleviate your symptoms.

Once we've found a drug that works, we generally continue it for a long time. How long is something on which doctors disagree. There are two philosophies. One is that we'll get as much response as we're going to get in about six months, so we should give the chemo for six months and then stop. The other philosophy is to give it continuously until the patient becomes resistant to it, and then move on to something else. There are arguments for both schools. Most of the studies suggest improved quality of life and better symptom control with continuous therapy, but again this may not be best for every woman. It's something you should discuss with your doctor and be clear about before you start treatments.

Dr. Hayes tells his patients that four things can happen with treatment for metastatic disease:

1. Terrible toxicity; it is the wrong drug and should be stopped and something else tried
2. Obvious disease progression; it is the wrong drug or the cancer has become resistant and it is time to stop that drug and try something else
3. A stable situation; it is not clear whether the drug is holding the disease in check or not; continue the drug with monitoring of disease and side effects
4. Improvement with little toxicity; it is the right drug and should be continued

It is not hard to figure out which of the four categories you are in—you can see how you feel, what your physical exam reveals, and data from X rays and markers. For this reason many oncologists monitor your X rays every 3–4 cycles of chemotherapy with the same tests you had in the beginning—comparing apples to apples. In addition they do routine blood tests for liver function and tumor markers (Ca 15-3, 27, 29 and CEA). More recent studies have shown that we can measure specific tumor cells known as *circulating tumor cells (CTC)* in the blood of women with metastatic disease.[30] If there is an increase in circulating tumor cells, you probably are on the wrong drug and should switch. A new study now taking place will examine whether this strategy actually improves survival.

It might seem that combining chemotherapy and hormone therapy would work better than either one alone. But it doesn't. In women with hormone-sensitive tumors, adding chemotherapy to hormones doesn't increase the disease-free or overall survival and they get side effects. However, chemotherapy works just as well after hormone therapy has been used.

Any woman with metastatic disease needs to investigate the available clinical trials. New drugs and/or new combinations of drugs and biologic agents are being tested continuously and may be the best choice for someone with metastatic disease. It's important to talk with your doctor and get clear, precise information about what drugs are best for you, how long and in what sequence you can take them, and what their side effects are.

For a while it was popular to use high dose chemotherapy with stem cell rescue to treat metastatic disease. As I explained in Chapter 18, we now have two randomized controlled studies examining its use in women with metastasis and neither has shown a benefit over standard chemotherapy. Although there's always a temptation to go for what appears to be the most aggressive therapy, in this case the benefit isn't worth the increased side effects for most women. I would not recommend a stem cell transplant outside of a clinical trial.

TARGETED THERAPY

We have always dreamed of finding something distinctive about the cancer cell and developing a therapy specific to it. We would then give the antibody, kill or control all of the cancer cells, and do little or no harm to the rest of the body. Recently several drugs have been developed to target other molecules that might be specific to the cancer cells. Two of these are monoclonal antibodies that target Her-2 (trastuzumab) or new blood vessels that are necessary for the cancer to grow (bevacizumab). About 20 percent of women with breast cancer have too many copies of the Her-2/neu oncogene. This particular oncogene tells the cell to grow: harder, stronger, and longer. Trastuzumab is an antibody to that oncogene, which blocks it in its tracks.

There are now several trials suggesting that trastuzumab, either by itself or with chemotherapy, is very effective in Her-2/neu overexpressing breast cancer. In one larger randomized controlled trial, women who received chemotherapy plus trastuzumab had not only an increase in relapse-free survival and time to progression but also an increase in overall survival. However, trastuzumab can cause heart failure. This is uncommon (less than 5 percent of cases) when it is used alone or with non-anthracycline therapy, but when it was given with doxorubicin the rate of congestive heart failure rose to about 20 percent. Thus it should not be given with doxorubicin or other anthracyclines outside of a clinical trial. So all women with Her-2/neu-overexpressing metastatic breast cancer should receive trastuzumab either alone or with chemotherapy unless they have preexisting heart failure. When or if breast cancer progresses on trastuzumab, it is not clear the antibody should be continued. This is currently being addressed in a randomized clinical trial.

As we were in the final draft of this book, data came out on the second monoclonal antibody to be used for metastatic breast cancer. The antiangiogenesis drug bevacizumab (Avastin) is an antibody to VEGF, a growth factor responsible for inducing new blood vessels to grow and feed the tumor. Angiogenesis is the cancer's attempt to develop new blood vessels to support its growth. With drugs that block this function, the cancer theoretically will not be able to get enough nourishment from its inadequate blood vessels and will die. In this study bevacizumab was given with paclitaxel to women with metastatic disease and showed an improvement in progression-free survival.[31] This is indeed big news because, as with trastuzumab, the next step will be to see if it has any benefit in women who are newly diagnosed.

Other forms of immunotherapy such as vaccines are also being tested. Although we commonly think of a vaccine as prevention, such as the one used for polio or measles, it can also be used in treatment. These vaccines are made by training immune cells to hone in on a certain target found on breast cancer cells. It sounds great, but problems have prevented it from being effective so far. For one thing, not every cancer cell is the same. This means that a vaccine against one element such as Her-2 will kill only the cells that express it, leaving the others behind. Vaccines for metastatic breast cancer are being tested in clinical trials and may be useful in the near future.

BISPHOSPHONATES

Most of the treatments we have considered involve killing or controlling the cancer cell. The other approach is to alter the tissue that the cancer is trying to grow in. A bisphosphonate is a drug that blocks the resorption (breakdown) of bone. It has been shown to be very effective in treating bone metastasis. When there is cancer in the bone, there is an increase in resorption—one of the reasons the bone gets weaker and often fractures. Several studies have shown that women who take pamidronate (Aredia) or zolendronic acid (Zometa) every four weeks will have a decrease not only in the resorption of the bone but also in the number of new bone metastases that develop and the incidence of bone fractures.[32] One study also suggested that it decreased other sites of metastatic disease, although this has not been confirmed yet by other studies. It certainly is worth taking for any woman with bone metastasis. In 2003 the American Society of Clinical Oncology stated that "bisphosphonates provide a supportive albeit expensive and non-life-prolonging benefit to many patients with bone metastases." Unfortunately we do not have data on the optimal drug, dosing, route of delivery, duration of therapy, best time to start the drug, and how best to monitor toxicity.[33]

OTHER TREATMENTS

I've been discussing systemic therapies so far, but sometimes local treatment is called for. Certain kinds of metastatic disease respond best to local treatments because they're local problems.

Radiation, for example, works best if the cancer has spread to your eye. Spinal cord involvement with impending bone fracture (in which your bone is so weakened that it is about to break) also lends itself well to radiation, since it too is a local problem and there is only one spot to be treated. For impending bone fractures following spinal cord compression, surgical treatment is often needed to stabilize the bone before radiation.

Radiation for metastatic cancer is the same as for initial breast cancer, but its purpose is different—to alleviate pain or other symptoms. A couple of weeks usually pass before the pain noticeably lessens.

The timing is somewhat different too. There are usually 10–15 treatments, spread over two and a half to four weeks. A smaller dose of radiation is used. While a primary radiation treatment to your breast might use 6,000 centigrays of radiation over six and a half weeks, with 180 centigrays per treatment, the treatment for someone with, for example, bone metastasis in the hip might use 3,000 centigrays over 10 treatments of 300 centigrays each.

Surgery, as I mentioned earlier, is best if there is one spot in the lung or brain, for example, in a woman who has had a reasonably long interval between primary diagnosis and development of metastatic disease. If the cancer has recurred in several places, however, systemic treatment is best.

PAIN CONTROL

In terms of palliation—getting rid of symptoms so you feel better—treatments of the cancer itself aren't the only options. We've come an enormous way in pain control. If, for example, you're in severe pain because of bone metastasis, we now have ways of putting a catheter in the space along the spinal cord and dripping continuous low dose morphine to get rid of all the pain. Administered this way, it won't affect your mind the way it would if administered systemically. This won't cure you, but in your last three or four months of life, when systemic therapy is no longer working, it can give you quality time and reduce or eliminate suffering. There's now a whole specialty of pain control that includes psychiatrists, anesthesiologists, and internists. Since a thorough discussion of all the options is outside the scope of this book, suffice it to say that we have acquired a lot of knowledge about chronic pain and how to deal with it. Anybody who has chronic pain because of metastatic cancer and isn't getting relief should ask to be referred to a pain unit. Sometimes oncologists and people who work on cancer are so focused on treating and curing the disease that they forget about these ancillary things that can make an enormous difference in a patient's life. So ask to see a pain specialist; even if it means having to travel to the local medical school, it can make a big difference to you.

EXPERIMENTAL TREATMENTS

Throughout this book I have encouraged women to participate in phase 3 clinical trials (see Chapter 15)—trials of drugs or treatments that have been tested in earlier phases and shown not to harm the patient. There is a trickier area to consider with metastatic cancer, and that is phase 1 or phase 2 trials. These are much earlier stages in the testing of a drug, designed to determine first the toxicity of a possibly useful drug and then whether it works.

Since you know that traditional treatments, which were so helpful with your first diagnosis, offer only a slim chance of cure, an experimental treatment may be worth considering. Generally there is no harm in trying an innovative new therapy and postponing treatment with other standard therapies.

When is the best time to join an experimental trial? Classically, people do it when nothing else has helped and they've run out of options. However, by the time you run out of options you're least likely to be able to respond to the new treatment: you have no resources left. So the best time may be when you have been diagnosed with metastatic disease but are feeling well. You have a chest X ray or bone scan that shows a lesion but you actually have modest symptoms. At this stage, there's no rush to use chemotherapy or hormone therapy since, as I noted before, there's no evidence that treating with chemo earlier will give you better survival odds than waiting until you have symptoms. If you now try something experimental, you have an opportunity to see if it works; if it doesn't you can still get the usual chemotherapy if symptoms worsen.

Only a doctor who is working on the experiments is likely to offer such treatments routinely. The best way to find out about them is to go to your local cancer center and see what they're involved in, and you can also go to www.cancer.gov or call the National Cancer Institute (1-800-4-CANCER), for a computerized searching system. You can obtain a list of every clinical trial you're eligible for, either in your own geographical area or in the whole United States if you're willing and able to travel.

I think this is really worthwhile. It's a gamble, but sometimes the gamble pays off. For example, some of the women who first participated in the tests for docetaxel or trastuzumab had a remarkable response that lasted between 18 and 24 months.

There are exciting new experiments going on for metastatic disease. One example is antiangiogenesis drugs like bevacizumab (Avastin). Clinical trials are going on with this category of drugs.

While they may help you, these trials can involve side effects as well. But only you can decide what price in toxicity you are willing to pay. Some women want to try everything new and others don't. Don't let yourself be pushed by your doctor or family. Decide in your own heart what the best approach is for you.

TAKING CARE OF YOURSELF EMOTIONALLY

David Spiegel's study of women with metastatic disease who joined support groups (see Chapter 25) shows the importance of the mind–body connection. Not only did the women who participated in a support group live twice as long as those who did not, they also had a better quality of life.[34] Although this has been difficult to replicate, it still stands that a diagnosis of metastatic disease is a time to reorder your life and pay attention to what is most important to you. You may not be able to change the course of your disease, but you can improve how you deal with it.

Spiegel tells the story of a woman who had always wanted to write poetry and started after her diagnosis of metastatic disease. She had a book of her poems published before her death. One of my own patients, Susan Shapiro, was very distressed with the lack of analysis of breast cancer from a feminist political perspective. She wrote an article in the local feminist paper and called a meeting. From this she started the Women's Community Cancer Project in Boston a few months before she died. I'm certain she would be happy to know her work sparked a national movement that continues today.

A diagnosis of recurrence or metastasis will remind you that you do not have control over your body. But you certainly do have control over your mind, emotions, and spirit. This is a good time to revisit some of the complementary treatments such as visualization, self-hypnosis, and imagery (see Chapter 25). And find a doctor you can talk to and who will listen to you. Shop around if you have to. If you are in a small town and/or have an insurance plan with limited choice, then schedule an appointment with your oncologist so that you can talk about what you need, as well as what he or she expects from you. (See Appendix D for the patient's and doctor's rights.) You need to know as accurately as possible what to expect from your condition and your treatments so that you can plan. Ask for the information you need and tell your doctor if there are things you would rather not know. As in any relationship, frank communication about your needs will go far toward having them met.

There are two main fears that accompany a diagnosis of recurrent breast cancer: pain and death. As I discussed earlier in this chapter, pain is certainly not inevitable. Pain control has finally gone mainstream in the United States. There are pain centers, and many methods have been developed to deal with pain without clouding your mind and ruining your life.

Not everyone dies from a recurrence or metastatic breast cancer, but it is certainly a possibility. David Spiegel's book *Living Beyond Limits* is invaluable in addressing the needs of the heart and soul in confronting terminal illness.[35] You may not be able to avoid death, but you can control how you want to handle it. One of my patients was a great denier. From the first moment of her diagnosis she refused to let her cancer interfere with her life. When she developed metastatic disease, this pattern continued. She continued to hurl herself through life: sailing, traveling, and enjoying herself. My first reaction was to be a little critical of her inability to face the reality of the situation, until I realized that she *had* faced it. She knew exactly what she was doing and was determined to take control of whatever time she had left. She slipped into a coma on her sailboat among friends and died as she wanted, where she wanted, in control to the end.

WHEN TO STOP TREATMENT

When a patient would ask me, "How long do I have to live?" I'd never answer; not because I wanted to withhold information from my patient but because I simply didn't know. There are statistical likelihoods, but they do not tell what will happen to each individual. There are patients who, according to the statistics, should die in four months but live four years; there are others who should last four years but die in four months. I'm always amazed at the variations. One of my patients had a small cancer and negative nodes with what should have been a good prognosis, but when she finished her radiation we discovered the cancer had metastasized to her lungs, and she died in three months. Another patient, a Chinese woman who spoke no English, had a cancer that was very bad, and I privately thought she wouldn't live very long. I had to talk to her through her sons, who kept trying to get me to say how long she had. I wouldn't tell them. It's a good thing, because she was still alive seven years later. Sometimes I think she lived so long because she didn't know she was supposed to die.

At the same time, it's important for your doctor to be honest with you. I think it's sensible to say to a patient who has asked for a frank response, "This is serious, but we don't know how long you'll live until we see how you respond to treatment. You'll probably eventually die of breast cancer, and you probably won't live another 40 years, so you may want to plan your life with that in mind." If you insist on more specific predictions, a doctor may quote statistics—but you should always be reminded that there are exceptions to statistics. If 99 out of 100 patients in your condition die within a year, 1 out of 100 doesn't—and there's no reason to assume you won't be that one.

Eventually, however, there comes the hardest part. We've tried all the available treatments, and we know that you don't have much longer. Even then, we don't know if it's days or weeks, and there is still the possibility of a miracle. But there's a point at which you're clearly dying, and you have a right to know that. The prevailing belief used to be that it was better not to tell patients they were dying. But this sets up an unhealthy climate of denial. It's likely you'll sense it yourself, but since no one wants to talk about it you pretend it's okay in order to spare them, and they pretend it's okay in order to spare you. Such denial can keep you from finishing your business—clearing up relationships, saying good-bye, saying the things you won't get another chance to say to the people you love, giving them the chance to say those things to you. I think doctors make a great error in denying death: we tend to look at it too much as a defeat and get caught up in our own denial, at the patient's expense.

While you're still feeling fairly well, you might want to talk with your doctor, and with your family members or friends, about how you want to die when the time comes. Do you want to be kept alive at all costs, or not? Do you want to die at home, or in the hospital?

Often people die in a hospital or a nursing home, and many think of that as an inevitability. But it isn't, and it's important to consider whether it might be better for you to die in your own home or in the home of a loved one. For many people this is the best option, particularly if a loved one is able to stay with you full-time. Dying at home offers more control over your surroundings and a greater likelihood that you will die with loved ones around you. If this is an option you want to explore, there are many hospice programs that can help you. They are experienced in caring for both the patient and the family in a way that can make all the difference. I had firsthand experience when my cousin was dying of bile duct cancer, and I cannot say enough about how terrific they are.

For some women and their families, this is not possible. If it makes more sense for you to die in a hospital, there is much you and your loved ones can do to ensure that the environment is as comfortable as possible. Many hospitals have hospice rooms for dying patients, and even those that don't can be made homelike. You will want to discuss your wishes with the caregivers there, to be sure they are willing and prepared to follow them.

There are other issues you'll want to look into—perhaps even before you have decided that it's time to stop fighting your illness. When the time comes—whether in months or years—do you want to be heavily medicated or as alert as possible? No way is universally better, but one way might be better for you. If your wishes are clearly known—especially if they can be documented in a living will—you might be able to prevent those tragic situations in which doctors and family members are fighting over whether to keep you on a life-support system.

A living will is only part of an advance directive—a set of written instructions that also include a health care proxy. The living will spells out what medical treatment you do and don't want if the time arrives when you are unable to verbalize your own decisions. A health care proxy specifies a particular person you authorize to make decisions about your care when you no longer can.

Living wills vary from state to state, and in some cases you may need to add information to yours. As Dr. Daniel Tobin writes in *Peaceful Dying,* the language of the typical living will may not be specific enough.[36] If the document merely says you don't want life-prolonging measures if you have an "incurable or irreversible condition," your doctor may define such a condition differently than you. So you might want to add a specific "do not resuscitate" to your living will, and other additions concerning artificial nutrition and hydration. You need to spend some time thinking about what you *do* want when the time comes. Do you want to be tube-fed? Do you want to be given antibiotics to fight infections? Or do you prefer to die from the infection rather than to continue for a short time and die of your cancer? These things may not be fun to think about, but they're important.

Betsy Carpenter, a speaker and activist around issues of advance directives, emphatically agrees. You may or may not want life-extending treatment at some point, and you have a right to decide. It's important to make those decisions before you reach the point where you can no longer speak for yourself. Like Dr. Tobin, Carpenter stresses the importance of talking with your family and friends in advance, discussing the options open to you and how you feel about them, and listening respectfully to the feelings of your loved ones. Your illness and your ultimate death will affect those who love you deeply, and it's important to involve them in your decision-making process. Understanding your feelings and sharing theirs with you will make it far less likely that they'll go against your wishes when the time comes.

In deciding what you do and don't want, Carpenter advises, think about four areas in particular. What are your fears? Most people fear pain, loss of control, inappropriate prolongation of life, and becoming a burden to loved ones. Each of these fears should be explored fully, in terms of what is reasonable to think may happen and in terms of your own emotions.

Pick out your health care proxy carefully, she says, and spell out who you *don't* want involved in making health care decisions for you as well. "This doesn't have to be hostile," she says. "You can write, 'although I dearly love my son Jim, I don't wish him to have any part in decision making around my care.'" The agent you choose should be someone you love *and* fully trust to honor your wishes, who knows you well enough to make decisions that you haven't spelled out, in ways that you would want. "For example," she says, "my husband is my proxy agent, and he knows that I wouldn't want my life artificially prolonged. But suppose my daughter, who lives in London, wasn't here when I went into a coma. He might be certain that it was important for her to see me living and breathing one last time. So he might decide to keep me on life support for 24 hours until she could get back home. And he would know that, loving her, I would also want this for her." Because of such contingencies, she adds, while your living will should be specific, it shouldn't be too specific to preclude your agent from making judgments in such unforeseen circumstances. You may want to write out a declaration of precedence: "If a conflict arises between my list and my agent's decision, I give precedent to my agent over my own written word."

If there is someone you don't want visiting you when you're dying, this too should be spelled out, says Carpenter, in a priority of visitation statement. Such documents are important even for those not facing imminent death, she says. Healthy people are sometimes injured in accidents and lose the ability to verbalize their wishes.

These questions are important for every one of us to consider, since none of us is immortal, and death can come for anyone anytime. Of course, you may live another 10 or 20 years, but you lose nothing by having those discussions, and you might even gain some peace of mind.

PART EIGHT

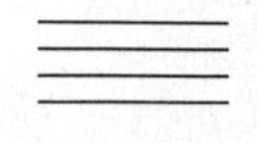

What Is Coming

28

The Future: From Lab to Bedside

Having reviewed state-of-the-art breast cancer treatment, I now get to peer into the future. I'll tell you what I think are the most interesting findings in biology and how they may translate into patient care. In the third edition of this book I included a whole chapter on molecular biology to get you ready for the advances I thought would be coming. Some of them are here, such as trastuzumab and the anti-VEGF bevacizumab (see Chapters 24, 27). Others, such as the interaction between the cells and their environment, are still evolving, and so I will discuss them here. The area I think has most promise is the one I am working on—preventing breast cancer by treating the ductal lining cells. But since I have already devoted a whole chapter to that, I will expand on other promising areas.

TUMOR STEM CELLS

One of the most exciting concepts in figuring out the biology of breast cancer has been that of *tumor stem cells*. You hear a lot about stem cells in the news, usually in relation to using healthy embryonic stem cells to grow new organs or treat diseases. This is the opposite approach. I guess you could call it "stem cells gone bad."

It all started when a group at the University of Michigan tried to transplant tumors into mice. Doing that requires a lot of tumor cells, and even then it doesn't always work. At first, researchers thought that it was just an inefficient process. But Michael Clarke and his group found that when they separated the cells into groups based on surface markers (like dividing up a group of people by what clothes they're wearing), one group was always very efficient (needing only 20 cells for the transplant), while another could not get the transplant to take with 20,000 cells.[1] It seemed that not every cell in the cancer was able to generate a new tumor when transplanted. This was counter to the prevailing view that any cancer cell can spread to other areas of the body and grow new tumors there. But if not all tumor cells could generate a cancer, which ones could? When researchers studied the new cancers, they found something interesting. The transplanted cells all had the same group of surface markers, but the resulting tumor had the usual variety of cells. This suggested that the original cells were able to self-renew (clone themselves) and also differentiate into less primitive cells. These characteristics are the fundamental properties of stem cells. When stem cells divide, the division can give rise to new stem cells as well as differentiated cells of the organ or tumor. (See Fig. 28-1.)Usually the number of normal stem cells present in an organ is tightly regulated, but cancer stem cells lose this regulation, giving them the ability to self-renew and constantly expand themselves. One of my favorite metaphors is that these cells are like the queen bee. They can make a new queen or they can make lots of worker bees that are not able to make a queen. And only a queen can set up a new hive.

Normal breast stem cells live in the milk ducts and are important in maintaining the ductal lining. Exactly where they are located in the ductal system and what they look like are not yet known. If the setup is like that of white blood stem cells versus leukemia stem cells, then the differences may be subtle. Both normal stem cells and tumor stem cells are tough: they are made to survive. After all, the organ depends on them to maintain it as cells die naturally. So the stem cells have the ability to pump out certain drugs to prevent them from causing harm, and they divide slowly and methodically to avoid errors. This would make them more resistant to irradiation and other DNA-damaging agents.

This new paradigm suggests what may be an important flaw in our approach to cancer treatment. We give drugs that are based on the idea that cells are dividing. But the stem cell actually doesn't divide very much. That means that we may see a tumor shrink but not be cured, which is exactly what happens in metastatic breast cancer. It's a bit like capturing a lot of drug dealers but not the leaders of the drug cartel. In addition, when we carefully study the tumor cells and compare them to normal cells in order to find ways to target them, we may be finding targets on the daughter cells and not the stem cells. Finally, when we

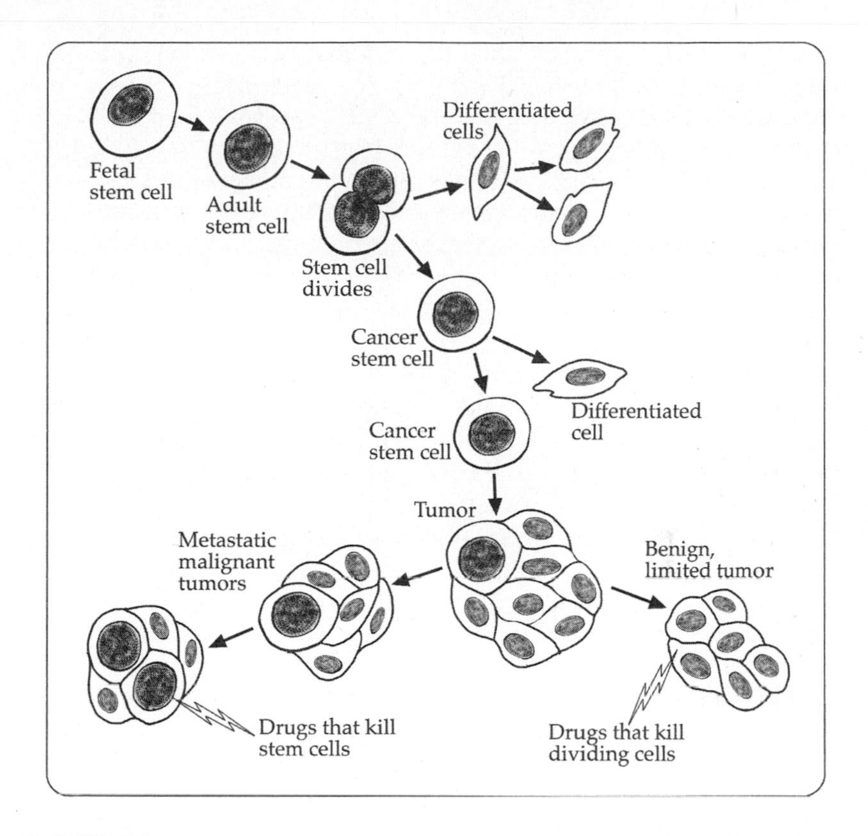

FIGURE 28-1

find cancer cells in the bone marrow of women with breast cancer, they do not reliably predict who will develop metastatic disease. This may be because some of the cells in the circulation are daughter cells that are not capable of setting up a new tumor.

Needless to say, researchers are feverishly trying to learn more about these stem cells, how to find them and eventually how to destroy them. It may be difficult to differentiate between the bad guys and the good guys, at least at first. But once we figure this out, we may be able to employ the intraductal approach (Chapter 13) to search and destroy these dangerous cells. It won't be tomorrow, but I am sure this new hypothesis will become more and more important in the future.

GENE–ENVIRONMENT INTERACTION

In parallel with the new thinking about cancer stem cells has come new thinking about the importance of the environment that the cells live in. All these years we've been studying cancer cells by looking at them in isolation. Scientists take cancer cells and grow them in petri dishes, then study their behavior. It's a little like taking a bee out of a hive and studying it in a glass jar. Since the bee is not in its natural environment, observing its behavior is difficult. We've begun to realize that if we study cancer cells in their own environment, we can learn a lot more, since they interact with the surrounding cells (stroma), and these cells have an effect on them.

Let's look at a hypothetical murderer. Maybe she's born with a sociopathic character—like the girl in *The Bad Seed.* But how is she raised, and in what environment? Let's say her parents are too busy with their social lives to pay much attention to her and there are no strong, loving family members; kind, responsible neighbors; solid school, or good community activities to offer positive behavioral guidance. There are drug dealers at her school and she's impressed by them. Nothing prevents her from hanging out with them, and soon she's in a world where she learns criminal skills. Each of these factors plays a part in the development of her criminal behavior. Had the original sociopathic tendencies been absent, the environment might not have made such a difference: she wouldn't be predisposed toward criminal acts. But even with the sociopathic tendencies, early training might have worked against the predisposition, developing a strong conscience that would prevent her from acting on her instincts. Finally, even with the sociopathic tendencies and the amoral background, she might not have learned the skills to become an efficient criminal. Of course, her basic predisposition might not be permanently countered by the wholesome influences in childhood. As an adult, away from those influences, she might find herself in circumstances that nourish her basic character—"fall in with a bad crowd." And so that good little girl grows into a middle-aged murderer.

The other element of the discussion about gene-environment interaction is the cell-environment interaction. We know that there is "cross talk" between the cells and the stroma they are suspended in. As the cells grow, they make certain proteins—growth factors, cytokines, enzymes—that are messengers telling the surrounding cells what to do. The surrounding cells then respond to these messages with messages of their own. This cross talk is called *epigenetic interaction.* It results in a change in a gene expression rather than structural alterations in the genes themselves. Epigenetic interaction is probably an important determinant of cancer cell growth and metastasis, and thus it is likely to respond to therapeutic intervention. For an analogy, let's say there is a certain plant that can be pollinated only if there is a particular kind of bee in the environment that will take pollen on its body to another plant. The original flower secretes a message in the form of a smell that attracts the bee. The bee then responds by cross-pollinating the plant. If you could block the flower's scent, that species might die out. Or you could change the environment to make it inhospitable for the bee but not the flower. This also would eliminate the species. We don't want to eliminate any species of flower, of course. But it would be wonderful to be able to eliminate any species of cancer cells by blocking this type of interaction.

This may be how it works with cancer. Mina Bissel, a researcher in Berkeley, California, has for the past few years been studying breast cancer cells in a breast tissue environment. She has taken breast cancer cells that have the mutations of breast cancer, and grown them in a culture made from the tissues that support the breast ducts (normal extracellular matrix). In that environment, the cancer cells behaved like normal cells—they made ducts and did the other things that healthy breast cells do.[2] The healthy influence of the surrounding cells caused the cancer cells, even though they were genetically altered, to conduct themselves properly—like the sociopath in the perfect environment. When Dr. Bissel and her associates put the same cells in a malignant environment, the cells went back to behaving like cancer. (See Fig. 28-2.)

Recently Charlotte Kuperwasser and her team did an elegant experiment demonstrating that breast cancer cells can be influenced in women as well.[3] They developed a mouse model that used human mammary cells from reduction mammoplasties (see Chapter 3) and human stroma with added growth factors. When they grew the "normal" epithelial cells in this "activated" stroma, it gave rise to hyperplasia and in one case DCIS. The researchers concluded that these

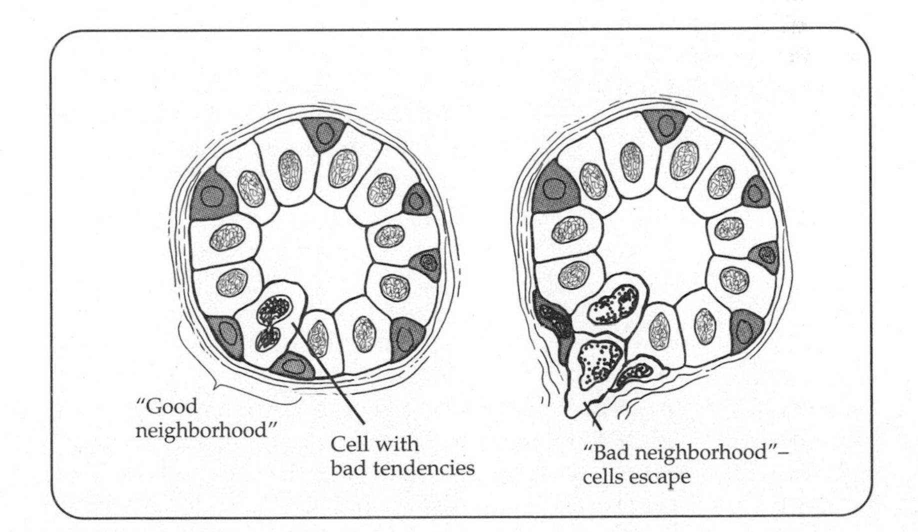

FIGURE 28-2

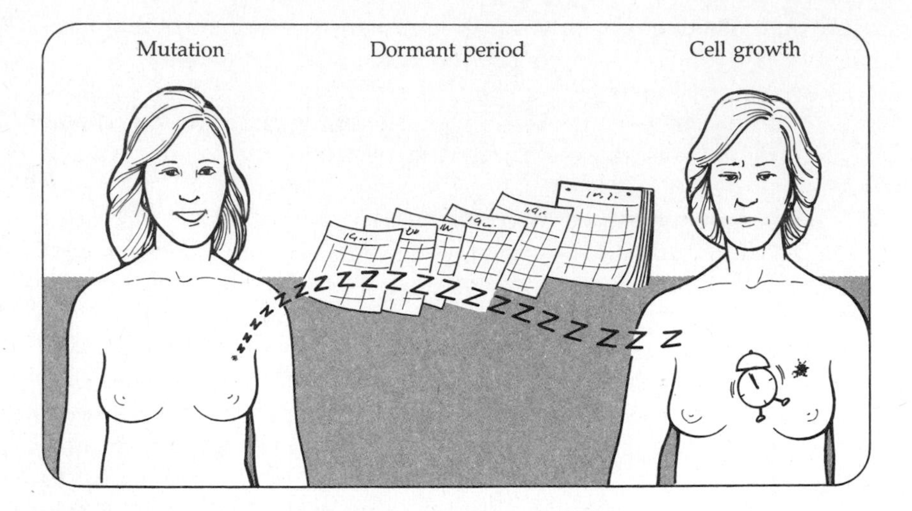

FIGURE 28-3

human epithelial cells had undergone one or several premalignant changes before they were put in the mice even though they looked perfectly normal under the microscope. They showed up only when placed in an environment that encouraged cancer. This means that if we knew the right environment, the reverse would be possible as well: we might be able to keep the cancer stem cells from misbehaving. The ability to control or reverse cancer may also explain a phenomenon known as *tumor dormancy* (see Fig. 28-3). This is thought to happen in women who appear to be cured at the end of treatment but have a recurrence ten years later. What were the cells doing for ten years? They were asleep. What put them to sleep? What woke them up?

In summary, all cancer is probably caused by a combination of genes that are altered by carcinogens stimulated by an environment conducive to growth and spread.

ANGIOGENESIS

Once the cancer cells get out of the breast duct (or any other organ) and start to grow, they need their own blood supply—the lifeline that gives them oxygen and nutrients. It's as if you started a new colony or a commune out in the desert. You've found this nice place, but you need roads to bring in your supplies and take out your garbage. Without such roads, your community will die off quickly. In the same way, cancer cells die off quickly if they don't have a blood supply. Tumors stop growing at about 2 millimeters unless they have more blood vessels.

At this point proteins send a message saying, "Let's grow new blood vessels."

These proteins are specific growth factors. When you're an embryo, for example, you need new blood vessels that can go all the way down your arms and legs, so you'll have fingers and toes. Later, if you have an injury, you need new blood vessels to grow and heal it. That's part of the reason an injury turns red. A protein that stimulates blood vessel growth (*VEGF: vascular endothelial growth factor*) is secreted by the cancer and then fits into a specific receptor on the blood vessels and tells them to make more.

This process is called *angiogenesis*: "angio" means vessels, and "genesis" means growth. If you look at tumors under a microscope, you see that some have more blood vessels than others. The more blood vessels you have, the greater blood supply you have. Thus there is a greater chance that the cancer will spread, since there are more "roads" to spread out on (see Fig. 28-4). Even in DCIS that is still trapped inside the duct, there is an increase in blood vessels around the outside of the duct. Those blood vessels can't do the DCIS cells any good, since they're too far away. But their presence means that the DCIS is secreting angiogenic factors such as VEGF to create new blood vessels even before the cells are there. This may be a clue that these are the cells that will eventually get out and invade. Some researchers think that per-

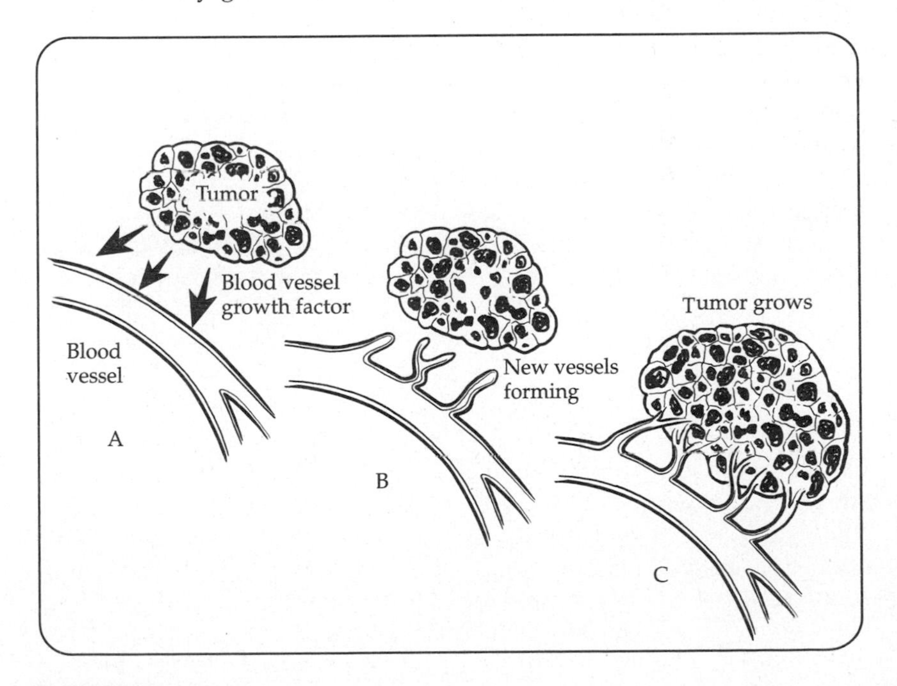

FIGURE 28-4

haps we can measure VEGF in the bloodstream or duct fluid to see if there are new blood vessels growing.

Or it may be something else. My own theory regarding the increase in blood vessels in cases of DCIS is that it may not mean the cells are any more likely to get out, but if they do get out, the cancer is likely to be aggressive. When there's a lot of bleeding with a biopsy, as I said earlier, the surgeon knows it's probably cancer, since benign tumors seldom have that many blood vessels. Surgeons have known this for years, but we never realized its implications till now.

Judah Folkman, a researcher in Boston, has made the startling discovery that cancer tumors actually secrete not only angiogenic factors but also angiogenic inhibitors (the factor that keeps metastasis under control). When the primary tumor is removed, the metastasis grows more because the angiogenic inhibitors have been removed.[4] This is interesting because there's always been a sort of folk belief that if you have surgery to remove a tumor, it "lets the air get into it" and causes the cancer to spread. It's unlikely that the air has anything to do with it, but this may be canny observers' way of interpreting something they realized was happening—that the cancer spread more quickly after the tumor was removed. Until we learned about this tumor-secreted angiogenesis inhibitor, there was no way to account for these observations.

It seems odd that the cancer would also secrete inhibitors when it "wants" to spread. It's fanciful, but I find myself thinking that the tumor doesn't like having rivals. It will grow in its own area but will keep any cells from growing in other organs. This isn't to suggest that if you have a tumor you should ignore it because it won't spread unless you have it removed. For one thing, this behavior probably isn't true of all tumors. For another, the process is far from absolute. The tumor doesn't stop the cancer from metastasizing; it only keeps the metastases already out there under control. The tumor wants to be king, and it sends out dukes to oversee the provinces, but it doesn't want the dukes to become as strong as it is. When the king dies, the dukes all take advantage of his absence to throw off his limitations and expand their own powers.

For this reason researchers have been looking for substances that inhibit angiogenesis. The first of the antiangiogenesis drugs (bevacizumab), an antibody to VEGF, has been shown to be beneficial in metastatic disease (see Chapters 16, 27).

TRANSLATIONAL RESEARCH

Tamoxifen and trastuzumab (Herceptin) are examples of how biological research actually works in practice. In the case of tamoxifen, we started out with a drug we were using and then tried to figure out the mechanism by which it worked. With Herceptin we started out with biological observations and made a drug to fit them.

Although tamoxifen and trastuzumab are good examples of this kind of research—*translational research*—they also point out how hard it is. Let's say we want to kill a stem cell. If we give an antibody intravenously, will it survive or will it get eaten up (metabolized) by the liver? Can it be swallowed? Injected into the tumor? Will it kill normal stem cells like those in the intestine and skin? Does it have to be specifically designed to kill only breast stem cells and are those cells all the same? The concept is good, but getting it to work takes a lot of steps. It's like saying, "Let's put on a production of *The Wizard of Oz.* We'll do it next Saturday night." But you need to hold auditions for the cast, find a crew, find a theater, do rehearsals . . . you need months to put it all together. And you'll encounter a lot of frustrations—30 women will audition for Dorothy and none will be right. Similarly, a lot of work—a lot of trial and error—goes with any medical discovery. Unfortunately, while the media are good at announcing a supposedly great discovery, they're not so good at reporting that it turned out not to work or needs a lot more honing. Most of the "breakthroughs" that get reported don't lead to changes in our therapies. One of the frustrating things with all this research is that while we're at the point of knowing how it works and realizing that it may be helpful, we're not at the point of knowing how to use most of it in patients. But the good thing is that these promising new findings are already in the pipeline. It's not fantasy; it's a question of how soon we'll know what to do with our knowledge.

In the future breast cancer may be as treatable as high blood pressure and diabetes are today. These diseases can be effectively treated by controlling the symptoms with medication without totally eliminating the underlying disease. The rehabilitation of the cancer cell may be an effective treatment so that the patient, while still having cancer, will be alive and well.[5]

Or even better, we will be able to stop breast cancer at its source—destroy the cells lining the milk ducts where all breast cancer starts. In this way, we will be able to prevent it all together. As I noted in the dedication of this book, "we are working hard toward the day when our daughters and nieces will never have to hear the words 'you have breast cancer.'"

APPENDICES

A

Drugs Used for Systemic Treatment of Breast Cancer

This list of drugs is not meant to be exhaustive. Check with your oncologist about your specific drugs. Unusual signs and symptoms should be reported to your doctor immediately.

I. CHEMOTHERAPY

capecitabine (Xeloda) oral
Use: for metastatic disease resistant to anthracyclines and paclitaxel
Method of action: converted to 5-FU in body; prevents DNA and RNA synthesis
Adverse effects: nausea, diarrhea, tingling hands and feet, fatigue, anemia, reduced immunity

cyclophosphamide (Cytoxan) IV or oral
Use: primary therapy and metastatic disease
Method of action: interferes with tumor cell growth
Adverse effects: temporary or permanent infertility, hair loss, cystitis, immune suppression

docetaxel (Taxotere) IV
Use: locally advanced or metastatic disease after failure of first treatment
Method of action: inhibits cell division
Adverse effects: fluid retention, suppressed immunity, hair loss, loss of feeling in hands and feet

doxorubicin (Adriamycin, Rubex) IV
Use: primary therapy and metastatic disease
Method of action: inhibits DNA synthesis
Adverse effects: nausea, hair loss, immune suppression, may cause heart damage, increased risk of leukemia

epirubicin (Ellence) IV
Use: primary therapy and metastatic disease
Method of action: inhibits DNA synthesis
Adverse effects: nausea, hair loss, immune suppression, may be less toxic to heart than doxorubicin, increased risk of leukemia

etoposide (VePesid) oral
Use: metastatic disease
Method of action: stops cell division
Adverse effects: immune suppression, nausea, diarrhea

5-Fluorouracil (5-FU) IV
Use: primary and metastatic disease
Method of action: prevents DNA and RNA synthesis
Adverse effects: nausea, diarrhea, tingling hands and feet, fatigue, anemia, reduced immunity, less hair loss than other drugs

methotrexate IV
Use: primary and metastatic disease
Method of action: interferes with DNA synthesis and repair
Adverse effects: immune suppression, nausea, gastrointestinal distress, flu-like symptoms

mitoxantrone (Novantrone) IV
Use: metastatic disease; may be less effective than doxorubicin and epirubicin
Method of action: inhibits DNA synthesis
Adverse effects: nausea, hair loss, immune suppression, may cause heart damage, increased risk of leukemia

mitomycin C (Mutamycin) IV
Use: metastatic disease
Method of action: inhibits DNA synthesis
Adverse effects: nausea, hair loss, immune suppression, may cause heart damage, increased risk of leukemia

paclitaxel (Taxol) IV
Use: metastatic disease
Method of action: inhibits cell division
Adverse effects: fluid retention, suppressed immunity, hair loss, loss of feeling in hands and feet

vinblastine (Velban) IV
Use: metastatic disease
Method of action: inhibits cell division
Adverse effects: nausea, diarrhea, tingling hands and feet, fatigue, anemia, reduced immunity

vinorelbine (Navelbine) IV
Use: metastatic disease
Method of action: inhibits cell division
Adverse effects: Nausea, diarrhea, tingling hands and feet, fatigue, anemia, reduced immunity

II. BIOLOGIC

bevacizumab (Avastin) IV
Use: metastatic disease with chemotherapy
Method of action: blocks VEGF and new blood vessels to grow to feed tumor
Adverse effects: gastrointestinal perforations, problems with wound healing, bleeding

trastuzumab (Herceptin) IV
Use: metastatic disease in patients who overexpress Her-2/neu
Method of action: blocks Her-2, a growth factor receptor, to inhibit tumor cell growth
Adverse effects: anemia, immune suppression, flulike symptoms

III. HORMONE THERAPY

anastrozole (Arimidex) oral
Use: for treatment of primary and metastatic disease in postmenopausal women
Method of action: inhibits production of aromatase—an enzyme that converts precursor hormones to estrogen in the breast
Adverse effects: fractures, muscular and joint pain, hot flashes

exemestane (Aromasin) oral
Use: for treatment of primary and metastatic disease in postmenopausal women
Method of action: inactivates aromatase
Adverse effects: fractures, muscular and joint pain, hot flashes

fulvestrant (Faslodex) IV
Use: in postmenopausal women to treat metastatic breast cancer
Method of action: blocks estrogen
Adverse effects: headaches, hot flashes, gastrointestinal distress

goserelin (Zoladex) IV
Use: advanced breast cancer, primarily in premenopausal women
Method of action: blocks release of luteinizing hormone and follicle stimulating hormone to shut down ovaries
Adverse effects: hot flashes, vaginal dryness

letrozole (Femara) oral
Use: for treatment of primary and metastatic disease in postmenopausal women
Method of action: nonsteroidal aromatase inhibitor that blocks production of estrogen
Adverse effects: fractures, muscular and joint pain, hot flashes

megestrol acetate (Megace) oral
Use: Advanced breast cancer in women whose disease has progressed after tamoxifen treatment
Method of action: uncertain; may prevent estrogen from reaching tumor
Schedule: 40-mg tablet, 4 times a day
Adverse effects: weight gain, PMS-like effects, increased risk of blood clots

tamoxifen (Nolvadex) oral
Use: breast-cancer prevention and treatment of primary and metastatic disease
Method of action: selective estrogen receptor modulator (SERM) that blocks estrogen in breast but not in uterus
Adverse effects: hot flashes, vaginal dryness, increased risk of blood clots, endometrial cancer

toremifene citrate (Fareston) oral
Use: metastatic disease in postmenopausal women with ER positive tumors
Method of action: selective estrogen receptor modulator (SERM) that blocks estrogen in breast
Adverse effects: hot flashes, vaginal dryness, increased risk of blood clots; risk of endometrial cancer still unknown

B

Resources

In past editions we have listed resources, references and books that may be of help. Because the Internet is so much more extensive and up-to-date than anything we can present here, we are limiting our recommendations to what we feel are the best websites for you to use. For those of you not adept at searching the web, remember that your local library will be happy to help

WEBSITES

www.drsusanloveresearchfoundation.org (Dr. Susan Love Research Foundation) Obviously we feel this is your best resource. We keep it up-to-date as new research data come along.

www.cancer.gov (National Cancer Institute) This is a very comprehensive site, with data for both doctors and patients. It lists clinical trials and is a good source of accurate, unbiased information.

www.cancer.org (American Cancer Society) This is also a good resource for the general public.

www.nccn.com (National Comprehensive Cancer Network) Here is where you can find the practice guidelines quoted throughout this book.

www.y-me.org (Y-ME) a national organization that is focused on support. They have a 24-hour hotline (800/221-2141 in English and 800/986-9505 in Spanish) to help answer and provide direction for clinical questions.

www.adjuvantonline.com (Adjuvant!) This is where your doctor can find a program that will calculate the benefit of various treatments in your individual case.

www.breastcancer.org (Living with Breast Cancer) This site is another good overall resource. It was created by Dr. Marisa Weiss, a radiation oncologist.

www.youngsurvival.org (Young Survival Coalition) is focused on young women diagnosed and living post breast cancer treatment.

www.stopbreastcancer.org (National Breast Cancer Coalition) The best national organization focused on political and policies issues.

www.facingourrisk.org (FORCE) Website for women at high risk to provide support and information.

www.nccam.nih.gov (National Center for Complementary and Alternative Medicine) Good starting place for scientific information regarding complementary and alternative therapies.

www.ibcsupport.org Inflammatory breast cancer site that provides accurate and helpful information for patients with IBC.

www.fertilehope.org Focuses on fertility issues in women with breast cancer.

www.lymphnet.org (National Lymphedema Network) Support for all kinds of lymphedema, including that caused by breast cancer.

www.nho.org (Hospice Resources) National Hospice Organization will provide a directory of hospice programs by state.

C

NCI-Designated Cancer Centers Listed by State

(http://www3.cancer.gov/cancercenters/centerslist.html)

Alabama

UAB Comprehensive Cancer Center
University of Alabama at Birmingham
1824 Sixth Avenue South, Room 237
Birmingham, Alabama 35293-3300
Tel: 205/934-5077
Fax: 205/975-7428
(Comprehensive Cancer Center)

Arizona

Arizona Cancer Center
University of Arizona
1501 North Campbell Avenue
Tucson, Arizona 85724
Tel: 520/626-7925
Fax: 520/626-2284
(Comprehensive Cancer Center)

California

Cancer Research Center
Beckman Research Institute, City of Hope
Needleman Bldg., Room 204
1500 East Duarte Road
Duarte, California 91010-3000
Tel: 626/256-HOPE (4673)
Fax: 626/930-5394
(Comprehensive Cancer Center)

Cancer Center, Salk Institute
10010 North Torrey Pines Road
La Jolla, California 92037
Tel: 858/453-4100 X1386
Fax: 858/457-4765
(Cancer Center)

The Burnham Institute
10901 North Torrey Pines Road
La Jolla, California 92037
Tel: 858/646-3100
Fax: 858/713-6274
(Cancer Center)

Rebecca and John Moores UCSD Cancer Center
University of California at San Diego
9500 Gilman Drive
La Jolla, California 92093-0658
Tel: 858/822-1222
Fax: 858/822-0207
(Comprehensive Cancer Center)

Jonsson Comprehensive Cancer Center
University of California Los Angeles
Factor Building, Room 8-684
10833 Le Conte Avenue
Los Angeles, California 90095-1781
Tel: 310/825-5268
Fax: 310/206-5553
(Comprehensive Cancer Center)

USC/Norris Comprehensive Cancer Center
University of Southern California
1441 Eastlake Avenue, NOR 8302L
Los Angeles, California 90089-9181
Tel: 323/865-0816
Fax: 323/865-0102
(Comprehensive Cancer Center)

Chao Family Comprehensive Cancer Center
University of California at Irvine
101 The City Drive
Building 23, Rt. 81, Rm. 406
Orange, California 92868
Tel: 714/456-6310
Fax: 714/456-2240
(Comprehensive Cancer Center)

UC Davis Cancer Center
University of California, Davis
4501 X Street, Suite 3003
Sacramento, CA 95817
Tel: 916/734-5800
Fax: 916/451-4464
(Cancer Center)

UCSF Cancer Center & Cancer Research Institute
University of California San Francisco
2340 Sutter Street, Box 0128
San Francisco, California 94115-0128
Tel: 415/502-1710
Fax: 415/502-1712
(Comprehensive Cancer Center)

Colorado

University of Colorado Cancer Center
University of Colorado Health Science Center
4200 East 9th Avenue, Box B188
Denver, Colorado 80262
Tel: 303/724-3155
Fax: 303/315-3304
(Comprehensive Cancer Center)

Connecticut

Yale Cancer Center
Yale University School of Medicine
333 Cedar Street, Box 208028
New Haven, Connecticut 06520-8028
Tel: 203/785-4371
Fax: 203/785-4116
(Comprehensive Cancer Center)

District of Columbia

Lombardi Cancer Research Center
Georgetown University Medical Center
3800 Reservoir Road, N.W.
Washington, DC 20007
Tel: 202/687-2110
Fax: 202/687-6402
(Comprehensive Cancer Center)

Florida

H. Lee Moffitt Cancer Center & Research Institute at the University of South Florida
12902 Magnolia Drive, MCC-CEO
Tampa, Florida 33612-9497
Tel: 813/615-4261
Fax: 813/615-4258
(Comprehensive Cancer Center)

Hawaii

Cancer Research Center of Hawaii
University of Hawaii at Manoa
1236 Lauhala Street
Honolulu, Hawaii 96813
Tel: 808/586-3013
Fax: 808/586-3052
(Cancer Center)

Illinois

University of Chicago Cancer Research Center
5841 South Maryland Avenue, MC 2115

Chicago, Illinois 60637-1470
Tel: 773/702-6180
Fax: 773/702-9311
(Cancer Center)

Robert H. Lurie Cancer Center
of Northwestern University
303 East Chicago Avenue
Olson Pavilion 8250
Chicago, Illinois 60611
Tel: 312/908-5250
Fax: 312/908-1372
(Comprehensive Cancer Center)

Indiana

Indiana University Cancer Center
Indiana Cancer Pavilion
535 Barnhill Drive, Room 455
Indianapolis, Indiana 46202-5289
Tel: 317/278-0070
Fax: 317/278-0074
(Cancer Center)

Purdue University Cancer Center
Hansen Life Sciences Research
Building
South University Street
West Lafayette, Indiana 47907-1524
Tel: 765/494-9129
Fax: 765/494-9193
(Cancer Center)

Iowa

Holden Comprehensive Cancer
Center at The University of Iowa
5970 "Z" JPP
200 Hawkins Drive
Iowa City, Iowa 52242
Tel: 319/3553-8620
Fax: 319/353-8988
(Comprehensive Cancer Center)

Maine

The Jackson Laboratory
600 Main Street
Bar Harbor, Maine 04609-0800
Tel: 207/288-6041
Fax: 207/288-6044
(Cancer Center)

Maryland

The Sidney Kimmel Comprehensive
Cancer Center at Johns Hopkins
401 North Broadway
Baltimore, Maryland 21231
Tel: 410/955-8822
Fax: 410/955-6787
(Comprehensive Cancer Center)

Massachusetts

Dana-Farber/Harvard Cancer Center
44 Binney Street, Room 1628
Boston, Massachusetts 02115
Tel: 617/632-4266
Fax: 617/632-2161
(Comprehensive Cancer Center)

Center for Cancer Research
Massachusetts Institute of
Technology
77 Massachusetts Avenue,
Room E17-110
Cambridge, Massachusetts 02139-
4307
Tel: 617/253-8511
Fax: 617/253-0262
(Cancer Center)

Michigan

Comprehensive Cancer Center
University of Michigan
6302 CGC/0942
1500 East Medical Center Drive
Ann Arbor, Michigan 48109-0942
Tel: 734/936-1831
Fax: 734/615-3947
(Comprehensive Cancer Center)

The Meyer L. Prentis Comprehensive
Cancer Center of Metropolitan
Detroit
Operated by The Barbara Ann
Karmanos Cancer Institute
Wayne State University
4100 John R. Street
Detroit, Michigan 48201-1379
Tel: 313/993-7777
Fax: 313/993-7165
(Comprehensive Cancer Center)

Minnesota

Univ. of Minnesota Cancer Center
MMC 806, 420 Delaware Street, S.E.
Minneapolis, Minnesota 55455
Tel: 612/624-8484
Fax: 612/626-3069
(Comprehensive Cancer Center)

Mayo Clinic Cancer Center
Mayo Clinic Rochester
200 First Street, S.W.
Rochester, Minnesota 55905
Tel: 507/284-3753
Fax: 507/284-9349
(Comprehensive Cancer Center)

Missouri

Siteman Cancer Center
Washington University School of Medicine
660 South Euclid Avenue, Campus Box 8109
St. Louis, Missouri 63110
Tel: 314/362-8020
Fax: 314/454-1898
(Comprehensive Cancer Center)

Nebraska

University of Nebraska Medical Center/Eppley Cancer Center
600 South 42nd Street
Omaha, Nebraska 68198-6805
Tel: 402/559-4238
Fax: 402/559-4652
(Cancer Center)

New Hampshire

Norris Cotton Cancer Center
Dartmouth-Hitchcock Medical Center
One Medical Center Drive, Hinman Box 7920
Lebanon, New Hampshire 03756-0001
Tel: 603/650-6300
Fax: 603/650-6333
(Comprehensive Cancer Center)

New Jersey

The Cancer Institute of New Jersey
Robert Wood Johnson Medical School
195 Little Albany Street, Room 2002B
New Brunswick, New Jersey 08901
Tel: 732/235-8064
Fax: 732/235-8094
(Comprehensive Cancer Center)

New York

Cancer Research Center
Albert Einstein College of Medicine
Chanin Building, Room 209
1300 Morris Park Avenue
Bronx, New York 10461
Tel: 718/430-2302
Fax: 718/430-8550
(Cancer Center)

Roswell Park Cancer Institute
Elm & Carlton Streets
Buffalo, New York 14263-0001
Tel: 716/845-5772
Fax: 716/845-8261
(Comprehensive Cancer Center)

Cold Spring Harbor Laboratory
P.O. Box 100
Cold Spring Harbor, New York 11724
Tel: 516/367-8383
Fax: 516/367-8879
(Cancer Center)

NYU Cancer Institute
New York University Medical Center
550 First Avenue
New York, New York 10016
Tel: 212/263-8950
Fax: 212/263-8210
(Cancer Center)

Memorial Sloan-Kettering Cancer Center
1275 York Avenue
New York, New York 10021
Tel: 212/639-2000 or 800/525-2225
Fax: 212/717-3299
(Comprehensive Cancer Center)

Herbert Irving Comprehensive Cancer Center College of Physicians & Surgeons
Columbia University
161 Fort Washington Avenue
11th Floor, Room 1153
New York, New York 10032
Tel: 212/305-5201
Fax: 212/305-6813
(Comprehensive Cancer Center)

North Carolina

UNC Lineberger Comprehensive Cancer Center
University of North Carolina Chapel Hill School of Medicine, CB-7295
102 West Drive
Chapel Hill, North Carolina 27599-7295
Tel: 919/966-3036
Fax: 919/966-3015
(Comprehensive Cancer Center)

Duke Comprehensive Cancer Center
Duke University Medical Center Box 3843
Durham, North Carolina 27710
Tel: 919/684-5613
Fax: 919/684-5653
(Comprehensive Cancer Center)

Comprehensive Cancer Center
Wake Forest University
Medical Center Boulevard
Winston-Salem, North Carolina 27157-1082
Tel: 336/716-7971
Fax: 336/716-0293
(Comprehensive Cancer Center)

Ohio

Case Comprehensive Cancer Center
Case Western Reserve University
11100 Euclid Ave., Wearn 151
Cleveland, Ohio 44106-5065
Tel: 216/844-8562
Fax: 216/844-4975
(Comprehensive Cancer Center)

Comprehensive Cancer Center
Arthur G. James Cancer Hospital & Richard J. Solove Research Institute
Ohio State University A458 Staring Loving Hall
300 West 10th Avenue
Columbus, Ohio 43210-1240
Tel: 614/293-7521
Fax: 614/293-7522
(Comprehensive Cancer Center)

Oregon

OHSU Cancer Institute
Oregon Health Sciences University
3181 S.W. Sam Jackson Park Rd., CR145
Portland, Oregon 97201-3098
Tel: 503/494-1617
Fax: 503/494-7086
(Cancer Center)

Pennsylvania

Abramson Cancer Center of the University of Pennsylvania
16th Floor Penn Tower
3400 Spruce Street
Philadelphia, Pennsylvania 19104-4283
Tel: 215/662-6065
Fax: 215/349-5325
(Comprehensive Cancer Center)

The Wistar Institute
3601 Spruce Street
Philadelphia, Pennsylvania 19104-4268
Tel: 215/898-3926
Fax: 215/573-2097
(Cancer Center)

Fox Chase Cancer Center
7701 Burholme Avenue
Philadelphia, Pennsylvania 19111
Tel: 215/728-2781
Fax: 215/728-2571
(Comprehensive Cancer Center)

Kimmel Cancer Center
Thomas Jefferson University
233 South 10th Street
BLSB, Room 1050
Philadelphia, Pennsylvania 19107-5799
Tel: 215/503-4645
Fax: 215/923-3528
(Cancer Center)

University of Pittsburgh Cancer Institute
UPMC Cancer Pavilion
5150 Centre Avenue, Suite 500
Pittsburgh, Pennsylvania 15232
Tel: 412/623-3205
Fax: 412/623-3210
(Comprehensive Cancer Center)

Tennessee

St. Jude Children's Research Hospital
332 North Lauderdale
P.O. Box 318
Memphis, Tennessee 38105-2794
Tel: 901/495-3982
Fax: 901/495-3966
(Cancer Center)

Vanderbilt-Ingram Cancer Center
Vanderbilt University
691 Preston Research Building
Nashville, Tennessee 37232-6838
Tel: 615/936-1782
Fax: 615/936-1790
(Comprehensive Cancer Center)

Texas

University of Texas
M.D. Anderson Cancer Center
1515 Holcombe Boulevard, Box 91
Houston, Texas 77030
Tel: 713/792-2121
Fax: 713/799-2210
(Comprehensive Cancer Center)

San Antonio Cancer Institute
University of Texas Health Science Center at San Antonio, Dept. Hematology
7703 Floyd Curl Drive
San Antonio, Texas 78229-3900
Tel: 210/567-4848
Fax: 210/567-1956
(Cancer Center)

Utah

Huntsman Cancer Institute
University of Utah
2000 Circle of Hope
Salt Lake City, Utah 84112-5550
Tel: 801/585-3401
Fax: 801/585-6345
(Cancer Center)

Vermont

Vermont Cancer Center
University of Vermont
149 Beaumont Ave, HRSF 326
Burlington, Vermont 05405
Tel: 802/656-4414
Fax: 802/656-8788
(Comprehensive Cancer Center)

Virginia

Cancer Center
University of Virginia, Health Sciences Center
Jefferson Park Ave., Room 617E
Charlottesville, Virginia 22908
Tel: 434/243-9926
Fax: 434/982-0918
(Clinical Cancer Center)

Massey Cancer Center
Virginia Commonwealth University
P.O. Box 980037
Richmond, Virginia 23298-0037
Tel: 804/828-0450
Fax: 804/828-8453
(Cancer Center)

Washington

Fred Hutchinson Cancer Research Center
P.O. Box 19024, D1-060
Seattle, Washington 98109-1024
Tel: 206/667-4305
Fax: 206/667-5268
(Comprehensive Cancer Center)

Wisconsin

Comprehensive Cancer Center
University of Wisconsin
600 Highland Ave., Room K4/610
Madison, Wisconsin 53792-0001
Tel: 608/263-8610
Fax: 608/263-8613
(Comprehensive Cancer Center)

D

The Wellness Community Physician/Patient Statement

In 1990, six prominent Los Angeles oncologists met with the staff of the Wellness Community over a period of six months to answer the question, What can cancer patients expect from their oncologists? The question was considered important since they believed that the relationship between the patient and the physician can affect the course of the illness. After many meetings they arrived at *The Wellness Community Patient/Oncologist Statement.* They then tested the statement with their patients and found that a great majority had confidence in their physician and considered their relationship "excellent." However, there was agreement among patients that the issues considered in the statement were important to a continuation of excellent relationships. The statement reproduced below was then published in the UCLA Jonsson Comprehensive Cancer Center Bulletin and is given by physicians to their patients.

The effective treatment of serious illness requires a considerable effort by both the patient and the physician. A clear understanding by both of us as to what each of us can realistically and reasonably expect of the other will do much to enhance the outlook. I am giving this "statement" to you as one step in making our relationship as effective and productive as possible. It might be helpful if you would read this statement and, if you think it appropriate, discuss it with me.

As your physician, I will make every effort to:

1. Provide you with the care most likely to be beneficial to you.
2. Inform and educate you about your situation, and the various treatment alternatives. How detailed an explanation is given will be dependent upon your specific desires.
3. Encourage you to ask questions about your illness and its treatment and to answer your questions as clearly as possible. I will also attempt to answer the questions asked by your family; however, my primary responsibility is to you, and I will discuss your medical situation only with those people authorized by you.
4. Remain aware that all major decisions about the course of your care shall be made by you. However, I will accept the responsibility for making certain decisions if you want me to.
5. Assist you to obtain other professional opinions if you desire, or if I believe it to be in your best interests.
6. Relate to you as one competent adult to another, always attempting to consider your emotional, social and psychological needs as well as your physical needs.
7. Spend a reasonable amount of time with you on each return visit unless required by something urgent to do otherwise, and give you my undivided attention during that time.
8. Honor all appointment times unless required by something urgent to do otherwise.
9. Return phone calls as promptly as possible, especially those you indicate are urgent.
10. Make available test results promptly if you desire such reports and I will indicate to you, at the time the test is given, when you can expect the results and who you should call to get them.
11. Provide you with any information you request concerning my professional training, experience, philosophy and fees.
12. Respect your desire to try treatment that might not be conventionally accepted. However, I will give you my honest opinion about such unconventional treatments.
13. Maintain my active support and attention throughout the course of the illness.

I hope that you as the patient will make every effort to:

1. Comply with our agreed-upon treatment plan.
2. Be as candid as possible with me about what you need and expect from me.
3. Inform me if you desire another professional opinion.
4. Inform me of all forms of therapy you are involved with.
5. Honor all appointment times unless required by something urgent to do otherwise.
6. Be as considerate as possible of my need to adhere to a schedule to see other patients.
7. Attempt to make all phone calls to me during the working hours. Call on nights and weekends only when absolutely necessary.
8. Attempt to coordinate the requests of your family and confidantes, so that I do not have to answer the same questions about you to several different persons.

E

Pathology Checklist

Your name ______________________________

Your age ______________________________

Your menopausal status:

Premenopausal ________

Postmenopausal ________

Your hospital number ______________________________

Your hospital ______________________________

Your doctors

Primary care ______________________________

Surgeon ______________________________

Medical oncologist ______________________________

Radiation oncologist ______________________________

Date of biopsy/surgery ______________________________

Place of biopsy/surgery ______________________________

Name of doctor doing procedure ______________________________

Place of pathological reading ______________________________

Name of pathologist ______________________________

Pathology reference number ______________________________

- Specimen type
  - Biopsy
    - Core (needle) ____________
    - Surgical _________________
  - Lumpectomy _______________
  - Mastectomy ________________
- Lymph node sampling
  - Axillary node dissection ___________
  - Sentinel node biopsy ______________
- Specimen size (for excisions less than total mastectomy)
  - Greatest dimension (cm) _____________________
  - Additional dimensions ______________________
- Side of tumor
  - Right ______
  - Left _______
- Tumor site
  - Upper outer quadrant _____________
  - Lower outer quadrant _____________
  - Upper inner quadrant _____________
  - Lower inner quadrant _____________
  - Central __________________________

MICROSCOPIC

- Invasive or in situ
  - In situ
    - Ductal carcinoma in situ (DCIS) __________
    - Lobular carcinoma in situ (LCIS) _________
    - Ductal and lobular in situ _______________
    - Paget's disease in the nipple ____________
  - Invasive/infiltrating
    - Ductal ___________________
      - Tubular _______________
      - Mucinous _____________
      - Adenoid cystic _________
      - Inflammatory ______________________

Secretory ___________

Medullary ___________

Papillary ___________

Undifferentiated ___________

Not otherwise specified (NOS) ___________

Lobular ___________

Size of invasive tumor in greatest dimension

Less than 2 cm

Less than 0.1 cm (microinvasion) ___________

Between 0.1 cm–0.5 cm ___________

Between 0.5 cm–1 cm ___________

Between 1 cm–2 cm ___________

Between 2 cm–5 cm ___________

Greater than 5 cm ___________

Any size with direct extension to

Chest wall ___________

Edema (swelling) ___________

Both chest wall and edema ___________

Inflammatory carcinoma ___________

Histology

Grade of tumor

Low ___________

Moderate ___________

High ___________

Differentiation

Low ___________

Moderate ___________

High ___________

Mitosis

Low ___________

High ___________

Lympho/vascular invasion

Positive ___________

Negative ___________

Extent of DCIS associated with the tumor (EIC) ___________

Margins

Negative

No tumor within 1 cm or no residual tumor __________

No tumor within 1 mm of margin ___________________

Tumor focally (at one spot) next to a margin __________

Positive

Invasive tumor involving the inked margin ___________

In situ tumor involving inked margin ________________

Markers

Hormones

Estrogen receptor positive/progesterone receptor positive ___________

Estrogen receptor positive/progesterone receptor negative___________

Estrogen receptor negative/progesterone receptor positive___________

Estrogen receptor negative/progesterone receptor negative__________

Her-2/neu

Negative ________

Positive _________

By IHC __________

By FISH _________

Others

P 53 positive ________

Ki 67 _______________

S phase _____________

Axillary lymph nodes

No lymph nodes ________________

Lymph nodes negative ___________

Negative on histology but positive on IHC ___________

Negative on histology but positive on RTPCR_________

Lymph nodes positive

1–3 nodes positive __________

4–9 nodes positive __________

10 or more positive _________

Glossary

abscess: Infection that has formed a pocket of pus.
adenocarcinoma: Cancer arising in gland forming tissue. Breast cancer is a type of adenocarcinoma.
adenine: A nucleotide base that pairs with thymine in forming DNA.
adjuvant chemotherapy: Anticancer drugs used in combination with surgery and/or radiation as an initial treatment before there is detectable spread, to prevent or delay recurrence.
adrenal gland: Small gland found above each kidney that secretes cortisone, adrenalin, aldosterone and many other important hormones.
alopecia: Hair loss, a common side effect of chemotherapy.
amenorrhea: Absence or stoppage of menstrual period.
amino acid: The building block of proteins.
androgen: Hormone that produces male characteristics.
angiogenesis (angiogenic): Stimulates new blood vessels to be formed.
anorexia: Loss of appetite.
apoptosis: Cell suicide.
areola: Area of pigment around the nipple.
aromatase inhibitors: A class of drugs that block an enzyme called aromatase, thereby reducing estrogen levels in the breast tissue.
aspiration: Putting a hypodermic needle into a tissue and drawing back on the syringe to obtain fluid or cells.
asymmetrical: Not matching.

ataxia telangectasia: Disease of the nervous system; carriers of the gene are more sensitive to radiation and have a higher risk of cancer.

atypical cell: Mild to moderately abnormal cell.

atypical hyperplasia: Cells that are not only abnormal but increased in number.

augmented: Added to such, as an augmented breast: one that has had a silicone implant added to it.

autologous: From the same person. An autologous blood transfusion is blood removed and then transfused back to the same person at a later date.

axilla: Armpit.

axillary lymph nodes: Lymph nodes found in the armpit area.

axillary lymph node dissection: Surgical removal of lymph nodes found in the armpit region.

basal type: triple negatives or ER negative PR negative and Her-2/neu negative.

base pairs: Two nucleic acids that bind together in DNA and RNA.

benign: Not cancerous.

bilateral: Involving both sides, such as both breasts.

biological response modifier: Usually natural substances such as colony stimulating factor that stimulates the bone marrow to make blood cells, that alter the body's natural response.

biomarker: A measurable biological property that can be used to identify women at risk.

biopsy: Removal of tissue. This term does not indicate how *much* tissue will be removed.

bone marrow: The soft inner part of large bones that produces blood cells.

bone scan: Test to determine if there is any sign of cancer in the bones.

brachial plexus: A bundle of nerves in the armpit that go on to supply the arm.

breast reconstruction: Creation of an artificial breast after mastectomy by a plastic surgeon.

bromocriptine: Drug used to block the hormone prolactin.

calcifications: Small calcium deposits in the breast tissue that can be seen by mammography.

carcinoembryonic antigen (CEA): Nonspecific (not specific to cancer) blood test used to follow women with metastatic breast cancer to help determine if the treatment is working.

carcinogen: Substance that can cause cancer.

carcinoma: Cancer arising in the epithelial tissue (skin, glands, and lining of internal organs). Most cancers are carcinomas.

cell cycle: The steps a cell goes through in order to reproduce itself.

cellulitis: Infection of the soft tissues.

centigray: Measurement of radiation absorbed dose, same as a *rad*.
checkpoint: Point in the cell cycle where the cell's DNA is checked for mutations before it is allowed to move forward.
chemotherapy: Treatment of disease with certain chemicals. The term usually refers to *cytotoxic* drugs given for cancer treatment.
chromosome: Genes are strung together in a chromosome.
cohort study: Study of a group of people who have something in common when they are first assembled and who are then observed for a period of time to see what happens to them
colostrum: Liquid produced by the breast before the milk comes in: pre-milk.
comedo: Type of DCIS where the cells filling the duct are more aggressive looking.
comedon: Whitehead pimple.
contracture: Formation of a thick scar tissue; in the breast a contracture can form around an implant.
core biopsy: Type of needle biopsy where a small core of tissue is removed from a lump without surgery.
corpus luteum: Ovarian follicle after ovulation.
cortisol: Hormone produced by the adrenal gland.
costochondritis: Inflammation of the connection between ribs and breast bone, a type of arthritis.
cribriform: Type of DCIS where the cells filling the duct have punched out areas.
cyclical: In a cycle like the menstrual period, which is every 28 days, or chemotherapy treatment, which is periodic.
cyst: Fluid filled sac.
cystosarcoma phylloides: Unusual type of breast tumor.
cytology: Study of cells.
cytologist: One who specializes in studying cells.
cytosine: A nucleotide base that pairs with guanine in DNA.
cytotoxic: Causing the death of cells. The term usually refers to drugs used in chemotherapy.
Danazol (danocrine): Drug used to block hormones from the pituitary gland, used in endometriosis and rarely in breast pain.
diethylstilbesterol (DES): Synthetic estrogen once used to prevent miscarriages, now shown to cause vaginal cancer in the daughters of the women who took it. DES is sometimes used to treat metastatic breast cancer.
DNA: Deoxyriboneucleic acid, the genetic code.
DNA microarray analysis: A way of analyzing the many mutations in many tumors at the same time.
dose dense: chemotherapy where the interval between two courses is shortened while the dose of each course may be increased, decreased

or made equivalent to a standard dose so that the dose per unit of time is higher.

double helix: The structure of DNA that allows it to be easily replicated.

doubling time: Time it takes the cell population to double in number.

ductal carcinoma in situ (DCIS): Ductal cancer cells that have not grown outside of their site of origin, sometimes referred to as precancer.

ductoscope: A tiny endoscope that is threaded through the nipple into a duct.

eczema: Skin irritation characterized by redness and open weeping.

edema: Swelling caused by a collection of fluid in the soft tissues.

electrocautery: Instrument used in surgery to cut, coagulate or destroy tissue by heating it with an electric current.

embolus: Plug or clot of tumor cells within a blood vessel.

engorgement: Swelling with fluid, as in a breast engorged with milk.

erb-b2: Another name for the Her-2/neu oncogene.

esophagus (esophageal): Organ carrying food from the mouth and the stomach.

estrogen: Female sex hormones produced by the ovaries, adrenal glands, placenta, and fat.

estrogen receptor: Protein found on some cells to which estrogen molecules will attach. If a tumor is positive for estrogen receptors, it is sensitive to hormones.

excisional biopsy: Taking the whole lump out.

extracellular matrix: The material that surrounds the cells.

fat necrosis: Area of dead fat usually following some form of trauma or surgery, a cause of lumps.

fibroadenoma: Benign fibrous tumor of the breast most common in young women.

fibrocystic disease: Much misused term for any benign condition of the breast.

fibroid: Benign fibrous tumor of the uterus (not in the breast).

flow cytometry: Test that measures DNA content in tumors.

fluoroscopy: Use of an x-ray machine to examine parts of the body directly rather than taking a picture and developing it, as in conventional X rays. Fluoroscopy uses more radiation than a single X ray.

follicle stimulating hormone (FSH): Hormone from the pituitary gland that stimulates the ovary.

follicles: In the ovaries, eggs encased in their developmental sacs.

frozen section: Freezing and slicing tissue to make a slide immediately for diagnosis.

frozen shoulder: Stiffness of the shoulder, which is painful and makes it hard to lift the arm over your head.

galactocele: Milk cyst sometimes found in a nursing mother's breast.

GCSF (granulocyte stimulating factor): A drug that stimulates the bone marrow to recover faster from chemotherapy.

gene: A linear sequence of DNA that is required to produce a protein.

genetic: Relating to genes or inherited characteristics.

genome: All of the chromosomes that together form the genetic map.

germ line: Cells that are involved in reproduction, i.e., sperm and eggs.

ghostectomy: Removal of breast tissue in the area where there was a previous lump.

GNRH agonist: A drug that blocks the pituitary production of hormones that stimulate the ovaries.

guanine: One of the base pairs that form DNA; pairs with cytosine.

gynecomastia: Swollen breast tissue in a man or boy.

hemangioma: A birth mark consisting of overgrowth of blood vessels.

hematoma: Collection of blood in the tissues. Hematomas may occur in the breast after surgery.

hemorrhage: Bleeding.

Her-2/neu: An oncogene that, when overexpressed, leads to more cell growth.

heterogeneous: Composed of many different elements. In relation to breast cancer, heterogeneous refers to the fact that there are many different types of breast cancer cells within one tumor.

homeopathy: System of therapy using very small doses of drugs, which can produce in healthy people symptoms similar to those of the disease being treated. These are believed to stimulate the immune system.

hormone: Chemical substance produced by glands in the body which enters the bloodstream and causes effects in other tissues.

hot flashes: Sudden sensations of heat and swelling associated with the menopause.

HRT: Hormone replacement therapy.

human choriogonadotropin (HCG): Hormone produced by the *corpus luteum.*

hyperplasia: Excessive growth of cells.

hypothalamus: Area at the base of the brain that controls various functions including hormone production in the pituitary.

hysterectomy: Removal of the uterus. Hysterectomy does not necessarily mean the removal of ovaries *(oophorectomy).*

immunocytochemistry: Study of the chemistry of cells using techniques that employ immune mechanisms.

immune system: Complex system by which the body is able to protect itself from foreign invaders.

incisional biopsy: Taking a piece of the lump out.

infiltrating cancer: Cancer that can grow beyond its site of origin into neighboring tissue. Infiltrating does not imply that the cancer has already spread outside the breast. Infiltrating has the same meaning as invasive.

informed consent: Process in which the patient is fully informed of all risks and complications of a planned procedure and agrees to proceed.

interstitial brachytherapy: Partial breast irradiation through tubes loaded with radioactive seeds.

intracavitary brachytherapy: Partial breast irradiation through a balloon filling the biopsy cavity.

in situ: In the site of. In regard to cancer, in situ refers to tumors that haven't grown beyond their site of origin and invaded neighboring tissue.

intraductal: Within the duct. Intraductal can describe a benign or malignant process.

intraductal papilloma: Benign tumor that projects like a finger from the lining of the duct.

intraoperative limited radiation therapy: Irradiation applied in the operating room to the bed of the tumor.

invasive cancer: Cancers that are capable of growing beyond their site of origin and invading neighboring tissue. Invasive does not imply that the cancer is aggressive or has already spread.

lactation: Production of milk from the breast.

latissimus flap: Flap of skin and muscle taken from the back used for reconstruction after mastectomy or partial mastectomy.

lidocaine: Drug most commonly used for local anesthesia.

lobules: Parts of the breast capable of making milk.

lobular carcinoma in situ: Abnormal cells within the lobule that don't form lumps. They can serve as a marker of future cancer risk.

lobular: Having to do with the lobules of the breast.

local treatment of cancer: Treatment of the tumor only.

lumpectomy: Surgery to remove lump with small rim of normal tissue around it.

luteinizing hormone: Hormone produced by the pituitary, which helps control the menstrual cycle.

lymphatic vessels: Vessels that carry lymph (tissue fluid) to and from lymph nodes.

lymphedema: Milk arm. This swelling of the arm can follow surgery to the lymph nodes under the arm. It can be temporary, or permanent and occur immediately, or any time later.

lymph nodes: Glands found throughout the body that help defend against foreign invaders such as bacteria. Lymph nodes can be a location of cancer spread.

macrophages: Blood cells that are part of the immune system.
malignant: Cancerous.
mastalgia: Pain in the breast.
mastitis: Infection of the breast. Mastitis is sometimes used loosely to refer to any benign process in the breast.
mastodynia: Pain in the breast.
mastopexy: Uplift of the breast through plastic surgery.
menarche: First menstrual period.
metastasis: Spread of cancer to another organ, usually through the blood stream.
metastasizing: Spreading to a distant site.
methylxanthine: Chemical group to which caffeine belongs.
microcalcification: Tiny calcifications in the breast tissue usually seen only on a mammogram. When clustered can be a sign of ductal carcinoma in situ.
micrometastasis: Microscopic and as yet undetectable but presumed spread of tumor cells to other organs.
micropapillary: Type of DCIS where the cells filling the duct take the form of 'finger' projections into the center.
mitosis: Cell division.
mutation: An alteration of the genetic code.
myocutaneous flap: Flap of skin and muscle and fat taken from one part of the body to fill in an empty space.
myoepithelial cells: The cells that surround the ductal lining cells and may serve to contain the cells.
necrosis: Dead tissue.
nodular: Forming little nodules.
nuclear magnetic resonance (NMR or MRI): Imaging technique using a magnet and electrical coil to transmit radio waves through the body.
nucleotide: One of the base pairs forming DNA.
observational study: A study in which a factor is observed in a group of people.
oncogene: Tumor genes are present in the body. These can be activated by carcinogens and cause cell to grow uncontrollably.
oncogenes: Altered DNA that can lead to cancerous growth.
oncology: Study of cancer.
oophorectomy: Removal of the ovaries.
osteoporosis: Softening of the bones, and bone loss, that occurs with age in some people.
oxytocin: Hormone produced by the pituitary gland, involved in lactation.
p53: A tumor suppressor gene.
palliation: Act of relieving a symptom without curing the cause.

partial breast irradiation: Radiation just to the bed of the tumor rather than to the whole breast.

pathologist: Doctor who specializes in examining tissue and diagnosing disease.

pectoralis major: Muscle that lies under the breast.

phlebitis: Irritation of a vein.

pituitary gland: A gland located in the brain that secretes many hormones to regulate other glands in the body: the master gland.

Poland's syndrome: A congenital condition in which there is no breast development on one side of the chest.

polychemotherapy: Chemotherapy with more than one drug at a time.

polygenic: Relating to more than one gene.

polymastia: Literally many breasts. Existence of an extra breast or breasts.

postmenopausal: After the menopause has occurred.

Premarin (conjugated estrogen): Estrogen from pregnant horses' urine that is sometimes given to women after the menopause.

progesterone: Hormone produced by the ovary involved in the normal menstrual cycle.

prognosis: Expected or probable outcome.

prolactin: Hormone produced by the pituitary that stimulates progesterone production by the ovaries and lactation.

prophylactic subcutaneous mastectomies: Removal of all breast tissue beneath the skin and nipple, to prevent future breast cancer risk.

prosthesis: Artificial substitute for an absent part of the body, as in breast prosthesis.

protein: Formed from amino acids, this is the building block of life.

protocol: Research designed to answer a hypothesis. Protocols often involve testing a specific new treatment under controlled conditions.

proto-oncogene: Normal gene controlling cell growth or turnover.

Provera (medroxyprogesterone acetate): Progesterone that is sometimes given to women in combination with Premarin after menopause.

pseudolump: Breast tissue that feels like a lump but when removed proves to be normal.

ptosis: Drooping, as in breasts that hang down.

punch biopsy: A biopsy of skin done that just punches a small hole out of the skin.

quadrantectomy: Removal of a quarter of the breast.

rad: Radiation absorbed dose, same as centigray. One chest X ray equals 1/10 of a rad.

radial scar: A benign lesion where glands are trapped in fibrous tissue often difficult to distinguish from cancer.

randomized: Chosen at random. In regard to a research study it means choosing the subjects to be given a particular treatment by means of a computer programmed to choose names at random.

randomized controlled study: A study in which the participants are randomized to one treatment or another.

recurrence: Return of cancer after its apparent complete disappearance.

recurrence score: Score developing from analyzing different mutations and predicting the risk of recurrence with tamoxifen or chemotherapy.

remission: Disappearance of detectable disease.

repair endonucleases: Enzymes that can repair mutations.

RNA: Ribonucleic acid; carries the message from the DNA into the cell to make proteins.

sarcoma: Cancer arising in the connective tissue.

scleroderma: An autoimmune disease that involves thickening of the skin and difficulty swallowing among other symptoms.

scoliosis: Deformity of the back bone that causes a person to bend to one side or the other.

sebaceous: Oily, cheesy material secreted by glands in the skin.

selenium: Metallic element found in food.

SERM: Selective estrogen receptor modulator: a compound that is estrogenic in some organs and anti-estrogenic in others.

seroma: Collection of tissue fluid.

side effect: Unintentional or undesirable secondary effect of treatment.

silicone: Synthetic material used in breast implants because of its flexibility, resilience and durability.

somatic: A cell that forms the organs of the body but is not involved in reproduction.

S phase fraction: A measure of how many cells are dividing at a time; if it is high it is thought to indicate an aggressive tumor.

stem cell: A primitive cells that is self renewing as well as capable of giving rise to daughter cells.

subareolar abscess: Infection of the glands under the nipple.

subcutaneous tissue: The tissue under the skin.

systemic treatment: Treatment involving the whole body, usually using drugs.

tamoxifen: Estrogen blocker used in treating breast cancer.

targeted therapy: An antibody directed to a specific molecular target, for example, Herceptin.

telomerase: An enzyme that reattaches the end of a chromosome when it divides.

telomere: The end of a chromosome, a bit of which is clipped off every time a cell divides.

thoracic: Concerning the chest (thorax).

thoracic nerves: Nerves in the chest area.

thoracoepigastric vein: Vein that starts under the arm and passes along the side of the breast and then down into the abdomen.

thymine: A nucleotide base that pairs with adenine in DNA formation.

titration: Systems of balancing. In chemotherapy, titration means using the largest amount of a drug possible while keeping the side effects from becoming intolerable.

trauma: Wound or injury.

triglyceride: Form in which fat is stored in the body, consisting of glycerol and three fatty acids.

tru-cut biopsy: Type of core needle biopsy where a small core of tissue is removed from a lump without surgery.

tumor: Abnormal mass of tissue. Strictly speaking a tumor can be benign or malignant.

tumor dormancy: Tumors that are present in a stable state.

tumor suppressor gene: A gene that prevents cells from growing if they have a mutation.

VEGF: Vascular epidermal growth factor; a protein that stimulates new blood vessels to grow.

virginal hypertrophy: Inappropriately large breasts in a young woman.

xeroradiography: Type of mammogram taken on a xerox plate rather than x-ray film.

Notes

1. THE BREAST AND ITS DEVELOPMENT

1. Cooper A. *On the Anatomy of the Breast.* London: Orme, Green, Brown & Longmans, 1840.

2. Love SM, Barksy SH. Anatomy of the nipple and breast ducts revisited. *Cancer* 2004; 101:1947–1957.

3. Al-Hajj M, Wicha M, Benito-Hernandez A, Morrison SJ, Clarke MF. Prospective identification of tumorigenic breast cancer cells. *Proceedings of the National Academy of Science* 2003; 100(7):3983–3988.

4. Ayalah D, Weinstock IJ. *Breasts,* vol. 1. New York: Summit, 1979.

5. Stanway A, Stanway P. *The Breast.* London: Granada, 1982.

6. New England Research Institute. *Women and their health in Massachusetts. Final report 1991.* Watertown, MA, 1991.

7. Sluijmer AV, Heineman MJ, DeJong FH, Evers JL. Endocrine activity of the postmenopausal ovary: The effects of pituitary down-regulation and oophorectomy. *Journal of Clinical Endocrinology and Metabolism* 1995; 80:2163–2167.

8. Ushiroyama T, Sugimoto O. Endocrine function of the peri- and postmenopausal ovary. *Hormone Research* 1995; 44:64–68.

9. Hreshchyshyn MM, Hopkins A, Zylstra S, Anbar M. Effects of natural menopause, hysterectomy, and oophorectomy on lumbar spine and femoral neck bone densities. *Obstetrics and Gynecology* 1988; 72:631.

10. Ayalah and Weinstock, *Breasts.*

2. GETTING ACQUAINTED WITH YOUR BREASTS

1. Kash K, Holland J, Halper M, et al. Psychological distress and surveillance behaviors of women with a family history of breast cancer. *Journal of the National Cancer Institute* 1992; 84:24.

3. VARIATIONS IN DEVELOPMENT AND PLASTIC SURGERY

1. Letterman G, Schurter MA. A history of mammoplasty with emphasis on correction of ptosis and macromastia. In: Goldwyn R, ed. *Plastic and Reconstructive Surgery of the Breast.* Boston: Little, Brown, 1976; 361.
2. Silverman BS, Brown SL, Bright RA, et al. A critical assessment of the relationship between silicone implants and connective tissue diseases (a review). *Regul Toxicology Pharmacology* 1996; 23(1 Pt 1):74–85.
3. Deapen DM, Brody GS. Augmentation mammaplasty and breast cancer: A 5-year update of the Los Angeles study. *Plastic Reconstructive Surgery* 1992; 89(4):660–665.
4. Berkel H, Birdsell DC, Jenkins H. Breast augmentation: A risk factor for breast cancer? *New England Journal of Medicine* 1992; 326(25):1649–1653.
5. Silverstein MJ, Gierson ED, Gamagami P, Handel N, Waisman JR. Breast cancer diagnosis and prognosis in women augmented with silicone gel-filled implants. *Cancer* 1990; 66(July 1):97.
6. Noone RB. A review of the possible health implications of silicone breast implants. *Cancer* 1997; 79(9):1747–1756.
7. Heuston JT. Unilateral agenesis and hypoplasia: Difficulties and suggestions. In: Goldwyn R, ed. *Plastic and Reconstructive Surgery of the Breast.* Boston: Little, Brown, 1976; 361.
8. Gifford S. Emotional attitudes toward cosmetic breast surgery: Loss and restitution of the "ideal" self. In: Goldwyn R, ed. *Plastic and Reconstructive Surgery of the Breast.* Boston: Little, Brown, 1976; 117.

4. "FIBROCYSTIC DISEASE" AND BREAST PAIN

1. Boyd NF, Lockwood GA, Byng JW, Tritchler DL, Yaffe MJ. Mammographic densities and breast cancer risk. *Cancer Epidemiology, Biomarkers & Prevention* 1998; 7(December):1133–1144.
2. Cancer Committee of the American College of Pathologists. Is "fibrocystic" disease of the breast precancerous? *Archives of Pathology and Laboratory Medicine* 1986; 110:173.
3. Preece PE, Hughes LE, Mansel RE, et al. Clinical syndromes of mastalgia. *Lancet* 1976; 2:670.
4. Mansel RE. Breast pain. *British Medical Journal* 1994; 309(1 October):866–868.
5. Wren BG. The breast and the menopause. *Bailliere's Clinical Obstetrics and Gynaecology* 1996; 10(3):433–447.
6. Barros AC, Mottola J, Ruiz CA, Borges MN, Pinotti JA. Reassurance in the treatment of mastalgia. *Breast Journal* 1999; 5(3):162–165.
7. Page JK, Mansel RE, Hughes SE. Clinical experience of drug treatments for mastalgia. *Lancet* 1985; 2:373.
8. Steinbrunn BS, Zera RT, Rodriguez JL. Mastalgia: Tailoring treatment to type of breast pain. *Postgraduate Medicine* 1997; 102(5):183–198.
9. Greenblatt RB, Dmowsky WP, Mahesh VB, et al. Clinical studies with an antigonadotropin-Danazol. *Fertility and Sterility* 1971; 22:102.

10. Mansel RE, Dogliotti L. European multicentre trial of bromocriptine in cyclical mastalgia. *Lancet* 1990; 335:190.

11. Fentiman IS, Caleffi M, Brame K, et al. Double-blind controlled trial of tamoxifen therapy for mastalgia. *Lancet* 1986; 1:287.

12. Steinbrunn et al. Mastalgia.

13. Hamed H, Chaudary MA, Caleffi M, Fentiman IS. LHRH analogues for treatment of recurrent and refractory mastalgia. *Annual Review College of Surg England* 1990; 72(4):221–224.

14. Boyd N, McGuire V, Shannon P, et al. Effect of low-fat high carbohydrate diet on symptoms of cyclical mastopathy. *Lancet* 1988; 2(8603):128.

15. Ghent WR, Eskin BA, Low DA, et al. Iodine replacement in fibrocystic disease of the breast. *Canadian Journal of Surgery* 1993; 36(453).

16. LeBan MM, Meerscharet JR, Taylor RS. Breast pain: A symptom of cervical radiculopathy. *Archives of Physical Medicine and Rehabilitation* 1979; 60:315.

17. Page et al. Clinical experience of drug treatments for mastalgia.

18. Maddox PR, Harrison BJ, Mansel RE, et al. Non-cyclical mastalgia: An improved classification and treatment. *British Journal of Surgery* 1989; 76(9):901–904.

19. Preece et al. Clinical syndromes of mastalgia.

5. BREAST INFECTIONS AND NIPPLE PROBLEMS

1. Thomsen AC, Espersen MD, Maigaard S. Course and treatment of milk stasis, noninfectious inflammation of the breast and infectious mastitis in nursing women. *American Journal of Obstetrics and Gynecology* 1984; 149:492.

2. Meguid MM, Oler A, Numann PJ, Khan S. Pathogenesis-based treatment of recurring subareolar breast abscesses. *Surgery* 1995; 118:775–782.

3. Maier WP, Berger A, Derrick BM. Periareolar abscess in the nonlactating breast. *American Journal of Obstetrics and Gynecology* 1982; 149:492.

4. Sartorius O. Personal communication.

5. Watt-Boolsen S, Ryegaard R, Blichert-Toft M. Primary periareolar abscess in the nonlactating breast: Risk of recurrence. *American Journal of Surgery* 1987; 153:571.

6. Love SM, Schnitt SJ, Connolly JL, Shirley RL. Benign breast diseases. In: Harris JR, Hellman S, Henderson IC, Kinne DW, eds. *Breast Diseases*. Philadelphia: Lippincott, 1987; 22.

7. Elzer MH, Perloff LJ, Kelley RI, et al. Significance of age in patients with nipple discharge. *Surgical Gynecology and Obstetetrics* 1970; 131:519.

8. Pritt B, Pang Y, St John T, Elhosseiny A. Diagnostic value of nipple cytology: Study of 466 cases. *Cancer* 2004; 102(4):233–238.

9. Cabioglu N, Hunt KK, Singletary SE, et al. Surgical decision making and factors determining a diagnosis of breast carcinoma in women presenting with nipple discharge. *Journal of the American College of Surgeons* 2003; 3:354–364.

10. Pereira B, Mokbel K. Mammary Ductoscopy: past present and future. *International Journal of Clinical Oncology* 2005; 2(Apr 10):112-116.

6. LUMPS AND LUMPINESS

1. Herrman JB. Mammary cancer subsequent to aspiration of cysts in the breast. *Annals of Surgery* 1971; 173:40.

2. Haagensen CD. The relationship of gross cystic disease of the breast and carcinoma. *Annals of Surgery* 1977; 185:375.

3. Haagenson CD. *Diseases of the Breast*. Philadelphia: Saunders, 1996.

4. Greenberg R, Skornick Y, Kaplan O. Management of breast fibroadenomas. *Journal of General Internal Medicine* 1998; 13(Sept):640–645.

5. Kaufman CS, Littrup PJ, Freman-Gibb LA, Francescatti D, et al. Office-based cryoablation of breast fibroadenomas: 12-month followup. *Journal of the American College of Surgeons* 2004; 198(6):914–923.

7. DIAGNOSTIC IMAGING: MAMMOGRAPHY, ULTRASOUND, MRI, AND OTHER TECHNIQUES

1. Sadowski N. Personal communication 1988.

2. Kornguth P, Rimer B, Conaway M, et al. Impact of patient-controlled compression on the mammography experience. *Radiology* 1993; 186(1):99.

3. Lewin JM, Hendrick RE, D'Orsi CJ, et al. Comparison of full-field digital mammography with screen-film mammography for cancer detection: Results of 4,945 paired examinations. *Radiology* 2001; 218(3):873–880.

4. Lewin JM, D'Orsi CJ, Hendrick RE, et al. Clinical comparison of full-field digital mammography and screen-film mammography for detection of breast cancer. *American Journal of Roentgenology* 2002; 179(3):671–677.

5. Gur D, Sumkin JH, Rockette HE, et al. Changes in breast cancer detection and mammography recall rates after the introduction of a computer aided detection system. *Journal of the National Cancer Institute* 2004; 96:185–190.

6. Elmore JG, Carney P. Computer-aided detection of breast cancer: Has promise outstripped performance? *Journal of the National Cancer Institute* 2004; 96:162–163.

7. Homer MJ. Nonpalpable breast microcalcifications: Frequency, management, and results of incisional biopsy. *Radiology* 1992; 185:411.

8. Berend ME, Sullivan DC, Kornguth PJ, et al. The natural history of mammographic calcifications subjected to interval follow-up. *Archives of Surgery* 1992; 127(November): 1309.

9. Stomper P, Kopans D, Sadowski N, et al. Is mammograph painful? A multicenter patient survey. *Archives of Internal Medicine* 1988; 148(3):521.

10. Kolb TM, Lichy J, Newhouse JH. Comparison of the performance of screening, mammography, physical examination, and breast US and evaluation of factors that influence them: An analysis of 27,825 patient evaluations. *Radiology* 2002; 225:165–175.

11. Kolb TM, Lichy J, Newhouse JH, et al. Occult cancer in women with dense breasts: Detection with screening US-diagnostic yields and tumor characteristics. *Radiology* 1998; 207:191–199.

12. Parker SH, Lovin JD, Jobe WE, et al. Stereotactic breast biopsy with a biopsy gun. *Radiology* 1990; 176(Sept.):741.

13. Petro J, Klein S, Niazi Z, Salzberg C, Byrne D. Evaluation of ultrasound as a tool in the follow-up of patients with breast implants: A preliminary, prospective study. *Annals of Plastic Surgery* 1994; 32(6):580.

14. Peters-Engl C, Medl M, Mirau M, et al. Color-coded and spectral Doppler flow in breast carcinomas: Relationship with the tumor microvasculature. *Breast Cancer Research and Treatment* 1998; 47:83–89.

15. Warner E, Plewes DB, et al. Comparison of breast magnetic resonance imaging mammography, and ultrasound for surveillance of women at high risk for hereditary breast cancer. *Journal of Clinical Oncology* 2001; 19:3524–3531.

16. van der Hoeven JJM, Krak NC, Hoekstra OS, et al. ^{18}F-2-Fluoro-2-Deoxy-D-Glucose Positron Emission Tomography in staging of locally advanced breast cancer. *Journal of Clinical Oncology* 2004: 22:1253–1259.

17. Waxman ADR, L, Memsic LD, Foster CE, et al. Thallium scintigraphy in the evaluation of mass abnormalities of the breast. *Journal of Nuclear Medicine* 1993; 34:18.

18. Akashi-Tanaka S, Fukutomi T, Miyakawa K, Uchiyama N, Tsuda H. Diagnostic value of contrast-enhanced computed tomography for diagnosing the intraductal component of breast cancer. *Breast Cancer Research and Treatment* 1998; 49:79–86.

19. Randal J. Researchers test hi-tech bra for detecting breast cancer. *Journal of the National Cancer Institute* 1997; 89(19):1400–1401.

20. Stojadinovic A, Nissan A, Gallimidi Z, et al. Electrical impedance scanning for the early detection of breast cancer in young women: preliminary results of a multicenter prospective clinical trial. *Journal of Clinical Oncology* 2005; Apr 2023;(12):2703-2701.

8. BIOPSY

1. Layfield LJ, Parkinson B, Wong J, Guiliano AE, Bassett LW. Mammographically guided fine-needle aspiration biopsy of nonpalpable breast lesions. *Cancer* 1991; 68: 2007.

2. Martelli G, Pilotti S, De Yoldi GC, et al. Diagnostic efficacy of physical examination, mammography, fine needle aspiration, cytology (triple-test) in solid breast lumps: An analysis of 1708 cases. *Tumori* 1990; 76:476.

3. Pass HA. Stereotactic biopsy of breast cancer. PPO Updates (*Principles & Practice of Oncology*) 1998; 12(12):1–7.

4. Martelli et al. Diagnostic efficacy, op cit.

9. RISK FACTORS: NONGENETIC

1. Newell GR, Vogel VG. Personal risk factors: What do they mean? *Cancer* 1988; 62:1695.

2. Cuzick J. Women at high risk of breast cancer. *Reviews on Endocrine-Related Cancer* 1987; 25:5.

3. Miller AB. Epidemiology and prevention. In: Harris JR, Hellman S, Henderson IC, Kinne DW, eds. *Breast Diseases*. Philadelphia: Lippincott, 1987.

4. Seidman H, Stellman SD, Mushinski MH. A different perspective on breast cancer risk factors: Some implications of the nonattributable risk. *CA: A Cancer Journal for Clinicians* 1982; 32:301.

5. Willett WC, Stampfer MJ, Colditz GA, Rosner BA, Hennekens CJ, Speizer FE. Moderate alcohol consumption and the risk of breast cancer. *New England Journal of Medicine* 1980; 316:1174.

6. Morris CR, Wright WE, Schlag RD. The risk of developing breast cancer within the next 5, 10, or 20 years of a woman's life. *American Journal of Preventive Medicine* 2001; 20(3):214–218.

7. Chlebowski RT, Chen Z, Anderson GL, et al. Ethnicity and breast cancer: Factors influencing differences in incidence and outcome. *Journal of the National Cancer Institute* 2005; 97:439–448.

8. Kelsey JL, Berkowitz GS. Breast cancer epidemiology. *Cancer Research* 1988; 48:5615.

9. Haynes S. Prevention and early detection of breast cancer in lesbians. National Gay and Lesbian Health Education Conference 1992.

10. Michels KB, Trichopoulos D, Robbins JM, et al. Birthweight as a risk factor for breast cancer. *Lancet* 1996; 348:1542–1546.

11. Potischman N, Troisi R. In utero and early life exposures in relation to risk of breast cancer. *Cancer Causes Control* 1999; 10:561–573.

12. Okasha M, McCarron P, Gunnell D, et al. Exposures in childhood, adolescence and early adulthood and breast cancer risk: A systematic review of the literature. *Breast Cancer Research and Treatment* 2003; 78:223–276.

13. Trichopoulos D. Hypothesis: Does breast cancer originate in utero? *Lancet* 1990; 335:939–940.

14. MacMahon B, Cole P, Brown J. Etiology of human breast cancer: A review. *Journal of the National Cancer Institute* 1973; 50:21.

15. Pike MC, Krailo MD, Henderson BE, et al. "Hormonal" risk factors, "breast tissue age" and the age-incidence of breast cancer. *Nature* 1983; 303:767–770.

16. Rosner B, Colditz GA, Willett WC. Reproductive risk factors in a prospective study of breast cancer: The Nurses' Health Study. *American Journal of Epidemiology* 1994; 139:819–835.

17. Melbye M, Wohlfahrt J, Olsen J. Induced abortion and the risk of breast cancer. *New England Journal of Medicine* 1997; 336:81–85.

18. Ye Z, Gao DL, Qin Q, et al. Breast cancer in relation to induced abortions in a cohort of Chinese Women. *British Journal of Cancer* 2002; 87:977–981.

19. Collaborative Group on Hormonal Factors in Breast Cancer. Breast cancer and abortion: Collaborative reanalysis of data of 53 epidemiological studies, including 83,000 women with breast cancer from 16 countries. *Lancet* 2004; 363:1007–1016.

20. Collaborative Group on Hormonal Factors in Breast Cancer. Breast cancer and breastfeeding: Collaborative reanalysis of individual data from 47 epidemiological studies in 30 countries, including 50,302 women with breast cancer and 96,973 women without the disease. *Lancet* 2002; 360:187–195.

21. Chubak J, Tworoger SS, Yasui Y. Associations between reproductive and menstrual factors and postmenopasual sex hormone concentrations. *Cancer Epidemiology and Biomarkers Prevention* 2004; 13(8):1296–1301.

22. Endogenous Hormones and Breast Cancer Collaborative Group. Endogenous sex hormones and breast cancer in postmenopausal women: Reanalysis of nine prospective studies. *Journal of the National Cancer Institute* 2002; 94:606–616.

23. The Writing Group for the PEPI Trial. Effects of estrogen or estrogen/progestin regimens on heart disease risk factors in postmenopausal women: The postmenopausal estrogen/progestin interventions (PEPI) trial. *Journal of the American Medical Association* 1995; 273(3):199.

24. Rosenberg L, Miller DR, Kaufman DW, et al. Breast cancer and oral contraceptive use. *American Journal of Epidemiology* 1984; 119:167.

25. Kelsey JL, Fischer DB, Holford TR, et al. Exogenous estrogens and other factors in the epidemiology of breast cancer. *Journal of the National Cancer Institute* 1981; 55:327.

26. Marchbanks PA, McDonald JA, Wilson HG, et al. Oral contraceptives and the risk of breast cancer. *New England Journal of Medicine* 2002; 346:2025–2032.

27. Narod SA, Dube MP, Klijn J, et al. Oral contraceptives and the risk of breast cancer in BRCA1 and BRCA 2 mutation carriers. *Journal of the National Cancer Institute* 2002; 94:1773–1779.

28. Greenberg ER, Barnes AB, Resseguie L, et al. Breast cancer in mothers given diethylstilbestrol in pregnancy. *New England Journal of Medicine* 1984; 311:1393.

29. Kelsey JL, Berkowitz GS. Breast cancer epidemiology. *Cancer Research* 1988; 48:5615.

30. Stone L. *The Family, Sex, and Marriage.* New York: Harper & Row, 1979.

31. Hale JR. *Renaissance Europe.* Berkeley: University of California Press, 1971.

32. Fraser A. *The Weaker Vessel.* New York: Vintage, 1984.

33. Chlebowski RT, Hendrix SL, Langer RD, et al. Influence of estrogen plus progestin on breast cancer and mammography in healthy postmenopasual women: The Women's Health Initiative randomized trial. *Journal of the American Medical Association* 2003; 289:3243–3253.

34. Collaborative Group on Hormonal Factors in Breast Cancer. Breast cancer and hormone replacement therapy: Collaborative reanalysis of data from 51 epidemiologic studies of 52,705 women with breast cancer and 108,411 women without breast cancer. *Lancet* 1997; 350:1047–1059.

35. The Women's Health Initiative Steering Committee. Effects of conjugated equine estrogen in postmenopausal women with hysterectomy: The Women's Health Initiative randomized controlled trial. *Journal of the American Medical Association* 2004; 291:1701–1712.

36. Ross RK, Paganini-Hill A, Wan PC, and Pike MC. Effect of hormone replacement therapy on breast cancer risk: Estrogen versus estrogen plus progestin. *Journal of the National Cancer Institute* 2000; 92:328–332.

37. Vachon CM, Sellers TA, Vierkant RA, et al. Case-control study of increased mammographic breast density response to hormone replacement therapy. *Cancer Epidemiology Biomarkers and Prevention* 2002; 11:1382–1388.

38. Ettinger B, Friedman GD, Bush T, Quesenberry CP, Jr. Reduced mortality associated with long-term postmenopausal estrogen therapy. *Obstetrics and Gynecology* 1996; 87(1):6–12.

39. Greendale GA, Reboussin BA, Slone S, et al. Postmenopausal hormone therapy and change in mammographic density *Journal of the National Cancer Institute* 2003; 95:30–37.

40. Hormone replacement therapy and the risk of breast cancer: Nested case-control study in a cohort of Swedish women attending mammography screening. *Cancer* 1977; 72(5):758–761.

41. The Collaborative Group on Hormonal Factors in Breast Cancer, 1997, op cit.

42. Million Women Study collaborators. Breast Cancer and hormone-replacement therapy in the Million Women Study. *Lancet* 2003; 362:419–427.

43. Chen CL, Weiss NS, Newcomb P, Barlow W, and White E. Hormone replacement therapy in relation to breast cancer. *Journal of the American Medical Association* 2002; 287:734–741.

44. Newcomer LM, Newcomb PA, Daling JR, et al. Postmenopausal hormone use and risk of breast cancer by histologic type. *American Journal of Epidemiology* 1999; 149:S79.

45. Li CI, Weiss NS, Stanford JL, and Daling JR. Hormone replacement therapy in relation to risk of lobular and ductal breast carcinoma in middle-aged women. *Cancer* 2000; 88:2570–2577.

46. Newcomb PA, Titus-Ernstoff L, Egan KM, et al. Postmenopausal estrogen and progestin use in relation to breast cancer risk. *Cancer Epidemiology, Biomarkers & Prevention* 2002; 11:593–600.

47. Wolff MS, Weston A. Breast cancer risk and environmental exposures. *Environ mental Health Perspectives* 1997; 105(Supplement 4):891–895.

48. Fowke JH, She XO, Dai QI, et al. Oral contraceptive use and breast cancer risk: Modification by NAD(P)H:Quinone Oxoreductase (NQ01) Genetic Polymorphisms. *Cancer Epidemiological Biomarkers & Prevention* 2004; 13(8):1308–1315.

49. Miller WR, Mullen P, Sourdaine P, et al. Regulation of aromatase activity within the breast. *Journal of Steroid Biochem and Molecular Biology* 1997; 61(3–6):193–202.

50. Hunter DJ, Hankinson SE, Larden F, et al. Plasma organochlorine levels and the risk of breast cancer. *New England Journal of Medicine* 1997; 337:1253–1258.

51. Van't Veer P, Lobbezoo IE, Martin-Moreno JM, et al. DDT and postmenopausal breast cancer in Europe: Case control study. *British Medical Journal* 1997; 315:81–85.

52. Lopez-Carillo L, Blair A, Lopez-Cervantes M, et al. Dicholorodiphenyltrichloroethane serum levels and breast cancer risk: A case control study from Mexico. *Cancer Research* 1997; 57:3728–3732.

53. Wolff MS, Zeleniuch-Jacquotte A, Dubin N, et al. Risk of breast cancer and organochlorine exposure. *Cancer Epidemiology Biomarkers & Prevention* 2000; 9:271–277.

54. Hunter DJ, Hankinson SE, Larden F, et al. Plasma organochlorine levels and the risk of breast cancer, op cit.

55. Holmes MD, Hunter DJ, Colditz GA, et al. Association of dietary intake of fat and fatty acids with risk of breast cancer. *Journal of the American Medical Association* 1999; 281(10):914–920.

56. Goldin BR, Adlercreutz H, Gorbach SL, et al. Estrogen excretion patterns and plasma levels in vegetarian and omnivorous women. *New England Journal of Medicine* 1982; 307:1542.

57. Yood MU, Johnson CC, Blount A, et al. Race and differences in breast cancer survival in a managed care population. *Journal of the National Cancer Institute* 1999; 91(17): 1487–1491.

58. Longnecker MP, Newcomb PA, Mittendorf R, et al. Risk of breast cancer in relation to lifetime alcohol consumption. *Journal of the National Cancer Institute* 1995; 87: 923–929.

59. Reichman ME, Judd JT, Longcope C, et al. Effects of alcohol consumption on plasma and urinary hormone concentrations in premenopausal women. *Journal of the National Cancer Institute* 1993; 85:722–727.

60. Ginsburg ES, Walsh BW, Gao XP, et al. The effect of acute ethanol ingestion on estrogen levels in postmenopausal women using transdermal estradiol. *Journal of Soc Gynecol Invest* 1995; 2:26–29.

61. Zhang S, Hunter DJ, Hankinson SE, et al. A prospective study of folate intake and the risk of breast cancer. *Journal of the American Medical Association* 1999; 281:1632–1637.

62. Sellers TA, Kushi LH, Cerhan JR, et al. Dietary folate intake, alcohol and risk of breast cancer in a prospective study of postmenopausal women. *Epidemiology* 2001; 12:420–428.

63. Zhang SM, Willett WC, Selhub J, et al. Plasma folate, vitamin B6, vitamin B12 and homocysteine and risk of breast cancer. *Journal of the National Cancer Institute* 2003; 95:373–380. Rohan TE, Jain MG, Howe GR, et al. Dietary folate consumption and breast cancer risk. *Journal of the National Cancer Institute* 2000; 92:266–269.

64. Tokunaga M, Land CE, Yamamoto T, et al. Breast cancer among atomic bomb survivors. In: Boice JD, Jr., Fraumeni JF, Jr., eds. *Radiation Carcinogenesis Epidemiology and Biological Significance,* vol. 45. New York: Raven, 1984.

65. Tokunaga M, Land CE, Tokuoka S, et al. Incidence of female breast cancer among atomic bomb survivors, 1950–1985. *Radiation Research* 1994; 138:209–223.

66. Land C. Epidemiology of radiation induced breast cancer. NAPBC Breast Cancer Etiology Working Group Workshop on Medical Ionizing of Radiation and Human Breast Cancer 1997.

67. Miller AB, Howe GR, Sherman GJ, et al. Mortality from breast cancer after irradiation during fluoroscopic examinations in patients being treated for tuberculosis. *New England Journal of Medicine* 1989; 321:1285.

68. Mettler FA, Hempelmann LH, Dutton AM, Pifer JW, Toyooka ET, Ames WR. Breast neoplasma in women treated with x rays for acute postpartum mastitis: A pilot study. *Journal of the National Cancer Institute* 1969; 43:803.

69. Hoffman DA, Lonstein JE, Morin MM, et al. Breast cancer in women with scoliosis exposed to multiple diagnostic x rays. *Journal of the National Cancer Institute* 1989; 81:1307.

70. Simon N. Breast cancer induced by radiation: Relation to mammography and treatment of acne. *Journal of the American Medical Association* 1977; 237(8):789.

71. Hildreth NG, Shore RE, Dvoretsky PM. The risk of breast cancer after irradiation of the thymus in infancy. *New England Journal of Medicine* 1989; 321:1281.

72. Boice JD, Day NE, Anderson A, et al. Second cancer following radiation treatment for cervical cancer: An international collaboration among cancer registries. *Journal of the National Cancer Institute* 1985; 74:955.

73. Tucker MA, Coleman CN, Cox RS, et al. Risk of second cancers after treatment for Hodgkin's disease. *New England Journal of Medicine* 1988; 318:76.

74. Li FP, Corkery J, Vawter G, et al. Breast carcinoma after cancer therapy in childhood. *Cancer* 1983; 51:521.

75. Wang J, Inskip PD, Bioce JDJ. Cancer incidence among medical diagnostic xray workers in China 1950 to 1985. *International Journal of Cancer* 1990; 45:889–895.

76. Vaughan TL, Lee JA, Strader CH. Breast cancer incidence of a nuclear facility: Demonstration of a morbidity surveillance system. *Health Phys* 1993; 64:349–354.

77. Pukkala E, Auvinen A, Wahberg G. Incidence of cancer among Finnish airline attendants. *British Medical Journal* 1995; 311:649–952.

78. Boice JDJ, Mandel JS, Doody MM. Breast cancer among radiologic technologists. *Journal of the American Medical Association* 1995; 274:394–401.

79. Goss PE, Sierra S. Current perspectives on radiation induced breast cancer. *Journal of Clinical Oncology* 1998; 16:338–347.

80. Demers PA, Thomas DB, Rosenblatt KA, et al. Occupational exposure to electromagnetic fields and breast cancer in men. *American Journal of Epidemiology* 1991; 134(4):340.

81. Stevens RG, Davis S. The melatonin hypothesis: Electric power and breast cancer. *Environmental Health Perspectives* 1996; 104(Suppl 1):135–140.

82. Bartsch C, Bartsch H, Buchberger A, et al. Serial transplants of DMBA-induced mammary tumors in Fischer rats as a model system for human breast cancer. VI. The role of different forms of tumor-associated stress for the regulation of pineal melatonin secretion. *Oncology* 1999; 56(2):169–176.

83. Graham C. EMF effects on melatonin in humans. NAPBC Etiology Working Group Workshop on Electromagnetic Fields, Light at Night and Human Breast Cancer 1997.

84. Ibid.

85. Loomis DP, Savitz DA, Ananth CV. Breast cancer mortality among female electrical workers in the United States. *Journal of the National Cancer Institute* 1994; 86(12):921.

86. *Environmental Health Perspectives* 1996; 104(Suppl 1):135–140.

10. RISK FACTORS: GENETIC

1. The Collaborative Group on Hormonal Factors in Breast Cancer. Familial breast cancer. Collaborative reanalysis of individual data from 52 epidemiological studies including 58,209 women with breast cancer and 101,986 women without the disease. *Lancet* 2001; 358:1389–1399.

2. Easton DF, Bishop DT, Ford D, Crockford GP, Consortium BCL. Genetic linkage analysis in familial breast and ovarian cancer: Results from 214 families. *American Journal of Human Genetics* 1993; 52:678.

3. Shattuck-Eidens D, Oliphant A, McClure M, at al. BRCA 1 sequence analysis in women at high risk for susceptiblity mutations: Risk factor analysis and implications for genetic testing. *Journal of the American Medical Association* 1997; 278:1242.

4. King MC, Marks JH, Mandell JB. Breast and ovarian cancer risks due to inherited mutations in BRCA 1/2. *Science* 2003; 302(5645):643–646.

5. Liede A, Karlan BY, Narod SA. Cancer risks for male carriers of germline mutations in BRCA 1 or BRCA 2: A review of the literature. *Journal of Clinical Oncology* 2004; 22:735–742.

6. Bergthorsson JT, Johannsdottir J, Jonasdottir A, et al. Chromosome imbalance at the 3pl4 region in human breast tumors: High frequency in patients with inherited predisposition due to BRCA 2. *European Journal of Cancer* 1998; 34(1):1544.

7. Dorum A, Moller P, Kamsteeg EJ, et al. A BRCA1 founder mutation, identified with haplotype analysis, allowing genotype/phenotype determination and predictive testing. *European Journal of Cancer* 1997; 33:2390.

8. Narod SA. Modifiers of risk of hereditary breast and ovarian cancer. *Nature Rev Cancer* 2002; 2:113–123.

9. Risch HA, et al. Prevalence and penetrance of germline BRCA 1/2 mutations in a population series of 649 women with ovarian cancer. *American Journal of Human Genetics* 2001; 68:700–710.

10. Olopade OI, Artioli G. Efficacy of risk-reducing salpingo-oophorectomy in women with BRCA 1/2 mutations. *The Breast Journal* 2004; 10(Suppl 1):S5-S9.

11. Scully R, Livingston DM. In search of the tumour suppressor functions of BRCA 1/2. *Nature* 2000; 408:429–432.

12. Iglehart JD, Miron A, Rimer BK, Winer EP, Berry D, Shildkraut JM. Overestimation of hereditary breast cancer risk. *Annals of Surgery* 1998; 228(3):375–384.

13. Ibid.

14. Newman B, Mu H, Butler LM, Millikan RC, Moorman PG, King M-C. Frequency of breast cancer attributable to BRCA 1 in a population-based series of American women. *Journal of the American Medical Association* 1998; 279:915–921.

15. Peto J, Collins N, Barfoot R, Seal S, Warren W, Rahman N, Easton DF, Evans C, Deacon J, Stratton MR. Prevalence of BRCA 1 and BRCA 2 gene mutations in patients with early-onset breast cancer. *Journal of the National Cancer Institute* 1999; 91(11):943–949.

16. Shattuck-Eidens D, Oliphant A, McClure M, at al. BRCA 1 sequence analysis in women at high risk for susceptiblity mutations: Risk factor analysis and implications for genetic testing. *Journal of the American Medical Association* 1997; 278:1242.

17. Frank TS, Manley SA, Olopade OI, et al. Sequence analysis of BRCA 1/2: Correlation of mutations with family history and ovarian cancer risk. *Journal of Clinical Oncology* 1998; 16:2417.

18. Meijers-Heijboer H, van Greel B, van Putten WL et al. Breast cancer after prophylactic mastectomy in women with a BRCA 1 or BRCA 2 mutation. *New England Journal of Medicine* 2001; 345:159–164.

19. Brekelmans CTM, Seynaeve C, Bartels CCMM, et al. Effectiveness of breast cancer surveillance in BRCA 1/2 gene mutation carriers and women with high familial risk. *Journal of Clinical Oncology* 2001; 19:924–930.

20. Komenaka IK, Ditkoff BA, Joseph KA, et al. The development of interval breast malignancies in patients with BRCA mutations. *Cancer* 2004; 100:2079–2083.

21. Kriege M, Brekelmans CTM, Boetes C, et al. Efficacy of MRI and mammography for breast cancer screening in women with a familial or genetic predisposition. *New England Journal of Medicine* 2004; 351:427–437.

22. Petricoin EF III, Ardekani AM, Hitt BA, et al. Use of proteomic patterns in serum to identify ovarian cancer. *Lancet* 359:572–577.

23. Jernstrom H, et al. Pregnancy increases the risk of early onset breast cancer in BRCA 1/2 carriers. *Lancet* 1999; 354:1846–1850.

24. Jernstrom H, et al. Breast feeding and the risk of breast cancer in BRCA 1/2 carriers. *American Journal of Human Genetics* 2001; 69:S418.

25. Olopade OI, Artioli G. Efficacy of risk-reducing salpingo-oophorectomy in women with BRCA-1 and BRCA-2 mutations, op. cit.

26. Piver MS, Jishi MF, Tsukada Y, et al. Primary peritoneal carcinoma after prophylactic oophorectomy in women with a family history of ovarian cancer. *Cancer* 1993; 71:2751–2755.

27. Rebbeck TR, Lynch HT, Neuhausen SL, et al. Prophylactic oophorectomy in carriers of BRCA 1 or BRCA 2 mutations. *New England Journal of Medicine* 2002; 346:1616–1622.

28. MacMahon B, Cole P, Brown J. Etiology of human breast cancer: A review. *Journal of the National Cancer Institute* 1973; 50:21.

29. Narod SA, et al. Tamoxifen and risk of contralateral breast cancer in BRCA 1/2 carriers. *Lancet* 2000; 356:1876–1881.

30. Temple W, Lindsay R, Magi E, Urbanski S. Technical considerations for prophylactic mastectomy in patients at high risk for breast cancer. *American Journal of Surgery* 1991; 161(4):413.

31. Hartmann LC, Schaid DJ, Woods JE, Crotty TP, et al. Efficacy of bilateral prophylactic mastectomy in women with a family history of breast cancer. *New England Journal of Medicine* 1999; 340(2):77–84.

32. Meijers-Heijboer H, van Geel B, van Putten WL, et al. Breast cancer after prophylactic bilateral mastectomy in women with a BRCA 1 or BRCA 2 mutation, op cit.

33. Rebbeck TR, Friebel T, Lynch HT, et al. Bilateral prophylactic mastectomy in carriers of BRCA 1/2 mutations. *Journal of Clinical Oncology* 2004; 22:1055–1062.

34. Metcalfe K, Lynch HT, Ghadrian P, et al. Contralateral breast cancer in BRCA 1/2 mutation carriers. *Journal of Clinical Oncology* 2004; 22:2328–2335.

35. Grann VR, Jacobson JS, Thomason D, et al. Effect of prevention strategies on survival and quality-adjusted survival of women with BRCA 1 and 2 mutations: An updated decision analysis. *Journal of Clinical Oncology* 2002; 15:2520–2529.

36. Herrinton LJ, Barlow WE, Yu O, Geiger AM, et al. Efficacy of prophylactic mastectomy in women with unilateral breast cancer: A Cancer Research Network Project. *Journal of Clinical Oncology* 2005; 23(19).

37. Eisen A, Weber BL. Prophylactic mastectomy: The price of fear (editorial). *New England Journal of Medicine* 1999; 340(2):137–138.

11. PREVENTION

1. Miller AB. Epidemiology and prevention. In: Harris JR, Hellman S, Henderson IC, Kinne DW, eds. *Breast Diseases*. Philadelphia: Lippincott, 1987.

2. Van Gils CH, Peeters PHM, BBM H, et al. Consumption of vegetables and fruits and risk of breast cancer. *Journal of the American Medical Association* 2005; 293:183–193.

3. Gaudet MM, Britton JA, Kabat GC, et al. Fruits, vegetables, and micronutrients in relation to breast cancer modified by menopause and hormone receptor status. *Cancer Epidemiology and Biomarkers Prevention* 2004; 13(9):1485–1494.

4. Wu AH, Wan P, Hankin J, et al. Adolescent and adult soy intake and risk of breast cancer in Asian Americans. *Carcinogenesis* 2002; 23(9):1491–1496.

5. Holmes MD, Willet WC. Does diet affect breast cancer risk? *Breast Cancer Research* 2004; 6:170–178.

6. Toniolo P, Van Kappel AL, Akhmedkhanov A, et al. Serum carotenoids and breast cancer. *American Journal of Epidemiology* 2001; 153:1142–1147.

7. Sato R, Helzlsouer KJ, Alberg AJ, et al. Prospective study of carotenoids tocopherols and retinoid concentrations and the risk of breast cancer. *Cancer Epidemiology Biomarkers Prevention* 2002; 11:451–457.

8. Kline K, Lawson KA, Yu W, et al. Vitamin E and breast cancer prevention: Current status and future potential. *Journal of Mammary Gland Biology and Neoplasia* 2003; 8(1).

9. Bernstein L, Henderson BE, Hanisch R, Sullivan-Halley J, Ross RK. Physical exercise activity and reduced risk of breast cancer in young women. *Journal of the National Cancer Institute* 1994; 86:1403.

10. Bernstein L, Ross RK, Lobo RA, Hanisch R, Krailo MD, Henderson BE. The effects of moderate physical activity on menstrual cycle patterns in adolescence: Implications for breast cancer prevention. *British Journal of Cancer* 1987; 55:681.

11. Thune I, Brenn T, Lund E, Gaard M. Physical activity and the risk of breast cancer. *New England Journal of Medicine* 1997; 336:1269–1275.

12. Frisch RE, Wyshak G, Albright N, et al. Lower lifetime occurrence of breast cancer and cancer of the reproductive system among former college athletes. *American Journal of Clinical Nutrition* 1987; 45:328.

13. Spicer DV, Pike MC, Pike A, Rude R, Shoupe D, Richardson J. Pilot trial of a gonadotropin hormone agonist with replacement hormones as a prototype contraceptive to prevent breast cancer. *Contraception* 1993; 47:427.

14. Spicer D, Ursin G, Parisky YR, et al. Changes in mammographic densities induced by a hormonal contraceptive designed to reduce breast cancer risk. *Journal of the National Cancer Institute* 1994; 86(6):431.

15. Fisher B, Costantino JP, Wickerham DL, Redmond CK, Kavanah M, et al. Tamoxifen for prevention of breast cancer: Report of the National Surgical Adjuvant Breast and Bowel Project P–1 study. *Journal of the National Cancer Institute* 1998; 90(18):1371–1388.

16. Gail MH, Brinton LA, Byar DP, et al. Projecting individualized probabilities of developing breast cancer for white females who are examined annually. *Journal of the National Cancer Institute* 1989; 81(24):1879–1886.

17. IBIS Investigators. First results from the International Breast Cancer Intervention Study (IBISOI): A randomized prevention trial. *Lancet* 2002; 360:817–824.

18. Gail MH, Brinton LA, Bryar DP, et al. Projecting individualized probabilities of developing breast cancer for white females who are being examined annually. *Journal of the National Cancer Institute* 1989; 81:1879–1886.

19. Gail M, Costantino JP, Bryant J, et al. Weighing the risks and benefits of tamoxifen treatment for preventing breast cancer. *Journal of the National Cancer Institute* 1999; 91:1829–1846.

20. Cummings SR, Eckert S, Krueger KA, Grady D, Powles TJ, et al. The effect of raloxifene on risk of breast cancer in postmenopausal women: Results from the MORE trial. *Journal of the American Medical Association* 1999; 281(23):2189–2197.

21. Veronesi U, DePalo G, Costa A. Chemoprevention of breast cancer with retinoids. NCI Monographs 1992; 12:93.

22. Veronesi U, DePalo G, et al. Randomized trial of fenretinide to prevent second breast malignancy in women with early breast cancer. *Journal of the National Cancer Institute* 1999; 91:1847–1856.

23. Terry MB, Gammon MD, Zhang FF, et al. Association of frequency and duration of aspirin use and hormone receptor status with breast cancer risk. *Journal of the American Medical Association* 2004; 291:2433–2440.

24. R. Kochhar, V. Khurana, H. Bejjanki, G. Caldito, C Fort. Statins reduce breast cancer risk: A case control study in U.S. female veterans, Abstract 514 2005 ASCO, Annual Meeting Proceedings Supplement to *Journal of Clinical Oncology*, vol. 23, pt. I of II, June 1, 2005.

12. PRECANCEROUS CONDITIONS

1. Dupont WD, Page DL. Risk factors for breast cancer in women with proliferative breast disease. *New England Journal of Medicine* 1985; 312:146–151.

2. Rubin E, Visscher DW, Alexander RW, et al. Proliferative disease and atypia in biopsies performed for nonpalpable lesions detected mammographically. *Cancer* 1988; 61:2077–2082.

3. Davis HH, Simons M, Davis JB. Cystic disease of the breast relationship to cancer. *Cancer* 1974; 17:957.

4. Marshall LM, Hunter DJ, Connolly JL, et al. Risk of breast cancer associated with atypical hyperplasia of lobular and ductal types. *Cancer Epidemiology, Biomarkers, and Prevention* 1997; 6:297–201.

5. Page DL, Dupont WD, Rogers LW, et al. Atypical hyperplastic lesions of the female breast: A long term follow up study. *Cancer* 1985; 55:2698–2708.

6. Dupont WD, Parl FF, Hartmann WH, et al. Breast cancer risk associated with proliferative breast disease and atypical hyperplasia. *Cancer* 1993:71:1258–1265.

7. Dupont WD, Page DL. Risk factors for breast cancer in women with proliferative breast disease. *New England Journal of Medicine* 1985; 312:146.

8. Page DL, Schuyler PA, Dupont WD, Jensen RA, Plummer Jr WD, Simpson JF. Atypical lobular hyperplasia as a unilateral predictor of breast cancer risk: A retrospective cohort study. *Lancet* 2003; 361:125–29.

9. Arpino G, Allred DC, Mohsin SK, Weiss HL, Conrow D, Elledge RM. Lobular neoplasia on core-needle biopsy: Clinical significance. *Cancer* 2004; 101:242–250.

10. Fisher B, Costantino JP, Wickerham DL, Redmond CK, Kavanah M, et al. Tamoxifen for prevention of breast cancer: Report of the National Surgical Adjuvant Breast and Bowel Project P–1 study. *Journal of the National Cancer Institute* 1998; 90(18):1371–1388.

11. Fisher ER, Land SR, Fisher B, Mamounas E, Gilarski L, Wolmark N. Pathological findings from the National Surgical Adjuvant Breast and Bowel Project: Twelve-year observations concerning lobular carcinoma in situ. *Cancer* 2004; 100:238–244.

12. Hwang ES, Nyante SJ, Chen YY, Moore D, et al. Clonality of lobular carcinoma in situ and synchronous invasive lobular carcinoma. *Cancer* 2004; 100:2562–2572.

13. Akashi-Tanaka S, Fukutomi T, Nanasawa T, Matuso K, Hasegawa T, Tsuda H. Treatment of non-invasive carcinoma: Fifteen year results at the National Cancer Center Hospital in Tokyo. *Breast Cancer* 2000; 7:341–344.

14. Ottesen GL, Gaversen HP, Blichert-Toft M, Christensen IJ, Anderson JA. Carcinoma in situ of the female breast: 10 year follow-up results of a prospective nationwide study. *Breast Cancer Research & Treatment* 2000; 62:197–210.

15. Goldstein NS, Kestin LL, Vicini FA. Clinical pathologic implications of E-cadherin reactivity in patients with lobular carcinoma in situ of the breast. *Cancer* 2001; 92:738–747.

16. Moran M, Haffty BG. Lobular carcinoma in situ as a component of breast cancer the long-term outcome in patients treated with breast conservation therapy. *Journal of Radiation, Oncology Biology & Phys* 1998; 40:353–358.

17. Abner AL, Connolly JL, Recht A, et al. The relation between the presence and extent of lobular carcinoma in situ and the risk of local recurrence for patients with infiltrating carcinoma of the breast treated with conservative surgery and radiation therapy. *Cancer* 2000; 88:1072–1077.

18. Sasson AR, Fowble B, Hanlon AL, et al. Lobular carcinoma in situ increases the risk of local recurrence in selected patients with stages I and II breast carcinoma treated with conservative surgery and radiation *Cancer* 2001; 91:1862–1869.

19. Carolin KA, Tekyi Mensah S, Pass HA. Lobular carcinoma in situ and invasive cancer: The contralateral breast controversy. *Breast Journal* 2002; 8:263–268.

20. Alpers CE, Wellings SR. The prevalence of carcinoma in situ in normal and cancer-associated breasts. *Human Pathology* 1985; 16:796.

21. Nielsen M, Jensen J, Andersen J. Precancerous and cancerous breast lesions during lifetime and at autopsy. *Cancer* 1984; 54:612.

22. Betsill WL, Rosen PP, Lieberman PH, et al. Intraductal carcinoma: Long-term follow-up after treatment by biopsy alone. *Journal of the American Medical Association* 1978; 239:1863.

23. Page DL, Dupont WD. Intraductal carcinoma of the breast. *Cancer* 1982; 49:751.

24. Sternlicht MD, Kadeshian P, Shao Z-M, Safarians S, Barsky SH. The human myoepithelial cell is a natural tumor suppressor. *Clinical Cancer Research* 1997; 3:1949–1958.

25. Gupta SK, Douglas-Jones AG, Fenn N, Morgan JM, Mansel RE. The clinical behavior of breast carcinoma is probably determined at the preinvasive stage (ductal carcinoma in situ). *Cancer* 1997; 80(9):1740–1745.

26. Anastassiades O, Iakovou E, Stavridou N, Gogas J, Karameris A. Multicentricity in breast cancer: A study of 366 cases. *American Journal of Clinical Pathology* 1993; 99(3):238.

27. Rosen P, Fracchia A, Urban J, et al. "Residual" mammary carcinoma following simulated partial mastectomy. *Cancer* 1975; 35:739.

28. Love SM, Barksy SH. Anatomy of the nipple and breast ducts revisited. *Cancer* 2004; 101:1947–57.

29. Holland R, Hendriks J, Verberek A, et al. Extent, distribution and mammographic/histological correlations of breast ductal carcinoma in situ. *Lancet* 1990; 335:519.

30. Noguchi S, Motomura K, Inaji H, Imaoka S, Koyama H. Clonal analysis of pre-

dominantly intraductal carcinoma and precancerous lesions of the breast by means of polymerase chain reaction. *Cancer Research* 1994; 54(April 1):1849–1853.

31. Ernster VL, Barclay J, Kerlikowske K, et al. Mortality among women with ductal carcinoma in situ of the breast in the population-based Surveillance, Epidemiology and End Results program. *Archives of Internal Medicine* 2000; 160:953–958.

32. Fisher B, Costantino J, Redmond C, et al. Lumpectomy compared with lumpectomy and radiation therapy for the treatment of intraductal breast cancer. *New England Journal of Medicine* 1993; 328:1581–1586.

33. Julien JP, Bijker N, Fentimean IS, et al. Radiotherapy in breast-conserving treatment for ductal carcinoma in situ: First results of the EORTC randomized phase III trial 10853. *Lancet* 2000; 355:528–533.

34. Houghton J, George WD, Cuzick J, et al. Radiotherapy and tamoxifen in women with completely excised ductal carcinoma in situ of the breast in the UK, Australia and New Zealand: Randomized controlled trial. *Lancet* 2003; 362:95–102.

35. Fisher B, Dignam J, Wolmark N, Wickerham DL, Fisher ER, et al. Tamoxifen in treatment of intraductal breast cancer: National Surgical Adjuvant Breast and Bowel Project B-24 randomized controlled trial. *Lancet* 1999; 353 (June 12):1993–2000.

36. Houghton J, George WD, Cuzick J, et al. Radiotherapy and tamoxifen in women with completely excised ductal carcinoma in situ of the breast in the UK, Australia and New Zealand: Randomized controlled trial. *Lancet*, op cit.

37. Allred DC, Bryant J, Land S, et al. Estrogen receptor expression as a predictive marker of effectiveness of tamoxifen in the treatment of DCIS: Findings from NSABP Protocol B-24. *Breast Cancer Research and Treatment* 2002; 76:Suppl1:S36.abstract.

38. Habel LA, Moe RE, Daling JR, Holte S, et al. Risk of contralateral breast cancer among women with carcinoma in situ of the breast. *Annals of Surgery* 1997; 225:65–75.

39. Finkelstein SD, Sayegh R, Thompson WR. Late recurrence of ductal carcinoma in situ at the cutaneous end of surgical drainage following total mastectomy. *American Surgeon* 1993; 59(July):410.

40. Fisher DE, Schnitt SJ, Christian R, Harris JR, Henderson IC. Chest wall recurrence of ductal carcinoma in situ of the breast after mastectomy. *Cancer* 1993; 71(10):3025.

41. Silverstein M, Waisman J, Gamagami P, et al. Intraductal carcinoma of the breast (208 cases). Clinical factors influencing treatment choice. *Cancer* 1990; 66(1):102.

13. THE INTRADUCTAL APPROACH: GETTING TO THE SOURCE

1. Leborgne R. Intraductal biopsy of certain pathologic processes of the breast. *Surgery* 1946; 19:47–54.

2. Papanicolaou GN, Holmquist DG, Bader GM, Falk EA. Exfoliative cytology of the human mammary gland and its value in the diagnosis of cancer and other diseases of the breast. *Cancer* 1958; II(2):377–409.

3. Buehring GC. Screening for breast atypias using exfoliative cytology. *Cancer* 1979; 43(5):1788–1799.

4. Sartorius OW, Smith HS, Morris P, Benedict D, Friesen L. Cytologic evaluation of breast fluid in the detection of breast disease. *Journal of the National Cancer Institute* 1977; 67:277–284.

5. Wrensch MR, Petrakis NL, King EB, et al. Breast cancer incidence in women with abnormal cytology in nipple aspirates of breast fluid. *American Journal of Epidemiology* 1992; 135:130–141.

6. Gertrude Buehring, personal communication.

7. Sauter E, Ross E, Daly M, et al. Nipple aspirate fluid: A promising non-invasive method to identify cellular markers of breast cancer risk. *British Journal of Cancer* 1997; 76(4):494–501.

8. Fabian C, Zalles C, Kamel S, et al. Correlation of breast tissue biomarkers with hyperplasia and dysplasia in fine-needle aspirates (FNAs) of women at high and low risk for breast cancer. *Proceedings of Annual Meeting of American Association of Cancer Researchers* 1994; 35(A1703).

9. Love SM, Barsky SH. Anatomy of the nipple and breast ducts revisited. *Cancer* 2004; 101:1947–1957.

10. Dooley WC, Ljung B, Veronesi U, et al. Ductal lavage for detection of cellular atypia in women at high risk for breast cancer. *Journal of the National Cancer Institute* 2001; 93:1624–1632.

11. King BL, Crisi GM, Tsai S, et al. Immunocytochemical analysis of breast cells obtained by ductal lavage. *Cancer Cytopathol* 2002:96.

12. Yamamoto D, Tanaka K. A review of mammary ductoscopy in breast cancer. *The Breast Journal* 2004; 10(4):295–297.

13. Papanicolaou et al. Exfoliative cytology of the human mammary gland, op cit.

14. SCREENING

1. Thomas DB, Gao DL, Self SG, et al. Randomized trial of breast self-examination in Shanghai: Methodology and preliminary results. *Journal of the National Cancer Institute* 1997; 89:355–365.

2. Ibid.

3. Shapiro S, Venet W, Strax P, et al. Ten- to fourteen-year effects of screening on breast cancer mortality. *Journal of the National Cancer Institute* 1982; 69:349.

4. Ibid.

5. Shapiro S. Periodic screening for breast cancer: The HIP Randomized Controlled Trial (Health Insurance Plan). *Journal of the National Cancer Institute* 1997; 22:27–30.

6. Miller A, Baines C, To T, Wall C. Canadian National Breast Screening Study: 2. Breast cancer detection and death rates among women aged 50–59 years. *Canadian Medical Association Journal* 1992; 147(10):1477.

7. Fletcher SW, Black W, Harris R, Rimer BK, Shapiro S. Report of the international workshop for screening for breast cancer. *Journal of the National Cancer Institute* 1993; 85(20):1644.

8. National Institutes of Health. Consensus Development Statement: Breast cancer screening for women ages 40–49. 1997 (January 21–23).

9. Kerlikowske K, Grady D, et al. Effect of age, breast density, and family history on the sensitivity of first screening mammography. *Journal of the American Medical Association* 1996; 276:33–38.

10. Kopans DB. NBSS Revisited-Again (response). *Journal of the National Cancer Institute* 1993; 85(21):1774.

11. Duffy SW, Tabar L, Chen H, et al. The impact of organized mammography service screening on breast carcinoma mortality in seven Swedish countries; a collaborative evaluation. *Cancer* 2002; 95:458–69.

15. INTRODUCTION TO BREAST CANCER

1. Perou CM, Sorlie T, Eisen MB, et al. Molecular portraits of human breast tumors. *Nature* 2000; 406:747–752.

2. Berry DA, Cirrincione C, Henderson IC, et al. Effects of improvements in chemotherapy on disease-free and overall survival of estrogen-receptor negative, node positive breast cancer: 20 year experience of the CALGB and US Breast Intergroup. *Breast Cancer Research and Treatment* 2004 88(S1):Abstract no. 29.

3. Bonadonna G. Evolving concepts in the systemic adjuvant treatment of breast cancer. *Cancer Research* 1992; 52:2127.

4. Veronesi U. Randomized trials comparing conservative techniques with conventional surgery: An overview. In: Tobias JS, Peckham MJ, eds. *Primary Management of Breast Cancer: Alternatives to Mastectomy Management of Malignant Disease Series.* London: E. Arnold; 1985.

5. Peters WP, Ross M, Vredenburgh JJ, et al. High-dose chemotherapy and autologous bone marrow support as consolidation after standard-dose adjuvant therapy for high-risk primary breast cancer. *Journal of Clinical Oncology* 1993; 11:1132–1143.

6. Tallman MS, Gray R, Robert NJ, et al. Conventional adjuvant chemotherapy with or without high-dose chemotherapy and autologous stem cell transplantation in high-risk breast cancer. *New England Journal of Medicine* 2003; 349:17–26.

7. Garcia-Carbonero R, Hidalgo M, Paz-Ares L, et al. Patient selection in high-dose chemotherapy trials: Relevance in high-risk breast cancer. *Journal of Clinical Oncology* 1997; 15:3178–3184.

8. Early Breast Cancer Trialists' Cooperative Group. Effects of chemotherapy and hormonal therapy for early breast cancer on recurrence and 15-year survival; an overview of the randomized trials. *Lancet* 2005; 1687–1717.

9. Lorde A. *A Burst of Light.* New York: Firebrand; 1988.

16. WHAT KIND OF CANCER IS IT?

1. Dixon JM, Anderson TJ, Page DL, et al. Infiltrating lobular carcinoma of the breast: An evaluation of the incidence and consequence of bilateral disease. *British Journal of Surgery* 1983; 70:513.

2. Mansi JL, Gogas H, Bliss JM, et al. Outcome of primary breast cancer patients with micrometastases: A long-term follow-up study. *Lancet* 1999; 354:197–202.

3. Diehl IJ, Kaufmann M, Goerner R, et al. Detection of tumor cells in bone marrow of patients with primary breast cancer: A prognostic factor for distant metastasis. *Journal of Clinical Oncology* 1992; 10:1534–1539.

4. Haagensen C. *Diseases of the Breast*. Philadelphia: Saunders, 1971.

5. Gotteland M, May E, May-Levin F, Contesso G, Delarue JC, Mouriesse H. Estrogen receptors (ER) in human breast cancer. *Cancer* 1994; 74(3):864.

6. Ewers SV, Attewell R, Baldetorp B, et al. Prognostic significance of flow cytometric DNA analysis and estrogen receptor content in breast carcinomas: A 10-year survival study. *Breast Cancer Research and Treatment* 1992; 24:115.

7. Slamon D, Godolphin W, Jones L, et al. Studies of the Her-2/neu proto-oncogene in human breast and ovarian cancer. *Science* 1989; 244(4905):707.

8. Cobleigh MA, Vogel CL, Tripathy D, et al. Multinational study of the efficacy and safety of humanized anti-Her-2 monoclonal antibody in women who have Her-2 overexpressing metastatic breast cancer that has progressed after chemotherapy for metastatic disease. *Journal of Clinical Oncololgy* 1999; 17:2639–2648.

9. Mass RD, Sanders C, Kasian C, et al. The concordance between the clinical trial assay (CTA) and fluorescence in situ hybridization (FISH) in the Herceptin pivotal trials. *Proceedings of the American Society of Clinical Oncologists* 2000; 19:75a (Abstract no. 291).

10. DeLaurentiis M, Arpino G, Massarelli E, et al. HER 2 as predictive marker of resistance to endocrine treatment for advanced breast cancer: A metaanalysis of published studies. *Breast Cancer Research & Treatment* 2002; 7:S68.

11. Love RR, Duc NB, Havighurst TC, et al. Her 2/neu overexpression and response to oophorectomy plus tamoxifen adjuvant therapy in estrogen receptor positive premenopausal women with operable breast cancer. *Journal of Clinical Oncology* 2003; 21:453–457.

12. Ellis MJH, Coop A, Singh B, et al. Letrozole is more effective neoadjuvant en-

docrine therapy than tamoxifen for ErbB-1 and/or Erb B-2 positive primary breast cancer: Evidence from a phase III randomized trial. *Journal of Clinical Oncology* 2001; 19:3808–3816.

13. Wong WW, Vijayakumar S, Weichselbaum RR. Prognostic indicators in node-negative early stage breast cancer. *American Journal of Medicine* 1992; 92:539.

14. Paik S, Shak S, Tang G, et al. A multigene assay to predict recurrence of tamoxifen-treated, node-negative breast cancer. *New England Journal of Medicine* 2004; 351(27): 2817–2865.

15. Paik S, Shak S, Tang G, et al. Expression of the 21 genes in the recurrence score assay and prediction of clinical benefit from tamoxifen in NSABP study B 14 and chemotherapy in NSABP study B 20. *Proceedings of San Antonio Breast Cancer Symposium* 2004; 24.

16. Piccart MJ, Loi S, van't Veer LJ, et al. Multi-center external validation study of the Amsterdam 70-gene prognostic signature in node negative untreated breast cancer: Are the results still outperforming the clinical-pathological criteria? *Breast Cancer Research and Treatment* 2004; 88:S17 (Abstract no. 38).

17. TREATMENT OPTIONS: LOCAL THERAPY

1. Veronesi U. Randomized trials comparing conservative techniques with conventional surgery: An overview. In: Tobias JS, Peckham MJ, eds. *Primary Management of Breast Cancer: Alternatives to Mastectomy Management of Malignant Disease Series.* London: E. Arnold; 1985.

2. Veronesi U, Cascinelli N, Mariani, L, et al. Twenty year follow-up of a randomized study comparing breast-conserving surgery with radical mastectomy for early breast cancer. *New England Journal of Medicine* 2002; 347:1227–1232.

3. Fisher B, Anderson S, Bryant J, et al. Twenty-year follow-up of a randomized trial comparing total mastectomy, lumpectomy, and lumpectomy plus irradiation for the treatment of breast cancer. *New England Journal of Medicine* 2002; 347:1233–1241.

4. Locker GY, Sainsbury JR, Cuzick J, ATAC Trialists' Group. Breast surgery in the "Arimidex, Tamoxifen Alone or in Combination" (ATAC) trial: American women are more likely than women from the United Kingdom to undergo mastectomy. *Cancer* 2004; 101(4):735–740.

5. Holland R, Veling S, Mravunac M, et al. Histological multifocality of Tis, T1-2 breast carcinomas: Implications for clinical trials of breast-conserving treatment. *Cancer* 1985; 56:979.

6. Fisher B, Anderson S, Bryant J, et al. 2002, op cit.

7. Golshan M, Fung BB, Wolfman J, et al. The effect of ipsilateral whole breast ultrasound on the surgical management of breast carcinoma. *American Journal of Surgery* 2003: 186:391. Tillman GF, Orel SG, Schnall MD, et al. Effect of breast magnetic resonance imaging on the clinical management of women with early-stage breast carcinoma. *Journal of Clinical Oncology* 2002; 20:3413.

8. Schnitt SJ, Abner A, Gelman R, et al. The relationship between microscopic margins of resection and the risk of local recurrence in patients with breast cancer treated with breast conserving surgery and radiotherapy. *Cancer* 1994; 74:1746.

9. Harris J, Morrow M. Local management of invasive cancer: breast. Chapter 43 from Harris JR, Lippman ME, Morrow M, Osborne CK, eds. *Diseases of the Breast*, 3rd ed. Philadelphia: Lippincott/Williams & Wilkins 2004; 731.

10. Okumura SO, Mitsumori M, Yamauchi C, et al. Feasibility of breast-conserving therapy for macroscopically multiple ipsilateral breast cancer. *International Journal of Radiation Oncology Biology and Physics* 2004; 59(1):146–151.

11. Fisher B, Anderson S, Bryant J, et al. Twenty-year follow-up of a randomized trial comparing total mastectomy, lumpectomy, and lumpectomy plus irradiation for the treatment of invasive breast cancer, op cit.

12. Harris J, Morrow M. *Diseases of the Breast*, 2004, 732.

13. Fyles AW, McReady DR, Manchul LA, et al. Tamoxifen with or without breast irradiation in women 50 years of age or older with early breast cancer. *New England Journal of Medicine* 2004; 351:963–970.

14. Hughes KS, Schnaper LA, Berry D, et al. Lumpectomy plus tamoxifen with or without irradiation in women 70 years of age or older with early breast cancer. *New England Journal of Medicine* 2004; 351:971–977.

15. Veronesi U, Luini A, Del Becchio M, et al. Radiotherapy after breast-preserving surgery in women with localized cancer of the breast. *New England Journal of Medicine* 1993; 328:1587.

16. Malmstrom P, Holmberg L, Anderson H, et al. Breast conservation, with and without radiotherapy in women with lymph node negative breast cancer: A randomized clinical trial in a population with access to public mammography screening. *European Journal of Cancer* 2003; 39:1690.

17. Harris J, Morrow M. *Diseases of the Breast*, 2004, op cit.

18. Ragaz J, Olivotto IA, Spinelli JJ, et al. Locoregional radiation therapy in patients with high-risk breast cancer receiving adjuvant chemotherapy: 20-year results of the British Columbia randomized trial. *Journal of the National Cancer Institute* 2005; 97(2):82–84.

19. Overgaard M, Hansen PS, Overgaard J, Rose C, et al. Postoperative radiotherapy in high-risk premenopausal women with breast cancer who receive adjuvant chemotherapy. Danish Breast Cancer Cooperative Group 82 b Trial. *New England Journal of Medicine* 1997; 337:949–955.

20. Overgaard M, Jensen MB, Overgaard J, et al. Postoperative radiotherapy in high-risk postmenopausal breast cancer patients given adjuvant tamoxifen: Danish Breast Cancer Cooperative Group DBCG 82c randomized trial. *Lancet* 1999; 353:1641–1648.

21. Giordano SH, Kuo YF, Freeman JL, et al. Risk of cardiac death after adjuvant radiotherapy for breast cancer. *Journal of the National Cancer Institute* 2005; 97(6):416–424.

22. Deutsch M, Land SR, Begovic M, et al. The incidence of lung carcinoma after surgery for breast carcinoma with and without postoperative radiotherapy: Results of National Surgical Adjuvant Breast and Bowel Project (NSABP) Clinical Trials B–04 and B–06. *Cancer* 2003; 98:1362–1368.

23. Zablotska LB, Neugut AI. Lung carcinoma after radiation therapy in women treated with lumpectomy or mastectomy for primary breast carcinoma. *Cancer* 2003; 97:1404–1411.

24. Harris JR, Halpin-Murphy P, McNeese M, et al. Consensus statement on postmastectomy radiation therapy. *International Journal of Radiation Oncology Biology and Physics* 1999; 44:989–990.

25. Recht A, Edge SB, Solin LJ, et al. Postmastectomy radiotherapy: Clinical practice guidelines of the American Society of Clinical Oncology. *Journal of Clinical Oncology* 2001; 19:1539–1569.

26. National Comprehensive Cancer Network. Clinical practice guidelines in oncology. http://www.nccn.org. Accessed 2004.

27. Fenn AJ, Wolf GL, Fogle RM. An adaptive microwave phased array for targeted heating of deep tumours in intact breast: Animal study results. *Journal of Hyperthermia* 1999; 15:45.

28. Dowlatshahi K, Fan M, Gould VE, et al. Stereotactically guided laser therapy of occult breast tumors: A work in progress. *Archives of Surgery* 2000; 135:1345.

29. Sabel MS, Edge SB. In-situ ablation of breast cancer. *Breast Disease* 2001; 12:131–140.

30. Orr RK. The impact of prophylactic axillary node dissection on breast cancer survival: A Bayesian meta-analysis. *Annals of Surgical Oncology* 1999; 6:109–116.

31. Louis-sylvestre C, Clough K, Asselain B, et al. Axillary treatment in conservative

management of operable breast cancer: Dissection or radiotherapy? Results of a randomized study with 15 years of follow-up. *Journal of Clinical Oncology* 2004; 22:97–101.

32. Giuliano AE, Jones RC, Brennan M, Statman R. Sentinel lymphadenectomy in breast cancer. *Journal of Clinical Oncology* 1997; 5:2345–2350.

33. Krag DN, Weaver OJ, Alex JC, Fairbank JT. Surgical resection and radiolocalization of the sentinel node in breast cancer using a gamma probe. *Surgical Oncology* 1993; 2:335.

34. Turner RR, Ollila DW, Krasne DL, Giuliano AE. Histopathologic validation of the sentinel lymph node hypothesis for breast carcinoma. *Annals of Surgery* 1997; 226:271–278.

35. Krag D, Ashikraga T. The design of trials comparing sentinel-node surgery and axillary resection. *New England Journal of Medicine* 2003; 349, 6:603–605.

36. Turner RR, Ollila DW, Krasne DL, Giuliano AE. Histopathologic validation of the sentinel lymph node hypothesis for breast carcinoma, op cit.

37. Moore KH, Thaler HT, Tan LK, et al. Immunohistochemically detected tumor cells in the sentinel lymph nodes of patients with breast carcinoma: Biological metastasis or procedural artifact? *Cancer* 2004; 100:929–934.

38. Hagen A, Hrushesky WJM. Menstrual timing of breast cancer surgery. *American Journal of Surgery* 1998; 104:245–261.

39. Hrushesky WJM, Bluming AZ, Gruber SA, Sothern RB. Menstrual influence on surgical cure of breast cancer. *Lancet* 1989; 2:94.

40. Love RR, Ba Duc N, Van Dinh N, et al. Mastectomy and oophorectomy by menstrual cycle phase in women with operable breast cancer. *Journal of the National Cancer Institute* 2002; 94(9):662–669.

41. Love SM, McGuigan KA, Chap L. The Revlon/UCLA Breast Center practice guidelines for the treatment of breast disease. *The Cancer Journal from Scientific American* 1996; 2(1):2–15.

42. Rosen P, et al. Contralateral breast carcinoma: An assessment of risk and prognosis in stage I (TINOMO and stage II (T1N1M0) patients with 20 year follow up. *Surgery* 1989:106(5):904–910.

43. Hislop T, et al. Second primary cancers of the breast: Incidence and risk factors. *British Journal of Cancer* 1984; 49:79–85

44. Herrington LJ, Barlow WE, Yu O, et al. Efficacy of prophylactic mastectomy in women with unilateral breast cancer: A Cancer Research Network Project. *Journal of Clinical Oncology* 2005; 23(19):July 1.

18. TREATMENT OPTIONS: SYSTEMIC THERAPY

1. Bonadonna G, Valagussa VE, Rossi A, et al. Ten-year experience with CMF-based adjuvant chemotherapy in resectable breast cancer. *Breast Cancer Research and Treatment* 1985; 5:95.

2. Wolmark N, Fisher B. Adjuvant chemotherapy in Stage II breast cancer: An overview of the NSABP clinical trials. *Breast Cancer Research Treatment* 1983; 3(Supplement):S19.

3. Early Breast Cancer Collaborative Trialists' Group. Polychemotherapy for early breast cancer: An overview of the randomized trials. *Lancet* 1998; 352(Sept. 19):930–942.

4. Osborne CK. Adjuvant endocrine therapy. In: Harris JR, Lippman ME, Morrow M, Osborne CK, eds. *Diseases of the Breast*, 3rd ed. Philadelphia: Lippincott/Williams & Wilkins, 2004; 868.

5. Osborne CK, Ravdin PM. Adjuvant systemic therapy of primary breast cancer. In: Harris JR, Lippman ME, Morrow M, Osborne CK, eds. *Diseases of the Breast*, 2nd ed. Philadelphia: Lippincott/Williams & Wilkins, 2000; 625.

6. Stearns V, Davidson N. Adjuvant chemotherapy and chemoendorcine therapy. In: Harris JR, Lippman ME, Morrow M, Osborne CK, eds. *Diseases of the Breast*, 3rd ed. Philadelphia: Lippincott/Williams & Wilkins, 2004.

7. Rajagopal S, Goodman PJ, Tannock IF. Adjuvant chemotherapy for breast cancer: Discordance between physicians' perception of benefit and the results of clinical trials. *Journal of Clinical Oncology* 1994; 12(6):1296.

8. Stearns V, Davidson N. Adjuvant chemotherapy and chemoendorcine therapy, In: Harris JR, Lippman ME, Morrow M, Osborne CK, eds. *Diseases of the Breast*, 3rd ed., op cit.

9. Hortobagyi GN, Buzdar AU, Theriault RL, et al. Randomized trial of high-dose chemotherapy and blood cell autografts for high-risk primary breast cancer. *Journal of the National Cancer Institute* 2000; 92:225–233.

10. Zander AR, Kroger N, Schmoor C, et al. High-dose chemotherapy with autologous hematopoietic stem-cell support compared with standard-dose chemotherapy in breast cancer patients with 10 or more positive lymph nodes: First results of a randomized trial. *Journal of Clinical Oncology* 2004; 22:2273–2283.

11. Citron ML, Berry DA, Cirrincione C, et al. Randomized trial of dose-dense versus conventionally scheduled and sequential versus concurrent combination chemotherapy as postoperative adjuvant treatment of node positive primary breast cancer: First report of Intergroup Trial C9741/Cancer and Leukemia Group B Trial 9741. *Journal of Clinical Oncology* 2003; 21:1431–1439.

12. Fisher B, Brown A, Mamounas E, et al. Effect of preoperative chemotherapy on local-regional disease in women with operable breast cancer: Findings from National Surgical Adjuvant Breast and Bowel Project B-18. *Journal of Clinical Oncology* 1997; 15:2483.

13. Hortobagyi G, et al. Invasive Lobular Carcinoma Classic Type: Response to Primary Chemotherapy and Survival Outcomes, *Journal of Clinical Oncology* 2005; 41–48.

14. Cortazar P, Johnson BE. Review of the efficacy of individualized chemotherapy selected by in-vitro drug sensitivity testing for patients with cancer. *Journal of Clinical Oncology* 1999; 17(5):1625–1631.

15. Early Breast Cancer Collaborative Trialists' Group. Effects of adjuvant tamoxifen and of cytotoxic therapy on mortality in early breast cancer: An overview of 61 randomized trials among 28,896 women. *New England Journal of Medicine* 1988; 319:1681.

16. Crivellari D, Price K, Gelber RD, et al. Adjuvant endocrine therapy compared with no systemic therapy for elderly women with early breast cancer: 21 year results of International Breast Cancer Study Group Trial IV. *Journal of Clinical Oncology* 2003; 21:4517–4523.

17. Fisher B, Dignam J, Bryant J, et al. Five versus more than five years of tamoxifen therapy for breast cancer patients with negative lymph nodes and estrogen receptor-positive tumors. *Journal of the National Cancer Institute* 1996; 88(21):1510–1512.

18. Fisher B, Dignam J, Bryant J, Wolmark N. Five versus more than five years of tamoxifen for lymph node-negative breast cancer: Updated findings from the National Surgical Adjuvant Breast and Bowel Project B-14 randomized trial. *Journal of the National Cancer Institute* 2001; 93:684–690.

19. Early Breast Cancer Trialists' Cooperative Group. Effects of chemotherapy and hormonal therapy for early breast cancer on recurrence and 15-year survival; an overview of the randomized trials. *Lancet* 2005; 1687–1717.

20. Taylor CW, Green S, Dalton WS, et al. Multicenter randomized clinical trial of goserelin versus surgical ovariectomy in premenopausal patients with receptor-positive metastatic breast cancer an intergroup study. *Journal of Clinical Oncology* 1998; March 16(3):994–999.

21. Kaufmann M, Jonat W, Blamey R, et al. Survival analyses from the ZEBRA study: Goserelin (Zoladex) versus CMF in premenopausal women with node-positive breast cancer. *European Journal of Cancer* 2003; 39:1711–1717.

22. Jakesz R, Hausmaninger H, Kubista E, et al. Randomized adjuvant trial of tamox-

ifen and goserelin versus cyclophosphamide methotrexate and fluorouracil: Evidence for the superiority of treatment with endocrine blockade in premenopausal patients with hormone-responsive breast cancer. Austrian Breast and Colorectal Cancer Study Group Trial 5. *Journal of Clinical Oncology* 2002; 20:4621–4627.

23. Davidson NE, O'Neill A, Vukov A, et al. Chemohormonal therapy in premenopausal node-positive, receptor-positive breast cancer: An Eastern Cooperative Oncology Group phase III intergroup trial (E5188, INT–0101). *Proceedings of the American Society of Clinical Oncology* 2003; 22:15a.

24. Santner SJ, Pauley RJ, Tait L, et al. Aromatase activity and expression in breast cancer and benign breast tissue stromal cells. *Journal of Clinical Endocrinology Metabolism* 1997; 82:200.

25. ATAC Trialists' Group. Results of the ATAC (Arimidex, Tamoxifen, Alone or in Combination) trial after completion of 5 years' adjuvant treatment for breast cancer. *Lancet* 2005; 365(9453):60–62.

26. Goss PE, Ingle JN, Martino S, et al. A randomized trial of letrozole in postmenopausal women after five years of tamoxifen therapy for early-stage breast cancer. *New England Journal of Medicine* 2003; 349:1793–1802.

27. Coombes RC, Hall E, Gibson LJ, et al. A randomized trial of exemestane after two to three years of tamoxifen therapy in postmenopausal women with primary breast cancer. *New England Journal of Medicine* 2004; 350:1081–1092.

28. Kakcsz R, Kaufmann M, Gnant M, et al. Benefits of switching postmenopausal women with hormone-sensitive early breast cancer to anastrozole after 2 years adjuvant tamoxifen: Combined results from 3,123 women enrolled in the ABCSG Trial 8 and the ARNO 95 Trial. *Breast Cancer Research and Treatment* 2004; 88(S1):Abstract 2.

29. Winer, EP, Hudis C, Burstein HJ, et al. Use of aromatase inhibitors as adjuvant therapy for postmenopausal women with hormone receptor-positive breast cancer: Status Report 2004, November 18, 2004, accessed April 23, 2005. http://www.asco.org/asco/shared/asco_print_view/1,1168,_12–00203.

30. Cobleigh MA, Vogel CL, Tripathy D, et al. Multinational study of the efficacy and safety of humanized anti-HER2 monoclonal antibody in women who have HER2-overexpressing metastatic breast cancer. *Journal of Clinical Oncology* 1999; 17:2639–26486.

31. Vogel CL, Cobleigh MA, Tripathy D, et al. Efficacy and safety of trastuzumab as a single agent in first-line treatment of HER2-overexpressing metastatic breast cancer. *Journal of Clinical Oncology* 2002; 20:719–772.

32. Herceptin Combined with Chemotherapy Improves Disease-Free Survival for Patients with Early-Stage Breast Cancer, http://www.cancer.gov/newscenter/pressreleases/HerceptinCombination2005; accessed May 30, 2005.

33. Bergh J, Holmquist M. Who should not receive adjuvant chemotherapy? International databases. *Journal of the National Cancer Institute Monograph* 2001:103–108.

34. Morrow M, Krontiras H. Who should not receive chemotherapy? Data from American databases and trials. *Journal of the National Cancer Institute Monograph* 2001:109–113.

19. SPECIAL CASES AND POPULATIONS

1. Lippman ME, Sorace RA, Bagley CS, et al. Treatment of locally advanced breast cancer in primary induction chemotherapy with hormonal synchronization followed by radiation therapy with or without debulking surgery. *NCI Monograph* 1986; 1:153–159.

2. Hortobagyi GN, Singletary SE, Strom EA. Locally advanced breast cancer. In: Harris JR, Lippman, ME, Morrow M, Osborne CK, eds. *Diseases of the Breast*, 3rd ed. Philadelphia: Lippincott/Williams & Wilkins 2004; 952–953.

3. Smith IC, Heys SD, Hutcheon AW, et al. Neoadjuvant chemotherapy in breast

cancer: Significantly enhanced response with docetaxel. *Journal of Clinical Oncology* 2002; 20:1456–1466.

4. National Surgical Breast and Bowel Project. The effect of primary tumor response of adding sequential Taxotere to Adriamycin and cyclophosaphamide: Preliminary results of NSABP protocol B-27. *Breast Cancer Research and Treatment* 2001; 69(3):210.

5. Hortobagyi GN, Blumenschein GR, Spanos W, et al. Multimodal treatment of locally advanced breast cancer. *Cancer* 1983; 51:763.

6. Low JA, Berman AW, Steinberg SM, et al. Long-term follow-up for locally advanced and inflammatory breast cancer patients treated with multimodality therapy. *Journal of Clinical Oncology*. 22:4067–4074.

7. Chang S, Buzdar AU, Hursting SD. Inflammatory breast cancer and body mass index. *Journal of Clinical Oncology* 1998; 16(12):3731–3735.

8. Liauw SL, Benda RK, Morris CG, et al. Inflammatory breast carcinoma: Outcomes with trimodality therapy for nonmetastatic disease. *Cancer* 2004; 1000(5):920–928.

9. Fourquet A, Meunier M, Campana. Occult primary cancer with axillary metastases. In: Harris JR, Lippman, ME, Morrow M, Osborne CK, eds. *Diseases of the Breast*, 3rd ed.; 1048.

10. Ellerbrock N, Holmes F, Singletary T, et al. Treatment of patients with isolated axillary nodal metastases from an occult primary carcinoma consistent with breast origin. *Cancer* 1990; 66:1461.

11. Van Ooijen B, Bontenbal M, Henzen-Logmans SC, Koper PC. Axillary nodal metastases from an occult primary consistent with breast carcinoma. *British Journal of Surgery* 1993; 80(10):1299.

12. Graham H. *The Story of Surgery*. New York: Doubleday, Doran, 1939.

13. Wood WS, Hegedus C. Mammary Paget's disease and intraductal carcinoma: Histologic, histochemical and immunocytochemical comparison. *American Journal of Dermapathology* 1988; 10:183–188.

14. Fu W, Mittel VK, Young SC. Paget disease of the breast: Analysis of 41 patients. *American Journal of Clinical Oncology* 2001; 24:397–400.

15. Kaelin C. Paget's Disease. In: Harris JR, Lippman, ME, Morrow M, Osborne CK, eds. *Diseases of the Breast*, 3rd ed.; 1008.

16. Marshall JK, Griffith KA, Haffty BG, et al. Conservative management of Paget disease of the breast with radiotherapy: 10–15 year results. *Cancer* 2003; 97:2142–2149.

17. Lagios MD, Westdahl PR, Rose MR, et al. Paget's disease of the nipple. *Cancer* 1984; 54:545.

18. Kister SJ, Haagensen CD. Paget's disease of the breast. *American Journal of Surgery* 1970; 119:606.

19. Lagios, et al., 1984.

20. Malak G, Tapolcsanyi L. Characteristics of Paget's carcinoma of the nipple and problems of its negligence. *Oncology* 1974; 30:278.

21. Guerrero MA, Ballard BR, Grau AM. Malignant phylloides tumor of the breast: Review of the literature and case report of stromal overgrowth. *Surgical Oncology* 2003; 12:27–37.

22. Haagensen CD. *Diseases of the Breast*. Philadelphia: Saunders, 1975.

23. Bartoli C, Zurridas C, Veronesi P, et al. Small sized phyllodes tumor of the breast. *European Journal of Surgical Oncology* 1990; 16:215–219.

24. Salvadori B, Greco M, Galluzzo D, et al. Surgery for malignant mesenchymal tumors of the breast: A series of 31 cases. *Tumori* 1982; 68:325–329.

25. Chaney AW, Pollack A, McNeese MD, et al. Primary treatment of cystosarcoma phyllodes of the breast. *Cancer* 2000; 89(7):1502–1511.

26. Intra M, Rotmensz N, Viale G, et al. Clinicopathologic characteristics of 143 patients with synchronous bilateral invasive breast carcinomas treated in a single institution. *Cancer* 2004; 101:905–912.

27. Thompson WD. Genetic epidemiology of breast cancer. *Cancer* 1994; 74:279.

28. Guinee VF, Olsson H, Moller T, et al. Effect of pregnancy on prognosis for young women with breast cancer. *Lancet* 1994; 343:1587.

29. Lambe M, Hsieh CC, Trichopoulos D, Ekbom A, Pavia M, Adami HO. Transient increase in the risk of breast cancer after giving birth. *New England Journal of Medicine* 1994; 331(1):5.

30. Dixon JM, Sainsbury JRC, Rodger A. Breast cancer: Treatment of elderly patients and uncommon conditions. *British Medical Journal* 1994; 309:1292–1295.

31. Henderson IC, Patek AJ. Are breast cancers in young women qualitatively distinct? *Lancet* 1997; 349:1488–1489.

32. McCormick B. Selection criteria for breast conservation: The impact of young and old age and collagen vascular disease. *Cancer* 1994; 74:430.

33. Lee CG, McCormick B, Mazumdar M, Vetto J, Borgen PI. Infiltrating breast carcinoma in patients age 30 years and younger: Long term outcome for life, relapse, and second primary tumors. *International Journal of Radiation, Oncology, Biology, and Physics* 1992; 23:969.

34. Oktay K, Erkan, B, Veeck L, et al. Embryo development after heterotopic transplantation of cryopreserved ovarian tissue. *Lancet* 2004; 363:837–840.

35. Oktay K, Buyuk E, Davis O, et al. Fertility preservation in breast cancer patients: IVF and embryo cryoperservation after ovarian stimulation with tamoxifen. *Human Reproduction* 2003; 8(1):90–95.

36. Silliman RA, Balducci L, Goodwin JS, Holmes FF, Leventhal EA. Breast cancer care in old age: What we know, don't know, and do. *Journal of the National Cancer Institute* 1993; 85(3):190.

37. Hughes KS, Schnapper LA, Berry D, et al. Lumpectomy plus tamoxifen with or without irradiation in women 70 years of age or older with early breast cancer. *New England Journal of Medicine* 2004; 351:971–977.

38. Margolese RG, Foster RS Jr. Tamoxifen as an alternative to surgical resection for selected geriatric patients with primary breast cancer. *Archives of Surgery* 1989; 124:548–550.

39. Horobin JM, Preece PE, Dewar JA, et al. Long-term follow-up of elderly patients with locoregional breast cancer treated with tamoxifen only. *British Journal of Surgery* 1991; 78:213–217.

40. Akhtar SS, Allan SG, Rodger A, et al. A 10 year experience of tamoxifen as primary treatment of breast cancer in 100 elderly and frail patients. *European Journal of Surgical Oncology* 1991; 17:30–35.

41. Eiermann W, Paepke S, Appfelstaedy J, et al. Preoperative treatment of postmenopausal breast cancer patients with letrozole: A randomized double-blind multicenter study. *Annals of Oncology* 2001; 12:1505–1506.

42. Lambe et al., 1994, op cit; Guinee, VF, et al., 1994, op cit.

43. Petrek JA. Childbearing issues in breast carcinoma survivors. *Cancer* 1997; 79(7):1271–1278.

44. Blakely LJ, Buzdarm AU, Lozada JA, et al. Effects of pregnancy after treatment for breast carcinoma on survival and risk of recurrence. *Cancer* 2004; 100:465–469.

45. Gelber S, Coates A, Goldhirsch A, et al. Effect of pregnancy on overall survival after the diagnosis of early-stage breast cancer. *Journal of Clinical Oncology* 2001; 19:1671–1675.

46. Mueller BA, Simon MS, Deapen D, et al. Childbearing and survival after breast carcinoma in young women. *Cancer* 2003; 98:1131–1140.

47. Deapen MD, Pike MC, Casagrande JT, et al. The relationship between breast cancer and augmentation mammoplasty: An epidemiologic study. *Plastic and Reconstructive Surgery* 1986; 77:361.

48. Jacobson GM, Sause WT, Thomson JW, Plenk HP. Breast irradiation following silicone gel implants. *International Journal of Radiation, Oncology, Biology and Physics* 1986; 12(5):835.

49. Cunningham JE, Butler WM. Racial disparities in female breast cancer in South Carolina: Clinical evidence for a biological basis. *Breast Cancer Research and Treatment* 2004; 88:161–176.

50. Kotwall CA, Brinker CC, Covington DL, et al. Prognostic indices in breast cancer are related to race. *American Surgeon* 2003; 5:372–376.

51. Jones BA, Kasl SV, Howe CL, et al. African American/white differences in breast carcinoma: p53 alterations and other tumor characteristics. *Cancer* 2004; 101:1293–1301.

52. Schwartz RM, Newell RB, Hauch JF, et al. A study of familial male breast carcinoma and a second report. *Cancer* 1980; 46:2629.

53. Jackson AW, et al. Carcinoma of the male breast in association with the Klinefelter syndrome. *British Medical Journal* 1965; 1:223.

54. Ikeda RE, Preston DL, Tokuoka S. Male breast cancer incidence among atomic bomb survivors. *Journal of the National Cancer Institute* 2005; 97(8):603–605.

55. Sorensen HT, Olsen ML, Mellemkjaer L, et al. The intrauterine origin of male breast cancer: A birth order study in Denmark. *European Journal of Cancer Prevention* 2005; 14(2):185–186.

56. Campbell JH, Cummins SD. Metastases simulating mammary cancer in prostatic carcinoma under estrogenic therapy. *Cancer* 1951; 4:303.

57. Port ER, Fey JV, Cody HS III, et al. Sentinel lymph node biopsy in patients with male breast carcinoma. *Cancer* 2001; 91(2):319–323.

58. Chakravarthy A, Kim CR. Post-mastectomy radiation in male breast cancer. *Radiotherapy Oncology* 2002; 65(2):99–103.

59. Zabolotny BP, Zalai CV, Meterissian SH. Successful use of letrozole in male breast cancer: A case report and review of hormonal therapy for male breast cancer. *Journal of Surgical Oncology* 2005; 90(1):26–30.

60. Giordano, SH, Valero V, Buzdar AU, et al. Efficacy of anastrozole in male breast cancer. *American Journal of Clinical Oncology* 25(3):235–237.

61. Hittmair AP, Lininger RA, Tavassoli FA. Ductal carcinoma in situ (DCIS) in the male breast. *Cancer* 1998; 83(10):2139–2149.

20. FEARS, FEELINGS, AND WAYS TO COPE

1. Rollin B. *First, You Cry*. New York: New American Library, 1976.

2. Kushner R. *Alternatives*. Cambridge, MA: Kensington, 1984.

3. Peters-Golden H. Breast cancer: Varied perceptions of social support in the illness experience. *Social Science Medicine* 1982; 16:483.

4. Kaspar A. Telephone interview.

5. Taylor SE, Lichtman RR, Wood JV. Attributions, beliefs about control and adjustment to breast cancer. *Journal of Perspectives on Sociology and Psychology* 1984; 46:489.

6. Wellisch DK, Gritz ER, Schain W, Wang HJ, Siau J. Psychological functioning of daughters of breast cancer patients. Part II: Characterizing the distressed daughter of the breast cancer patient. *Psychosomatics* 1992; 33(2):171.

7. Lichtman RR, Taylor SE, et al. Relations with children after breast cancer: The mother-daughter relationship at risk. *Journal of Psychosociology and Oncology* 1984; 2:1.

21. SURGERY

1. Silen W, Matory WE, Love SM. *Atlas of Techniques in Breast Surgery*. Philadelphia: Lippincott-Raven, 1996.

2. Troyan S. Personal communication.

3. Anderson BO, Masetti R, Silverstien MJ. Oncoplastic approaches to partial mastec-

tomy: An overview of volume-displacement techniques. *Lancet Oncology* 2005; 6(3):145–157.

4. Krishna C, Lewis J, Benoit C, et al. Oncoplastic techniques allow extensive resections for breast conserving therapy of breast carcinomas. *Annals of Surgery* 2003; 237(1):26–34.

5. Silen, et al., 1996, op cit.

6. Rosen PP, Lesser MT, Kinne DW, et al. Discontinuous or "skip" metastases in breast carcinoma: Analysis of 1228 axillary dissections. *Annals of Surgery* 1983; 197:276.

7. Siegel BM, Mayzel KA, Love SM. Level I and II axillary dissection in the treatment of early-stage breast cancer. *Archives of Surgery* 1990; 125:1144.

8. Moskovitz AH, Anderson BO, Yeung RS, Byrd DR, Lawton TJ, Moe RE. Axillary web syndrome after axillary dissection. *American Journal of Surgery* 2001; 181:434–439.

9. Lorde A. *The Cancer Journals.* New York: Spinsters, 1980.

22. RECONSTRUCTION AND PROSTHESIS

1. Metzger D. *Tree & The Woman Who Slept with Men to Take the War Out of Them.* Oakland, CA: Wingbow, 1983.

2. Rollin B. *First, You Cry.* New York: New American Library, 1976.

3. Kushner R. *Why Me?* Cambridge, MA: Kensington, 1982.

4. Johnson CH, van Heerden JA, Donohue JH, et al. Oncological aspects of immediate breast reconstruction following mastectomy for malignancy. *Archives of Surgery* 1989; 124:819.

23. RADIATION THERAPY

1. Whelan T, MacKenzie R, Julain Jim, et al. Randomized trial of breast irradiation schedules after lumpectomy for women with lymph node-negative breast cancer. *Journal of the National Cancer Institute* 2002; 94:1143–1150.

2. Dirbas FM, Jeffrey SS, Goffinet DR. The evolution of accelerated, partial breast irradiation as a potential treatment option for women with newly diagnosed breast cancer considering breast conservation. *Cancer Biotherapy and Radiopharmaceuticals* 2004; 19(6):673–705.

3. Vicini FA, Baglan KL, Kestin LL, et al. Accelerated treatment of breast cancer. *Journal of Clinical Oncology* 2001; 19:1993–2001.

4. Veronesi U, Orecchia R, Luini A, et al. A preliminary report of interoperative radiotherapy (IORT) in limited stage breast cancers that are conservatively treated. *European Journal of Cancer* 2001; 37:2178–2183.

5. Kurtz JM, Amalric R, Brandone H, et al. Contralateral breast cancer and other second malignancies in patients treated by breast-conserving therapy with radiation. *International Journal of Radiation, Oncology, Biology and Physics* 1987; 15:277.

24. SYSTEMIC THERAPY

1. Bonadonna G, Valagussa VE, Rossi A, et al. Ten-year experience with CMF-based adjuvant chemotherapy in resectable breast cancer. *Breast Cancer Research and Treatment* 1985; 5:95.

2. ASCO. American Society of Clinical Oncology recommendations for the use of hematopoetic colony stimulating factors: Evidence-based clinical practice guidelines. *Journal of Clinical Oncology* 1994; 12:247.

3. NCCN Practice Guidelines in Oncology 2004; v.1. High Emetic Risk Chemotherapy-Emesis Prevention.

4. Denmark-Wahnefried W, Winer EP, Rimer BK. Why women gain weight with adjuvant chemotherapy for breast cancer. *Journal of Clinical Oncology* 1993; 11(7):1418.

5. Goodwin PJ, Ennis M, Pritchard KI, Trudeau M, Hood N. Risk of menopause during the first year after breast cancer diagnosisis. *Journal of Clinical Oncology* 1999; 17(8):2365–2370.

6. Bines J, Oleske DM, Cobleigh MA. Ovarian function in premenopausal women treated with adjuvant chemotherapy for breast cancer. *Journal of Clinical Oncology* 1996; 14(5):1718–1729.

7. Cobleigh MA, Bines J, Harris D, LaFollette S, Lincoln ST, Walter JM. Amenorrhea following adjuvant chemotherapy for breast cancer. *Proceedings of the American Society of Clinical Oncology* 1995; 14:115.

8. Bryce CJ, Shenkier T, Gelmon K, Trevisan C, Olivitto I. Menstrual disruption in premenopausal breast cancer patients receiving CMF (V) vs AC adjuvant chemotherapy. *Breast Cancer Research and Treatment* 1998; 50:284.

9. Montz FJ, Wolff A, Cambone JC. Gonadal protection and fecundity rates in cyclophosphamide-treated rats. *Cancer Research* 1991; 51:2124.

10. Ataya K, Rao LV, Lawrence E, Kimmel R. Luteinizing hormone releasing hormone agonist inhibits cyclophosphamide induced ovarian follicular depletion in rhesus monkeys. *Biology of Reproduction* 1995; 52:365.

11. Fisher B, Rockette H, Fisher ER, et al. Leukemia in breast cancer patients following adjuvant chemotherapy or postoperative radiation: The NSABP experience. *Journal of Clinical Oncology* 1985; 3:1640.

12. Klewer SE, Goldberg SJ, Donnerstein RL, Berg RA, Hutter JJ, Jr. Dobutamine stress echocardiography: A sensitive indicator of diminished myocardial function in asymptomatic doxirubin-treated long-term survivors of childhood cancer. *Journal of the American College of Cardiologists* 1992; 19(2):394.

13. Lucca, Gianni. Abstract no. 255. *American Society of Clinical Oncology* 1999.

14. Siegel BS. *Love, Medicine and Miracles.* New York: Harper & Row, 1986.

15. Loprinski CL, Dugler J, Sloan JA, et al. Venlafaxine alleviates hot flashes: An NCCTG Trial. Abstract 4, Proceedings of ASCO, vol. 19, 2000.

16. Saphner T, Tormey DC, Gray R. Venous and arterial thrombosis in patients who received adjuvant therapy for breast cancer. *Journal of Clinical Oncology* 1991; 9(2):286.

17. Fisher B, Costantino JP, Wickerham DL, et al. Tamoxifen for the prevention of breast cancer: Report of the National Surgical Adjuvant Breast and Bowel Project P-1 Study. *Journal of the National Cancer Institute* 1998; 90:1371–1388.

18. Chalas E, Costantino JP, Wickerham DL, et al. Benign gynecological conditions among participants in the Breast Cancer Prevention Trial. *American Journal of Obstetrics and Gynecology* 2005; 192(4):1230–1237.

19. Caleffi M, Fentiman IS, Clark GM, et al. Effect of tamoxifen on oestrogen binding, lipid and lipoprotein concentrations and blood clotting parameters in premenopausal women with breast pain. *Journal of Endocrinology* 1988; 119(2):335.

20. Kristensen B, Ejlertsen B, Dalgaard P, et al. Tamoxifen and bone metabolism in postmenopausal low-risk breast cancer patients: A randomized study. *Journal of Clinical Oncology* 1994; 12(5):992.

21. Budzar AU, Marcus C, Holmes F, Hug V, Hortobagyi G. Phase II evaluation of Ly156758 in metastatic breast cancer. *Oncology* 1988; 45(5):344–345.

22. Gradishar WJ, Glusman JE, Vogel CL, et al. Raloxifene HCl: A new endocrine agent is active in estrogen receptor positive metastatic breast cancer. *Breast Cancer Research and Treatment* 1997; 46(53) (Abstract no. 209).

23. ATAC Trialists' Group Results of the ATAC (Arimidex, Tamoxifen, Alone or in

Combination) trial after completion of 5 years' adjuvant treatment for breast cancer. *Lancet* 2005; 365:60–62.

25. COMPLEMENTARY AND ALTERNATIVE TREATMENTS

1. Cousins N. *Anatomy of an Illness.* New York: Bantam Books, 1979.

2. Chvetzoff G, Tannoci IF. Placebo effects in oncology. *Journal of the National Cancer Institute* 2003; 95:19-29

3. Spiegel D. Effects of psychotherapy on cancer survival. *Nature Reviews: Cancer* 2002; 2:383-388

4. Spiegel D, Bloom JR, Kraemer HC, Gottheil E. Effect of psychosocial treatment on survival of patients with metastatic breast cancer. *Lancet* 1989; 2:888.

5. Duckro P, Magaletta PR. The effect of prayer on physical health: Experimental evidence. *Journal of Health and Religion.*

6. Dossey L. *Healing Words: The Healing Power of Prayer.* San Francisco: Harper, 1993.

7. Simonton OC, Matthews S, Creighton JL. *Getting Well Again.* New York: Bantam Books, 1992.

8. Cousins N. *Anatomy of an Illness.* New York: Bantam Books; 1979.

9. Benson H. *Beyond the Relaxation Response.* New York: Berkley Books, 1985.

10. Mella DL. *The Legendary and Practical Use of Gems and Stones.* Albuquerque, NM: Domel, 1979.

11. Navo MA, Phan J, Vaughan et al. An Assessment of the Utilization of Complementary and Alternative Medication in Women with Gynecologic or Breast Malignancies. *J Clin Oncol* 2004; 22:671–677.

12. Sparreboom A, Fox MC, Acharya MR, Figg WD. Herbal Remedies in the United States: Potential Adverse Interactions with Anticancer Agents. *J Clin Oncol* 2004; 22: 2489–2503.

13. Roffe L, Schmidt K, Ernst E. Efficacy of Coenzyme Q10 for Improved Tolerability of Cancer Treatments: A Systematic Review. *J Clin Oncol* 2004; 22:4418–4424.

14. Cassileth BR. Evaluating complementary and alternative therapies for cancer patients. *CA-A Cancer Journal for Clinicians* 1999; 49:362–375.

15. Sun AS, Ostadal O, Ryznar V, et al. Phase I/II study of stage III and IV non-small cell lung cancer patients taking a specific dietary supplement. *Nutrition and Cancer* 1999; 34:62–69.

16. Kennedy D. Food and Drug Administration's warning on laetrile.

17. Gonzalez NJ, Isaacs LL. Evaluation of pancreatic protoleolytic enzyme treatment of adenocarcinoma of the pancreas with nutrition and detoxification support. *Nutrition and Cancer* 1999; 33:117–124.

18. Bruzynski SR, Kubove E. Initial clinical study with antineoplaston A2 injections in cancer patients with five years' follow-up. *Drugs Exper Clinical Research* 1987; 13:1–11.

19. Green S. Antineoplastons: An unproven cancer therapy. *Journal of the American Medical Association* 1992; 267:2924–2928.

20. Harrison LE, Wojciechowicz DC, Brennan MF, Paty PB. Phenylacetate inhibits isoprenoid biosynthesis and suppresses growth of human pancreatic carcinoma. Surgery 1998; 124:541–550.

21. Miller DR, Anderson GT, Stark JJ, et al. Phase I/II trial of the safety and efficacy of shark cartilage in the treatment of advanced cancer. *Journal of Clinical Oncology* 1998; 16:3649–3655.

22. Trull L. *The CanCell Controversy: Why is a possible cure for cancer being suppressed?* Norfolk, VA: Hampton Roads, 1993.

23. Bennett LM, Montgomery JL, Steinberg SM, et al. Flor-Essence herbal tonic doses

not inhibit mammary tumor development in Sprague Dawley rats. *Breast Cancer Research and Treatment* 2004; 88:87–93.

24. Grossarth-Maticek R, Kiene H, Baumgartner SM, Ziegler R. Use of Iscador, an Extract of European mistletoe (Viscum Album), in Cancer Treatment: Prospective Nonrandomized and Randomized Matched-Pair Studies Nested within a Cohort Study. *Alternative Therapies* May/June 2001; 7(3):57–77.

25. Lorde A. *A Burst of Light*. New York: Firebrand Books, 1988.

26. AFTER TREATMENT

1. Joseph E, Hyacinthe M, Lyman GH, et al. Evaluation of an intensive strategy for follow-up and surveillance of primary breast cancer. *Annals of Surgical Oncology* 1998; 5:552–528.

2. Ganz PA, Desmond KA, Leedham B, et al. Quality of life in long-term, disease-free survivors of breast cancer: A follow-up study. *Journal of the National Cancer Institute* 2002; 94:39–49.

3. Robbins GF, Berg JW. Bilateral primary breast cancers: A prospective clinical pathological study. *Cancer* 1964; 17:1501.

4. Haagensen CD, Lane N, Bodian C. Coexisting lobular neoplasia and carcinoma of the breast. *Cancer* 1983; 51:1468.

5. Grunfeld E, Mant D, Yudkin P, et al. Routine follow up of breast cancer in primary care: Randomised trial. *British Medical Journal* 1996; 313:665–669.

6. Insa A, Lluch A, Prosper F, et al. Prognostic factors predicting survival from first recurrence in patients with metastatic breast cancer: Analysis of 439 patients. *Breast Cancer Research and Treatment* 1999; 56(1):67–78.

7. Chang J, Clark GM, Allred C, et al. Survival of patients with metastatic breast carcinoma: Importance of prognostic markers of the primary tumor. *Cancer* 2003; 97(3): 545–553.

8. Stierer M, Rosen HR. Influence of early diagnosis on prognosis of recurrent breast cancer. *Cancer* 1989; 64:1128.

9. Smith TJ, Davidson NE, Schapira DV, et al. American Society of Clinical Oncology 1998 update of recommended breast surveillance guidelines. *Journal of Clinical Oncology* 1999; 17:1080–1082.

10. Carlson RW, Anderson BO, Bensinger W, et al. Clinical Practice Guidelines in Oncology, Breast Cancer v 1.04 National Comprehensive Cancer Network, 2004; available at http://www.nccn.org. Accessed February 2005.

11. Ganz PA, Kwan L, Stanton AL, et al. Quality of life at the end of primary treatment of breast cancer: First results from the moving beyond cancer randomized trial. *Journal of the National Cancer Institute* 2004; 96(5):376–387.

12. Tasmuth T, Kataja M, Blomqvist C, von Smitten K, Kalso E. Treatment-related factors predisposing to chronic pain in patients with breast cancer: A multivariate approach. *Acta Oncology* 1997; 36(6):625–630.

13. Wallace MS, Wallace AM, Lee J, Kobke MK. Pain after breast surgery: A survey of 282 women. *Pain* 1996; 66(Aug):2–3.

14. Tasmuth T, Blomqvist C, Kalso E. Chronic post-treatment symptoms in patients with breast cancer operated in different surgical units. *European Journal of Surgical Oncology* 1999; 25(1).

15. Crawford JS, Simpson J, Crawford P. Myofascial release provides symptomatic relief from chest wall tenderness occasionally seen following lumpectomy and radiation in breast cancer patients [letter]. *International Journal of Radiation, Oncology, Biology and Physics* 1996; 34(5): 1188–1189.

16. Eija K, Tiina T, Pertti NJ. Amitriptyline effectively relieves neuropathic pain following treatment of breast cancer. *Pain* 1996; 64(2):293–302.

17. Petrek JA, Senie RT, Peters M, et al. Lymphedema in a cohort of breast carcinoma survivors 20 years after diagnosis. *Cancer* 2001; 92:1368–1377.

18. Blanchard DK, Donohue JH, Reynolds C, et al. Relapse and morbidity in patents undergoing sentinel lymph node biopsy alone or with axillary dissection for breast cancer. *Archives of Surgery* 2003; 138:482.

19. Martin GM, Dowlatshahi K. Sentinel lymph node biopsy lowers the rate of lymphedema when compared with standard axillary lymph node dissection. *Annals of Surgery* 2003; 69:209.

20. Sener SF, Winchester DJ, Martz CH, et al. Lymphedema after sentinel lymphadectomy for breast carcinoma. *Cancer* 2001; 92:748.

21. Petrek JA, Heelan MC. Incidence of breast carcinoma-related lymphedema. *Cancer* 1998; 83:2776.

22. Kasserollen RG. The Vodder School: The Vodder method. *Cancer* 1998; 83:2840.

23. Foldi E. The treatment of lymphedema. *Cancer* 1998; 83:2883.

24. Bernas M, Witte M, Kriederman B, et al. Massage therapy in the treatment of lymphedema. Rationale, results and applications. *IEEE Engineering in Medicine and Biology Magazine* 2005; 24(2):58–68.

25. Casley-Smith JR, Morgan RG, Piller NB. Treatment of lymphedema of the arms and legs with 5,6-Benso(alpha)-pyrone. *New England Journal of Medicine* 1993; 329:1158.

26. Loprinzi CL, Kugler JW, Sloan JA, et al. Lack of effect of coumarin in women with lymphedema after treatment for breast cancer. *New England Journal of Medicine* 1999; 340(5):346–350.

27. Wieneke MH, Dienst ER. Neuropsychological assessment of cognitive functioning following chemotherapy for breast cancer. *Psychooncology* 1995; 4:61–66.

28. Schagen SB, Van Dam FSAM, Muller JM, et al. Cognitive deficits after postoperative adjuvant chemotherapy for breast carcinoma. *Cancer* 1999; 85:640–650.

29. Wefel JS, Lenzi R, Theriault RL, et al. The cognitive sequelae of standard-dose adjuvant chemotherapy in women with breast carcinoma: Results of a prospective, randomized, longitudinal trial. *Cancer* 2004; 100:2292–2299.

30. Wefel JS, Lenzi E, Theriault, et al. "Chemobrain" in breast carcinoma? *Cancer* 2004; 101:466–475.

31. Schagen SB, Muller MJ, Boogerd W, et al. Late effects of adjuvant chemotherapy on cognitive function: A follow up study in breast cancer patients. *Annals of Oncology* 2002; 13:1387–1397.

32. Ahles TA, Saykin AJ, Furstenberg CT, et al. Neuropsychological impact of standard-dose systemic chemotherapy in long-term survivors of breast cancer and lymphoma. *Journal of Clinical Oncology* 2002; 20:485–493.

33. Tannock IF, Ahles TA, Ganz PA, et al. Cognitive impairment associated with chemotherapy for cancer: Report of a workshop. *Journal of Clinical Oncology* 2004; 22(1): 2233–2239.

34. Irvine D, Vincent L, Graydon JE, Bubela N, Thompson L. The prevalence and correlates of fatigue in patients receiving treatment with chemotherapy and radiotherapy. Comparison with the fatigue experienced by healthy individuals. *Cancer Nursing* 1994; 17(5):367–378.

35. Johnston E, Crawford J. The hematologic support of the cancer patient. In: Berger A, Portenoy R, Weissan D, eds. *Principles and Practice of Supportive Oncology.* Philadelphia: Lippincott-Raven, 1998; 549.

36. Friendenreich C, Courneya KS. Exercise as rehabilitation for cancer patients. *Clinical Journal of Sports Medicine* 1996; 6:237

37. Young-McCaughon S, Sexton DL. A retrospective investigation of the relationship

between aerobic exercise and quality of life in women with breast cancer. *Oncology Nursing Forum* 1991; 18:751

38. Schwartz A. Patterns of exercise and fatigue in physically active cancer survivors. *Oncology Nursing Forum* 1998; 25:485.

39. Huntington M. Weight gain in patients receiving adjuvant chemotherapy for carcinoma of the breast. *Cancer* 1985; 65:572.

40. Herbert JR, Hurley TG, Ma Y, Hampl JS. The effect of dietary exposure on recurrence and mortality in early stage breast cancer. *Breast Cancer Research and Treatment* 1998; 51:17.

41. Sverrisdottir A, Fornander T, Jacobsson H, et al. Bone mineral density among premenopausal women with early breast cancer in a randomized trial of adjuvant endocrine therapy. *Journal of Clinical Oncology* 2004; 22:3694–3699.

42. Lonning PE, Geisler LE, Krag L, et al. Changes in bone metabolism after 2 years' treatment with exemestane (E) in postmenopausal women with early breast cancer (EBC) at low risk: Follow up (FU) results of a randomized placebo-controlled study. *Journal of Clinical Oncology* 2005; Annual Meeting Proceedings 23(16S), Part I of II, Abstract 531.

43. Cummings SR, Black DM, Thompson ED, et al. Effect of alendronate on risk of fracture in women with low bone density but without vertebral fractures: Results from the Fracture Intervention Trial. *Journal of the American Medical Association* 1998; 280: 2077–2082.

44. Holmberg L, Anderson H, et al. HABITS (hormonal replacement therapy after breast cancer): Is it safe?, a randomized comparison: Trial stopped. *Lancet* 2004; 363: 453–455.

45. Morrow M, et al. San Antonio; 2004.

46. The Writing Group for the PEPI Trial. Effects of estrogen or estrogen/progestin regimens on heart disease risk factors in postmenopausal women: The postmenopausal estrogen/progestin interventions (PEPI) trial. *Journal of the American Medical Association* 1995; 273(3):199.

47. Cialli AR, Fugh-Berman A. Is Estriol Safe? *Alternative Therapies in Women's Health* 2002; 14(10):73–74.

48. Boothby LA, Doering PL, Kipersztok S. Bioidentical hormone therapy: A review. *Menopause* 2004; 11(3):356–367.

49. Wren BG. Progesterone creams: Do they work? *Climacteric* 2003; 6:184–187.

50. Million Women Study Coordinators. Breast cancer and hormone replacement therapy in the Million Women Study. *Lancet* 2003; 362:419–427.

51. Million Women Study Collaborators: Endometrial cancer and hormone-replacement therapy in the Million Women Study. *Lancet* 2005; 365:1543–1545.

52. Lieberman S. A review of the effectiveness of cimicifuga racemosa (black cohosh) for the symptoms of menopause. *Journal of Women's Health* 1998; 7(5):525–529.

53. Anon. Meeting summary, American Society for Clinical Oncology 1998.

54. Kronenberg F, Fugh-Berman A. Complementary and alternative medicine for menopausal symptoms: A review of randomized, controlled trials. *Annals of Internal Medicine* 2002; 137:805–813.

55. Albertazzi P, Pansini F, Bonaccorsi G, Zanotti L, Forini E, De Aloysio D. The effects of dietary soy supplementation on hot flushes. *Obstetrics and Gynecology* 1998; 91(1):6–11.

56. Potter SM, Baum JA, Teng H, Stillman RJ, Shay NF, Erdman JWJ. Soy protein and isoflavones: Their effects on blood lipids and bone density in postmenopausal women. *American Journal of Clinical Nutrition* 1998; 68(6 Suppl):1375S–1379S.

57. Shao Z-M, Wu J, Shen Z-Z, Barsky SH. Genistein exerts multiple suppressive effects on human breast carcinoma cells. *Cancer Research* 1998; 58:4851–4857.

58. Ito A, Goto T, Okamoto T, Yamada K, Roy G. A combined effect of tamoxifen

(TAM) and miso for the development of mammary tumors induced with MNU in SD rats. *Proceedings of the American Association for Cancer Research* 1996; 37(March).

59. Hilakivi-ClarkeL, Cho E, Cabanes A, et al. Dietary modulation of pregnancy estrogen levels and breast cancer risk among female rat offspring. *Clinical Cancer Research* 2002; 8:3601–3610.

60. Teede HJ, Dalais FS, Mc Grath BP. Dietary soy containing phytoestrogens does not have detectable estrogen effects on hepatic protein synthesis in postmenopausal women. *American Journal of Clinical Nutrition* 2004; 79(3):396–401.

61. Sartippour MR, Rao JY, Apple S, et al. A pilot clinical study of short-term isoflavone supplements in breast cancer patients. *Nutrition and Cancer* 2004; 49(1):59–65.

62. Bodinet C, Freudenstein J. Influence of Cimicifuga racemosa on the proliferation of estrogen receptor positive human breast cancer cells. *Breast Cancer Research and Treatment* 2002; 76:1–10.

63. Amato P, et al. Estrogenic activity of herbs commonly used as remedies for menopausal symptoms. *Menopause* 2002; 9:145–150.

64. Liu J, et al. Evaluation of estrogenic activity of plant extracts for the potential treatment of menopausal symptoms. *Journal of Agriculture and Food Chemistry* 2001; 49:2472–2479.

65. Dixon-Shanies D, Shaikh N. Growth inhibition of human breast cancer cells by herbs and phytoestroges. *Oncology Reports* 1999; 6:1383–1387.

66. Zierau O, et al. Antiestrogenic activities of Cimicifuga racemosa extracts. *Journal of Steroid Biochemical Molecular Biology* 2002; 80:125–130.

67. Jacobson JS, et al. Randomized trial of black cohosh for the treatment of hot flashes among women with a history of breast cancer. *Journal of Clinical Oncology* 2001; 19:2739–2795.

68. Liske E, et al. Physiological investigation of a unique extract of black cohosh (Cimicifugae racemosae rhizoma): A 6 month clinical study demonstrates no systemic estrogenic effect. *Journal of Women's Health and Gender Based Medicine* 2002; 11:163–174.

69. Pokaj BA, Loprinzi CL, Sloan JA, et al. Pilot evaluation of black cohosh for the treatment of hot flashes in women. *Cancer Investigation* 2004, 22(4):515–521.

70. Loprinzi CL, Peethambaram PP. Management of menopausal symptoms in breast cancer patients. *Annals of Medicine* 1995; 27(6):653–656.

71. Stearns V, Beebe KL, Iyengar M, et al. Paroxetine controlled release in the treatment of menopausal hot flashes: A randomized controlled trial. *Journal of the American Medical Association* 2003; 289(21):2827–2834.

72. Stearns V, Ullmer L, Lopez JF, et al. Hot flushes. *Lancet* 2002; 360:1851–1861.

73. Guttusp T Jr, Kurlan R, Mc Dermott MP, et al. Gabapentin's effects on hot flashes in postmenopausal women: A randomized controlled trial. *Obstetrics and Gynecology* 2003; 1:337–345.

74. Chebowski RT, Aiello E, McTiernan A. Weight loss in breast cancer patient management. *Journal of Clinical Oncology* 2002; 20(4):1128–1143.

75. Goodwin PJ, Boyd NF. Body size and breast cancer prognosis: A critical review of the evidence. *Breast Cancer Research and Treatment* 1990; 16(3):205–214.

76. Chlebowski RT, Blackburn GL, Elashoff RE, et al. Dietary fat reduction in postmenopausal women with primary breast cancer: Phase III Women's Intervention Nutrition Study (WINS) *Journal of Clinical Oncology* 2005; Annual Meeting Proceedings 16S (Part I of II): Abstract no. 10.

77. Holmes MD, Chen WY, Feskanich D, et al. Physical activity and survival after breast cancer diagnosis. *JAMA* 2005; 293:2479-2486.

78. Rock CL, Denmark-Wahnefried W. Nutrition and survival after the diagnosis of breast cancer: A review of the evidence. *Journal of Clinical Oncology* 2002; 20:3302–3316.

79. Segal R, Evans W, Johnson D, et al. Structured exercise improves physical

functioning in women with stages I and II breast cancer: Results of a randomized controlled trial. *Journal of Clinical Oncology* 2001; 19:657–665.

80. Weuve J, Kand JH, Manson JE, et al. Physical activity, including walking, and cognitive function in older women. *Journal of the American Medicine Association* 2004; 292: 1454–1461.

81. Knoops KT, de Groot LCPGM, Kromhout D, et al. Mediterranean diet lifestyle factors, and 10-year mortality in elderly European men and women. *Journal of the American Medical Association* 2004; 292:1433–1439.

82. Stampfer MJ, Hu FB, Manson MJ, et al. Primary prevention of coronary heart disease in women through diet and lifestyle. *New England Journal of Medicine* 2000; 343:16–22.

83. Kitzinger S. *Woman's Experience of Sex*. New York: Putnam's, 1983.

84. Wellisch DK, Jamison KR, Pasnau RO. Psychosocial aspects of mastectomy. II. The man's perspective. *American Journal of Psychiatry* 1978; 135:543.

85. Baider L, Kaplan-DeNour A. Couples' reactions and adjustments to mastectomy: A preliminary report. *International Journal of Psychiatry and Medicine* 1984; 14:265.

86. Ganz PA, Rowland JH, Desmond K, et al. Life after breast cancer: Understanding women's health related quality of life and sexual functioning. *Journal of Clinical Oncology* 1998; 16:501.

87. Mignot L, et al. Breast cancer and subsequent pregnancy. *American Society of Clinical Oncology Proceedings* 1986; 5:57.

88. Peters M. The effect of pregnancy in breast cancer. *Prognostic Factors in Breast Cancer* 1968; 65.

89. Maunsell E, Drolet M, Brisson J, et al. Work situation after breast cancer: Results from a population-based study. *Journal of the National Cancer Institute* 2004; 96:1813–1822.

27. WHEN CANCER COMES BACK

1. Solin LJ, Harris EER, Orel SG, Glick JH. Local-regional recurrence after breast conservation treatment or mastectomy. In: Harris JR, Lippman ME, Morrow M, Osborne CK, eds. *Diseases of the Breast*, 3rd ed. Philadelphia: Lippincott Williams & Wilkins, 2004; 1068–1069.

2. Rutgers E, van Slooten E, Kluck H. Follow up after treatment of primary breast cancer. *British Journal of Surgery* 1989; 76:187–190.

3. Kurtz J, et al. The prognostic significance of late local recurrence after breast conserving therapy. *International Journal of Radiation Oncology, Biology and Physics* 1990; 18:87–93.

4. Kuerer HM, Arthur DW, Haffty BG. Repeat breast-conserving surgery for in-breast local breast carcinoma recurrence: The potential role of partial breast irradiation. *Cancer* 2004; 100:2269–2280.

5. Solin LJ, Harris EER, Orel SG, Glick JH. Local-regional recurrence after breast conservation treatment of mastectomy. In: Harris JR, Lippman ME, Morrow M, Osborne CK, eds. *Diseases of the Breast*, 3rd ed. Op cit, p. 1072.

6. Gilliland MD, Barton RM, Copeland EM. The implications of local recurrence of breast cancer as the first site of therapeutic failure. *Annals of Surgery* 1983; 197:284–287.

7. Slavin SA, Love SM, Goldwyn RM. Recurrent breast cancer following immediatereconstruction with myocutaneous flaps. *Plastic and Reconstructive Surgery* 1994; 93(May):1191.

8. Borner M, Bacchi A, Goldhirsch A, et al. First isolated locoregional recurrence following mastectomy for breast cancer: Results of a phase III multicenter study comparing systemic treatment with observation after excision and radiation. *Journal of Clinical Oncology* 1994; 12:2071.

9. Hortobagyi G. Can we cure limited metastatic breast cancer? *Journal of Clinical Oncology* 2001; 20(3):620–623.

10. Halverson KJ, Perez CA, Kuske RR, et al. Locoregional recurrence of breast cancer: A retrospective comparison of irradiation alone versus irradiation and systemic therapy. *American Journal of Clinical Oncology* 1992; 15:93–101.

11. Recht A, Pierce S, Abner A, et al. Regional nodal failure after conservative surgery and radiotherapy for early-stage breast carcinoma. *Journal of Clinical Oncology* 1991; 9:988.

12. Seidman AD. Sequential single-agent chemotherapy for metastatic breast cancer: Therapeutic nihilism or realism? *Journal of Clinical Oncology* 2003; 21(4):577–579.

13. Hortobagyi GN. Can we cure limited metastatic breast cancer? Op cit.

14. Falkson G, Gelman RS, Leone L, et al. Survival of premenopausal women with metastatic breast cancer: Long term follow-up of Eastern Cooperative Group and Cancer and Leukemia Group B studies. *Cancer* 1990; 66:1621.

15. Ibid.

16. Chia S, Speers C, Kang A, et al. The impact of new chemotherapeutic and hormonal agents on the survival of women with metastatic breast cancer in a population based cohort. *Proceedings of the American Society of Clinical Oncology* 2003; 22:6a.

17. Giordano SH, Budzar AU, Smith TL, et al. Is breast cancer survival improving? *Cancer* 2004; 100(1):44–52.

18. Hamaoka T, Madewell JE, Podoloff DA, et al. Bone imaging in metastatic breast cancer. *Journal of Clinical Oncology* 2004; 22:2942–2953.

19. Hillner BE, Ingle JN, Chlebowski RT, et al. Update on the role of bisphosphonates and bone health issues in women with breast cancer. *Journal of Clinical Oncology* 2003; 21:4042–4057.

20. Patchell RA, Tibbs PA, Walsh JW, et al. A randomized trial of surgery in the treatment of single metastases to the brain. *New England Journal of Medicine* 1990; 322(8): 494–500.

21. Bonnaterre J, Budzar A, Nabholtz JM, et al. Anastrozole is superior to tamoxifen as first-line therapy in hormone receptor positive advanced breast carcinoma. *Cancer* 2001; 92:2247.

22. Nabholtz JM, Bonneterre J, Budzar A, et al. Anastrozole (Arimidex) versus tamoxifen as first-line therapy for advanced breast cancer in postmenopausal women: Survival analysis and updated safety results. *European Journal of Cancer* 2003; 39:1684

23. Slamon D, Leyland-Jones B, Shak S, Paton V, Bajamonde A, et al. Addition of Herceptin (humanized anti-HER2 antibody) to first line chemotherapy for HER2 overexpressing metastatic breast cancer (HER2+/MBC) markedly increases anticancer activity: A randomized, multinational controlled Phase III trial. *American Society of Clinical Oncology Proceedings* 1998; 17:98a.

24. http://www.nci.nih.gov/newscenter/pressreleases/AvastinBreast. Accessed on May 5, 2005.

25. Howell A, Robertson JFR, Abram P, et al. Comparison of gulvestrant versus tamoxifen for the treatment of advanced breast cancer in postmenopausal women previously untreated with endocrine therapy: A multinational double-blind, randomized trial. *Journal of Clinical Oncology* 2004; 22(9):1605–1613.

26. Robertson JF, Osborne CK, Howell A, et al. Fulvestrant versus anastrozole for the treatment of advanced breast carcinoma in postmenopausal women: A prospective combined analysis of two multicenter trials *Cancer* 2003; 98(2):229–238.

27. Osborne CK, Pippen J, Jones SE, et al. Double-blind, randomized trial comparing the efficacy and tolerability of fulvestrant versus anastrozole in postmenopausal women with advanced breast cancer progressing on prior endocrine therapy: Results of a North American trial. *Journal of Clinical Oncology* 2002; 16(August):3386–3395.

28. Saeki T, Takashima S. Capecitiabine plus docetaxel combination chemotherapy for metastatic breast cancer. *Breast Cancer* 2004; 11(2):116–120.

29. Colomer R. Gemcitabine and paclitaxel in metastatic breast cancer: A review. *Oncology (Huntingt)* 2004; 14(Supp)l: 8–12.

30. Critofanilli M, Budd T, Ellis MJ, et al. Circulating tumor cells, disease progression and survival in metastatic breast cancer. *New England Journal of Medicine* 2004; 351:781–791.

31. http://www.nci.nih.gov/newscenter/pressreleases/AvastinBreast. Accessed on May 5, 2005.

32. Lipton A, Theriault RL, Hortobagyi GN, et al. Pamidronate prevents skeletal complications and is effective palliative treatment in women with breast carcinoma and osteolytic bone metastases: Long term follow-up of two randomized, placebo- and controlled trials. *Cancer* 2000; 88(5):1082–1090.

33. Hillner BE, Ingle JN, Chlebowski RT, et al. Update on the role of bisphosphonates and bone health issues in women with breast cancer; Op cit.

34. Spiegel D, Bloom JR, Kraemer HC, Gottheil E. Effect of psychosocial treatment on survival of patients with metastatic breast cancer. *Lancet* 1989; 2(8668):888.

35. Spiegel D. *Living Beyond Limits: New Hope and Help for Facing Life-Threatening Illness.* New York: Times Books, 1993.

36. Tobin DR, with Lindsey K. *Peaceful Dying.* Reading, MA: Perseus, 1999.

28. THE FUTURE: FROM LAB TO BEDSIDE

1. Al-Hajj M, Wicha MS, Benito-Hernandez A, et al. Prospective identification of tumourigenic breast cancer cells. *Proceedings of the National Academy of Science USA* 2003; 100:3983–3988.

2. Weaver VM, Peterson OW, Wang F, et al. Reversion of the malignant phenotype of human breast cells in three-dimensional culture and in vivo by integrin blocking antibodies. *The Journal of Cell Biology* 1997; 137(1):231–245.

3. Kupperwasser C, Chavarria T, Wu M, et al. Reconstruction of functionally normal and laignant human breast tissues in mice. *Proceedings of the National Academy of Science* 2004; 101(14):4966–4971.

4. O'Reilly MS, Holmgren L, Shing Y, et al. Angiostatin: A novel angiogenesis inhibitor that mediates the suppression of metastases by a Lewis lung carcinoma. *Cell* 1994; 79(2):315–328.

5. Reynolds T. Researchers slowly unveil where cancer cells hide. *Journal of the National Cancer Institute* 1998; 90(22):1690–1691.

Index

Page numbers in **bold** indicate glossary terms. Page numbers in *italics* indicate illustrations.

ABOUT THE AUTHORS

Susan Love, MD, MBA, is an author, surgeon, researcher, entrepreneur, and mother. She is Clinical Professor of Surgery at UCLA, President and Medical Director of the Dr. Susan Love Research Foundation, and a founder and Director of the National Breast Cancer Coalition. She is the author of *Dr. Susan Love's Breast Book,* one of the first books for the lay public that explained the scientific information and options for treatment in an accessible manner. Updated every five years, it has been termed the "bible" for women with breast cancer by the *New York Times.* Her second book, *Dr. Susan Love's Menopause and Hormone Book* was the first to sound the alarm about the dangers of long-term use of hormone replacement therapy in postmenopausal women. She served a six-year term as a presidential appointee to the National Cancer Advisory Board and continues to advise both for profit and not-for-profit organizations regarding breast cancer and women's health. In addition to her media appearances, speaking, and political activities, she dedicates her time through her foundation to research on the intraductal approach to breast cancer in her quest to eradicate breast cancer once and for all within ten years. Her website, www.drsusanloveresearchfoundation.org is a place where women can find out how to become part of the solution as well as find answers to all their health care questions. She shares her home in Southern California with her life partner, Helen Cooksey MD, their daughter Katie, and their companions, two dogs, two cats, and eight fish.

Karen Lindsey is the author of *Divorced, Beheaded, Survived: A Feminist Reinterpretation of the Wives of Henry VII; Friends as Family;* and *Falling Off the Roof;* and co-author of *Dr. Susan Love's Menopause and Hormone Book* and, with Dr. Daniel Tobin, *Peaceful Dying.* She has co-authored *Shelter from the Storm: Caring for a Child with a Life-Threatening Condition,* with Drs. Joanne Hilden and Daniel Tobin. Her articles have appeared in *Ms., The Women's Review of Books, Sojourner, International Figure Skating,* and many other publications and anthologies. She teaches women's studies at the University of Massachusetts/Boston, and writing and literature at Emerson College.